ANTHOLOGY
OF MEDICAL DISEASES

ANTHOLOGY
OF MEDICAL DISEASES

Valiere Alcena, MD., M.A.C.P.

authorHOUSE®

AuthorHouse™ LLC
1663 Liberty Drive
Bloomington, IN 47403
www.authorhouse.com
Phone: 1-800-839-8640

Published by AuthorHouse   10/22/2013

ISBN: 978-1-4918-2260-9 (sc)
ISBN: 978-1-4918-2261-6 (e)

Library of Congress Control Number: 2013918035

For further information, contact the author at:
LE NERGE PULISHING
Alcena Medical Communication, Inc
37 Davis Avenue
White Plains, NY 10605
(914) 682-8020
Fax (914) 682-8066
dralcena@aol.com
www.prestigemedialnews.com
www.Dr Alcena.com

CONTENTS

PREFACE

Many important advances have been made in basic sciences and clinical medicine in the twentieth and the twenty first centuries. The human genome has been deciphered the molecular genetic abnormalities of diseases such as

Chronic myelocytic leukemia (CML)
Breast cancer BRACA 1 and BRACA 2
Polycythemia Vera
Essential thrombocythemia
Myelofibrosis
Chronic lymphocytic leukemia (CLL)
Sickle cell disease
Certain types of prostate cancer
Essential hypertension
Alzheimers's disease,
Cystic fibrosis,
Color blindness
Neurofibromatosis
Polyccystic kidney disease
Down syndrome
Primary hemochromatosis
Hemophilia
Turner syndrome etc;

Molecular phamarcology of many diseases has allowed for specific medications to treat diseases such as CML, (gleveec), CLL, (Retuxan), polycythemia Vera (hydroxy urea), Sickle cell disease (hydroxyl urea), myelofibrosis (Rutolitinid a JAK 1 and JAK 2 inhibitor), essential hypertension (thiazide diuretics) etc;

While progress, breakthroughs and advances have been made both the diagnoses, treatments and cure of many diseases, much remains to be done to reaseach the genetic bases for many diseases, to diagnose and to find curable medications for thousands of disesases that remain in need of diagnoses, treatments and cures.

INTRODUCTION

Many changes have taken place in medicine both in the twenthieth and in the twenty first centuries. Physicians all over the world are able to do procedures and tests such as

CAT scan
MRI
MRA
Ultrasound
ERCP
Angiogram
Bone scan
PET scan
Fine needle biopsy under CAT scan visualization
Minimal invasive surgical procedures using ultrasound
Nuclear cardiac stress test
Echocardiogram
24 hour holter monitor
Place stents in coronary arteries
Open heart surgery
Coronary bypass
Reparing or replacing heart valves
Endoscopy
Colonoscopy
Biopsy of different organs
Robatic prostatectomy
Kee replacement
Hip replacement
Brain surgery
Cesarian section
Respirator
General anesthesia
Epidural anesthesia
New technics to remove cataracts
New technics to diagnose glaucoma and treat glaucoma
Blood tests to diagnose different diseases
Bone marrow specimen to diagnose different diseases
Urine samples to diagnose different diseases
Stool sample to diagnose different diseases
Sperm sample to diagnose different diseases
Sperm samples for use in IVF

Sperm bank to store sperm
Harvesting human eggs
Blood, siliva, urine, hair, etc; for DNA testing
Organs transplantation

New antibiotics to treat infections
New anti-viral medications to treat influenza, HIV/AIDS etc,
New medications to cancer
New medications to to treat anemia
New medications to treat coronary heart disease
New medications to treat heart failure
New medications to treat Rheumatoid arthritis
New medications to treat osteoarthritis
New medications to treat osteoporosis
New medications to treat ulcer of the stomach
New medications to treat migraine head ache
New medications to treat glaucoma and other diseases of the eyes
Chemotherapy
Radiotherapy
Bone marrow transplant
New medications to treat skin diseases etc;

These new technics and treatments to both diagnose and treat diseases have changed the ways physicians treat patients and have in many instances have relieved sufferings and prolonged lives in meaningful ways.

This book seeks to bring to light some of the diseases that are causing sufferings in some many people around the world and how best to evaluate and treat these diseases.

Chapter 1
HIGH CHOLESTEROL

World wide the incidence of high cholesterol is the highest in Europe (54% for both sexes), Americas (48% for both sexes), Africa 22.6%, and Asia 29.0 %. Source: WHO

Approximately 106,700 million individuals in the U.S. have high cholesterol: 50,800,000 males and 55,900,000 females have high cholesterol; 47.9% white males and 49.7% white females have high cholesterol; 44.8 black males and 42.1 black females have high cholesterol. Seven million children/adolescents in the U.S. have high cholesterol.

High cholesterol is one of the leading risk factors for coronary artery heart disease. The different types of abnormal lipids that can be found in the blood of people are:

1. Hyperlipidemia
2. High cholesterol
3. High triglycerides/high cholesterol
4. High low-density cholesterol (LDL)
5. Low high-density cholesterol (HDL)
6. High cholesterol/LDL ratio
7. High VLDL cholesterol

All these abnormal lipids are genetically transmitted from parents to their children to one degree or another.

According to a recent report that appeared in the New England Journal of Medicine, Vol. 342 No. 12 (March 23, 2000), four new markers of inflammation were found to be predictors of future development of coronary heart disease. These are hs-CRP, serum amyloid A., interleukin-6, and sICAM-1. According to the authors, the hs-CRP was the most sensitive predictor when found to be elevated.

Hyperlipidemia (too much fat in the blood) is, generally speaking, a genetically transmitted disease. If a person's mother or father has too much fat in his or her blood, this trait is likely to be transmitted to his or her children, resulting in hyperlipidemia, which can lead to the development of coronary heart disease resulting in heart attack and possible early death. Hyperlipidemia is categorized as:

1. High blood cholesterol

2. High blood triglycerides
3. High low-density lipoprotein
4. Low high-density lipoprotein
5. Cholesterol/HDL ratio, which is LDL/HDL, greater than 7.13.

In a man, if the LDL/HDL ratio is greater than 7.13, that is a high risk factor. In a woman, if the LDL/HDL ratio is greater than 5.57, that is a high risk factor.

Each one of these different components of hyperlipidemia represents an independent risk factor when abnormal, resulting in coronary heart disease.

Normal blood cholesterol is from 130 to 200 mg/dl. A normal blood triglyceride level is 60-150 mg/dl. Normal HDL is 35-80 mg/dl. Normal LDL is less than 130 mg/dl. Normal cholesterol/HDL is less than 3.4. Normal LDL/HDL is less than 2.8 these ratios are for men. In women, normal cholesterol /HDL ratio is less than 3.27 and the LDL/HDL less than 2.34.

Most people believe that blood cholesterol level is the only thing that matters when addressing abnormal fat levels in the blood. This is wrong because a person may have perfectly normal total blood cholesterol and yet have significant hyperlipidemia, predisposing that person to coronary artery disease. One must be aware that the quick cholesterol test may be misleading if normal. Normal blood cholesterol by itself is not enough to tell if a person has abnormal genetically transmitted lipid. There are five basic cholesterols in the blood:

1. Total cholesterol
2. High-density lipoprotein (HDL)
3. LDL cholesterol
4. Triglycerides
5. VLDL (Very low-density lipoprotein)

HDL is the cholesterol that takes the regular cholesterol from the blood, carries it into the bowel and the colon, mixes it with stool, and carries it out of the body. If the HDL is low—less than 45 mg/dl—then there is not enough of it in the blood to complex with bad cholesterol to remove it from the body. This is a genetic abnormality transmitted from parents to children. More appropriately, these lipid abnormalities are called hyperlipoproteinemias. When both the fasting total cholesterol and the LDL are elevated, this is type 2a hypercholesterolemia.

When the fasting total cholesterol, the LDL cholesterol, and the triglycerides are elevated, this is type 2b hypercholesterolemia. When the total cholesterol is high and when the level of triglycerides is very high, that is type 3 hyperlipidemia. When the triglycerides are very high and the VLDL is high, that is type 4 hyperlipidemia.

High chylomicrons, high VLDL, high triglycerides, and cholesterol manifest type 5 hyperlipidemia.

Type 1 hyperlipoproteinenemia is manifested by high chylomicrons.

Secondary hyperlipoproteinemia is seen in association with several medical conditions, such as diabetes mellitus, hypothyroidism, uremia, and nephrotic syndrome, alcoholism with acute or chronic pancreatitis, ingestion of oral contraceptive, etc.

First, high triglycerides and VLDL may be evident on the skin and under the eyes as deposits (xantomas). Second, VLDL, triglycerides, and high cholesterol may be high in diabetic women who develop ketoacidosis. Third, high triglycerides, high cholesterol, diabetes mellitus, and hypertension may be present persistently in obese people (Syndrome X).

The use of birth control pills or ingestion of any estrogen-containing pills can raise the level of VLDL and triglycerides. One of the dangers of taking estrogen-containing pills is the possibility of high level of lipids. It is important to know the lipid level in a person before he or she starts taking estrogen pills. If a woman has an elevated lipid level, estrogen-containing medication may be harmful to her health by increasing the blood lipid further, predisposing her to heart attack, stroke, phlebitis, pulmonary embolism, etc.

Alcohol abuse is also associated with elevated lipids in the blood, such as triglycerides and, in particular, a high level of very-low-density lipoprotein and chylomicrons. In addition, Type 5 hyperlipidemia and sometimes Type 4 hyperlipidemia may be associated with increased alcohol abuse. Type 5 hyperlipidemia may cause acute pancreatitis, which is a very serious medical condition and if left untreated can be fatal.

Hyperlipidemia causes coronary artery disease because in a high lipid state, lipid is deposited within the lumen of coronary arteries, causing gradual narrowing of these vessels and resulting in coronary occlusive heart disease. When the vessels around the heart become narrowed, the condition called angina pectoris frequently develops. Angina pectoris is manifested by chest pain because of lack of oxygen delivery to the heart muscle.

As just stated, the pain occurs when tissue is deprived of oxygen, causing a series of substances, called kinins, to be secreted in and around that tissue, which causes the burning pain to occur. A good example of what kinins are is what one develops in a blister in one's finger or toe. If one bursts the blister right away, the liquid that forms within it causes a burning sensation to occur in the finger or toe because this liquid contains kinins.

High lipoprotein A is also associated with coronary heart disease. A high level of homocysteine level is also associated with coronary heart disease. Both these conditions are genetically transmitted and can cause thrombosis to occur anywhere in the body.

When one is having a heart attack, what happens frequently is that the clot forms acutely because of the plaque within the vessels that cracks or a fissure within the vessel that develops, resulting in the crack. The result is that bleeding occurs acutely within that vessel, causing a clot to develop. The clot closes the vessel, acutely cutting off blood flow to the part of the heart muscle for which this vessel is responsible for delivering oxygen, and the result is an acute heart attack. The muscle that is damaged may die acutely due to lack of flow of blood to that muscle.

Cardiac dysrhythmias can develop, resulting in all sorts of rhythm disturbances such as atrial arrhythmias, ventricular tachycardia and ventricular fibrillation, etc., which can lead to the death of the individual who just had the heart attack. If a person presents to the emergency room with acute chest pain and a physician administers tPA acutely to dissolve the clot based on the symptoms and the EKG findings, the death of the involved muscle can be prevented.

This can frequently result in the survival of the patient by preventing the heart attack from occurring. It is safe to say that from the time that the patient presents with the symptoms up to several hours later, in certain circumstances, the tPA can still be of value if administered.

In 2011, coronary artery disease claimed the lives of of 7.5 million people in the world and 425,425 people in the United States. There is a high rate of cardiovascular-associated deaths in people due to the following factors: Sources: WHO and CDC

1. High blood pressure
2. Obesity
3. High lipids in the blood
4. Smoking
5. Diabetes mellitus
6. Poor diet with too much fat, carbohydrates, and salt. Two-third of people is obese/overweight in the United States and obesity is a major risk factor for coronary artery disease.
7. Genetic predisposition, gender, stress, poverty, poor education, poor economic status, marital problems, raising children and caring for a family, etc.

All these factors together play a major role in the causation of an increased rate of coronary artery disease.

The following is a list of some factors that can decrease the incidence of coronary occlusive disease secondary to high lipids:

1. Maintainance of an ideal weight.
2. Regular exercise.
3. Non-abuse of alcohol.
4. A diet of plenty fruits and vegetables.
5. Preparation of foods only with vegetable oils.
6. Avoidance of butter.
7. Use of skim milk.
8. Removal of the skin from the chicken to remove as much fat as possible.
9. Use of margarine that is low in fat.
10. Avoidance of red meat as much as possible.
11. Decreased ingestion of pork, bacon, cheese, sausages, egg yolk, all foods that are too rich in fat.
12. Avoidance of too much simple carbohydrate-containing foods because simple carbohydrates are converted into fat in the liver, which ultimately results in fat deposition in the tissues in the human body resulting in obesity.
13. Decreased consumption of foods with a high sugar content such as cakes and pies.
14. Avoidance of fast foods as much as possible because they contain too many fat and simple carbohydrates.
15. Minimization of the ingestion of high cholesterol foods such as lobster, crabs, shrimps, and oysters by individuals who already have high cholesterol.
16. Avoidance of cooking foods with coconut oil because coconut is too rich in cholesterol.
17. Eating foods with high fiber, such as collard greens when prepared without ham, hocks, hock tails, and bacon. Vegetable oil, a little bit of hot sauce, and a little bit of wine make the greens taste just as good.
18. Eating foods with complex carbohydrates, such as yams, plantain, sweet potato, green bananas, and pasta. These foods are very high in cellulose which turns into fiber which is good for the body. These foods also contain good vitamins and satisfy hunger. Yet, they will not result in gain weight because the human body is not capable of breaking down complex carbohydrates. People in the underdeveloped world eat these types of food and they, by and large, do not suffer from the same degree of obesity as people in the United States. The incidence of high lipids is quite low in the underdeveloped world because a lot of vegetables and fruits are consumed instead of fast foods frequently consumed in the so-called "developed world". Fat-containing foods that are a great part of the diet in the United States and other developed countries predispose their

inhabitants to all sorts of diseases such as cancer, coronary artery disease, and diabetes.

19. Using vegetable oils and olive oil that contain polyunsaturated fat in cooking.
20. Sparing use of mayonnaise which is very rich in cholesterol.

Treatments of hyperlipidemia:

The rate limiting enzyme that controls the synthesis of cholesterol in the liver is 3-Hydroxy-Methyl-glutaric—Co enzyme A (HMG-CoA). Once this enzyme is blocked, LDL receptors increase, preventing the re-absorption of cholesterol from the blood.

The medications in use to treat high cholesterol are called Statins and they include:

1. Zocor
2. Lipitor
3. Lescol
4. Mevacor
5. Crestor
6. Niacin
7. Pravastatin
8. Livalo

Some of the most important parts of the treatment of high cholesterol, high triglycerides and hyperlipidemia in general are diet, exercise and weight loss. However, once the cholesterol reaches a level at which the diet is not sufficient, then the clinical thing to do is to provide the patient with medication.

Medications in use to treat high triglycerides are:

1. Lopid (gemfibrozil)
2. Tricor (fenofibrate)
3. Cholestyramine
4. Colestipol (bile acid rasins)
5. Trilipix
6. Lipofen

The usual dose of Cholestyramine is 8-12 grams 2 or 3 times per day by mouth. The usual dose of Colestipol is 10-15 grams 2 or 3 times per day by mouth. Lopid (gemfibrozil) decreases triglycerides and VLDL (very low-density lipoprotein) and increases HDL. The usual dose of Lopid is 600 mg by mouth 2 times per day. The usual dose of Tricor is 145 mg or 43 mg daily by mouth.

The usual dose of Trilipix is 135 mg by mouth nightly and the usual dose of Lipofen is150 mg by mouth nightly.

It is important that these fat-lowering medications and, in particular, the Statin be taken one half hour after dinner every night and the reason is that fat is circadian, which means there is more fat in the blood at night. The more fat there is in the blood at the time the Statin is being taken, the better the chance of removing the most fat from the bloodstream.

It is important to realize that these medications work best when given in the evening because cholesterol works via the circadian system. That is to say, that cholesterol level is highest in the evening in the body. The usual doses of these medications are 10-20 mg a half hour after dinner nightly for Lovastatin, 10-40 mg for Provestatin, and 5-20 mg for Simvastatin. The maximum dose of Lovastatin can go as high as 80 mg daily, Provestatin as much as 40 mg and the Simvastatin as high as 40 mg. These medications are quite expensive, but they are very effective in bringing down the total cholesterol, LDL, and triglycerides and raising the HDL, thereby decreasing incidence of coronary disease and arterial occlusive disease all over the body.

All these medications, and in particular the HMG CoA reductase inhibitors, can cause mild liver function test abnormality and for that reason it is important to monitor the liver function tests every six weeks to two months. It is very important to emphasize that these medications must be used in conjunction with a low-fat, low simple-carbohydrate diet along with a good exercise program.

Another known side effect of these medications is muscle and joint pain. This occurs because of muscle breakdown and secondary inflammation. In some cases, this can lead to rhabdomyolysis, which, if not recognized quickly and treated, can lead to kidney failure. If these symptoms are persistent and severe, the medication ought to be stopped and the patient's doctor contacted.

The test to do to confirm this problem is serum CPK. When muscles are swollen, the CPK level in the blood goes up. Niacin is also a very good medication to treat high cholesterol. The usual starting dose is 500 mg at bedtime. The maximum dose of Niacin is 2000 mg at bedtime. Niacin has many side effects and prominent among them are flushing and diarrhea, etc.

Along the same line, it has been shown that drinking one or two glasses of wine at night, either red or white, with dinner, increases the level of the HDL (the good cholesterol). It is not advisable that people drink or abuse alcohol, but these studies clearly show that moderate ingestion of alcohol, in particular red wine, seems to have a significant advantage in increasing the level of the HDL cholesterol.

Diet plays a major role in the prevention of obesity and the prevention and control of hypertension. Diet also plays a major role in both preventing and controlling the levels of cholesterol and triglycerides in the blood. The so-called soul food that blacks like to eat so much is a legacy of slavery that began 500 hundred years ago in the United States.

However, soul foods have too much fat, simple carbohydrates, and salt, and are too spicy. These foods taste good, but they are unhealthy. Therefore, it is fine to eat them every now and then; but when a person eats them on a daily basis, it increases his or her chances of becoming obese and raising his and her blood pressure and cholesterol.

A combination of obesity, high blood pressure, and high level of fat in the blood is responsible in part for the high incidence of coronary artery disease and deaths of people in the United States. To prevent this high occurrence of coronary artery disease and deaths, the diet of most people must clearly be modified. Diet is very ethnic in its origin. People of different ethnic backgrounds have different tastes for different foods, and that is fine, except that one has to understand that everything has to be done in moderation.

If a person eats fat and simple carbohydrate and salt-laden foods too often, that person is likely to pay the consequences with an increased incidence of coronary artery disease, hypertension, diabetes, and stroke. Poor people in large measure suffer from these conditions because of poor education, poor living conditions, poor diet, and overall poor economic conditions.

An understanding of these issues and doing the things that are necessary either to modify or change them will go a long way to prevent the high incidence of high cholesterol, coronary heart disease, diabetes mellitus, micro vascular systemic arterial occlusive disease, macrovascular systemic arterial occlusive disease, and stroke seen in people in the world.

Chapter 2
OBESITY

"YOU DON'T HAVE TO BE WEALTHY TO EAT HEALTY
YOU DON'T HAVE TO BE WEALTHY TO BE HEALTHY"
VALIERE ALCENA, MACP.

Obesity is a serious medical problem and has reached epidemic proportion in the world. World wide, 200 million adults men, and 300 million adults women are obese. There are 73 million or 34% of adults who are obese and 12.5 million or 17% of children and teenagers who are obese in the U.S.

Blacks and other minorities are affected disproportionately by obesity compare to whites and other racial groups in the world. Seventy percent of Black women are obese and thirty eight percent of Black men are obese in the U.S. But obesity is also extremely prevalent in Hispanic men and women and all other racial groups. Asians as a rule are less obese.

Two-thirds of the U.S. population is overweight / obese. In 2007-2008, 32.2 % of adult men and 35.5 % of women in the U.S. were obese. Source: JAMA January 20, 20010, Vol 303, No 3.

According to a recent report from Columbia University that came out 8/15/2013
"Obesity Kills More Americans Than Previously Thought. One in five Americans, Black and white, dies from obesity".

Worldwide, there are an estimated 1 billion total obese people, and three million people die annually in the world because overweight/obesity. 440,000 deaths occur annually because of obesity in the U.S. Obesity if the fith leading cause of deaths in the world annually.

According to the WHO, by 2015 there will be 2.3 billion overweight people in the world and 700 million individuals will be obese. Annually, obesity is responsible for 440,000 deaths in the U.S. and costs $270 billion dollars per year.

In attempt to help curb the obesity epidemic in the U.S. the FAD approved to new medications to treat obesity. Qsymia (Phentermine plus topiramate extended—release) and Belviq (Lorcaserin) were approved in 2012.

Obesity, when it is not associated with malfunction of the endocrine system, is always the result of eating too much. Eating too much is a major psychological disorder.

The most effective diet is a diet that is low in carbohydrates, fats, and high in protein. Source: THE THIRD WORLD TROPICAL DIET HEALTH MAITENANCE AND MEDICAL MAGEMENT PROGRAM WRITTEN BY VALIERE ALCENA M.D. F.A.C.P PUBLISHED BY ALCENA MEDICAL COMMUNICATION INC, Copyright© 1994, ISBN 0-9633365-0-9

A diet that is low in fat and high in protein is good and will lower both weight and cholesterol. The same is true of a diet that is low in simple carbohydrates and high in protein. This raises the question: can these two types of diets help people maintain the weight they have lost on a long term basis?

When a person eats foods that have too much fat and carbohydrates, and the body is unable to break them all down, the remaining fat and carbohydrates are stored in the liver where they are distributed to different tissues of the abdomen, hips, thighs, and other parts of the body. The fat and carbohydrates that are broken down are used as fuel to provide needed energy for proper functions of the body.

In order for this process to work properly, one needs a well-functioning basal metabolism. The basal metabolism is a process through which the body burns calories that are ingested in the body. If the basal metabolism is high, one burns calories too fast and stays thin. If the basal metabolism is too low, one burns calories too slow and stays fat. Slow basal metabolism, when not associated with medical problems such as hypothyroidism, is always the result of a genetically transmitted abnormality, which is passed on from parents to offspring. There are several medical conditions that are associated with obesity, among them are:

1. Hypothyroidism
2. Synrdome X
3. Cushing's disease (when the adrenal gland secretes too much adrenal hormone)
4. Gigantism a condition where a person becomes overgrown, too big and too large, due to hyperfunctioning of the pituitary gland.

When a person is obese and the aforementioned endocrine conditions have been ruled out as a cause, he or she is not taking steroids or estrogen replacement medication, then he or she is obese because of a combination of low basal metabolism associated with ingestion of too much foods containing fat and simple carbohydrates.

Prevalence of obesity in the United States

Seventy percent of black women are obese/overweight and thirty eight percent of black males are obese/overweight. Sixty percent white females and Thirty two percent white males are obese. Sventy eight Hispanic percent women and eighty one percent of Hispanic men are obese. Nine percent of Asian Americans are obese and thirty two percent of American Indians/Alaska Natives are obese.

Obesity is defined as being 20% over one's ideal weight and a BMI >30. This represents an example of a 125-pound 5-foot—4-inch woman.

IDEAL WEIGHT FOR WOMEN

HEIGHT				
FEET	INCHES	SMALL FRAME	MEDIUM FRAME	LARGE FRAME
4	10	102-111	109-121	118-131
4	11	103-113	111-123	120-134
5	0	104-115	113-126	122-137
5	1	106-118	115-129	125-140
5	2	108-121	118-132	128-143
5	3	111-124	121-135	131-147
5	4	114-127	124-138	134-151
5	5	117-130	127-141	137-155
5	6	120-133	130-134	140-159
5	7	123-136	133-147	143-163
5	8	126-139	136-150	146-167
5	9	129-142	139-153	149-170
5	10	132-145	142-156	152-173
5	11	135-148	145-159	155-176
6	0	138-151	148-162	158-171

Weight in pounds, based on ages 25-59 with the lowest mortality rate
(indoor clothing weighing 5 pounds and shoes with 1" heels)

IDEAL WEIGTHS FOR MEN

HEIGHT				
FEET	INCHES	SMALL FRAME	MEDIUM FRAME	LARGE FRAME
5	2	128-134	131-141	138-150
5	3	130-136	133-143	140-153

5	4	132-138	135-145	142-156
5	5	134-140	137-148	144-160
5	6	136-142	139-151	146-164
5	7	138-145	142-154	149-168
5	8	140-148	154-157	152-172
5	9	142-151	148-160	155-176
5	10	144-154	151-163	158-180
5	11	146-157	154-166	161-184
6	0	149-160	157-170	164-188
6	1	152-164	160-174	168-192
6	2	155-168	164-178	172-197
6	3	158-172	167-182	176-202
6	4	162-176	171-187	181-207

Weight in pounds, based on ages 25-59 with the lowest mortality rate
(indoor clothing weighing 5 pounds and shoes with 1" heels)

Table II—Modified classification of overweightness on obesity by BMI		
	Obesity Class	**BMI kg/m2**
Underweight		<18.5
Normal		18.5-24.9
Overweight		25.0-29.9
Obese	I	30.0-34.9
	II	35.0-39.9
Extremely Obese	III	>40

In the United States of America, many factors interplay in causing this high degree of obesity. For instance, the diet industry spends somewhere from 40 to 50 billion dollars a year selling different products and types of dietary programs. The medical profession devotes very little time and resources in the prevention and treatment of obesity. The food industry spends somewhere around 36 billion dollars a year advertising the different food products and agricultural materials they produce and encouraging people to eat more.

The main reason that the medical profession in the United States spends very little time in the prevention and management of obesity is because insurance companies could not care less about obesity and will not pay the medical profession the monies that are necessary to prevent and treat obesity.

The federal and state governments are not doing very much either, because those two governments spend somewhere around 50 thousand dollars a year on nutritional and other educational programs addressing obesity, which is a pitiful type of gesture considering that 68.8 billion dollars were spent in 1990 to treat the different complications associated with obesity.

These complications include breast cancer, colon cancer, cancer of the uterus, heart disease, adult-onset diabetes, Gall Stones, Cholocystitis, Pancreatitis secondary to Gall Stones hypertension, strokes, high cholesterol, deep vein thromphlebitis, pulmonary embolism secondary to deep vein thrombophlebitis, etc.

Many factors interplay in the excessive degree of obesity. The main factor is low basal metabolism. Low basal metabolism is inherited from parents to offspring. Genetic traits are adaptable, penetrating, and "transmittable". Obese women the world over inherited the obesity gene from their African ancestry. This gene is disseminated among people and their children. The human race and all its original DNA genetic traits began in Africa around 4.4 million years ago. Source: Ardipithecus (Ardi) Fossils, reported by a group from the University of Minnesota.

Another factor that plays a significant role in the development of obesity in people is diet. People who live in the third world who, by necessity, are forced to eat a meager diet are less obese than people who live in the developed countries, such as the United States. In the under-developed world, people eat plenty of fresh fruits, green vegetables, grains, yams, plantains, bananas, and less red meat, and plenty of fish.

People in the so-called "third world" exercise more because they often have to walk long distances to the farm or marketplace and walk to the river to fetch water, etc. Some of them spend long hours working under the hot sun in the farms and some work long hours in sweatshops. Still others work at home doing all sorts of chores around their houses. All these activities cause them to lose calories, which is quite important in maintaining their weights.

A combination of these factors leads to less obesity/overweight in people who live in the under-developed world. Nevertheless, they still carry the gene and are able to pass it on, even though they themselves manage to work off the extra fat that was to be deposited into their tissues as predetermined by their hereditary trait.

In addition, it must be understood that fat people are likely to give birth to fat babies. Babies born to fat parents are destined to become fat children, fat adolescents, and fat adults. The low basal metabolism gene which is responsible for obesity is always passing on to the offspring of obese people.

Typically, diet in the under-developed world is a diet that is high in protein, low in fat, high in vitamins and fibers, and low in simple carbohydrates. This combination of foods contains high complex carbohydrates. Examples of high complex carbohydrates foods include brown rice, pretzels, pasta, yams, sweet plantains, potatoes, dumpling, corn, cereals, breads, grains, tortillas, waffle grits, millet, oats, wheat germs, granola, cornmeal, shredded wheat flour, etc.

High complex carbohydrates when eaten, is broken down very slowly in the body and provides a lower but longer level of energy. That is what makes them ideal food products, in that a person can eat high complex carbohydrates to satisfy hunger and also to provide vitamins and fiber for regular gastrointestinal functioning, particularly for proper bowel movements. Therefore, they do not lead to an increased level of calories, which can cause a person to become obese.

On the other hand, simple carbohydrates, such as sugar-containing foods, when eaten can be broken down in the liver and some of them distributed into the tissues and muscles, resulting in obesity in individuals who consume them in large quantities.

Examples of simple carbohydrates include refined sugar, sodas, cake, white bread, white rice, mayonnaise, candies, syrup, etc. Examples of fat containing foods include red meats, pork, lobsters, shrimps, crabs, oysters, goat meat, ham, sausages, bacon, eggs, butter, avocados (the fat in avocados is monoglyceride and is good fat), coconuts, etc.

The afore-outlined foods, when prepared in vegetable oil, either boiled or broiled and not fried, satisfy hunger, provide needed vitamins such as Vitamin A, Vitamin K, the B Vitamins, including B6, B12, etc. All of them are important nutrients for the body.

Breast cancer, uterine cancer, colon cancer, cancer of the stomach, and cancer of the pancreas, cancer of the kidney, cancer of the rectum and cancer of the esophagus are all associated with eating too much fatty, spicy, and smoked foods.

The following diseases are associated with obesity.

1. Diabetes mellitus type 2
2. Atherosclerotic heart disease
3. Hypertension
4. Stroke
5. Arthritis
6. Depression

7. High cholesterol
8. Breast cancer
9. Uterine cancer
10. Colon cancer
11. Cancer of the pancreas
12. Stomach cancer
13. Rectal cancer
14. Prostate cancer
15. Sleep apnea
16. Cardiac arrhythmia
17. Gall bladder disease etc;

The first disease on the list, adult-onset diabetes mellitus, is closely associated with obesity.

What is the relationship between the onset diabetes mellitus and obesity?

When a person is obese, his or her fat cells are resistant to the effect of insulin, creating an insulin-resistant state in his or her body. In this setting, the insulin cannot penetrate these fat cells to bring about the metabolism of sugar. Consequently, blood sugar rises. The rising blood sugar creates all sorts of symptoms which are very disturbing to the affected person. Since the insulin has difficulty entering into the fat cells, it remains elevated in her bloodstream.

The high insulin level, in turn, forces the obese person to crave for sweets-containing foods to satisfy him or her, resulting in a vicious cycle. The more obese a person is, the higher the level of insulin in his or her bloodstream. The higher the level of insulin in his or her bloodstream, the more he or she craves sweets-containing foods which are high in simple carbohydrates and rich in calories. The more he or she eats these calorie-rich foods, the fatter he or she becomes, raising his or her blood sugar even higher.

What is the relationship between atherosclerotic heart disease and obesity?

Obesity is associated with atherosclerotic heart disease, in that the persistent high level of insulin that is present in the bloodstream of the obese person causes plaques to develop within vessels throughout his or her body, including the coronary arteries around the heart. When these arteries are occluded, blood flow is impeded, preventing proper oxygen delivery to the muscles of the heart, causing pain in the chest to occur. Because there are plaques in the coronary arteries, sudden closure of one or several of these coronary arteries can result in a heart attack and, frequently, death.

Obesity as just outlined is quite common in blacks in the U.S. Obesity is very highly associated with hypertension, which is also quite common in blacks. When a person is obese, the obesity is frequently associated with diabetes mellitus, hyperlipidemia, and hypertension.

This combination of diseases is frequently referred to as syndrome X, or more recently renamed as metabolic hypertension. (Syndrome W is used as well to refer to this condition.) Blacks retain more salt in their bodies than other people do, and as a result, blacks retain more fluid, and the fluid retention causes elevation in their blood pressures. When a person who is obese loses weight, frequently, his or her blood pressure decreases, and the need for medication decreases proportionately.

Obesity is also commonly associated with stroke. Many of the conditions that are frequently seen in people who are obese, such as diabetes mellitus, hypertension and hyperlipidemia, are also seen in people who suffer from stroke, and frequently the underlying reason for the stroke seen in these people is the obesity. The reason why obesity, diabetes, hyperlipidemia, and hypertension are associated with stroke is because all these conditions can cause atherosclerosis to occur.

Once vessels in the brain develop plaques, these vessels become narrowed, thereby preventing the proper flow of blood and oxygen to the brain tissues. When one of these vessels becomes acutely closed, a stroke is usually the result.

Obesity is frequently associated with breast cancer in women. In particular, there is a frequent association of breast cancer in obese in women ages 38 to 49. The type of breast cancer seen in this group of women is extremely aggressive and very resistant to treatments, resulting in a high percentage of deaths.

Obesity is also associated with uterine cancer in a high percentage of women and prostate cancer in men.

Osteoarthritis of the shoulders, lower back, knees, and ankles is frequently seen in obese women. The obesity causes a great deal of mechanical stress on these areas of the body, resulting in wear and tear, causing severe pain, and suffering.

Obese people also feel the pressure of society, which seems to favor thinner people. This negative attitude causes some obese people to become depressed a great deal of the time. Depression is more common in obese people. Obese people have difficulty in finding boyfriends and girlfriends and experience more difficulties in finding suitable employment, frequently facing discriminations of all sorts in a society obsessed with thinness and beauty. Obesity is a serious medical problem with significant impact on the overall health of people who are afflicted with the condition.

Because of obesity, these people suffer from psychosocial deprivation, economic deprivation and the interplay of these problems results in unnecessary early death from heart disease, cancer, hypertension, diabetes mellitus, stroke, kidney failure, and suicide.

People are pre-disposed to obesity either from genetics or behavior, must fight against the disease by having a diet that is low in fat, salt, and simple carbohydrates, high in protein, green vegetables, fruits, non-shellfish, chicken, veal, and low in red meats, sausages, bacon, pork, ham, egg yolks, white breads, and cakes.

The poorer economic situation of poor people in the U.S. and the world makes it almost impossible to carry out these recommendations to eat healthier foods. The unemployment rate of blacks is now 15.8% compared to 8.3% for whites.

In general, fast foods are not healthy because they contain too much fat, salt, and simple carbohydrate, all of which can contribute to obesity when eaten in excess.

It is important for people to exercise at least three times per week. It is not necessary to spend money going to expensive gymnasiums to exercise. These exercise centers charge a lot of money which are largely unaffordable for most poor people. For those who can afford the cost, they are likely to benefit from going regularly.

However, walking one hour daily also helps to burn off significant calories. Aerobic exercise, push-ups, bicycling, gardening, walking the dog, and other forms of exercise can all result in weight loss without incurring the cost of an expensive gymnasium. Batiatric surgery is an effective treatment modality in many instances.

Paying to join the so-called diet programs is frequently useless and dangerous. These programs are expensive and, according to the U.S. Government, have questionable motives in saying that they are trying to help people to lose weight.

In addition, these programs may be medically dangerous if entered into without proper medical supervision.

Learning a new way to prepare foods and a change in eating habits by eating smaller portions of foods is important. Decreasing the consumption of the so-called soul foods, and eating less fast food, will go a long way in decreasing the rate of obesity among people in the U.S. and in the world.

People ought to pay attention to the basics and adhere closely to a healthy lifestyle of frequent exercise, good diet, low alcohol consumption, and frequent visits to the physician's office for proper health screening. In addition, people must change their mind set and develop a better understanting of their circumstances by doing the things that are necessary to get a good education.

Education is the only guaranteed **FORMULA** to achieving financial success and a better life in American Society. Education not only allows a person to feel better about himself or herself, but it increases an individual's self steem and allows him or her to understand better the pitfalls that exist in society, thus being better able to avoid them. As part of the package of education, is the attainment of professional skills that are necessary to facilitate people to get jobs that good salaries to get jobs that pay good wages.

Understanding these facts, following them and taking the necessary precautions are the best ways to go about solving the problems associated with obesity and its devastating consequences on people. Consider that the annual cost of obesity in the U.S. may exeed $215 billion. Source: The Brooking Instutition, May 3, 2011 and, $270 billion according to some reports in 2012

Chapter 3
DIABETES MELLITUS

World wide in 3012, 347 million people had diabetes mellitus, and of that number, 22 million have type 1 diabetes. About 10% of pregnant women world wide develops gestational diabetes. Source: WHO

There are 26 million people in the U.S. with diabetes mellitus; 1.7 million of them have type 1 diabetes and the rest have type 2 diabetes.

Gestational diabetes mellitus is the third form of diabetes. Each year 130,000 women develop Gestational diabetes in the U.S.

Type 1 diabetes accounts for 5% of all cases of diabetes mellitus. Type 1 diabetes is an autoimmune disease in which the body develops antibodies against the beta cells that produce insulin in the pancreas. There are 2 types of type 1 diabetes. Juvenile diabetes occurs mainly in children mainly and Latent Autoimmune Diabetes occurs mainly in Adults.

Both forms of type 1 diabetes can be seen in children as well as in adults. I addition, because of the epidemic of obesesity many adolescent have developed type diabetes as well.

The tests that are available to diagnose type 1 diabetes are
  "C peptide
  Diabetes mellitus autoantibodies panel
  Islet cell antibodies tests
  Glutamic acid Decarboxylase antibodies tests
  Insulin antibodies tests"

There are 79 million people with pre-diabetes: 13% or 2.8 million Blacks in the U.S. have diabetes mellitus. Diabetes mellitus is tow to three times more common in blacks compared to whites. According to the CDC, there are 7 million undiagnosed diabetics in the U.S.

As a consquense of obesity, 3,700 young people under the age of 20 are diagnosed every year with adult onset type diabetes. Source: CDC.

Diabetes mellitus has increased 600% in the United States since 1958 and it is estimated that the incidence of diabetes mellitus will rise by 35% in the next ten years. The genetics of diabetes mellitus Type II works out this way.

Roughly, one-half of the first-degree relatives of diabetics are said according to recent reports to have or will develop abnormal glucose tolerance, and about one-fourth will become diabetic. Another way of stating the genetics is that about 4/10 of siblings of diabetics and 1/3 of the offspring of diabetics have the propensity to become diabetic.

Type I diabetes is a different disease altogether from Type II diabetes and it is said to be caused by either an autoimmune disease or some sort of a viral disease, but no one is quite sure. Type I diabetes usually starts in childhood but, it can also be seen in young adults. According to the latest figures in 2012, the cost of diabetes in the U.S. was 245 billion dollars. Source: American Diabetics Association. World wide, $465 billion were spent for the treatments of diabetes mellitus in 2011. $65.2 billion were spent for treatment of diabetes in Latin America and the Carribbean in 2011.

The risk of death is roughly two times higher in black diabetics than in non-diabetic other racial groups. Diabetes is the sixth leading cause of death in the U.S. Every year, 3.2 million people die in the world because of diabetes.

What is diabetes mellitus?

Diabetes mellitus is a condition in which the body is incapable of using sugar as a fuel due to lack of insulin. Three basic abnormalities cause diabetes mellitus.

1. Lack of insulin secretion from the pancreas,
2. Abnormal insulin secretion from the pancreas, and
3. Insulin resistance.

In the first instance, the beta cells of the Islets of Langerhans of the pancreas have been destroyed either by an autoimmune process or by a viral organism resulting in a total lack of insulin in the body, sometimes since early infancy or childhood, resulting in juvenile diabetes. In the second instance, the pancreas still has the ability to produce insulin, but needs to be forced to secrete it. In the third instance, the pancreas simply cannot make any more insulin, period. That is Type II diabetes. In the third instance, insulin has to be given either subcutaneously or intravenously. This is called insulin-requiring diabetes mellitus type II.

The normal blood glucose is from 65 to about 109 mg/dL. Diabetes mellitus is a condition in which the blood glucose is higher than normal, when the blood glucose is drawn following a period of fasting for about 8 to 12 hours. As just mentioned, the normal blood glucose is between 65 to 109 mg/dL.

If the fasting blood sugar is 110 to 124, this is pre-diabetes. If the fasting blood sugar is 125 or higher, this is frank diabetes. If the screening hemoglobin A1C is 5-6, diabetes is not present. If the hemoglobin A1C is 6.2-6.5, pre-diabetes is present. If the hemoglobin is A1C is 6.6 or greater, frank diabetes is present. In diabetes mellitus, when the blood sugar is well controlled from 5-6 weeks, the A1C is normal.

However, if the blood sugar remains poorly controlled for up to 90 days, the A1C is abnormally high. A1C is hemoglobin A with glucose attached to a terminal amino acid of the beta chains of the molecule.

Another way to test the blood of an individual to see if she or he is diabetic is for the physician to order what is called a two-hour post-prandial glucose test (Post-prandial means after eating). Two hours after eating a meal containing sugar, a tube of blood is drawn from the individual and if the blood glucose is elevated, between 140 mg/dL and 190 milligrams per deciliter or (mg/dl), then that individual is said to have glucose intolerance or early diabetes mellitus. Except for evaluation of pregnant women and screening patients for episodic hypoglycemia, glucose tolerance test will no longer be carried out to diagnose diabetes mellitus.

By the time a person with type II diabetes becomes abnormally elated, he or she has been diabetic for about 10 years and he or she has already lost 80% the beta cells in his or her pancreas. In addition, if the blood sugar is not well controlled, he or she is using fat as fuel. When fat is used in the body as fuel, ketone bodies (broken down products of fat) are produced which further damages the remaining 20% of beta cells in his or her pancreas, making the situation worse.

The genetic locus for insulin-dependent diabetes mellitus is on chromosome 6. The genetic locus for non-insulin diabetes mellitus is unknown. Usually insulin-dependent diabetes (juvenile diabetes) or type I diabetes, occurs before age 40. On the other hand, non-insulin-dependent diabetes (Type II diabetes) occurs after 40, although there are exceptions. However, most of the time insulin-dependent diabetes mellitus appears before age twenty but it can also occur later in life. Non-insulin-dependent diabetes can also occur in the late teens and early adulthood.

It is not an absolute rule, but age 35 to 40 is usually the cut-off point for someone to present with Type I diabetes mellitus. If a person is age 35 or over, the diagnosis is most likely going to be adult-onset diabetes, or Type II diabetes. If a person is between childhood and age 35, the diagnosis is most likely going to be insulin-dependent diabetes or type I. Again, there are crossovers and there are exceptions.

Recently, a group of obese adolescents ages 10-19 has been reported to have Type II diabetes mellitus.

There are different types of Type II diabetes mellitus. The most common type is due to the inability of the pancreas to secrete sufficient insulin. Other types are due to insulin resistance because of obesity. Often, in people who have chronic pancreatitis, the pancreas may ultimately fail, resulting in Type II diabetes mellitus. Primary hemochromatosis always leads to type II diabetes. Cushing's disease can cause chemically induced secondary diabetes, although it can be transient.

Another common form of diabetes is gestational diabetes seen in pregnancy. It is more common in black, Hispanic, Asian American, Pacific Islander, and Native American women than in white women. It is very important to control the blood sugar very tightly in pregnant women using insulin to prevent complications in the infant. A multitude of birth defects is known to occur in infants born to diabetic mothers.

Diabetic mothers are known to give birth to large babies and sometimes, some of these babies can be born with a very large head, making vaginal delivery difficult, if not impossible. About 10% of women with gestational diabetes go on to continue to have type II diabetes after delivery. Some 20-50% of women who had gestational diabetes will become diabetic 5-10 years later.

Endocrine pancreatic failure occurs in obese individuals resulting in type II diabetes. This happens because the pancreas over secretes insulin due to insulin resistance, which the obese state causes. In obesity, the insulin is not able to penetrate the fat cells effectively; the result is that the pancreas keeps secreting insulin as though there is a need for it, and after an extended period, it uses up its store of insulin.

Steroids can cause blood sugar to rise in people who have occult or pre-diabetes. Alcoholics who suffer from chronic pancreatitis can also develop diabetes mellitus as result of pan-pancreatic failure.

People who have occult diabetes mellitus or pre-diabetes can develop overt diabetes with markedly elevated blood sugars when under stress or in the case of infection.

Stress causes an excess secretion of adrenalin, which works counter to the effect of insulin, allowing a rise in blood sugar. (Adrenalin is an anti-insulin hormone).

Individuals, who are known diabetics, when under stress, experience a constant rise in their blood sugars, necessitating an increase in the doses of their insulin or oral hypoglycemic medications.

Since blacks and other minorities live under constant racial discrimination, their blood sugars are harder to control. This, plus many other factors causes Black, Hispanic and Native American diabetics to develop a higher rate of complications compared to whites and other racial groups.

What is happening in the bodies of people that causes her to become diabetic?

The pancreas is an organ that is located on the left side of the abdomen. The pancreas has several functions to perform within the body for proper health. Among these functions is the production of insulin.

What is insulin?

Insulin is a hormone that is produced by the pancreas. The beta cells of the pancreas produce insulin in the Islands of Langerhans.

How is the pancreas able to produce insulin?

The pancreas is able to produce insulin by means of a group of cells located within the area of the pancreas referred to as the Islands of Langerhans. These cells have the ability to produce the hormone called insulin. Once produced, the insulin is secreted into the bloodstream.

What is the role of the insulin in the body?

The job of the insulin is to metabolize breakdown sugar (Glucose) so that the body can use it as fuel. The insulin actually forces the glucose into cells where it is used for the multitude of functions that are necessary for the body to function properly.

Glucose plays many roles in the human body under the influence of insulin.

1. Sugar is used as a fuel for the body to function properly. The human body gets the bulk of its energy from the breakdown of sugar under the influence of insulin.

2. Sugar is needed in order for the blood to carry oxygen to the different tissues and organs of the human body, most importantly—the brain. Without sugar, human beings cannot carry the appropriate amount of oxygen to the brain,

which is needed to remain alert. Insulin is needed to push the sugar into these tissues and organs for proper body functions.

When the body is not able to use sugar because of lack of insulin, it is forced to use fat for fuel. Fat is a very bad fuel to be used for energy because it is not effective. When one uses fat it produces breakdown products called ketones, bodies that are very toxic when dumped into the bloodstream. The accumulation of these ketone bodies in the body because of the inability to use sugar is a condition known as ketoacidosis, which can be life-threatening if it goes unrecognized and untreated.

There exists another common reason for diabetes mellitus Type II diabetes which is hemochromatosis. Hemochromatosis is a condition described in the chapter on Anemia. Hemolytic anemias cause iron overload and secondary hemochromatosis. The gene for primary hemochromatosis is located on the long arm of chromosome 6 on the HLA locus.

Recently, several more genes have been discovered that cause primary hemochromatosis. In addition, deficiency of hepcidin causes hemochromatosis/iron over load. (See Chapter 13). More recently, a genetic test has been developed that identifies the gene called C282Y. This gene is known to cause hemochromatosis. Many individuals who have Type II diabetes believe that they inherited the diabetic gene that was passed on to them by their parents, when, in fact, it is the hemochromatosis gene that was passed on to them, which results in their iron overload.

The excess iron accumulates in the pancreas, damaging the area where the beta cells are produced and preventing it from being able to make enough insulin, resulting in hyperglycemia and a form of Type II diabetes.

The percentage of blacks and other minorities who have hemochromatosis is not well known. However, it used to be thought that primary hemochromatosis was a disease seen mainly in European Caucasians and Scandinavians, which turned out not to be altogether the case.

Many blacks and other minorities have genetically transmitted primary hemochromatosis, although most blacks are negative for the C282Y gene. The C282Y gene that causes hemochromatosis has been identified in a black woman by the author. (See Valiere Alcena, MD, FACP, "Prevalence of Iron Overload in African-Americans: A Primary Care Experience; A Clinical Observation," Prestige Medical News, Feb. 7, 2003.

The serum ferritin test when elevated may mean that a person has hemochromatosis, costs about $18.00, and is routinely available.

Clinically, hemochromatosis is manifested the same way in non-Caucasians as it is in Caucasians, and the severity of the clinical disease is as intense in Caucasians as it is in blacks. What used to be called African Iron Overload Syndrome is, in fact, real primary hemochromatosis in blacks due to hepcidin deficiency. There is no such thing as African Iron Over load Syndrome. This syndrome never existed.

Some of the early signs of diabetes mellitus include:

Recurrent fungal vaginal infection
Recurrent fungal toenails infection
Recurrentfingernail infection, (paronychia infection in the bed of the nails)
Recurrent groin fungal infection
Infection in the foreskin of the penis
Blurry vision
Thirst
Recurrent infection under the breasts (especially in women with large breasts)
Infertility
Lack of libido
Numbness and tingling in toes and fingers
Frequent spontaneous abortions
Erectile dysfunction etc;

All of these symptoms may also be due to occult or overt diabetes, etc. Some of the overt signs of diabetes, in addition to those listed above are urinary frequency, excessive consumption of fluid, dryness of the mouth, weight loss and frequent urinary tract infection.

Diabetes is a very complicated and complex disease that affects all organs in the human body one way or another. However, the organs that suffer most from the devastation of diabetes are the so-called end organs. These end organs consist of:

1. The eyes
2. The heart
3. The kidneys
4. The brain
5. The peripheral vascular system
6. The peripheral nervous system
7. The general nervous system

Other organ systems that are frequently affected by diabetes mellitus, causing severe pain and suffering, are the nervous system, causing peripheral neuropathy with pain, numbness, and coldness in the toes, feet, and fingers. If severe enough, diabetic neuropathy can cause affected blacks to be unable to walk. The skin is one of the most frequently affected organs in patients with diabetes. Diabetes affects the colon by causing constipation. Diabetes affects the stomach by causing gastro paresis with frequent indigestion, bloating, and burning in the stomach. Diabetes affects the urinary system by causing urinary retention.

The eyes are affected by diabetes because of the damage that the elevated blood sugar causes to take place inside the eyes. This damage results in bleeding within the eyes, a condition called diabetic retinopathy (see figures 1 and 2). Diabetic retinopathy is a condition that, if left untreated, can lead to blindness. The treatment for diabetic retinopathy is laser surgery.

The heart is affected by diabetes by causing hardening of the arteries, known as atherosclerosis. Atherosclerosis causes narrowing of the coronary arteries, resulting in ischemic heart disease which causes angina pectoris, and frequently results in myocardial infarction (heart attack).

The kidneys are affected by diabetes through damage to the kidney tubules and glomureli, resulting in diabetic nephropathy of different degrees. Diabetic nephropathy can cause protein loss, microalbuminuria and, ultimately, nephrotic syndrome. The result of this constellation of abnormalities is elevated serum BUN, creatinine, potassium, and renal insufficiency, which usually results in end-stage renal failure. End-stage renal failure is treated with dialysis. Forty nine percent of blacks with end stage kidney failure needing dialysis are receiving dialysis because of the effects of diabetes.

The brain is affected by diabetes by way of atherosclerosis of the arteries inside the brain, causing narrowing of these vessels, and preventing easy flow of blood and oxygen which can result in strokes.

The following are some of the acute symptoms that may signify that a person is diabetic:

1. Weight loss
2. Thirst
3. Blurred vision
4. Urinary frequency
5. Frequent tiredness and a feeling of unwellness, which, if very nonspecific, may be due to diabetes mellitus.

If these symptoms are not recognized, and the diagnosis is established and treatment is begun, then the patient may go on to develop diabetic ketoacidosis, which can lead to a comatose state and, ultimately, death.

There is a subgroup of diabetes called hyperosmolar nonketotic diabetes mellitus: a condition in which the individual loses so much water that the blood sugar can exceed 1,000. In addition, sometimes the blood sugars can go up to 1,500 to 2,000.nanogram/ dL. because the person has lost so much water that the brain becomes dehydrated, and the patient can go into a coma without having diabetic ketoacidosis. This is a very serious condition and if it is not recognized right away and treatment given with appropriate and careful fluid replacement and insulin, then the person may develop acute kidney failure because of marked dehydration, and death can result.

Some of the late signs and symptoms of diabetes are.

1. Blindness
2. Chronic kidney failure
3. Coronary artery disease
4. Recurrent leg and feet ulcers with frequent loss of lower limbs
5. Peripheral neuropathy
6. Sexual impotence
7. Loss of libido
8. Gastroparesis.
9. Infertility
10. Constipation
11. Recurrent fungal infections of the skin, sinuses, etc.

Another frequent problem that develops is urinary tract infection because diabetes damages the smooth muscle and nerves within the bladder, causing poor contraction of the bladder, preventing complete excretion of urine. The residual urine that stays in the bladder serves as a culture medium allowing for bacterial growth, and the result is recurrent urinary tract infection and all its many potential complications.

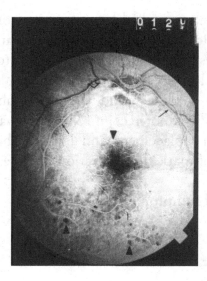

Figure 3.1-Showing different degrees of abnormalities in the eye of a patient with diabetes mellitus (diabetic retinopathy); Fluorescein angiogram shortly after injection of dye in patient's eye. Dye in arteries (white) and just starting to enter veins (large arrow). White area off NH is neovascular tuff (open arrow). White spots are hemorrhages (arrow heads). Tiny white dots are microaneurysms (small arrow).

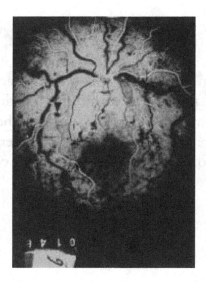

Figure 3.2-Showing different degrees of abnormalities in the eye of a patient with diabetes mellitus (diabetic retinopathy). Large arrows showing dilated veins. Arrowheads showing hemorrhages inside the eye.

Why is the incidence of diabetes mellitus so high?

The answer lies partly in the fact that obesity is more common in Blacks Hispanics, and Native Americans are more obese than Whites and Asians are, and obesity has a high association with diabetes mellitus.

Both obesity and certain forms of adult-onset diabetes mellitus are genetically transmitted diseases and it is therefore not surprising that these two diseases are so closely linked and so highly prevalent in blacks. Obesity causes a state of insulin resistance to exist, meaning that in the natural situation, the insulin that the obese person's pancreas secretes has a great deal of difficulty penetrating the fat cells to carry out proper metabolism (breaking down) of sugar. When that happens, the blood sugar stays above normal in the blood, causing a state of glucose intolerance, which is the earliest form of diabetes mellitus.

Another possible explanation for this high incidence of diabetes mellitus in Blacks Hispanics and Native Americans is stress. When added to the underlying obesity, stress associated with racial discrimination and its multitude of related problems, as well as the problems of daily living in the United States, it becomes clear why the blood sugar of many blacks is so much higher and so much more difficult to bring under control compared to their white counterparts. When an individual is under stress, that person secretes adrenalin in excess, and adrenalin is an anti-insulin hormone.

Another way of saying this is that the adrenalin prevents the insulin from doing its work, which is to break down sugar. The result is that the sugar level rises. Any other type of stressful situation, such as an acute heart attack, an acute infection such as urinary tract infection, pneumonia, or any accident can cause the level of adrenalin to go up, resulting in an elevation of blood sugar.

The dietary habits of some Blacks, Hiapanics, and Native Americans play a major role in their being overweight and play a major role in their being insulin-resistant. These blacks have a diet that is rich in fat and simple sugars. Poverty plays a major role in most blacks' inability to afford better foods. Therefore, they eat the foods they can afford. The types of foods that they can afford are frequently of poor quality. Even when the food is of very good quality, the manner in which it is prepared makes it too rich in fat and carbohydrates.

Food tends to be very ethnic in character. The foods that many blacks like to eat, so called "soul food", has its origin in Africa and the legacy of slavery. During slavery, slaves were not able to eat high-quality foods. Therefore, they compensated by preparing the foods in a way to make it more palatable by curing it with a fruit called "sour". This fruit is very juicy and is a bitter orange. When plenty of salt, hot pepper and other spices are added, the food is more palatable and its taste improves but not necessarily its quality. This is the legacy of the so-called "soul food", which is frequently eaten by some blacks, but is detrimental to their health. Whites and Asians eat these foods less frequently and when they do, they eat them as delicacies.

Fast foods like hamburgers, cheeseburgers, hot dogs, fried chicken, spareribs, pizza, pancakes, waffles, donuts etc; have proliferated in U.S. society and are easy to purchase. People, young and old, eat these types of foods very often, they are getting fat and many of them are developing type II diabetes. Those foods, although popular, are definitely not very nutritious and certainly not particularly healthy.

It is perfectly fine to eat fast foods if done infrequently, but if one makes it a habit to feast on these foods on a regular basis, then the health consequences can be dire indeed.

Obesity and diabetes are intertwined, and as just outlined, they are both genetically transmitted diseases and interact together. When they interact together in the same individual, it makes it much more difficult to provide medical care for such a person who is both obese and diabetic.

Insulin is a hormone that the body needs in order to break down glucose, to provide energy, and to carry oxygen to the brain and tissues in the body. Stress causes a person to secrete a series of other hormones called counter-regulatory hormones, which includes adrenalin and nor-adrenalin, and other catecholamines. When secreted in large amounts as described above, adrenalin and nor-adrenaline can negate the effect of insulin, making it much more difficult to lower a person's blood sugar. Most of these counter-regulatory hormones, including Cortisol, have effects that would counter the insulin's ability to do its work properly in the body.

An obese person has a good deal of difficulty using insulin because the obesity state renders his and or her insulin-resistant. Individuals who are obese and diabetic and living under stressful conditions have a constant interplay of over-secretion of adrenalin as well as an inability for insulin to penetrate the fat cells in order to lower their blood sugars. All these factors make the management of their diabetes extremely difficult.

What can people do to decrease their incidence of diabetes and what can those people who are genetically pre-determined to develop diabetes do to delay the onset of this disease?

The first thing for people to do is to learn about their family health history. They should ask questions about their parents and their grandparents who might have been diabetic. They should also find out if their siblings are diabetic. If their mothers or fathers died at an early age, they ought to inquire from their aunts and uncles whether diabetes existed in their immediate families.

If they have access to the treating physicians who cared for their parents, they ought to inquire as to the health records of their parents to ascertain whether the physicians treated their parents for diabetes. Knowing the family history may in many instances save lives. If either parent has diabetes, or more so, if both parents are diabetic, then these blacks must be ever so careful and must see their physicians for frequent evaluation of their blood sugars. Having this knowledge can go a long way in helping these blacks take the necessary precautions to delay the onset of diabetes and its devastating complications.

Some of the precautions that people need to take to decrease their chances of becoming diabetics and, if already diabetics, to better control their blood sugars include:

1. A diet rich in fruits, vegetables, protein, high in complex carbohydrates, and low in fat, simple sugar, and salt.
2. Regular exercise to burn calories, thereby decreasing weight and increasing insulin-sensitivity, which in turn decreases blood sugar.

The increase in insulin sensitivity decreases the level of insulin in the blood, which in turn decreases obese people's appetite and decreases the craving for carbohydrate-containing foods. High insulin levels in the blood of obese individuals are part of the reason why these individuals have such a craving for carbohydrates, resulting in a vicious cycle. The more obese people are, the more insulin-resistant they become, and the more insulin-resistant they are, the more they feel a need to eat simple carbohydrate-containing foods.

Insulin is an anabolic hormone, meaning that the more insulin is injected exogenously into the obese diabetics, the more the obese diabetics consume, and the more obese they become. The only way to break this vicious cycle is to treat the obese diabetics with a strict dietary program that can decrease their weight and thereby increases the insulin sensitivity. If possible, the best way to treat obese diabetics is with oral hypoglycemic agents and diet. Insulin should be used to treat obese diabetics only when it is necessary. Using a combination of oral hypoglycemia and insulin is used frequently to treat diabetics to bring down their blood sugars.

There is a long list of oral hypoglycemic agents available on the market to treat blacks with type II diabetes.

The following is a partial list of these medications.

1. DiaBeta
2. Glucotrol

3. Glucotrol XL
4. Amaryl
5. Avandia
6. Actos
7. Glucophage
8. Glucophage XR
9. Glucovance
10. Diabinese
11. Januvia
12. Onglyza
13. Kombiglyze XR etc.

Type I diabetes is treated only with insulin because the pancreas of diabetics with type I diabetes is not able to secrete any insulin at all.

The following oral hypoglycemic agents, Glucophage, Glucophage XR, Avandia and Actos and Januvia, work to lower blood sugar by increasing insulin sensitivity and uptake from the blood to cells and tissues. Glucovance, which is a combination of Glucophage and Glyburide on the other hand, works by both stimulating the pancreas to secrete insulin while facilitating insulin uptake in the blood to cells and tissues to lower the blood sugar. Because of that, these oral hypoglycemic agents can be used in conjunction with insulin, as well as with other oral agents to control blood sugar.

Diabeta, Glucotrol, Glucotrol XL, Amaryl, and Diabinese work to lower blood sugar by stimulating the pancreas to secrete insulin into the bloodstream to control blood sugar. In addition to controlling blood sugars, all these agents work to allow the body to use sugar properly as fuel for normal body functions.

Some Type II diabetics are insulin-requiring, meaning that they need to be given insulin in order to survive. In this sub—group of diabetics, the pancreas is no longer able to produce insulin in any amount.

There is another group of diabetics who are non-insulin-requiring, meaning that they still have enough beta cells left in their pancreas that can be stimulated by oral agents to secrete insulin into the bloodstream to break down the glucose as just described. The way one finds out which group of diabetics is insulin-requiring and which group is not, is by trial and error.

The different doses of oral hypoglycemic agents used to treat diabetics are as follows: The usual starting dose of Diabeta (glyburide) is 2.5 mg-5 mg each morning with breakfast; a maximum dose of 20 mg per day divided into 10 mg twice per day can be used.

The usual dose of Glucotrol (glipizide) is 5 mg each morning with breakfast, but a maximum dose of 40 mg can be given per day in divided doses. The usual dose of Glucotrol is 5 mg with breakfast each morning, but a maximum dose of 20 mg per day can be given in divided doses to control the blood sugar. The usual starting dose of Amaryl is 1-2 mg per day with breakfast. A maximum dose of 8 mg per day may be used in divided doses to control the blood sugar.

The usual starting of Avandia is 4 mg per day with breakfast. A maximum dose of 8 mg of Avandia can be used in two divided doses to control the blood sugar. The usual dose of Actos is 15-30 mg per day.

A maximum dose of 45 mg can be used to control the blood sugar. The usual dose of Glucophage (metformin) is 500 mg three times per day, but a maximum dose of 2550 mg per day can be used to control the blood sugar.

The usual dose of Glucophage XR (metformin) is 500 mg with supper, but up to 2000 mg with supper may be used to control the blood sugar. The usual starting dose of Glucovance is 1.25 mg Diabeta with 250 mg of Glucophage (1.25/250 mg), but 5/500 mg twice per day of Glucovance may be used to control the blood sugar. The usual dose of Diabinese is 250 mg per day, but up to 500 mg per day can be used to control the blood sugar.

The dose of these hypoglycemic agents must be decreased significantly in elderly people to prevent hypoglycemia, because elderly people are more likely to have fewer fats in their body and are less likely to have a good diet. These two factors, along with the long-acting effects of the agents, can cause severe and prolonged hypoglycemia in elderly women if the doses of these medications are not well monitored.

Another important factor to consider when treating elderly people with oral hypoglycemic agents is the status of their kidney functions. Renal insufficiency is very likely in an older individual which dictates that less insulin is needed to maintain the normoglycemic state. This is so because 15% of the body's sugar is metabolized (made in the kidneys), and as the kidneys become sick and insufficient, the less able they are to produce that amount of sugar, making the need for insulin less, therefore the need for oral hypoglycemic agents also much less.

There are many different insulin preparations available to treat diabetes mellitus, some of them, such as Humulin N or NPH, are long-acting, and some of them, such as Humulin R regular insulin, are short-acting. Some insulin preparations are intermediate-acting. There is also a mixture of regular insulin with long-acting insulin called 70/30. The patient's physician and the patient determine the types of insulin that are appropriate for her.

The following is a list of some of the insulin preparations in use to treat Diabetes Mellitus.

1. Humulin N
2. Lantus
3. Humulin R
4. NovoLog
5. Novolog 70/30
6. Bydureon once weekly injection (is GLP-1 receptor antagonist newly approved by the FDA)

In the acute setting, in a person who presents with elevated blood sugar, dehydration, thirst and other associated acute symptoms of diabetes, she must be treated inside a hospital with fluid replacement, electrolyte replacement, and either IV regular insulin drip or subcutaneous insulin to bring the blood sugar down and correct the dehydration and the electrolyte abnormalities. If he or she presents in diabetic ketoacidosis, he or she must be treated with IV fluid, and regular insulin either intravenously or subcutaneously. If he or she is in shock, and cannot perfuse his or her skin well, the regular insulin must be given intravenously to assure its entry into the bloodstream to bring down the blood sugar and correct the ketoacidosis.

The management of diabetes mellitus and its associated problems is very complex and it takes an experienced physician to properly treat them. A diet poor in simple sugar, carbohydrates, in association with exercise and weight management are crucial and necessary parts in the treatment of diabetes mellitus.

Type I diabetes mellitus (juvenile diabetes) is treated with insulin, diet, exercise, and weight management. Oral agents that work to control the blood sugar by stimulating the pancreas are not appropriate in the treatment of juvenile diabetes because there is no insulin in the pancreas for these oral agents to secrete in the bloodstream.

In the hospital setting, blood sugar is tested several times per day and insulin dosages are adjusted according to the level of sugar in the blood.

At home, there are different types of blood sugar meters available commercially for patients who are diabetic to test their blood sugar, which allow them to adjust their insulin dosages or the dosages of their oral hypoglycemic agents on instructions from their physicians.

Diabetics ought to have their eyes examined to be certain that they do not have diabetic retinopathy. They also ought to see the podiatrist in order to have proper foot care and avoid cuts in their toes that can lead to diabetic ulcers with the potential for the loss of a limb.

The reason that diabetics do not heal very easily is due in part to poor circulation, which is secondary to the damage that diabetes causes to veins, arteries, and smaller vessels in their feet, which results in poor blood and oxygen delivery to tissues in their extremities.

Another reason why diabetics do not heal easily is that when a cut occurs, the polynuclear white blood cells of the diabetics do not migrate well towards the site of the infection. The result is that the infection is much more difficult to treat.

It is a good idea also for diabetics to get in contact with the American Diabetic Association to become familiar with all the different programs that are available to them. In addition, wearing an arm bracelet identifying themselves as diabetics is a very good idea so that they can be easily identified as diabetics in the event they become ill in the street or on the job, either because of hypoglycemia (low blood sugar) or hyperglycemia (high blood sugar).

In such a case, the bracelet will show that the wearer is diabetic and can be quickly given a piece of candy, a glass of orange juice or soda while waiting for medical help to arrive. It is also a good idea for diabetics always to carry in their pocketbooks a candy bar. In the event they feel dizzy and weak or feel like they are going to develop a hypoglycemic episode, which consists primarily of dizziness, sweatiness, or a feeling of impending doom, they can prevent the hypoglycemic episode by eating the candy bar.

Hypoglycemia (low blood sugar) that occurs on a repeated basis is very dangerous because sugar is needed to carry oxygen into the brain. When the patient is having repeated episodes of hypoglycemia, the brain is being deprived of oxygen. In other words, when the diabetic person feels sick, it is best for him or her to ingest sugar because it is an easy way to raise the level of the blood sugar.

In addition, during each episode of hypoglycemia high level of adrenalin is secreted resulting stumilation of the heart which, can lead to ischemia resulting in heart attacks and cardiac arrhythmia and death.

Therefore, thightly control blood sugar is no longer recommended.

On the other hand, it is much more difficult to treat the condition of low blood sugar or hypoglycemia if it is the result of medications such as oral anti-diabetic medications. In particular, hypoglycemia associated with oral agents that the diabetic might be taking must be treated in a hospital setting because it could take days to raise the level of the blood sugar. This is because the half-life of some of these hypoglycemic agents can be quite long.

Recent literature supports the approach that it makes no sense to over treat diabetics with Insulin or oral hypoglycemic medications to control blood sugar tightly. There is no proof that this over treatment reduces vascular damage in diabetics. On the other hand, clear evidence exists to show that recurrent hypoglycemic episodes damage the brain which can lead to dementia.

Diabetes mellitus, while not a curable disease, is definitely a treatable disease. There are plans underway for pancreatic transplants and if these become successful, then the disease can, at that point, be considered curable. Insulin pumps are also already in use. These pumps add a great deal to the treatments of diabetics requiring insulin.

There is also research underway to try to determine the cause of Type I diabetes and the hope is that someday, the answer will be found. Meanwhile, it is important for diabetics to learn as much about diabetes mellitus as they can, and in the case of obese diabetics, it is important that they make every effort to get the excess weight under control to help better control their diabetes, decrease the multitudes of end organs damage, and thereby prolong their lives.

Chapter 4
HEART DISEASES

Cardiovascular disease (CVD) is a combination of hypertension, coronary heart disease, and stroke. 34% of individuals in the U.S. have CVD. 16 million have coronary artery disease. 5.8 millon have stroke, 73 million have hypertension and 5.3 million have congestive heart failure. CVD is the leading cause of deaths in the U.S. Every year, more than 900,000 individuals die of CVD in the U.S. Worldwide, 17,000,000 people die from CVD every year and hypertension is the cause of 8,000,000 of these deaths. The annual cost of CVD in the U.S. is $450 billion. The total annual cost of CVD worldwide is $863 billion.

Heart disease is the leading cause of death in the U.S. 12,900,000 million individuals who have coronary heart disease in the U.S., costing 130 billion dollars per year. About 7,600,000 million of these individuals have had heart attacks. Every year, there are 1.1 million heart attacks in the U.S. and 450,000 of them are recurrent heart attacks (Source: Morbidity and Mortality: 2002 Chart Book on Cardiovascular, Lung and Blood Diseases. Bethesda, Maryland National Heart, Lung and Blood Institute, May 2002). Some 6,600,000 individuals in the U.S. suffer from angina pectoris (chest pain). Every day 2,600 people die of cardiovascular disease in the U.S.; this represents on an average one death every 33 seconds.

In the year 2000, there were 2,400,000 deaths in the U.S. from different causes and 1,415,000 of these deaths were due to cardiovascular disease of different types. Each year over 600,000 people die from coronary heart disease in the U.S. Cardiovascular heart disease is the number one killer in the U.S.

The incidence of cardiovascular disease is much higher in blacks than it is in whites and other racial groups. In 2005, 44.6 percent of black males and 37.2 of white males had CVD and 35 percent of white females and 49 per cent of black females had CVD.

Every day, 2,400 people in the U.S. die of CVD. This is an average of one death every 37 seconds. The death rates from CVD are much higher for blacks than for whites and other racial groups.

Source: NCHS. Compressed mortality files underlying cause of death. Coronary heart disease is much more common in blacks than in whites and other non-blacks in the U.S.

In 2006, 81,100,000 individuals in the U.S. had CVD: 17,600,000 had Chronic Heart Disease (CHD), 8,500,000 had acute heart attack, 10,200,000 had angina pectoris, 6,400, 000 had stroke, 73,600,000 had high blood pressure, and 5,800,000 had congestive heart failure.

In 2012, 16.8 million Americans have CHD, 8.7 million men and 8.1 million women. In 2012, 1.2 million Americans had a new or recurrent heart attack. 770,000 had a new heart attack and 430,000 had a recurrent heart attack.

About 17,600,000 individuals living today have a history of heart attack or angina pectoris or both. This represents 9,200,000 males and 8,400,000 females.

The incidence of CHD and deaths from CHD are higher in blacks, Hispanics, American Indians, Alaska Natives than in Asians and whites and other racial groups.

The black community is not homogenous: about 10% of blacks in the U.S. were born outside the U.S. and as such have different dietary habits.

Blacks, Hispanics, Asians and Whites born outside the U.S. have a healthier diet than Blacks, Hispanics, Asians and Whites born in the U.S. do. A good example of that is the French; they have less CHD than Americans do.

Every 37 seconds some one has a heart attack and every 60 seconds some dies of a heart attack in the U.S.

Every year, 295,000 cardiac arrests occurred out of the hospital in the U.S. In 2006, 425,425 deaths resulted from CHD in the U.S. making CHD the leading yearly killer in the United States.

Although Black Americans, Hispanics and other minorities are less likely to be diagnosed with CHD, they die more frequently of CHD compared to White Americans.

In 2006, the death rates from CHD per 100,000 people were 206.4 Black American Males vs. 176.3 White American males and 130.0 Black American females vs. 101.5 White American females. Source: American Heart Association.

In 2011, 450,000 people died of CHD in the U.S. World wide, CHD is the leading cause of deaths, responsible for 1 in 5 men and 1 in 6 women deaths, totaling 7.2 million deaths.

In 2006, 5,800,000 individuals had congestive heart failure in the U.S. (water in the lungs) and there are 500,000 new cases of congestive heart failure every year. World wide 22 million people have CHF with 2 million new cases every year.

The rates of congestive heart failure are several times more common in American Blacks than in Whites and other racial groups. In addition, congestive heart failure occurs at an earlier age in Blacks compared to Whites and other racial groups.

"African Americans between the ages of 45 and 65 have a 70% higher rate of CHF, with mortality rates of 2.5 times more than the Caucasian population" Source: CDC, 2011

Why is there such a high incidence of coronary artery heart disease (CAD) and deaths from CAD in blacks in the USA?

Obesity contributes to CAD. Over all, 76% of African Americans are over weight/overweight; fifty three percent of African American women are obese and 77% of them are overweight; about 38% of African American men are obese. 75.7% of Hispanic women are overweight/obese. 59.5 % of white women are overweight/obese. 81.7 % of Hispanic males are overweight/obese. 69.9% of white males and 74.0% of black males are overweight/obese. See chapter on obesity above.

Hypertension also contributes to CAD in blacks: In 2010, there were 736, 000,000 people with hypertension in the USA. While forty percent of African Americans have hypertension, blacks are more likely to ignore their symptoms of hypertension. World wide 1 billion have hypertension. See chapter on hypertension.

The symptoms of hypertension are:

Head ache
Dizziness
Shortness of breath
Chest pain
Palpitations
Tiredness
Blurry vision, etc,

Blacks and other minorities are less likely to get proper medical attention when presenting to the emergency room seeking medical help because some of the health care professionals working in the ER believe that most blacks complain of vague and hysterical symptoms when they present in the ER. (Of course, more often than not, this assumption is false).

Blacks are less likely to be offered cardiac catheterization to evaluate them for the possibility of coronary artery disease. When blacks are found to have coronary occlusive disease, they are less likely to be offered coronary bypass to treat their coronary artery disease. Blacks live under conditions that oftentimes are more stressful than whites are. These multitudes of stresses predispose blacks to conditions that create a perfect formula for the development of CAD heart attacks and sudden death.

The combination of obesity, hypertension, diabetes mellitus, high cholesterol and insulin resistance, referred to as syndrome X or metabolic syndrome plays a major role in the causation of coronary artery disease in blacks in the USA.

The diet of African Americans is, for the most part, less healthy than that of whites, due partly to deprived economic circumstances. Because, generally, blacks are poorer than whites, the result is a lifestyle that predisposes them to poorer cardiac health.

The diet of most blacks and other minorities is too rich in fats, simple carbohydrates, salt, and too poor in protein, fibers, fruits and vegetables. The poor diet of most blacks is guaranteed to give rise to many serious medical problems including heart disease.

The cholesterol level of people of color is usually higher than that of whites. The higher rates of obesity seen in blacks compared to whites predispose them to higher rates of morbidity and mortality.

Stress as a psychological state is generally more prevalent in blacks and other minorities than in whites. The higher rate of stress seen in blacks and other minorities predisposes them to a much higher incidence of CAD.

The incidence of cigarette smoking is generally higher in blacks and other minorities than in whites. The higher rate of smoking as seen in blacks and other miorities predisposes them to higher incidence of CAD.

The incidence of alcohol abuse, percentage-wise, is higher in whites than in whites, but all the chronic medical problems associated with alcohol abuse is seen more frequently in blacks compared to their white counterparts. Chronic alcohol abuse is associated with an increased incidence of CAD.

The incidence of IV drug abuse is higher in blacks and other minorities than in whites. IV drug abuse is a major risk factor for overall poor heart health. The result is that the overall rate of heart disease morbidity/mortality is higher in blacks and other minorities than in whites.

When blacks and other minorities present to emergency rooms as previously mentioned with symptoms of heart disease, they are less likely to be taken seriously compared to white patients. Their pain is usually attributed to other factors. They are less likely to be admitted to a coronary care unit and they are less likely to be offered cardiac catheterization, angioplasty, or coronary bypass.

The individuals who receive the quickest attention and the highest priority in the health care system in the USA are white males. This is so, in part, because more often than not, the physicians making the decisions as to who gets what type of care are white male doctors in training (interns, residents, and fellows). These young physicians work at the front line in the emergency rooms and inside the hospitals.

It is a well known secret of the profession, white Physicians are more attentive to white patients than they are to black and other minority patients. Racism quite frequently enters into life and death decisions made by physicians who take an OATH to provide needed health care for all.

Not too long ago, the American Medical Association apologized for one hundred twelve years of racial discrimination towards black Americans.

The availability of health insurance also plays a major role in the type of care that is offered to blacks when they present seeking health care. The number of uninsured in the U.S. in 2010 is 47 million. When the number of people unemployed is factored in, the actual number of people uninsured in the U.S. is closer to 50 million.

The percentage of uninsured is higher in black and other minoritiy Americans than in white Americans. Thirty six percent of black Americans ages 19-29 are uninsured while twenty three percent of white Americans of the same ages are uninsured.

Many people who are uninsured are working. Economic status determines insurance status. In May 6, 2011, the unemployment number in the U.S. was 9.0%. During that same time, the unemployment rate for black Americans was 16.1% and 8.0% for whites. The unemployment for black males was 17.3%, compared to 7.8% for white males, 12.8% for black females, and 6.6% for white females.

Many people live below the poverty line. In fact, 24.7% black Americans live below the poverty line.

Risk factors for coronary heart disease include:

1. Hypertension
2. Obesity
3. Diabetes mellitus
4. Poor dietary habits

5. Hyperlipidemia (high cholesterol, high triglycerides, high LDL, low HDL, high cholesterol / HDL ratio)
6. High lipoprotein A in the blood
7. High lipoprotein A in conjunction with high LDL in the blood
8. High homocysteine level in the blood
9. Alcohol abuse
10. Stress
11. Type A personality
12. Tobacco smoking
13. Hereditary predisposition
14. Racial discrimination
15. Poverty
16. Lack of health insurance
17. Sickle cell disease
18. Hemochromatosis/Iron overload
19. Sleep apnea, etc.

How does hypertension cause heart disease?

Hypertension takes various routes in causing heart disease. First, the fact of having a high pressure within vessels while the blood passes through those vessels causes the lumen of the vessels to get damaged. The areas of the blood vessels' lumen that get damaged trap debris as the blood passes through them and platelets and lipid particles settle onto the damaged areas inside the vessels, resulting in the formation of a nidus.

Once a nidus is formed, then more of such materials are deposited on these areas, resulting in formation of plaques. The plaques grow larger and larger, causing narrowing of the vessels, particularly in the coronary arteries. The narrowed coronary arteries prevent blood and oxygen delivery to heart muscle, causing symptoms of coronary heart disease.

Another mechanism through which hypertension causes cardiovascular heart disease is sustained high blood pressure which lasts for a long time and remains untreated for a long time, resulting in a hypertrophied (enlarged) heart muscle. The enlarged heart, in time, becomes unable to pump blood properly and fails resulting in congestive heart failure. The reason that the enlarged heart fails is that muscle fibers have a finite stretching ability, and once the muscle fibers of the heart are stretched to the maximum, then the heart becomes like a big floppy bag with very poor function, resulting in the development of many serious and disabling symptoms of cardiovascular disease, including cardiac rhythm abnormalities.

Diabetes mellitus also has a high association with coronary artery heart disease.

How does diabetes mellitus cause heart disease?

The high level of blood sugar in the circulating blood damages blood vessels, including the vessel around the heart, namely the coronary arteries. Once the effects of diabetes damage the lumen of the coronary arteries, then plaques easily form, resulting in coronary disease and the symptoms of coronary heart disease. Sorbitol is a sugar whose level becomes quite elevated in uncontrolled diabetes and Sorbitol has a very toxic effect on different vessels in the body as well as different peripheral nerves in the body, causing a multitude of vascular and nerve damage. Obesity also has a high association with the development of coronary artery heart disease.

How does obesity cause heart disease?

Obesity is associated with coronary heart disease by being associated with diabetes mellitus, hyperlipidemia, and hypertension. Some prefer to call this metabolic syndrome, metabolic hypertension, syndrome W or syndrome X. A sedentary life style is highly associated with obesity, increasing the evidence of coronary heart disease. In addition, obesity is associated with coronary heart disease because obesity creates a state of insulin resistance in the human body.

The insulin resistance results in an elevated level of insulin in the circulation of the human body. This excess insulin works in a negative way to cause more plaques to develop in arterial vessels of these obese patients. In other words, too much insulin in the circulation is atrogenic. The higher the level of circulating insulin is in the blood, the higher the likelihood that affected people might develop coronary occlusive disease. The more obese a person is, the more insulin-resistant he or she is likely to be, the more insulin-resistant he or she is, and the higher the level of circulating insulin in his or her blood.

Once plaques form in these arteries, the vessels' narrowing process begins, leading to all the possible problems associated with this process.

How does a poor diet contribute to a high incidence of atherosclerotic heart disease in blacks?

A fat-rich diet leads to higher lipid levels and its propensity to cause coronary artery heart disease. The higher carbohydrate-containing diet results in obesity and its propensity to the development of heart disease.

The high salt in the diet of many people contributes to the development of hypertension and all of its associated problems. The average black eats about 7 grams of salt per day. "The average white eats 3.436 mg of salt per day. The recommended daily salt intake is 1.5 grams of salt per day. Decreasing the salt intake to 1.5 grams of salt per day can save more 100,000 lives per year in the U.S."

Moreover, according to a report by the AMA issued in April of 2010, most of the salt eaten by Americans comes from processed foods and, as a result, the health care system can save 24 billion dollars per year by decreasing the salt intake to 1.5 grams per day. Decreasing salt intake will result in the decreased occurrence of hypertension, coronary artery disease, heart attacks, congestive heart failure, stroke, and kidney failure.

The high carbohydrate content in the diet of many people is also associated with both the development and poor control of diabetes mellitus, which ultimately contributes to the development of coronary artery heart disease.

Having high cholesterol and high triglycerides (hyperlipidemia) is a genetically transmitted condition from parent or parents to their children. However, diet plays a major role in how high the level of cholesterol, triglycerides, and low-density lipoprotein goes. The high-density lipoprotein (HDL) goes up with exercise and moderate intake of wine—2-3 glasses of red or white wine or 1-2 drinks of hard liquor per day.

Alcohol in wine causes a decrease in coronary artery disease by raising HDL cholesterol. Substances found in the skin of the grapes that are used to make wine such as polyphenoles and flavonoids and other antioxidants decrease the incidence of coronary heart disease. These substances are also found in olives and green peas. Apparently, these substances play some role in preventing local inflammatory reaction within coronary arteries, which is an important factor in reducing the formation of coronary occlusive disease. The French, however, show that the effect of alcohol on decreasing the stickiness of the platelets is important in preventing clot formation. It is not altogether clear whether white wine has a similar effect.

How does high cholesterol cause heart disease?

One hundred and two million American adults have high cholesterol: 44.8% of black men and 47.9% of black women have high cholesterol in the U.S. The number of blacks dying of CAD yearly in the U.S. is approximately 104,000 and high cholesterol plays a significant role in causing these deaths. Therefore, it is very important that blacks have their cholesterol level tested on a regular basis.

There are five parts to the clinically lipid profile:

1. Cholesterol
2. Triglycerides
3. High-density lipoprotein
4. Low-density lipoprotein
5. HDL/cholesterol ratio

Each one of these five parts of the lipid profile, when abnormal, is a risk factor for the development of coronary heart disease. The cholesterol is abnormal when it is too high, greater than 200 (there are certain situations in clinical medicine when too low cholesterol is also abnormal, in particular in malabsorption). The triglycerides are abnormal when the level is too high. The HDL is abnormal when it is too low. The low-density (LDL) is abnormal when it is too high. The ratio of HDL to cholesterol is abnormal when it is too high.

Poor and lower-middle-class individuals in the U.S. and in the world have limited income, so their food-buying power is also limited to purchasing foods that are poor in quality. Consequently, the health benefit of these foods is limited. These foods satisfy hunger, but have very little nutritional value. Foods such as bologna, bacon, sausages, pig's feet, cow's feet, cheeseburgers, pizza, hamburgers, chitterlings, and collard greens cooked with ham hogs are greasy and too rich in fats and salt to have any substantial nutritional value. As just stated, these foods do satisfy hunger, and that is a positive thing, but in the long run they can cause high cholesterol.

In addition, they can contribute to obesity, high blood pressure, all of which can lead to the development of coronary artery disease, heart attacks, congestive heart failure, stroke, kidney failure, glaucoma, and other lethal consequences.

Foods such as pork, beef, goat meat, eggs, ham, lobster, shrimp, crabs, oysters, cheeses, avocado, coconut, etc., are rich in cholesterol and when eaten in large quantities and too frequently can cause elevation in blood cholesterol.

Once the lipid level is high in the blood, regardless of how it gets there, it causes plaque to form. Once plaque is formed, coronary arteries become narrowed, resulting in coronary artery heart disease, all its associated symptoms, and other consequences.

How can a high level of lipoprotein-A in the blood cause a heart attack to occur?

Lipoprotein-A is a large lipoprotein which is made by the liver and secreted into the blood. When the level of lipoprotein-A is elevated in the blood, if the LDL cholesterol is also elevated, the two work synergistically to bring about the development of plaques within the coronary arteries around the heart, resulting in coronary artery heart disease. In addition, the elevated lipoprotein-A by itself can cause a clot to develop in the coronary arteries without the formation of plaques, resulting in an acute myocardial infarction.

This reaction occurs because lipoprotein-A competes with plasminogen, displaces it, overwhelms it and renders it helpless in preventing clots from forming. (The main role of plasminogen is to prevent fibrin/clot from forming.) In addition, lipoprotein-A attaches itself to heparin, cells, and tissues creating a state of hypercoagulability making clot formation occur spontaneously, which can result in death.

Elevated lipoprotein-A can also cause a clot to form in the low pressure (venous system) resulting in Deep Vein Thrombophlebitis/Pulmonary Embolism.

About 20% of the U.S. population has elevated lipoprotein-A, but the percentage of lipoprotein—A is much higher in blacks than whites. The percentage of Lipoprotein-A is higher in Jamaicans and other Caribbean blacks than in black Americans and other racial groups. Overall, 20% of the U.S. population have high lipoptrotein-A. Elevated lipoprotein can also cause multiple stroke syndromes in the brain causing TIA, seizures and dementia.

High homocysteine level in the blood is toxic to blood vessels and can cause plaques to form inside vessels in both the high pressure and low pressure systems in the human body.

Alcohol abuse can cause coronary artery occlusive disease to develop, because when alcoholics are drunk, they frequently become agitated. The agitated state creates a hyperdynamic situation, resulting in rapid heart rate and elevation of blood pressure. This transient but frequent high blood pressure causes two things to happen: first, the high blood pressure damages the inside of coronary arteries, resulting in plaque formation and eventual narrowing of these vessels; and second, the frequent elevation of blood pressure causes enlargement of the heart, resulting in hypertensive heart disease, which in time causes congestive heart failure.

Another form of heart disease that frequently develops in alcoholics is alcoholic cardiomyopathy—enlargement of the muscles and different chambers of the heart. The toxic effect of alcohol itself causes damage to muscles of the heart. The result of alcohol-associated heart disease is congestive heart failure and cardiac arrhythmias of different types and severities.

Stress can cause heart disease to develop via several mechanisms: first, stress causes the level of adrenalin in the blood to rise; second, the rise in the level of adrenalin causes the blood pressure to rise; third, the rise in adrenalin can also cause both acute heart attack as well as cardiac arrhythmias to develop, with lethal consequences.

Blacks live under constant racism associated stress in America and this kind of stress increases the incidence of hypertension, coronary artery heart disease, stroke, kidney failure, high cholesterol, obesity, diabetes mellitus, alcoholism, drug addiction, tobacco smoking, depression, poverty, increased rate of suicide, etc.

Type A personality (an aggressive and restless person who is always on the go) is also associated with the development of coronary heart disease via some of the mechanisms just outlined.

Tobacco smoking can cause coronary occlusive disease because of the effects of nicotine on the coronary vessels resulting in the development of plaques inside these vessels.

Heredity is associated to a very high degree with coronary heart disease because if a woman's mother or father has coronary heart disease or died of a heart attack, chances are she also is at a high risk of encountering the same fate, if appropriate medical care is not sought by her to forestall the possibility of her developing CAD.

Poverty is associated with an increased incidence of coronary artery heart disease because all the factors just outlined are seen in greater numbers in poor blacks than in people of higher financial means.

A large percentage of the 47 million or so people in the USA who have no health insurance are blacks and other minorities. Many of these individuals are employed and yet they have no health insurance because they simply do not have enough money to pay for it.

According to recent reports, there are 18 million children in this country living below the poverty line; a good percentage of these children are black children, other minority children and white children. Tragically, roughly 14 million children in the USA go to bed hungry every night.

When people are poor, they are concerned about being able to find the bare necessities of daily living, such as where to find food to eat, and they will eat any food that is edible regardless of its nutritional value.

The quality of the food does not enter into the equation of their lives; they are more concerned about being able to afford the rent and utility bills—electric, oil and gas—to keep a roof over their heads and their homes warm in the winter. These are important and essential factors in the overall lives of poor people in the U.S. and the world.

Poverty is associated with a greater number of poor health habits, all of which can lead to the development of major medical problems such as hypertension, high cholesterol, obesity, diabetes mellitus, cancer, atherosclerotic heart disease, heart attack, congestive heart failure, stroke, osteoarthritis, etc. People of better financial means also suffer from these same medical problems but because they are more likely to have health insurance and can see a physician with ease, these problems are dealt with more quickly and more efficiently.

Blacks and other minorities tend to go to physicians with diseases of all sorts when these diseases are already in their advanced stages. They frequently ignore their symptoms and go to physicians when the medical problems are frequently more challenging to address. Symptoms of coronary artery disease and a heart attack in women are quite different than they are in men. Most women, when they are having a heart attack, do not have chest pain but often describe their symptoms of myocardial infarction as an aching, pressure, tightness in the chest, nausea, vomiting, and indigestion.

Other acute symptoms of heart attack are weakness, shortness of breath, fatigue, dizziness and cold sweat (Source: Circulation, 2003; 108: 2619-2623).

Typical symptoms of acute coronary syndrome include:

1. Chest pain often the most common symptom of arteriosclerotic heart disease.
2. Shortness of breath.
3. Pain in the left shoulder radiating down the left arm, associated with numbness and shortness of breath.
4. A combination of the three symptoms mentioned above and worsening of these symptoms on exertion. This complex of symptoms is often referred to as Angina Pectoris.
5. Irregular, rapid heartbeats and too slow heartbeats also known as Bradycardia / Tachycardia
6. Chest pain associated with dizziness, sweating, and shortness of breath which can often mean not just angina but often that the patient is in the process of having an acute heart attack.
7. Shortness of breath along with accumulation of fluid in the lungs and ankles can be a result of cardiovascular disease and a particular condition known as Congestive Heart Failure.

How to diagnose cardiovascular heart disease:

In order to arrive at a diagnosis of cardiovascular heart disease, the physician must:

1. Take a good medical history.
2. Carry out a good physical examination.
3. Perform an electrocardiogram (EKG).
4. Follow up with a chest x-ray.

Based on these tests, the physician may institute a treatment protocol involving beta-blocker, nitroglycerin, and aspirin, if there is no contraindication to aspirin. Then, arrangements can be made for the person to undergo a stress test, provided the person is not having active chest pain. If the cardiac stress test, along with the echocardiogram, suggests the possibility of a coronary occlusive disease, i.e., arteriosclerotic heart disease, then the patient may be referred to a cardiologist for a cardiac catheterization.

In the acute setting, when the patient presents to an emergency room, all of the steps just listed, namely the history, the physical exam, the EKG, and the chest x-ray can be done in an emergency room setting to begin the process of evaluating the patient's symptoms for an acute cardiac event.

In evaluating the patient with chest pain in the ER, a new blood test (troponin-1) can be done. Troponin-1 is a substance that is secreted by heart muscle that has just become damaged. This test becomes elevated within six hours of an acute myocardial infarction, and remains elevated for about two weeks. The troponin-1 is therefore quite sensitive to help the physician pick up an acute myocardial infarction. The normal troponin-1 is 0-0.4NG/ml.

The other blood tests available to assist the physician to ascertain whether the patient has had a myocardial infarction or is having a myocardial infarction, are the creatinine phosphokinases, known as CPK, in particular the total CPK and the MB CPK.

In acute heart attack where there is heart muscle damage, the total CPK and MB CPK are elevated. In most laboratories, the normal MB is as high as 4-5%. Most hospital laboratories are set up to do electrophoresis on the CPK MB fraction. The CPK MB electrophoresis is read as either positive or negative. If it is positive for MB, then you get the total MB level to follow. The first cardiac enzyme to rise when an acute heart attack has occurred is the troponin-1; it rises 1-6 hours after heart muscle damage. Ordinarily the CPK is tested three times during an acute hospitalization for an acute heart attack. Usually the total and MB CPK go up between 12 and 24 hours and start coming back down in about 24-48 hours.

The blood levels of lactic dehydrogenase (LDH) and the (SGOT) Serum Glutamic Pyruvic Transaminase go up after a heart attack. The first enzyme to go up following a heart attack is the troponin-1; follow by the CPK, then the SGOT and then the LDH. The first to go down after a heart attack is the CPK, followed by the SGOT, followed by the LDH and the troponin-1. It usually takes the troponin-1 about two weeks to go down to normal.

Elevated B-type Natriuretic Peptide (BNP) "Myocardial ischemia is a strong trigger of B-type natriuretic peptide (BNP) release. As ischemia precedes necrosis in acute myocardial infartction, we hypothesized that BNP might be useful in the early diagnosis and risk stratification of patients with acute chest pain." Source: The Amemerican Journal of Medicine May 2011, Volume 124, Number 5.

There are classic abnormalities that are seen on the EKG tracing when an acute myocardial infarction is about to occur, or has just occurred, hours before the person presents either to the emergency room or to the doctor's office. What is often seen is what is referred to as coronary insufficiency. The EKG might show what is called inversion of the T-wave on different parts of the EKG along with ST depression. A more classic example is called ST elevation, an elevation of the ST segment of the EKG from the base line.

Physicians are able to map out the circulation of the heart, as it relates to coronary artery, based on the 12-lead EKG. For instance, in a myocardial infarction occurring in the inferior wall of the heart, one expects to see abnormalities in leads 2, 3 and AVF. If it is happening in the lateral wall, then one sees abnormalities in leads 1, AVL and maybe V1, V2. If it is taking place in the anterior wall of the heart, then one can see findings in lead leads V1-V6. The right coronary artery supplies blood and oxygen to the inferior wall of the heart and the left anterior descending coronary artery supplies blood and oxygen to the left part of the heart, etc., etc.

It is very important for a physician to know how to read an EKG properly in order to know if a person is just about to have a heart attack or just had it hours before. This is very important because by infusing tPA (tissue plasminogen activator) in an individual's blood, the clot that is occluding the involved coronary artery causing the myocardial infarction can be dissolved, thereby preventing the heart attack from taking place.

In fact, up to six hours after a heart attack has occurred, if the patient presents to the emergency room, tPA can still dissolve the clot that has caused the heart attack, thereby opening up the vessel and preventing further muscle damage.

Limiting the severity of the heart attack, by infusing tPA can in many instances help to save the life of a patient. Often, the history regarding when the patient started to experience chest pain, shortness of breath, sweating or just severe pressure in the chest, along with the EKG finding, is all that is needed to prevent a heart attack from occurring.

If the EKG findings and history are not consistent with a myocardial infarction, then the person is said to be having angina, unstable angina, or pre-infarction angina or acute myocardial syndrome. A physician is able to determine if a person has had or is having a myocardial infarction, angina, unstable angina, or pre-infarction angina based strickly on the experience and clinical judgment of the physician, along with the findings on the EKG and the cardiac enzyme blood tests.

Every year, a significant percentage of people are admitted to intensive coronary care units complaining of chest pain, which, in fact, were not cardiac-related chest pain or myocardial infarctions. On other hand, many people get sent home because the physicians, either in the emergency rooms or in their offices, saw these people and did not believe they had heart-related chest pain, resulting in them having heart attacks at home and sometimes dying.

The literature amply confirms that blacks and other mionorities receive less attention when they present to an emergency room with chest pain compared to their white counterparts. As described above, blacks and other minorities also get referred less often for invasive cardiac tests, such as cardiac catheterization, to determine whether they have coronary occlusive disease to explain their complaints of chest pain.

To underline this issue even more strongly, the recent literature shows that the lifetime risk of heart attacks at age 40 is 1 in 2 for men and 1 in 3 for women. Even as late as age 70, the incidence of coronary artery disease and heart attacks is 1 in 3 for men and 1 in 4 for women.

These statistics are much worse in blacks and other minorities. It is also important to realize that cardiovascular disease is the number one cause of death in blacks and other poor people, and the number one cause of death in the U.S. and in the world.

Several possible scenarios exist when a black person presents to the emergency room with chest pain:

1. Blacks and other minorities may be seen in the emergency room for the complaint of chest pain, evaluated and sent home.
2. Whites may be seen in the emergency room for complaint of chest pain, evaluated and admitted for further evaluation and observation on a telemetry unit.
3. Whites may be seen in the emergency room for chest pain, evaluated and the physician may think that the patients have pre-infarction or unstable angina and are admitted for treatments in the coronary care unit. In this case, he or she will be treated with heparin, aspirin, nitroglycerine, a Beta-blocker and oxygen.
4. In addition, three sets of cardiac enzymes and troponin-1 tests are ordered. An EKG is taken also for three days to be sure that a myocardial infarction has

not occurred. In the setting of number 1 and 2 above, an echocardiogram may be done to rule out other causes of chest pain such as mitral valve prolapse, myocarditis, pericarditis, etc.

5. A person who presents to the emergency room with chest pain and other symptoms of a heart attack and is found to be having a heart attack by EKG findings and sometimes by the first elevated CPK value or the troponin-1 value will be admitted to the coronary care unit.

6. In the coronary care unit, IV nitroglycerine or nitroglycerine paste will be given.

7. In addition, Beta blocker, angiotensin inhibitor/or angiotensin receptor blocker along with nasal oxygen, Aspirin, pain medication and tPA will be given if there is no contraindication. As mentioned above, in this particular setting, the tPA can be lifesaving in that it can dissolve the clot that is causing the heart attack, thereby allowing blood flow and oxygen to go to the muscle of the heart and preventing further damage. Depending on the clinical circumstances, cardiac catheterization may be carried out.

The clinical scenarios outlined above unfortunately are not always afforded to blacks and other minorities in the U.S. and in the wolrd.

Across the USA in the world blacks and other minorities get worse medical care when they present to emergency rooms with complaints of heart disease than do whites.

Once a myocardial infarction has been ruled out, after three sets of enzymes and an EKG that is unremarkable, then further decision has to be made as to how to proceed in evaluating this person. One common approach is to do a nuclear Adenosine or MIBI stress test, Persantine MIBI test or a stress echocardiogram. If any one of these tests is found to be negative, then the assumption is that the patient does not have severe coronary occlusive disease. That patient is frequently sent home and taken off acute myocardial-type medications such as beta-blockers and nitrates. These tests, although they are excellent, are not 100% full-proofs.

There have been situations when a nuclear imaging test of the heart was normal, and yet the patient went on in a matter of days or weeks to have a heart attack. What can be said is that if the nuclear stress test or the stress echocardiogram is negative, the patient probably does not have major occlusive coronary heart disease. These stress tests can miss a 30-40% occlusion of a coronary artery. For several reasons, a fissure or crack can occur in a 30-40% plaque inside a coronary artery, causing bleeding and clot formation resulting in closure of that vessel and an acute heart attack. Human beings carry in their mouths anaerobic bacteria that produce enzymes that can cause this fissure or crack to occur in a coronary.

It is said that certain species of mycoplasma bacteria can contribute to the development of coronary artery disease. It may be wise to test the blood for the presence of the antibody to mycoplasma. In addition, if the antibody test is positive, then erythromycin can be used to treat these patients. When a person has only a 30-40% occlusion of a coronary vessel, this vessel has not had sufficient time to develop collateral vessels, so when this person suffers an occlusive incident, there are no collateral vessels in the immediate vicinity to protect the affected myocardium and keep it alive.

So, in this setting a 30-40% coronary occlusive disease is worse than an 80% occlusion in that the 80% occlusion has had plenty of time to develop collateral vessels, which can protect the heart muscle in the event of a heart attack to keep the heart muscle alive.

The other scenario is that if the patient continues to have chest pain and yet there is no clear evidence of acute myocardial infarction, then that patient is a candidate to be taken immediately to cardiac catheterization in order to visualize the vessels around the heart, to see if indeed the patient has major coronary occlusive disease. It is not safe to do a stress test on someone who is having active chest pain.

Doing the regular treadmill stress test in evaluating someone for coronary insufficiency has some value, but because it has such a high incidence of false positivity and also such a high incidence of false negativity, it has become less and less appropriate in the setting of acute evaluation of chest pain. Especially in women, there is a very high incidence of false negative treadmill stress test. For that reason, nuclear cardiac imaging has replaced the treadmill stress test.

The regular treadmill stress test is appropriate for a younger individual in the 35-to-40-year-old bracket who is being evaluated to fly planes, or race a car, starting a jogging program or something of that sort.

As just mentioned there are several sensitive stress tests available to evaluate the heart:

1. The MIBI Myoview stress test.
2. IV Persantine or IV Adenosine.
3. IV Dobutamine
4. Resting Thallium distribution stress test.
5. Stress echocardiogram

Any one of these tests can be used to evaluate the heart. In certain circumstances, a gated blood pool, known also as MUGA, is done in evaluating the heart.

The Persantine MIBI stress test and Adenosine stress test are suitable for individuals who are able to exercise. Roughly two days prior to having these stress tests, certain medications and certain beverages have to be stopped. Among them are beta-blocker medications to name a few, Tenormin, Atenolol, Metoprolol, Propanolol, Coreg, etc. Some calcium channel blockers need to be stopped as well such as Cardizem, Nifedipine, and Verapamil, etc. Certain medications such as Aminophylline and Theophylline must be stopped. Beverages such as coffee, tea, and any caffeine or decaffeinated beverages also ought to be stopped prior to having these tests done.

The cardiac nuclear department has a long list of things that people cannot do that they distribute prior to having these tests done, so patients know precisely what not to do. This is done because it is important that the heart is able to pump forcefully without interference. The higher the heart rate during exercise, the more stress there is on the heart, and the more stress there is on the heart the better the evaluation of the heart.

Anything that suppresses the contractile effort of the heart has a negative impact on the evaluation of the result of the stress test.

Individuals who are going to have the Persantine stress test also ought to take certain precautions as mentioned above. If the patient is taking Dipyridamole, which is still being used in certain settings, this medication must be stopped before undergoing a Persantine stress test.

The MIBI nuclear stress test or the Adenosine stress test is done in such a way as to be able to tell both angina and/or previous myocardial muscle damage. The Sestamibi test or the thallium test has the same clinical properties as potassium. That being the case, potassium will only be picked up by live heart muscle as a physiological fact.

Taking advantage of this known fact, the physician injects the MIBI substance into the blood of the person being tested, and after it mixes with his or her own blood, this minute nuclear material functions as a tracer in her blood to allow the stress test to be carried out. The entire process is computerized, allowing color pictures of the heart to be taken along with a lot of other important values such as the ejection fraction of the heart.

These nuclear cardiac stress tests enable cardiologists to differentiate between normal heart muscles, scarred heart muscles and heart muscles that are not receiving sufficient blood and oxygen. During the exercise, the area of the heart that is supplied by the plaque-containing coronary artery does not receive sufficient blood and oxygen, resulting in an area of emptiness or lightness compared to the rest of the pictured heart muscles.

Because at rest the oxygen demand is less, that same area when pictured again normalizes; then this is an area of poor blood flow made worse by the stress of the work imposed on the heart, simulating the natural phenomenon referred to as angina or coronary insufficiency. Physicians can, in fact, tell exactly which coronary artery or arteries are diseased with plaques based on the result of the MIBI stress test.

On the other hand, if the abnormal area remains unchanged, both at rest and during exercise when pictured, it means that this person has had a previous myocardial infarction, either known or unknown. The reason that the area remains unchanged, showing an area of defect, is that the muscle that is showing as a defect is scarred and is dead muscle. Dead tissue cannot pick up potassium, and Sestamibi and thallium have some of the same chemical properties as potassium, as previously mentioned.

Another nuclear stress test that is frequently employed to diagnose occlusive coronary artery disease is the Persantine MIBI stress test. This test is suitable for individuals with infirmities that prevent them from being able to exercise on a treadmill. Some of these individuals are women who suffer from arthritis of the lumbar spine or arthritis of the knees, who are markedly obese, have had a stroke or are somewhat more advanced in age and so are not able to exercise.

The difference between the regular MIBI stress test and the Persantine MIBI stress test is that Persantine is given to the person undergoing the test to dilate the coronary arteries acutely. The acute dilatation causes the heart to beat very fast, resulting in a stressful situation for the heart. The result is the same as exercising on the treadmill to raise the heart rate. Another advantage of the Persantine stress test is that Beta-blockers and calcium channel blocker medications can be continued while the patient is having the test.

The findings discussed under the heading Sesta MIBI stress test are the same as the Persantine stress test and have the same meaning. If the stress MIBI is negative, that is evidence that the woman who was tested probably does not have significant occlusive coronary artery disease. This is, however, not always the case; although these stress tests are very sensitive tests, every now and then there can be a false negative test.

If the person continues to have chest pain, then the right thing to do is first to do an abdominal ultrasound to evaluate the gall bladder, because gall bladder disease, such as gallstones, can cause chest pain that is similar to chest pain seen in coronary heart disease. Interestingly, medications such as nitroglycerin, which relieves angina chest pain, can also relieve gall bladder disease pain, confusing the whole situation. Gall bladder disease due to gallstones is quite common among women, in particular black and other minority women who are 30-40 years old, obese, and fertile.

Blacks and other minorities are more likely to develop obesity and therefore more prone to develop gallstones. In addition, blacks and other minorities are more likely to be carrying abnormal hemoglobins, which predispose them to a higher propensity to the formation of gallbladder disease. They are more likely to form bilirubin stones.

Sickle cell hemoglobin, hemoglobin C, beta thalassemia, alpha thalassemia, and different combinations of these abnormal hemoglobins cause hemolysis, resulting in the formation of bilirubin gallstones. It is the dumping of bilirubin in the bloodstream that ultimately leads to bilirubin gallstones causing gall bladder disease to be so frequently seen in this subgroup of women who suffer from hemolytic anemia of different types.

If the abdominal sonogram is negative, ruling out gallstones, then an upper G.I. series must be done to look for diseases such as hiatal hernia with or without reflux esophagitis or ulcers of different types and degrees in the stomach. Any one of these can cause chest pain similar to the chest pain caused by coronary artery heart disease. Hiatal hernia with reflux is frequently seen as a cause of severe chest pain. This particular condition is called GERD (gastroesopgeal reflux disease).

Frequently, the physician does not have the luxury of waiting to do an evaluation of the gallbladder or the stomach in a person who is having pain in the chest with a negative stress test. In this case, she must go directly for a coronary angiogram to be certain that coronary artery disease is not the cause of the pain.

It would be rather dangerous to wait to do a prolonged G.I. work-up while the patient is having pain that could be risking the possibility of a heart attack while the patient is waiting for these tests to be done. As just stated, before undertaking this invasive procedure, however, the physician must be sure that all other possible causes of chest pain have been ruled out, including mitral valve prolapse, which can be seen on an echocardiogram, and a costochondritis, which can be detected on physical examination.

Pulmonary embolism must also be ruled out by doing an ultrasound of the extremities, with d-Dimer blood test or by doing a lung scan. Other tests to conduct are the ESR and ANA to rule out inflammatory processes such as myocarditis, pericarditis and pleuritis. A chest x-ray ought to be done to rule out pneumonia which can also cause chest pain.

If the patient has a fever, then a series of viral blood tests ought to be done to rule out viral disease as a cause of the fever and chest pain.

Costochondritis is a condition that causes pain in the ribs and upper chest wall. When the physician touches these areas with the examining finger, they are tender. Conditions such as arthritis or bursitis of the left or right shoulder with radiating pain down the arm must also be considered. Chest pain can also be due to cancer of the lung, and therefore a chest x-ray must be done to rule out that possibility.

Many other conditions that can cause chest pain, but the point is that the physician must keep an open mind and properly evaluate for these possibilities before proceeding to more invasive tests to explain the chest pain. It is neither too expensive nor too time consuming to conduct these evaluations. As just stated, before offering a patient cardiac catheterization, a thorough medical evaluation must first be completed, unless she continues to have chest pain and the clinical impression is that she faces an impending myocardial infarction. In such a case, naturally the physician ought to proceed immediately to do a cardiac catheterization.

Ordinarily, cardiac catheterization for the possibility of coronary occlusive disease is undertaken when a patient has a positive stress test and he/she has failed medical management and the patient is of an age where cardiac catheterization will not be contraindicated. In addition, if the patient has major risk factors such as smoking, hypertension, hyperlipidemia, diabetes mellitus, obesity and a family history of coronary artery disease, in conjunction with the aforementioned factors, then this patient should be offered cardiac catheterization.

If a patient agrees to undergo a cardiac catheterization to determine whether there is an impending myocardial infarction and/or to determine whether the chest pain in question is due to coronary insufficiency, he or she must be given informed consent, to explain the risks and benefits of the procedure.

Cardiac catheterization is a procedure done by highly qualified cardiologists who do this procedure as a subspecialty of cardiology. The procedure is done in a special operating room, which is well equipped with all sorts of modern equipment to provide care for the heart under different circumstances.

The procedure is done by a making a large needle-size puncture in the groin, where the femoral artery is located. The area is shaved and properly cleansed with Betadine, and then appropriate local anesthetic is injected in the area. Time is allowed for the anesthetic to take effect, and then a puncture is made with a needle through which a catheter is threaded that goes to the heart, where it can be moved to different parts of its chambers. A dye is then injected through the catheter, which is able to display the coronary arteries around the heart.

A multitude of very important information is obtained during the cardiac catheterization including the displaying of the coronary arteries.

The displaying of the coronary arteries may show evidence of plaques and narrowing in the coronary arteries. If the cardiac catheterization is negative for occlusive coronary disease, it means no gross coronary artery disease is present. Other conditions can cause chest pain that can be seen during cardiac catheterization. Coronary spasm can be seen or induced during cardiac catheterization. Coronary spasm can cause chest pain and when it occurs acutely, it can cut off blood and oxygen flow to the heart muscle, sometimes resulting in acute myocardial infarction.

Recently, a new condition has been described in which people who suffer from long-time hypertension can develop this type of hypertensive cardiovascular disease with enlargement of the left ventricle and increased end diastolic pressure, suggesting that these people have what is called "small vessels myocardial disease" causing chest pain. Obese people, because of their greater propensity for having hypertension, are quite prone to having this particular condition.

During the cardiac catheterization, abnormalities of the valves of the heart can be discovered. Several other muscular abnormalities of the heart can also be discovered.

After completion of the cardiac catheterization, the results are evaluated and the determination is made as to whether the abnormalities found can explain a person's symptoms. In the case of chest pain, the key finding is coronary artery narrowing due to plaques of different degrees.

Normal and abnormal cardiac catheterization photographs

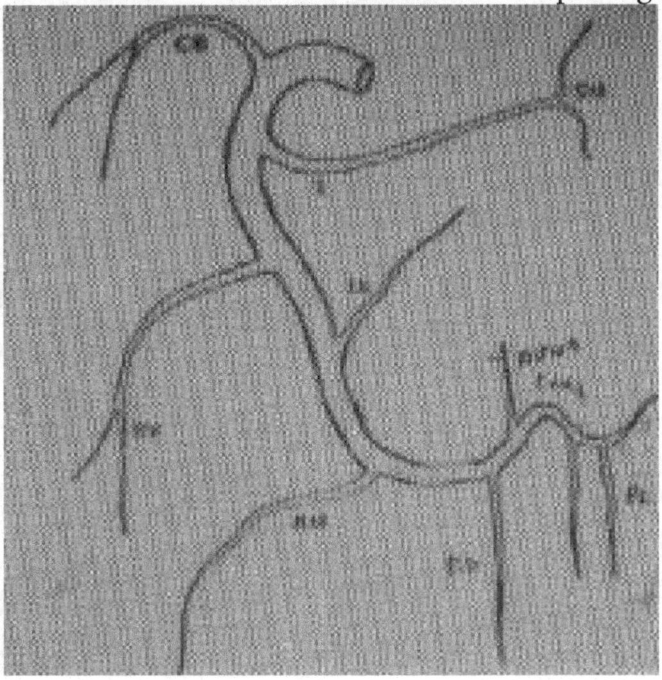

Figure 4.1-A normal right coronary artery in a person.

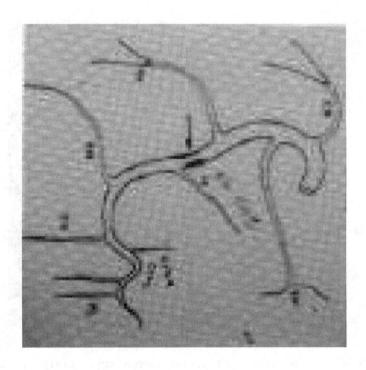

Figure 4.2-Big arrow shows 50-60% occlusion in the mid-portion of a right coronary artery of a person.

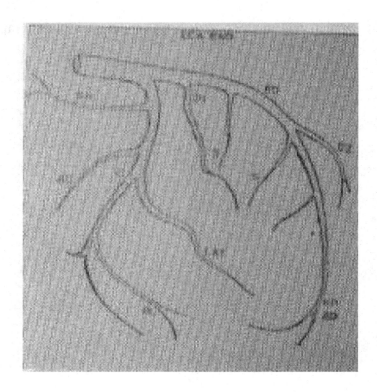

***Figure 4.3*-**A normal left coronary artery in a person.

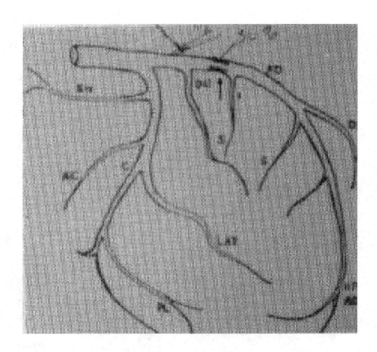

***Figure 4.4*-**A 50% occlusion of a left anterior descending coronary artery, in patient with both high cholesterol and hypertension.

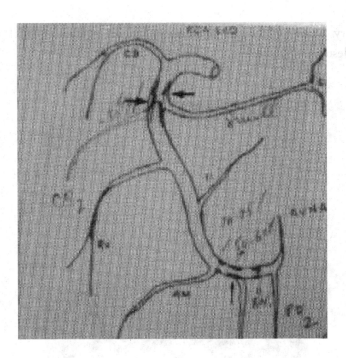

Figure 4.5-Big arrow showing 40-50% of the proximal portion of the right coronary artery in a person. Small arrow showing 70-75% occlusion of the distal right coronary artery. This right coronary artery has diffused atherosclerotic changes in other areas.

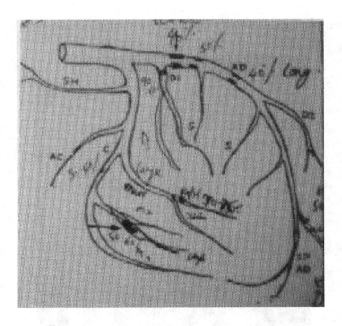

Figure 4.6-Small arrow shows 40% occlusion of the proximal left anterior descending artery. There is a 30% occlusion of the LAD in its proximal portion just before the first major septal artery and there is a 40% occlusion in the mid-portion of the LAD. Big arrow shows 50-60% occlusion of the epical diagonal branch of the left coronary artery. There are several areas of diffused atherosclerotic changes involving this left

coronary artery. Occlusive changes of coronary arteries in a patient with hypertension and high cholesterol who smoke.

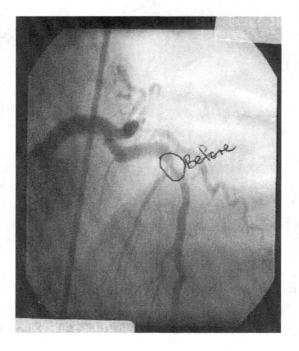

Figure 4.7-Stent placement of narrowed LAD (before) in a patient.

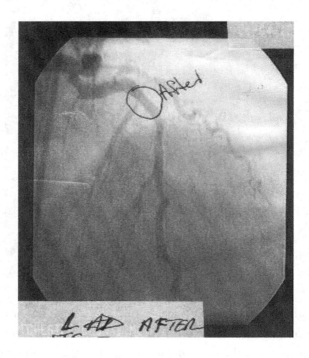

Figure 4.8-Showing how stent placement opens the LAD (after)in a patient.

Based on the findings of the cardiac catheterization just mentioned, recommendations are made as to what course of action to follow. If, for example, the coronary arteries are found to have plaques in them, then the following possibilities exist:

1. The patient can be offered angioplasty.
2. The patient can be offered cardiac bypass.
3. The patient can be offered medications assuming that the disease cannot be approached surgically and/or the patient refuses to have the angioplasty or cardiac catheterization.

There are sometimes contraindications to both angioplasty and cardiac bypass.

Angioplasty is simpler than coronary bypass, but it also has a higher rate of recurrence of disease. The very act of going through the vessels to push aside the plaques can damage the inside of the vessels, creating an area for new plaque formation. Sometimes a stent is placed inside a vessel to try to keep it open, which decreases the possibility of new plaque formation. These patients are frequently placed on anti-platelet medications such as Ticlid or Plavix in conjunction with aspirin to prevent platelet aggregation and closure of the coronary artery. Angioplasty is done in the cardiac catheterization lab and the same cardiologist who performs the cardiac catheterization usually performs it.

On the other hand, coronary bypass requires open-heart surgery which is performed by a heart surgeon. It is considered major surgery; the hospital stay is longer and it costs more money. The success of coronary artery bypass surgery is quite good, though some might say, in the aggregate, that coronary bypass relieves symptoms but does not prolong life compared to medical management. It has been reported that some people suffer some degree of dementia after coronary bypass surgery, and it is believed that micro-particles that break off from the coronary plaques during surgery lodge into the brain and may be responsible for the dementia.

It is important to stress that after angioplasty or coronary bypass, heart medications are continued for life. The list of medications used in cardiovascular disease is very long. The following is a partial list of different heart medications that are presently in use:

1. Aspirin.
2. Ticlid.
3. Plavix
4. Nitroglycerin.

5. Beta-blockers
6. Calcium channel blockers
7. Alpha channel blockers
8. Digitalis
9. Diuretics
10. Aldosterone
11. Angiotesin converting enzyme inhibitor (ACE)
12. Angiotensin ll receptor blocker (ABR)
13. Calcium channel blockers
14. Beta pace
15. Antiarrhythmic such as Lidocaine, Quinidine, Procainamide, Amiodarone IV Vasotec, IV Verapamil, IV Cardizem, Adenosine, etc.
16. Pacemakers also play a major role in the management of patients with heart disease.
17. Sometimes, a pacemaker is used in the setting of an acute myocardial infarction, and sometimes it is used to treat heart blockage of different types to treat sinus disease, or bundle branch blocks.
18. There are special pacemakers that are used to treat arrhythmias of different types and severity. These pacemakers can, on demand, shock the heart to eliminate rhythm abnormalities as they occur, without the patient being aware of what is happening. Moreover, these special pacemakers keep a record for the cardiologist to print out and evaluate management of patients. It is very important for people who are having unexplained cardiac arrhythmias to undergo electrophysiological studies to determine both the source and the cause of the arrhythmia, so that specific and appropriate anti-arrhythmic treatments can be prescribed for the affected patients.

How do these medications work to treat heart disease?

Aspirin, Ticlid, and Plavix work to treat heart disease because these three medications are able to prevent clot formation within the lumen of the vessels around the heart. They do so by preventing platelet clumping, and in so doing they prevent aggregation of platelets, which is necessary for clots to form. Aspirin works both in the prevention of coronary artery disease and in the acute treatment of coronary artery disease.

When a patient presents to the hospital in the process of having a heart attack, if the patient is given two aspirins to chew and swallow, and, added to that, heparin, that patient frequently can lessen the amount of damage that is done to the heart. On top of that, if tPA is injected into the patient within the first hour or so while the patient is about to have a heart attack, a great deal of heart muscle can be spared.

Beta-blockers are a group of medications that are very useful in the treatment of cardiovascular heart disease of different types. Among the most commonly used beta-blockers are the following:

1. Inderal
2. Lopressor
3. Tenormin
4. Toprol XL
5. Coreg
6. Bystolic
7. Betapace, etc

Beta-blockers work to improve the function of the heart via different mechanisms. Beta-blockers have their main effect on the sympathetic system of the body to decrease stimulation of the heart. They also decrease the forcefulness of the pumping of the heart, thereby sparing the need for greater oxygen delivery. Beta-blockers are also anti-arrhythmic and they prevent arrhythmia from occurring. The long-acting beta-blockers in the Lopressor-type family actually cut down on the amount of adrenalin that the body can secrete, and this decreases the incidence of death from myocardial infarction.

This is the reason that long-acting beta blockers are used to protect the heart when a person is sleeping, so that in the early morning hours of the day, when the adrenalin is being secreted in large amounts to prepare the body for the upcoming day's work, protection will continue. By cutting down on the amount of adrenalin that is being secreted, the heart is spared the stimulation from the excess adrenalin, thereby cutting down on the incidence of sudden death.

The harder the heart pumps, the more blood and oxygen are needed to keep up with the needs of the heart muscle and if the vessels around the heart are narrowed by plaques, then that demand cannot be met. So it is in that manner that beta-blockers are effective in the treatment of angina pectoris, also known as chest pain. Beta-blockers also work in another way in the treatment of heart disease; that is, they slow the heart rate or make the heart beat in a regular fashion, thereby preventing what are called cardiac arrhythmias from occurring.

These arrhythmias are frequently the reason that the heart stops after a heart attack or as a result of a complex abnormal rhythm which prevents proper pumping activities of the heart that are needed for sustaining life. In fact, using long-acting beta blockers as just mentioned, especially a dose that has a 24-hour effect on the heart, not only can prevent these abnormalities, but also may in fact prevent heart attacks that frequently occur in the early hours of the morning.

Another group of medications that are frequently used in coronary disease is the nitrates. Nitroglycerin, which is a well-known medication, is in the family of nitrates. Nitrates come in different forms, from sublingual nitroglycerin to nitroglycerin capsules, nitroglycerin patches, nitroglycerin paste, to nitroglycerin liquid that can be used intravenously. Nitroglycerin works to relieve symptoms of angina pectoris by dilating the smooth muscles inside the coronary arteries, allowing for better blood and oxygen flow to go around the heart.

Calcium channel blockers are excellent medications that have multiple uses in the treatment of cardiovascular disease. Calcium channel blockers, such as Nifedipine, Cardizem, Verapamil, Norvasc, etc. work to relieve some symptoms associated with coronary artery disease by blocking the effects of calcium to the smooth muscle inside the coronary arteries around the heart.

Calcium is needed for muscle contraction to occur at the cellular level. Muscle contraction is associated with vasoconstriction.

Vasoconstriction means that the inside of the blood vessel becomes narrowed. The narrowing of the blood vessel prevents proper circulation of blood and thereby prevents proper delivery of oxygen to the heart muscles. When oxygen fails to reach the heart muscle in sufficient amount, the result is chest pain. Another important function of calcium channel blockers is to decrease blood pressure. Increase in blood pressure is a major cause of cardiovascular disease.

Calcium channel blockers work to decrease blood pressure by blocking the effect of calcium on the muscle, resulting in relaxation of smooth muscle and that relaxation of smooth muscle causes the blood pressure to come down. In blacks, these medications must be used in combination with diuretics, assuming that the person is not in renal failure, for effective control of blood pressure.

Calcium channel blockers are frequently used to treat cardiac arrhythmias and they are very effective. In particular, Verapamil IV or Cardizem IV is used extensively in the emergency room setting to treat different types of ventricular cardiac dysrhythmias.

Diuretics are very important medications in the treatment of cardiovascular disease. When the heart has been damaged, it frequently fails, and heart failure causes fluid to be accumulated in the lungs, the abdomen, the legs, and the ankles.

The so-called loop diuretics, such as Lasix, Bumex, etc., are used to remove the fluid from the body, thereby improving heart function and relieving the symptoms of fluid overload from the body.

Salt plays a major role in causing fluid accumulation in the body; therefore the intake of salt must be curtailed significantly in the treatment of heart failure. Any person, who has chronic congestive heart failure, by definition, has a total body salt that is elevated. The daily salt intake ought not to exceed 1.5 grams per day. By genetics, blacks and Asians retain more salt in their bodies than any other racial groups.

Heart failure can occur because of acute damage to the heart. Heart failure can complicate heart attack and it frequently does. However, heart failure most frequently occurs because of damage that has occurred to the heart due to longstanding hypertension that was either not properly treated or left untreated. Because the muscles of the heart have been stretched to the limit, the heart enlarges and becomes incapable of pumping properly.

Once the heart loses its proper pumping ability then fluid backs up in the body, causing the person to be unable to breathe properly and unable to lie down flat. This person must use several pillows to sleep. Heart failure can also occur because of chronic damage that has occurred to the heart because of multiple previous heart attacks, whereby heart muscles have been damaged, and the scarred muscles lose their ability to pump properly. A combination of an enlarged heart, a condition referred to as Cardiomegaly, and hypertrophy of the muscles of the heart, can result in heart failure.

People with cardiomyopathy and congestive heart failure who eat too much salt in their foods can cause their heart failure to be worse. It is very important to make the point that in the process of using these diuretics to remove fluids from the body, a proper level of potassium must be maintained in order to prevent potassium deficiency, which can cause serious complications to develop.

Potassium must be given by mouth for those who are able to take it by mouth in an outpatient setting and it can be given intravenously when necessary for those who are in the hospital and cannot take it by mouth because they are acutely sick.

About 550,000 individuals are diagnosed with heart failure every year. Currently, 5.5 million people in the U.S. have heart failure.

The incidence of heart failure is much higher in blacks compared to whites.
Three percent of blacks have congestive heart failure compared to two per cent of whites. In addition, heart failure occurs earlier in blacks compared to whites.

"One in 100 African-American men and women developed heart failure at an average age of 39, 20 times the rate in Caucasians." Source: New England Journal of Medicine Vol 360, March 19, 2009, Number 12.

The higher rate of congestive heart failure seen in blacks is not related to past heart attacks, but is related to the higher incidence of hypertension and diabetes mellitus seen in this sub-group according to an article in the Archive of Internal Medicine, 2008, 168(19):2138-2145.

The death rate from congestive heart failure is also higher in blacks compared to whites. Of the individuals who develop heart failure, 10% die within one year and 50% die within five years. The yearly cost of congestive heart failure, direct and indirect, was 37.2 billion dollars in 2008. Source: 2009 Update, American Heart Association Scientific American Session.

What are the causes of chronic congestive heart failure?

The causes of chronic congestive heart failure include:

1. Hypertension
2. Ischemic heart disease
3. Cardiomyopathy
4. Anemia
5. Myocardial infarction
6. Cardiac arrhythmias
7. Valvular heart disease
8. Bacterial endocarditis
9. Myocarditis
10. Hyperthyroidism(Thyrotoxicosis)
11. Pulmonary embolism
12. Acute intracranial hemorrhage with intracranial pressure
13. Infection with high fever, fast heart rate superimposed on a sick heart
14. Low vitamin D in the body
15. Hypothyroidism

Low vitamin causes congestive heart failure because it allows the Renin Angiotensin Aldosterone System to become activated thereby causing the retention of salt and water resulting in congestive heart failure. Source: Cleveland Clinic Journal of Medicine Volume 77, Number 5, May 2010.

What are the symptoms of congestive heart failure?

The symptoms of congestive heart failure include:

1. Shortness of breath (dyspnea and orthopnea) left sided heart failure
2. Orthopnea or paroxysmal nocturnal dyspnea (right sided heart failure)
3. Lassitude
4. Irritability

5. Insomnia
6. Chest pain
7. Head ache
8. Restlessness
9. Tiredness
10. Weakness
11. Abdominal pain due to swollen liver
12. Nausea
13. Anorexia
14. Poor memory due to poor blood flow to the brain
15. Head ache

What are the clinical signs of congestive heart failure?

1. Rapid respiration
2. Labored respiration
3. Rapid pulse rate
4. Bulging neck veins
5. Rapid or irregular heart
6. Swollen ankles
7. Swollen legs
8. Swollen abdomen
9. Palpable liver
10. Tender liver to palpation
11. Swollen face
12. Third and fourth heart sounds when listening to the heart with the Stethoscope
13. Rales heard when listening to the lung with the stethoscope
14. Weight gain
15. Using several pillows under the chest to sleep (nocturnal Dyspnea)
16. Raising the head of the bed in order to sleep
17. Jaundice
18. Renal insufficiency (abnormal kidney function)

What is Acute Congestive heart failure? (Pulmonary edema)

Pulmonary edema is an accumulation of fluid in the lungs because of failure of the left side of the heart. As this happens, more blood enters into the pulmonary circulation than can be removed.

What are the causes of cardiac pulmonary edema?

The causes of pulmonary edema include:

1. Acute myocardial infarction(heart attack) resulting in severe muscle damage with heart losing significant pumping ability, thereby causing fluid to back up into the lungs;
2. Acute ischemic episode (angina pectoris) superimposed on an already sick heart;
3. Decompensated chronic congestive heart failure due to too much salt in the diet and/or failure to take prescribed diuretic;
4. Sinus tachycardia (rapid heart rate);
5. Cardiac arrhythmias;
6. Heart blocks;
7. Pulmonary embolism;
8. Acute bacterial endocarditis;
9. Acute rupture of a heart valve;
10. Acute intracranial hemorrhage, etc.

What are the symptoms of pulmonary edema?

The symptoms of pulmonary edema include:

1. Severe dyspnea
2. Severe tachypnea
3. Severe wheezing
4. Diaphoresis (sweating)
5. Tachycardia
6. A feeling of doom
7. Cold feeling over the body, etc.

What are the clinical and physical signs of pulmonary edema?

The clinical signs of pulmonary edema include:

1. Severe dyspnea (marked shortness of breath)
2. Severe tachypnea (very rapid respiration)
3. Severe diaphoresis (Severe sweating)
4. Marked inability to lie flat
5. Distended neck veins
6. Rapid heart rate or rapid an irregular heart rate
7. Rales and wheezings in both lungs

8. Swollen ankles, legs, abdominal walls and scrotum or groins
9. Chest x ray evidence of pulmonary edema involving both lungs with fluid in them
10. EKG evidence of acute myocardial infarction
11. EKG evidence of acute ischemia of the heart
12. EKG evidence of complete heart block
13. EKG evidence of rapid atrial fibrillation or other cardiac arrhythmias, etc.

Recommended methods of treating pulmonary edema include the following:

1. IV Lasix
2. 100% oxygen via re-breather mask
3. IV digitalis if there is no bradycardia or significant AV heart block
4. Application of nitro paste to chest wall or IV nitroglycerin (if the blood pressure is normal)
5. Administer Dobutrex or Dopamine in drip form if the patient is hypotensive
6. Administer IV Lopressor if the patient's pulse is not too low or there is no significant AV heart block
7. Administer IV Vasotec or an ARBs if the blood pressure is not to low
8. Administer IV nitroglycerine if the patient is having chest pain
9. Adminsiter IV morphine
10. Insert a Foley catheter to monitor urine output
11. Monitor oxygen saturation
12. Monitor serial portable chest x-ray
13. Continue treatment as per chronic congestive heart failure once the acute pulmonary edema is brought under control
14. Do Serum BNP

How do physicians diagnose chronic congestive heart failure?

To diagnose congestive heart failure, conduct the following examinations:

1. History of shortness of breath by the patient
2. History of swollen ankles by the patient
3. History of needing several pillows to sleep
4. History of recurrent coughing when lying down
5. History of difficulty breathing when walking upstairs
6. Enlarged heart seen on chest x-ray with the presence of fluid in the lungs
7. Abnormal left ventricular function seen on Echocardiogram
8. Low Ejection Fraction on Echocardiogram, Rest Muga or Nuclear stress test
9. The presence of S3, S4 galop on listening to heart using the stethoscope

10. Rales heard on listening to the lungs using the stethoscope
11. Elevated Beta naturatic peptibe BNP
12. Swollen ankles
13. Swollen abdomen etc

How to treat congestive heart failure

1. Lasix IV or by mouth
2. Bumex IV
3. Aldactone
4. Beta Blocker such as Coreg, Lopressor, Toprol XL, Tenormin etc
5. Nitro paste on the chest wall or IV nitroglycerin
6. Digitalis IV or by mouth if the heart is enlarged
7. Nasal oxygen
8. Low salt diet
9. Daily weight when in the hospital
10. BiDil is said to be effective in the treatment of congestive heart failure in blacks

This is a controversial issue because although this medication works to treat congestive heart failure, it is a good medication in all racial groups to treat heart failure. The research was to done on this medication only in blacks. No white, no Asians, and no Hispanic patients were included and treated with BiDil during the research.

The two most important medications in BiDil namely hypresoline and isosorbide have been used in the treatment of patients with congestive heart failure for many years individually and in combination in some settings.

How does BiDil work to treat congestive heart failure?

BiDil works to treat congestive heart failure by

1. Isosorbide one of the two medications in BiDil is a vasodilator which on the venous system causes venous dilation and it also causes the release of nitric oxide which in turn activates guanylyl cyclase resulting in relaxation of the vascular smooth muscle.

Hydralazine, the other medication in BiDil is an arterial smooth muscle dilator; it also prevents the degradation of nitric oxide. It is said that blacks have lower level of nitric oxide than whites do. BiDil works to treat congestive heart failure in all patients with congestive heart failure, without regards to race. Medications that cause vasodilatation help to ease the load off the heart and help to perfuse the kidneys allowing for increase urine excretion which is essential in the treatment of congestive heart failure.

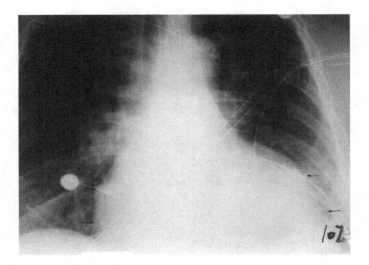

Figure 4.9: Chest x-ray of a patient with ischemic myocardial disease with associated congestive heart failure.

Digitalis is a medication that has been around for many years and it still is a very effective medication in the treatment of cardiovascular disease. If the heart is enlarged, the ejection fraction is low, and the person has congestive heart failure, digitalis is quite effective in helping the heart to pump well and thereby relieving the symptoms of congestive heart failure.

If the rhythm of the heart is irregular, such as in atrial fibrillation, digitalis is the drugs that can be used to regulate the heart rhythm. Digitalis has other uses also in the treatment of coronary heart disease, such as in the treatment of paroxysmal atrial tachycardia, and it is quite effective when used for that particular condition.

Other medications that are very important in the treatment of congestive heart failure include Beta blockers, Angiotensin converting enzyme inhibitors, Angiotensin ll receptor blockers, Aldactone, Lasix, Bumex etc.

Medications in use to treat congestive heart failure are

Lasix
Bumex
Aldactone
Cozaar
Diovan
Avapro

Atacand
Benicar
Micardis
Teveten
Zestril
Capoten
Vasotec
Altace
Lopressor
Coreg
Toprol XL
Bystolic
Sectral
Tenormin
Kerlone
Zebetal
Brevibloc
Hydralazine
Nitropaste
Isosorbide
Nitro-Dur etc

Cardiovascular diseases require a multitude of different medications, frequently used in combination in order to make the heart function properly.

Another common technique that is frequently used to help the heart to function better is the insertion of a pacemaker. Pacemakers are inserted for different reasons. Clinically when a man has sick sinus disease, that is when the area of the heart where the electrical system is located has become degenerated and a person develops heart block, a pacemaker has to be inserted in order to take over the proper electrical functioning of the heart. Heart block occurs usually in the aged or because of an acute myocardial infarction. Pacemakers are used in different sets of circumstances in different age groups for different reasons.

Some of the reasons for which a pace maker may be inserted are

2. Third degree AV black
3. Symptomatic left ventricular block
4. Symptomatic Right ventricular
5. Symptomatic bifascicular block

It is important to realize that the pacemaker, once inserted, must be tested periodically to assure that it is functioning properly. The pacemaker can be tested, even if the man in whose heart the pacemaker is inserted is away in a foreign country. It can be tested using a telephone. It is very important to realize that these things are being modified frequently and the technology has improved remarkably in the last few years. Pacemakers can do wonders to keep people alive who have different types of cardiovascular disease. Insertion of a mechanical pump is being frequently used in the treatment of medications resistant congestive heart failure with great success.

Another common problem that individuals with cardiovascular disease have to deal with is cardiac arrhythmias.

Some of the most common cardiac arrhythmias are

1. Sinus tachycardia
2. Atrial fibrillation
3. Atrial flutter
4. Premature ventricular contraction (VPC's)
5. Premature atrial contraction (APC's)
6. Paroxysmal supraventricular tachycardia
7. Ventricular tachycardia (V Tach)
8. Ventricular fibrillation

What are the most common causes of cardiac arrhythmias?
The most common causes of cardiac arrhythmias are

1. Arthrosclerotic heart disease
2. Myocardial infarction
3. Cardiomyopathy
4. Congestive heart failure
5. Ischemic valvular heart disease
6. Congenital heart disease
7. Pulmonary embolism
8. Hyperthyroidism etc.

How to diagnose cardiac arrhythmias?

1. Patient's history of irregular heart beats
2. Examination of the heart using the stethoscope
3. 12 lead EKG
4. 24 hour Holter monitor

5. Monitoring the patient's heart rhythm on telemetry in the hospital
6. Echocardiogram
7. Nuclear cardiac stress test
8. Thyroid blood tests etc,

How to treat cardiac arrhythmias?

Each arrhythmia is treated differently and according to the underline heart disease

The different medications used to treat cardiac arrhythmias are

1. Lidocaine
2. Tocainide
3. Digitalis
4. Quinidine
5. Procainamide
6. Amiodarone
7. Dronedarone (Multag)
8. Beta blockers
9. Adenosine
10. Verapamil
11. Diltiazem
12. Vasotec
13. Aspirin
14. Coumadin
15. Heparin
16. Lovenox
17. Pradaxa etc

Severe and life threatening ventricular arrhythmias are treated with implantable cardio ventricular defibrillation (ICD)

Atrial fibrillation must be treated with Coumadin, Lovenox, Pradaxa, or aspirin long term to prevent the development of stroke.

Another aspect of cardiovascular disease, which ought to be mentioned, is heart valve replacement. The different valves of the heart can get damaged because of infection and because of the aging process. The heart valves can also get damaged because of congenital problems. In any event, cardiac valve replacement is being done all over the country and all over the world.

Cardiovascular surgeons are using different materials; some of them are prosthetic materials to replace heart valves to make the heart function better. Sometimes, acutely, in the process of a heart attack, a man's heart valve can become damaged and the result can be acute heart failure.

The acute heart muscle damage that occurs when a man suffers a heart attack can also cause acute congestive heart failure to develop. Cardiac catheterization can be done to document which coronary artery vessel or vessels is or occluded to have caused the heart attack and which heart valve if any is damaged by the acute myocardial infarction.

Following cardiac catheterization, angioplasty, bypass surgery with or without valve replacement may be carried out, depending on the particular clinical situation. The chordae tendineae are little strands cordlike structures that keep the heart valves together. They can become ischemic resulting in damages. They can also get damaged because of a heart attack, the aging process. When the chordae tendineae are ruptured, frequently acute heart failure develops.

One of the most common symptoms of sick sinus disease is dizziness, tiredness and a general feeling of unwellness and, fainting spells. A person may at times, actually lose consciousness. That happens because the person's pulse has become too slow, sometimes less than 30 beats per minute, so that the heart cannot pump enough blood to the brain, resulting in the loss of consciousness or blackout spells.

On EKG, different degrees of heart block can be seen to explain the person's symptoms. Third-degree heart block is the heart block most associated with the symptom complex just outlined. In the acute setting, the cardiologist can insert a temporary pacemaker to try to get the patient through the acute period. Sometimes, these patients will need a permanent pacemaker and sometimes they will not. As their hearts recover, the problem that causes the slow pulse may resolve itself and then the pacemaker may not be needed.

That usually occurs as part of an acute heart attack. In the setting of sick sinus disease and third-degree heart block, a permanent pacemaker is inserted by a chest surgeon. Sometimes, in an acute setting, the so-called bundle branch block can occur, and that bundle branch block can necessitate the insertion of a permanent pacemaker.

Be that as it may, if a person has a slow heart rate, a condition referred to as bradycardia, and the heart cannot pump well enough to perfuse the brain, it is very important that a temporary pacemaker be put in, in order to allow for better cardiovascular function.

Another common cause of severe bradycardia is elderly people on Beta-Blocker containing eye drops for the treatment of glaucoma. These medications can slow their heart rates. Beta-Blockers are used to treat various medical conditions. This combination of medications frequently leads to life threatening bradycardia that can cause congestive heart failure and syncope, because of the inability of the heart to pump forcefully to prevent fluid accumulation in the lungs.

A problem that affects the heart quite often is infection:

The different infections that can affect the heart are
1. Infective endocarditis
2. Myocarditis
3. Pericarditis

What is endocarditis?

Endocarditis is when a heart valve becomes infected with a microorganism. There are three different types of infective endocarditis.
1. Native valve endocarditis
2. Prosthetic valve endocarditis
3. Intravenous drug addicts endocarditis

The most bacteria that cause endocarditis in native valve endocarditis are Streptococci, Enterococci, Staphylococci, and many gram negative, as well as different fungi. The different types of native heart valves that that become infected in endocarditis are

1. Normal heart valve
2. Congenital heart valve
3. Degenerative heart valve
4. Rheumatic heart valve

The mechanism through which endocarditis develops is different in different heart valves and in different clinical settings. In an individual with normal heart vale, infective endocarditis can occur, and if the individual becomes either bacteremic or septic (bacteria circulating in the blood stream) and the bacteria settle on the heart valve leading to either sub-acute or acute bacterial endocarditis.

In congenital bacterial endocarditis the same situation exists as above, except that in this instance, the abnormal valve makes it easier for bacteria that are circulating in the blood to get trapped on causing endocarditis. The same situation occurs in degenerative heart valve and rheumatic heart valve.

Prosthetic valve endocarditis is responsible for about 20% of all cases of infectious endocarditis. Most of the individuals in this category are patients 60 years of age or older.

The different microorganisms that cause prosthetic endocarditis are, Staphylococci epidermidis, Staphylococcus Aureus, gram negative bacteria, and fungi. Prosthetic endocarditis can develop 1 year, 2 years or many years after the prosthetic valves were placed. Bacterial endocarditis in intravenous drug addicts occurs usually on normal heart valves most of the time and in young adults.

The skin is the usual site of entry and the valves most frequently affected are tricuspid valve 52% of the time, the aortic is involved 25% of the time, the mitral valve is involved 20% of the time and 3% of the time, multiple valves are involved.

The microorganisms most often involved in causing infectious endocarditis are Staphylococci, Streptococci, Enterococci, Gram negative bacteria, and fungi such as Candida and aspergillus.

The symptoms and clinical signs of endocarditis are:

1. Fever
2. Chills
3. Joints pain
4. Muscle pain
5. Heart murmur
6. Enlarged Spleen
7. Head ache
8. Weakness

Skin lesions such as Janeway lesions, Roth's spots and Osier's nodes, splinter hemorrhages that can be seen in endocarditis.

Abnormal blood tests findings frequently seen in infectious endocarditis are:

1. Elavated white blood cell count
2. Low red blood cell count
3. Low platelets count
4. The Prothrombin time may be high which may indicate Desseminated intravascular coagulopathy (DIC)

5. There maybe red blood cells in the urine, due to emboli to the kidneys from the heart valves
6. There is protein in the urine
7. The erythrocyte sedimentation rate is quite high
8. The blood cultures are positive growing the responsible bacteria
9. The serum BUN and creatinine are usually high due to emboli and immune complexes to the kidneys
10. The rheumatoid factor is frequently positive
11. There may be circulating immune complexes
12. Serum Complement is usually is decreased
13. Elevated C-reactive protein

The cardiology tests that may be abnormal in infectious are:

1. Echocardiogram may show vegetation on heart valve or abscesses in the heart muscle
2. In addition, cardiac arrhythmias may develop
3. Myocarditis and pericarditis may develop
4. 24 hour Holter monitor
5. Cardiac Telemetry monitoring
6. Echocardiogram
7. Transesophageal echocardiogram (TEE)
8. Transthoracic echocardiogram (TTE)

The following are the different antibiotics that used to treat bacterial endocarditis

1. Penicillin G
2. Vancomycin
3. Cubicin
4. Ceftriaxone
5. Nafcillin
6. Gentamicin
7. Ceftazidime
8. Piperacillin
9. Cefotaxime
10. Levaquin
11. Ciprofloxacin
12. Erythromycin
13. Zoszyn
14. Xyvox etc

These different antibiotics are used in different dosages based on the patient's sizes, ages and renal function and clinical settings for 6-8weeks IV.

Individuals who are at risks to develop endocarditis because of valvular heart diseases or heart murmurs of different types and in individuals who have received prosthetic implants such as heart valves and hip prostheses etc, of one kind or an other, the following antibiotics are used prophylactically when invasive procedures are being done in the body of the affected person.

The invasive procedures that require prophylactic antibiotics are:

1. **Intravaginal and intrapelvis surgical procedures**
2. **Any intraabdominal surgical procedures**
3. **Intraoral procedures of any kind**
4. **Any serious skin infection**
5. **Before colonoscopy etc**

Erythromycin by mouth or IV

Amoxicillin by mouth or IV

Ceftriaxone IM or IV

Vancomycin IV

Cleocin by moth or IV

If acute bacterial endocarditis develops, a cardiothoracic surgeon must be brought to take the patient to operating room to replace the damaged heart vale. In addition, if it is discovered that on either TEE or echocardiogram that there is vegetation on the heart vale or abscesses on the heart muscle, a cardiothoracic surgeon must be brought in to surgically remove the infected part of the heart vale or muscle to save the patient's life and to prevent infected emboli from being thrown to multiple organs in the body.

Two other significant infectious conditions frequently affect the human heart. **Infectious myocarditis and Infectious pericarditis.**

Infectious myocarditis develops when the muscles of the heart become infected by a microorganism.

The most common bacteria are Staphylococcus aureus, Streptococcus and Enterococcus, Staph epedipermidis, Pseudomonas, Proteus, E Coli, Klebsellia pneumonia, etc

The most common viruses that cause infection of the myocardium is coxsackieviruses,

Influenza virus,

The AIDS virus can also cause myocarditis.

Lyme disease can also affect the myocardium of the heart causing myocarditis etc.

The symptoms of myocarditis are:

1. Chest pain
2. Shortness of breath
3. irregular heart beats
4. Tiredness etc.
5. Although the physical examination is frequently normal, signs of CHF and irregular Cardiac rhythm can be heard
6. Heart murmur

The EKG findings may be similar to that seen when the person is having an acute myocardial infarction. The cardiac enzymes such as the CPK, LDH, and SGOT might be elevated as well.

The erythrocytes sedimentation rate is usually elevated.
The tests that are used to diagnose myocarditis are

1. **CBC**
2. **SMA 20 and cardiac enzymes**
3. **ERS**
4. **ANA, rheumatoid factor, double stranded DNA to rule out collagen vascular diseases such as Lupus or Rheumatoid arthritis as a possible cause of the myocarditis**
5. **Blood cultures**
6. **Urine analysis**
7. **Viral titers for coxsackievirus B**
8. **Lyme disease blood tests**
9. **HIV blood test**
10. **Chest x-ray**
11. **EKG**
12. **24 hour cardiac monitoring**
13. **Echocardiogram**
14. **Myocardial biopsy when appropriate**

The treatment of myocarditis is based on the clinical profile and presentation of the affected individual and the best judgment of the treating physician.

At presentation, the patient ought to be treated with broad spectrum antibiotics that cover both for gram positive and gram negative bacteria. When bacterial myocarditis is ruled out, then other treatment modality may be considered based on viral titers or collagen vascular test results, such as the ANA, or Rheumatoid factor or other blood tests for Lupus etc. Supportive care with bed rest, nasal oxygen, pain medication, and antipyretics to control fever needs to be provided.

Infectious pericarditis is a condition that occurs when the pericardium becomes infected by micro organism such as bacteria, virus, or a fungus.

Although any microorganism can cause infection in the pericardial sac of the heart if it were to find its way there, the most common bacteria that cause acute infectious pericarditis are:

1. **Streptococcus**
2. **Pneumococcus**
3. **Staphylococcus**
4. **Tuberculous etc**

The most common viruses that cause acute pericarditis are:

1. **Coxsackievirus A**
2. **Coxsackievirus B**
3. **Adenovirus**
4. **Hepatitis viruses**
5. **HIV /AIDS etc;**

The most common fungi that cause acute pericarditis are:

1. **Candida**
2. **Histoplasma**
3. **Blastoplasma**
4. **Coccidiomycosis**

The most common symptoms of acute infectious peircarditis are:

1. **Chest pain that is made worst by coughing**
2. **Chest pain that is made worst by lying in a supine position**
3. **Chest pain that is made worst by taking a deep breath**
4. **Chest pain that is relieved by leaning forward**
5. **Chest pain that is relieved by sitting up**

The clinical findings of pericarditis on physical examination are:

1. **Distant heart sounds**
2. **Pericardial friction rub**

3. Irregular heart sounds may be heard secondary to different rhythm abnormalities that may develop because of the infection.

Many different abnormal findings may be seen on EKG, chest x-ray, in blood tests and echocardiogram in infectious pericarditis.

The most common tests done to diagnose infectious pericarditis are:

1. CBC and blood cultures
2. ESR
3. SMA20
4. Cardiac enzymes
5. Viral titers for Coxsackieviruses A and B
6. Adenovirus titer
7. Hepatitis A, B, and C
8. HIV virus blood test
9. Histoplasma titer
10. Blastoplasma titer
11. Coccidiomycosis titer
12. Blood for Candida culture
13. Pericardial tap and biopsy to obtain specimens for these different cultures including gram stain and AFB stain and culture for mycobacterium tuberculosis
14. Blood test for syphilis (VDRL)
15. EKG
16. Echocardiogram

17. Cardiac Telemetry monitoring
18. Chest x-ray etc.
19. A complete collagen vascular blood profile must always be drawn and sent to the laboratory such as ANA, Rheumatoid factor, double stranded DNA. Blood for Angiotensin—1-Coverting Enzyme ought to be sent to the laboratory as well to rule out the possibility of sarcoidosis as the cause of the pericarditis.

The treatments of infectious pericarditis include:

1. Broad spectrum antibiotics covering for both gram negative and gram positive bacteria pending the results of blood cultures, pericardia fluid, and pericardial biopsy if one was done.
2. Anti fungal IV Amphotericin B if there is a strong suspicion of fungal infection and or if the patient is immunosuppressed.
3. Nasal oxygen
4. Antipyretics to control fever
5. Bed rest and general supportive care

In infectious percarditis, pericardial fluid can build up inside the pericardial sac resulting in pericardiac temponade. If pericardial temponade develops in a patient, if it can cause sudden death.

The best way to diagnose pericardial is physical examination and echocardiogram;
The best way to treat pericardial temponade is surgical intervention by a cardiothoracic surgeon.

Infectious pericarditis can develop into chronic as well as constrictive pericarditis which can be markedly debilitating to affected individuals.

Pericarditis can be caused by

1. Trauma
2. Acute myocardial infarction,
3. Lupus,
4. Rheumatoid
5. Arthritis
6. Cancer
7. Kidney failure
8. Hypothyroidism with myxedema and many more.

The following measures can help to lessen the incidence of cardiovascular heart disease in blacks:

1. Eat a low-fat, low-carbohydrate, low-salt, and high-protein diet to prevent weight gain.
2. Exercise regularly.
3. Visit the doctor frequently to have the blood pressure checked, so that hypertension can be detected and properly treated.
4. Take chest pain seriously and have it evaluated with an EKG and a stress test.
5. Stop smoking.
6. Don't abuse alcohol.
7. If diabetic, lose weight and control the blood sugar tightly.

If a person has family members who suffer from heart disease, it is very important that he or she mentions that to his or her physician, so that that fact can be entered into the clinical equation to ensure that he is properly evaluated to detect the existence of heart disease.

The incidence of coronary heart disease in and the incidence of deaths from coronary heart diseases in blacks are several time higher in blacks than in whites. The reasons for this blatetent health disparity in blacks in the U.S. have its root cause in racial discrimination. Racism against blacks in the U.S. leads to wide spread poor education, low economic status, poverty, and poor education.

In addition, racism causes minorities to experience stress, poor diet, obesity, hypertension, diabetes mellitus, coronary heart disease, stroke, kidney failure, AIDS, depression, alcoholism, high infant mortality, high prenatal maternal death rates, drug addiction, high crime rates, high homicide rates in black Americans against black Americans, high suicide rates, low self esteem and over all poor health, and lower life expectancy.

America is the greatest country in the world, and if a cure can be found for the disease of of racism against blacks and other minorities, millions of unproductive black American and other minority citizens can be put to work and the general economic situations of black Americans and other minorities would improve almost over night and in the process, and the overall U.S. economy would improve as well.

The billion of dollars being spent by the Federal government and states governments every year to pay for Medicaid, food stamps and a multitude of other programs would no longer be necessary because poor folks who are receiving these benefits would be fully employed and paying taxes which would help to solve their economic problems in the U.S. and in the world.

Understanding these facts and paying close attention to them, would help poor folks to turn around their negative experiences brought on in part by racial discrimination and become positive about themselves. The negative effects of racism against blacks and other minorities can be turned around in a positive direction if white people and other ethnic groups would make the necessary efforts to get to know black people other minorities and their cultures. This would be a motivating experience for blacks and other minorities to become successful human beings and in so doing, the high incidence and death rates from coronary heart disease and other deadly diseases that they are suffering from would decrease accordingly.

Chapter 5
CANCER

As of 2013, there were 315. 961. 515 people in the U.S. population and according to the Census bureau there were 42 million Black Americans, 52 million Hispanics, 17.3 million Asians, and 5.1 million American Indians, /Alaska Natives in the U.S.

The world population in 2013 was 7,113,968,427.

In 2013, there were 13.7 million Americans alive who had cancer and 1,660,290 new cancers are expected to be diagnosed in the U.S. and 12.5 million new cancers will be diagnosed in the world in 2013. Sources: ACS Facts and Figures 2013 and WHO

In 2013, 580,350 people are expected to die of cancer in the U.S. and 7.6 million people die every year from caner in the world. Sources: ACS, Facts and Figures 2013 and WHO.

Both the incidence and death rates of cancer are higher in Blacks, Hispanics and American Indians/Alaska Natives than in whites in the U.S. In 2010-2011, 168,900 blacks were diagnosed with cancer and 65.540 blacks died of cancer in the U.S. Source: ACS, Cancer Facts and Figures for African Americans 2011-2012. In 2012, 62 million people died of cancer in the world. WHO

"Racial disparities in lung cancer rates still exist in the U.S." According to the CDC, "The highest incidence rates of lung cancer diagnosis annually were observed among blacks. There were 1,433,172 lung cancer diagnoses in the U.S. during the study period, which ran from 1998 to 2006. The overall annual incidence rate was 69.3 per 100,000 populations. When broken down by race, the annual rates per 100,000 were as follows:

76.1 Among blacks
69.7 Among whites
48.4 Among American Indians or Alaska Natives
38.4 Among Asians or Pacific Islanders
37.3 Among Hispanics
71.9 Among non-Hispanics "(Source: HemOnc today: December 10, 2010)

The most common cancers in males in the U.S. in 2010-2011 were:

Prostate

Lung
Colorectal
Kidney
Urinary bladder
Pancreas
Liver
Head and neck
Non-Hodgkin lymphoma
Leukemia

The most common cancers seen in women in the U.S. are
Breast cancer
Lung cancer
Colon cancer

The most common top 5 cancers in the world in 2012 were
Lung cancer 1, 608,823
Breast cancer 1, 383,523
Colorectal cancer 1, 233,711
Stomach cancer 989, 598
Prostate cancer 903, 454
Source: WHO

In 2010-2011, 88,860 black men had cancer in the U.S. 35,110 black men had prostate cancer. 12,930 black males had lung cancer. 7,940 black males had colorectal cancer. 2,490 black males had cancer of the pancreas. 2,550 black males had head neck cancer. 4,210 black males had cancer of the kidney. 1,990 had multiple myeloma. 2,240 black males had cancer of the urinary bladder. 2,780 black males had cancer of the liver and gall bladder. 2,850black males had Non-Hodgkin lymphoma and 2,030 black males had leukemia.

The most common cancers in black women in the U.S. in 2010-2011 were:

Breast
Lung
Colorectal
Uterus
Ovary
Cervix
Pancreas
Kidney
Thyroid
Myeloma

Non-Hodgkin lymphoma

In 2010-2011, 80,040 black women had cancer in the U.S. 19, 540, black women had breast cancer. 9,730 black women had lung cancer. 8,540 black women had colorectal cancer.3.780 black women had cancer of the uterus. 2,480 black women had cancer of the kidney. 2,360 black women had cancer of the thyroid. 2, 490, black women had cancer of the pancreas. 1,990 black women had cancer of the cervix. 1,990 black women had multiple myeloma, and 2,310 black women had Non—Hodgkin lymphoma.

The death rates from cancer of all types are higher in blacks than in whites in the U.S.
In 2010-2011, 65,540 blacks died of cancer in the U.S.

In 2010-2011, 9,740 black men died of lung cancer. 5,300 black men died of prostate cancer. 3,520 black men died of colon-rectal cancer. 2,000, black men died of cancer of the pancreas. 1,810 black men died of liver and gall bladder cancer. 1,109 black men died of cancer of the stomach.760 black men died of cancer of the esophagus. 900 black men died of multiple myeloma. 980 black men died of leukemia. Fifty percent more blacks died of head and neck cancer than do wihtes.

In 2010-2011, 31,640 black women died of cancer in the U.S. 7,050 black women died of lung cancer. 6,040 black women died of breast cancer. 3,530 of black women died of colon-rectal cancer. 1,320 black women died of cancer of the ovary. 1,450 black women died of cancer of the uterus. 890 black women died of myeloma. 880 black women died of head and neck cancer. 880 black women died of cancer of the esophagus. 860 black women died of cancer of leukemia. 2,320 black women died of cancer of the pancreas. 760 black women died of cancer of the liver and gall bladder and 740 black women died of cancer of the stomach.
Source: ACS Cancer Facts and Figures for African Americans 2010-2011

Overall, according to figures published by the American Cancer Society, the death rate for cancer of all types is 33% higher in black males and 16% higher in black females as compared to white males and females in the U.S. These astonishingly high figures further demonstrate the large health disparity that exists among blacks vs. whites in both diagnosis and treatments of cancer in the U.S. Cancer is the second leading cause of deaths in the United States next to cardiovascular heart diseases.

What is cancer?

Cancer develops when a cell loses its ability to grow and multiply in a normal growth pattern. A good example of this is contact inhibition. When a normal cell is placed in contact with a hard surface in a Petri dish, the normal cell stops growing. However, in the case of an abnormal cell, it continues to grow because it has lost its contact inhibition ability, which allows it to grow uncontrollably, developing into a cancer growth.

The cancer cells fail in the process of cell-to-cell interactions. The development of cancer is a multi-step and multi-factorial process. In the multi-step and multi-factorial processes, there is normally a balance between growth-promoting genes (proteins) and growth-suppressive genes (proteins). Once mutation occurs for one reason or another, the growth-promoting genes (oncogenes) stop the suppressive effects of the suppressor genes.

The growth-promoting genes take control and promote abnormal cell growth, resulting in the formation of a cancerous clone of cells, resulting in cancer, as it is known. This is an out-of-control process of cell growth whose ultimate goal is to take over the body in which it is growing and destroys it.

The first step in the genesis of cancer is the process of oncogene. Oncogenes can be brought about by a hereditary or familial transmission of a protein from parent or parents to fetus at the time of conception. This protein (oncogene or oncogenes) can then enter over many years into a multi-step process, interactions, and reactions that can cause a cell or group of cells to mutate. Once this mutation occurs, then the cell or group of cells loses their ability to grow and multiply normally. The abnormal growth of cells then becomes a cancer mass. Many causative effects can bring about the damage that occurs to the cell or cells that cause this mutation to occur.

All of the following can damage the DNA/RNA materials inside a cell, resulting in malignant mutations: The different risks for cancer are:

1. Transmission of a hereditary cancer oncogene
2. Exposure to oncogenic viruses such as Epstein bar virus, which can cause nasopharyngeal carcinoma
3. Exposure to human papilloma virus, causing cervical cancer
4. Exposure to either hepatitis B or C virus, causing cancer of the liver
5. Exposure to HTLV-I and HTLV-II, causing T cell leukemia/lymphoma
6. Sun exposure causing basal cell carcinoma of the skin
7. Exposure to carcinogens such as tobacco smoking, causing lung cancer, cancer of the mouth, throat, head and neck, etc.
8. Exposure to ionizing radiation, causing leukemia, lymphoma and other cancers
9. Exposure to toxic chemicals such as benzene, etc., causing malignancies of different types.

10. Consumption of excessive alcohol, resulting in cancer of the mouth, throat, and esophagus.

11. Exposure to estrogen, causing increased incidence of breast cancer and uterine cancer in women

12. Consumption of too much red meats, resulting in increased incidence of breast, uterine and colon cancer

13. Alcohol abuse and tobacco smoking, associated with increase incidence of cancer of the esophagus.

14. 14. Long-term exposure to toxic pollutants and chemical solvents in the work place, resulting in the development of different types of cancer

15. HIV-I and II causing AIDS with its high propensity to cause lymphoma and Kaposi's sarcoma

16. Non-acquired immunodeficiency and its propensity to cause malignancy of different types

17. A newly discovered risk for cancer is chronically elevated white blood cells count. Elevated white blood cells count causes increase development of colon cancer, endometrial cancer, breast cancer and lung cancer in post menopausal women.

Source : Archive of Internal Medicine Vol. 167 NO, 17 Sep 24, 2007

Cancer genetics

Following are examples of cancers that develop because of oncogene activation:

Multiple endocrine neoplasia (MEN) type 2a and type 2b. MEN 2a include medullary carcinoma of the thyroid, pheochromocytoma and hyperparathyroidism.

MEN 2b include medullary carcinoma of the thyroid, pheochromocytoma, mucosal neuromas and bony abnormalities. Other cancers that occur as a result of damaged DNA and failure of DNA repair include:

Hereditary nonpolyposis colon cancer (HNPCC). This abnormality is responsible for about 10-15% of colon cancers and is associated with ovarian, endometrial and urinary tract cancers.

Other genetically associated cancers include neurofibromatosis 1 and 2, hereditary Wilm's tumor, Li-Fraumeni syndrome, and familial adenomatous polyposis of the colon. The percentage of colon cancer in familial adenomatous polyposis is 100%. Treatment usually requires the affected individual to undergo total removal of the colon by 20 to 30 years of age.

In breast cancer, the BRAC 1 and the BRAC 2 genes have been discovered. Women who inherited these genes have an 85% susceptibility to developing breast cancer in their lifetime. The BRAC 1 and BRAC 2 genes also associated with ovarian cancer are referred to as the breast-ovarian cancer syndrome. Some women who have breast cancer may also develop ovarian and colon cancer, because they inherited the BRAC1 gene from their parents.

There are many more genes that have been discovered that have association with many other cancers, which in the future will be better clarified. Gene therapy is being actively investigated and the hope is that these investigations will add immeasurably to the treatment of cancer in the future.

Breast cancer:

The incidence of breast cancer is 13% lower in black women as compared to white women. However, the incidence of breast cancer is higher in black women younger than 40 year old as compared to white women. Over all, one in eight women develops breast cancer.

While the death rate from breast cancer went down in the period from 2001-2005 in white American women, it went up 37% higher in black American women during that period. The 5 year survival for breast cancer is 77% in black American women and is 90% in white American women.

In 2013 there were more than 100 million people with breast cancer in the world and 600,000 women around the world died of breast cancer in 2013. Source: WHO

In the U.S. 234,580, 2,290 males and 232, 340 females had breast cancer in 2013.
In 2013, 40,030 people, 410 males and 39,620 females died of breast cancer in the U.S. Source: ACS, Facts and Figures 2013.

The factors that account for the differences in survival rates from breast cancer in black and other minority women as compared to white women are:

1. Black and other minority women have less access to health care
2. Black and other minority women go to see doctors less often
3. Black and other minority women usually present to doctors with more advanced stage breast cancer
4. Black and other minority women are more obese than white women are
5. Black and other minority women have more estrogen receptor and progesterone receptor negative breast cancer than do white women. (ER negative 41% black women vs. 31% white women, PR negative 56% vs. 44% white women) Source: HemOnc today,: July 25, 2010

Some of the risk factors for breast cancer are:

1. Genetic predisposition
2. Mother with breast cancer
3. A sister with breast cancer
4. A grandmother with breast cancer
5. A maternal aunt with breast cancer
6. A father with prostate cancer
7. A father with colon cancer
8. Having ovarian cancer
9. A woman with colon cancer
10. Carrying the BRAC1 or BRAC2 gene
11. Early menarche (age 8-9 years)
12. Childlessness
13. Late menopause
14. Exposure to toxic materials
15. Taking birth control pills may cause breast cancer
16. Taking estrogen-containing post menopausal hormone may cause breast cancer
17. Menarche (first menstruation episode) at an early age (8-9 years)
18. Late menopause
19. Childlessness
20. Obesity
21. Ingestion of too much red meats or too much fatty foods in general
22. Exposure to birth control pills or any estrogen-containing medications
23. Exposure to carcinogens are all additional risk factors for breast cancer

These different risk factors cause development of breast cancer through these mechanisms:

1. Heredity. This plays a role in the causation of breast cancer by mothers transmitting the breast cancer genes to their daughters. Ten to fifteen percent of women have this form of breast cancer.
2. Early menarche. This causes a predisposition to the development of breast cancer because the earlier a girl begins to menstruate, the earlier her breast tissue gets exposed to the effects of estrogen.
3. Childlessness. When a woman is pregnant, the breast tissues are less exposed to the effects of estrogen, giving these tissues a rest from estrogenic effect. Nuns, because they do not have children, have a higher incidence of breast cancer.
4. Obesity. This increases the incidence of breast cancer because too much estrogen is produced when a woman is obese. The increased production of estrogen comes from the cholesterol portion of fat. Estrogen is a hormone and cholesterol is the first step that is necessary in the production of any hormone. Further, when an obese woman becomes menopausal, her breast tissues do not get any

rest from the effects of estrogen because the excess fat is converted to estrogen under the influence of the adrenal glands. Under the influence of the adrenal glands, fat is then converted into estrone, which is a precursor of estrogen. In this way, estrone is converted into estrogen, which in turn over stimulates the breast tissues, increasing the incidence of breast cancer in obese women.

5. In the U.S., 60% of black females are obese, 32% white females are obese, and 41% Hispanic females are obese. 300 million women around the world are obese.

6. Consumption of the excessive amounts of red meats and other fatty foods increases not only the incidence of breast cancer, but colon cancer as well as cancer of the uterus.

7. Birth control pills and other estrogenic medications increase the incidence of breast cancer because the estrogen contained in these medications over stimulates breast tissue, thereby increasing the risk of breast cancer in women who take these estrogenic pills. Post-menopausal women who take estrogen-replacement medication also have a high risk of developing breast cancer.

8. Exposure to carcinogens in the air, in the water and in food can cause DNA damage, which in turn can lead to increased incidence of breast cancer.

It is important women whose mothers, grandmothers, sisters, and aunts have breast cancer be very vigilant about the health of their breasts. All women, and in particular those women who are at high risk for breast cancer, learn how to do breast self-examinations. These women must have their breasts examined two to three times per year by physicians who are proficient in examining breasts, such as gynecologists, surgeons, oncologists, internists, and primary care physicians.

Women who are at risk for breast cancer ought to have their breasts examined starting in their twenties. Other women ought to undergo regularly breast examinations starting in their mid-thirties. Women who have fibrocystic disease (benign cysts of the breast) should have their breasts examined two to three times per year because these cysts can and frequently cause confusion as it relates to the presence of breast cancer.

This is so because a cyst can at times feel like cancer on palpation. These cysts are not cancer and do not develop into cancer. However, there are published reports that there an increased incidence of breast cancer in women who have cystic breasts. The problem is the confusion that these cysts cause on examining the breasts and on mammograms. Fibrocystic disease of the breasts tend to be found in women on birth control pills and other estrogenic-containing medications, making fibrocystic nodules in the breasts worse. Caffeine and chocolate also make these cystic nodules worse.

When a woman is premenstrual or is menstruating, these cysts get larger often because of the effects of estrogen on the breast tissue.

Genetic testing for women who are at high risk for breast cancer is a good idea. Women who carry the hereditary mutations BRCA1 and BRCA2 genes are at very high risk for developing breast cancer and should consider prophylaxis mastectomy for prevent breast cancer. The BRCA1 and BRCA2 gene are seen less commonly in black women.

One in eight women in the United States will have breast cancer in their life times. Therefore, it is important for women to be vigilant in breast self-examination and have frequent mammograms starting at age 40 for black women with no known risk factors. Starting at age 50, all women should have a mammogram every year. Women in their late twenties and early thirties, whose mothers or sisters had breast cancer, placing them at an increasing risk for developing breast cancer, ought to have an MRI of the breast because a breast MRI is more likely to detect cancer in their breasts than mammogram.

Signs and symptoms of breast cancer include:
Lump in the breast
Tenderness in the breast
Pain in the breast
Discharge in the nipple
Pain in the nipple
Lump under the arm
Skin retraction in the breast etc;

How to evaluate a lump in a woman's breast

First thing is to take a complete history from the woman, including a thorough family history. It is important to determine whether she is taking any estrogen-containing medication.

It is also important to find out if she has any pain and how long ago she discovered the lump in her breast. Following the history and examination, a mammogram is to be done and if the breast is very cystic, it is important to do a sonogram of the breast at the same time.

The most up-to-date test to evaluate a woman's breast that has a high risk of developing breast cancer because of her family history is to do an MRI of the breast. In particular, if the woman is between 20 and 35 years old, because it is very difficult to pick up cancer in the breast of women this young, because the breast tissue is too dense, and therefore an MRI is most appropriate in this setting.

Once the presence of a lump is confirmed in a woman's breast, by mammogram, digital mammogram, sonogram, or MRI, the next step is to refer the woman to a surgeon for evaluation of the breast lump. The surgeon will proceed by scheduling the woman for a breast biopsy.

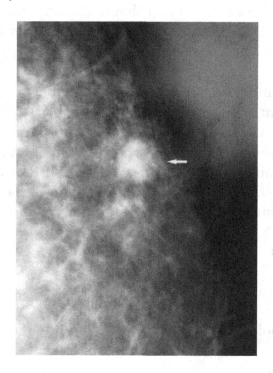

Figure 5.1-X-ray picture of positive mammogram for cancer in a woman.

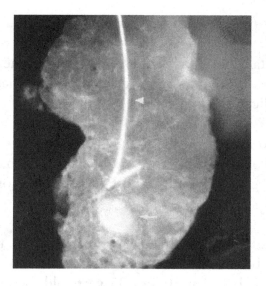

Figure 5.2-Needle biopsy of a breast cancer mass in a woman

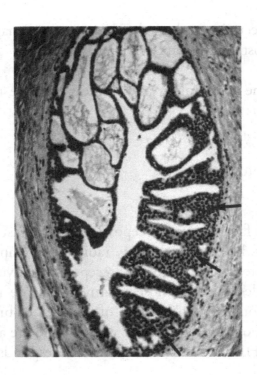

Figure 5.3-Intraductal carcinoma of the breast (arrow) in a woman

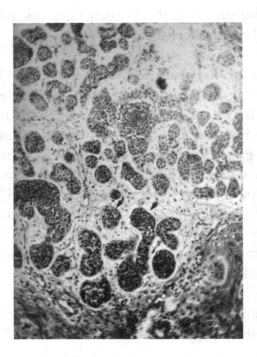

Figure 5.4-Lobular carcinoma of the breast (arrow) in a woman

In evaluating the breast cancer, it is important to know the different pathological and histological characteristics of the cancer. These characteristics have major significance in the treatment modalities that are chosen to treat the breast cancer. It is also important to know certain markers that breast cancer may have or may not have, which have major prognostic significance in breast cancer.

These are some of the most important markers that are used to characterize and treat breast cancer:

1. Estrogen receptor
2. Progesterone receptor
3. HER-2

As a matter of clinical fact, estrogen receptor-positive breast cancer seems to respond better to such treatments like chemotherapy, radiation therapy, or hormonal therapy. The reverse is true in breast cancer that is receptor-negative. Breast cancer is more aggressive and responds less well to those treatments. More recently, a gene product called HER-2 has been found on the surface of 25-30% of breast cancer cells, which, when present, denotes a poorer prognosis for women who are afflicted with this type of breast cancer. However, HER2 positive breast cancer responds extremely to treatment Herceptin.

Once it is determined that a woman has tissue-proven breast cancer, an evaluation must be undertaken to be sure that the woman does not have metastatic disease. A metastatic evaluation for breast cancer includes:

1. Complete blood count, liver function tests (LDH, SGOT, SGPT, bilirubin, and alkaline phosphatase). If the alkaline phosphatase is elevated, it may mean that cancer has gotten into the liver or the bone or it may mean that the patient has some other problem that causes her alkaline phosphatase to be elevated, such as chronic hepatitis, gall bladder disease, or Paget's disease of the bone. To know whether the elevated alkaline phosphatase is coming from the liver or the bone, a test called gamma glutamine transpeptidase (GGTP) is done. If the GGTP is high, it means that the elevated alkaline phosphatase is coming from the liver. If the alkaline GGTP phosphatase is normal, it means that the alkaline phosphatase is coming from the bone, which may mean that the breast cancer has already involved the bones.
2. Bone scan.
3. Abdominal CT scan or abdominal sonogram to look at the liver
4. Chest x-ray or chest CT scan.
5. PET scan

If all these tests are normal, indicating that the breast cancer is localized, then the woman is now ready for either a lumpectomy with axillary node dissection or a modified radical mastectomy. The decision as to whether a lumpectomy with axillary node dissection or a modified radical mastectomy is done is based on the size of the tumor, the choice of the woman or whether the cancer has spread or is localized.

Stages of breast cancer:

Stage 0
Stage I
Stage IIA
Stage IIB
Stage IIIA
Stage IIIB
Stage IV

Stage 0 breast cancer is ductal carcinoma in situ, lobular carcinoma in situ, tubular carcinoma in situ, Paget's disease of the nipple.

Stage I breast cancer is a breast cancer that is 2 cm or less in greatest dimension with no regional lymph node metastasis and no distant metastasis.

Stage IIA breast is a tumor that is greater than 2 cm and less than 5 cm and has metastasized to the lymph node or nodes in the same side of the breast that has the malignancy.

Stage IIB breast cancer is a tumor that is greater than 2 cm and less than 5 cm and metastasis is found in node or nodes on the side of the malignant breast, or a tumor that is greater than 5 cm in size with no metastasis to regional or distant nodes.

Stage IIIA breast cancer has multiple possible scenarios.

1. Metastasis to node, nodes, or other structures on the same side of the tumor.
2. Tumor no greater than 2 cm with positive lymph node or nodes on the same side of the tumor.
3. Tumor greater than 2 cm with metastasis to node or nodes on the same side of the cancer.
4. Tumor greater than 5 cm with metastasis to node or nodes on the same side of the tumor.

Stage IIIB. Is tumor with direct extension to the chest wall with metastasis to the lymph node.

Stage IV is distant metastasis to other parts of the body such as the lungs, liver, bones, or brain.

Evaluation and different treatments for breast cancer:

A biopsy can also be done via needle-guided technique, or an open biopsy can be done. In either case, the specimen is sent to the pathology lab for histological evaluation. If the pathological report comes back showing evidence of breast cancer, then a decision has to be made on what type of surgical approach to use to treat the patient.

Essentially there are several approaches. One approach is lumpectomy with axillary node dissection with employment of the sentinel node technique to be sure that nodes that contain cancer are removed during the axillary dissection. Another approach is modified radical mastectomy.

According to recent reports in the literature, HER2 positive breast cancer responds best to anthracycline based chemotherapy. HER2 negative breast cancer doest not respond as well to chemotherapy and in fact may be better off not receiving chemotherapy, thereby spearing the side effects of chemotherapy.

Different stages of breast cancer are treated differently. For patients who choose to have a lumpectomy with axillary node dissection with sentinel node evaluation, post-surgical treatment with two cycles of chemotherapy either with CMF (Cytoxan, Methotrexate and 5FU) or with CAF (Cytoxan, Adriamycin and 5FU) followed by radiation therapy, then followed by four more cycles of chemotherapy, seems to be the best approach.

Following modified mastectomy or lumpectomy with axillary node sampling, if it is decided, based on the extent of the disease, that adjuvant chemotherapy is needed, then the following chemotherapy protocols are frequently used. If a woman is premenopausal and has estrogen receptor-negative tumor, CAF is the preferred protocol Cytoxan, Adriamycin and 5FU is used in a 28-day cycle.

The most common protocol for women who have estrogen receptor-positive tumor is CMF Cytoxan, Methotrexate and 5FU. This protocol is also used in a 28-day cycle. Based on the extent of disease, these chemotherapies are used either for six months for Stage I tumor or for one year for a Stage II, III or IV tumor.

Other protocols that are commonly used are CMFVP Cyclophosphamide, Methotrexate, 5Fluorouracil, Vincristine and Prednisone. Cisplatin, Etoposide, Mitomycin, and Vinblastine are included at times in different protocols to treat more advanced breast cancer.

In metastatic breast cancer Taxol is also used at a dose of 90 mg/m2 as a continuous IV drip for 96 hours monthly. For women who are HER-2 positive, Herceptin is used to treat them and the results so far have been excellent. The recommended loading dose of Herceptin is 4 mg/Kg IV over 90 minutes followed by a weekly dose of 2 mg/Kg over 30 minutes.

According to recent literature, women with Her2 positive breast cancer (human epidermal growth factor-2) respond best to Adriamycin and Taxol based chemotherapy combination treatment.

Adjuvant Tamoxifen, Lotrezole, or Arimidex are used in estrogen receptor-positive postmenopausal women. All can be used while patients are receiving chemotherapy. They are all commonly used for 5 years and the results so far have been very good in preventing recurrence of breast cancer. The benefit of these medications in premenopausal women or in women with estrogen receptor-negative tumor is not conclusive and seems to be marginal at best.

There is an increased risk of endometrial cancer in women taking Tamoxifen. This is so because Tamoxifen is an estrogen-like medication and its stimulation of the lining of the uterus increases the development of endometrial cancer. The risk of endometrial cancer seems to be less when Lotrizole and Amiridex are used. There is also an increase in clot formation in the legs in women on these anti estrogen hormones.

Estrogen causes a decrease in anti-thrombin III, which then causes a hypercoagulation state resulting in possible clot formation and the end result can be DVT deep vein thrombophlebitis. Other side effects of these hormones include break through vaginal bleeding, easy bruising, and hypercalcemia (high serum calcium).

Alternatively, Letrozole or Amiridex can be used in estrogen receptor-positive post—menopausal women with breast cancer, either after 5 years of Tamoxifen or instead of Tamoxifen as adjuvant treatment. Letrozole can also be used in metastatic breast cancer with very good results.

According to a recent report published in the New England Journal of Medicine, Exemestane (Aromasin) given to 4, 560 post menopausal women from the United States, Canada, France, and Spain showed a 65% decrease in invasive breast cancer. "Exemestine works by blocking the production of estrogen which fuels tumor growth." Source: NEJM June 4, 2011 at NEJM.org 10.1056/NEJM oa 1103507

Exemestane has fewer side effects than Tomaxifen, Letrozole, and Amiridex. Source:

Radiotherapy, either alone or sandwiched between chemotherapy treatments, plays a major role in the treatment of breast cancer and is an important treatment modality.

Chemotherapy treatments used in breast cancer and their major side effects: injection, cardiac toxicity, which can lead to heart failure if too much Adriamycin is given over time. It is recommended a test called REST MUGA is done before starting Adriamycin to evaluate the ejection fraction of the heart (what the heart is capable of doing by way of work in any one second). REST MUGA is done periodically during the treatment with Adriamycin and if the ejection fraction is shown to be dropping significantly indicating cardiac malfunction, the Adriamycin is stopped. The same applies to Herceptin.

Some of the common side effects of the chemotherapeutic agents used in treating breast Cancer include

1. **Cytoxan:** Bone marrow suppression with low white blood cells, low platelets, low red blood cells, hematuria (blood in urine), alopecia (hair loss), nausea, and vomiting.
2. **Methotrexate:** Bone marrow suppression with low white blood cells, low red blood cells and Low platelets, nausea, vomiting and sores in the mouth.
3. **5-Fluorouracil:** Bone marrow suppression with low white blood cells, low red blood cells, and low platelets, nausea, vomiting, sores in the mouth, alopecia (hair loss), darkness of the skin of the back of hands and nails and chest pain.
4. **Adriamycin:** Bone marrow suppression with low white blood cells, low red blood cells and low platelets. Sores in the mouth, nausea, vomiting, darkening of the skin
5. **Herceptin:** The main side effects of Herceptin are cardiac toxicity, anemia, and leukopenia. That being the case, a REST MUGA and CBC must be done before Herceptin is started and periodically during its usage.
6. **Taxol:** The main side effect of Taxol is low white blood cells count; other frequent side effects of Taxol are low platelet count, peripheral neuropathy, and loss of hair.
7. **Docetaxel:** Is also being used to treat breast cancer. The side effects of Docetaxel are similar to that of Taxol.
8. **Amifostine:** Can be used in conjunction with these cytotoxic agents to decrease the incidence of peripheral neuropathy.
9. **Neurontin** 300 mg. by mouth every 8 hours is effective in the treatment of chemotherapy-associated peripheral neuropathy.
10. **Lyrica** 50mg by mouth every 8 hours is effective in the treatment of chemotherapy associated peripheral neuropathy.

Lung Cancer:

Lung cancer is the most common cancer in the world and accounting for 1.62 million of all cancers annually and kills 1.35 million people die every year in the world.

In the U.S. in 2013, 228,190 people had lung cancer 118,080 males and 110,110 females. 159,480 people died of lung cancer in 2013, 87,260 males and 72,220 females.

The number one reason that causes people to develop lung cancer is tobacco smoking. "An estimated 443000 deaths occur in the United States each year from tobacco-related diseases." Forty million Americans smoke in the U.S.

Blacks and other minorities have the third highest rate of tocabacco smoking in the U.S. and the tobacco companies target blacks and other minorities by putting mentol in the cigarettes because they know that minorities like the taste of mentol.
Tobacco related diseases cost $ 150 billion per year.

Other risk factors for lung cancer include:
Genetic predisposition to cancer
Industrial exposure to toxic fumes
Asbestosis
Scar from pulmonary tuberculosis
HIV/AIDS
Chronic fungal infection/ other inflammatory diseases of the lung
Exposure to coal in the mines, (black lung disease) arsenic, air pollution
Second hand smoke etc;

Some of the symptoms of lung cancer include:

1. Chronic cough
2. Coughing with streaks of blood
3. Coughing up blood
4. Chest pain
5. Shortness of breath
6. Weight loss, etc.
7. Recurrent pneumonia and/or pneumonia that fail to respond to treatment over a long period of time etc;

Sometimes lung cancer is discovered on a chest x-ray without any symptoms. Early detection is crucial in order to increase the chance of curing lung cancer; a chest x-ray is the first test in the diagnosis of lung cancer. The chest x-ray is done either as part of a routine examination or because the patient presents with symptoms such as those described earlier here. Things that can be seen on the chest x-ray or CT when a person has lung cancer include:

1. A mass
2. Effusion (fluid in the lung)

3. An infiltrate and in some cases, calcification mass (mesothelioma due to exposure to asbestos)

There are two broad types of lung cancer, large-cell lung cancer and small-cell lung cancer. Large-cell lung cancer may consist of adenocarcinoma of the lung, squamous cell carcinoma of the lung, or scar carcinoma of the lung. Mesothelioma is a form of lung cancer associated with asbestos exposure. Another name for small-cell carcinoma is oat cell carcinoma.

Once cancer of the lung is suspected on chest x-ray, the next test to be done is a CT scan of the chest.

See CT scan of the chest lesion in inferior segment of the lower lobe of the lung. Squamous cell carcinoma (cancer) in a smoker (Figure 5.5 [arrows]).

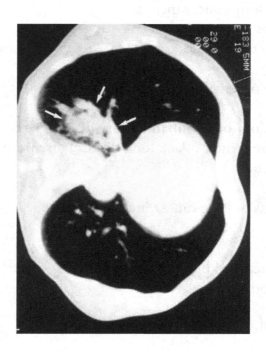

***Figure 5.5**-*See CT scan of the chest showing lobulated mass (cancer) in the right upper lung in a patient who smokes.

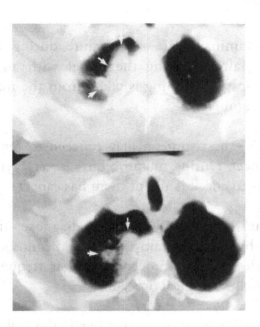

Figure 5.6 CT scan of the lung in smoker showing a cancerous mass (see arrows)

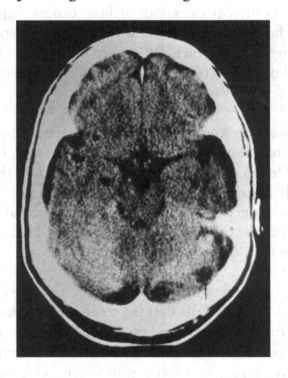

Figure 5.7-CT scan of brain: Hypodense mass left cerebellar hemisphere Metastatic
cancer to the brain from a lung primary cancer in a smoker (arrow).

Following the CT scan of the lung, the next step is to refer the patient to a
pulmonary specialist for a bronchoscopic examination. Another approach is to refer the
patient to a chest surgeon based on the location of the mass. Some masses of the lung
are located so peripherally that it cannot be reached via bronchoscopy.

The bronchoscopic examination is a procedure during which an instrument is introduced into the lung after spraying the throat with an anesthetic. During the bronchoscopy, either a biopsy or washing is taken from the mass in the lung and send to the pathology lab for examination.

If it is cancer, then the chest surgeon may proceed to remove the segment of the lung that contains the cancer. During the procedure, several lymph nodes are taken out from the surrounding area to check if any of them has cancer.

Another method that is frequently used to diagnose lung cancer is CAT—or sonogram-guided needle biopsy to obtain tissue for diagnosis. An invasive radiologist with great precision carries out this procedure and it frequently saves the patient a bronchoscopy or an open-chest surgical procedure.

It is very important to know in advance what is the cell type of lung cancer the patient has in order to know how to proceed with further treatment. As just stated, there are essentially two different categories of lung cancer, large cell carcinoma, and small cell carcinoma. The importance of knowing whether a person has small cell lung cancer, or large cell lung cancer. Small-cell cancer or oat-cell lung cancer usually has already spread by the time a mass is seen on the chest x-ray regardless of how small the mass is.

That being the case, the entire approach to the evaluation and treatment of small-cell cancer is different from any other lung cancer. In fact, it is almost a given that by the time a coin-size lesion is found in the lung of a patient that turns out to be oat cell, the cancer probably has already spread to the brain and possibly the liver and other organs as well. Frequently, once the cell type is known to be oat cell because of biopsy, the question as to whether the cancer should or should not be resected becomes a major clinical decision because the prognosis is poor.

On the other hand, once a tissue diagnosis is made that the cancer in the lung is of the large-cell type, and if the cancer is deemed respectable, based on the size, location, and overall physical status of the patient, the decision usually is to resect the cancer because the chances of cure are better. Though it must be remembered that 20-25% of people with large-cell-type lung cancer frequently present with metastasis to the brain at the time of diagnosis.

Evaluation of lung cancer includes:
1. History and physical examination
2. Chest x-ray
3. Chest CT scan
4. Sputum for cytology

5. Lung biopsy
6. Abdominal CT scan to look at the liver
7. Bone scan to be sure that the cancer has not spread to the bone
8. Brain CT scan with contrast because a brain CT without contrast will likely miss metastatic disease of the brain if its there or brain MRI can also be done.
9. In certain difficult cases a PET scan can be done.
10. Brain CT scan with contrast because a brain CAT without contrast will likely miss metastatic disease of the brain if it is there, or, brain MRI can also be done.
11. PET scan

Treatment of lung cancer includes:

1. Surgical resection of the cancerous mass
2. Adjuvant radiation therapy, after surgical resection
3. Adjuvant chemotherapy

Some frequently used chemotherapeutic agents in large-cell lung cancer include:

Cytoxan
Doxorubicin
Cisplatin
Etoposide
Taxol
Docetaxel
Carboplatin
Gemcitabine
Vinorelbine
Irinotecan

These are used in different combinations.
Some of the commonly used chemotherapeutic agents in small-cell lung cancer care consist of:

Cyclophosphamide
Doxorubicin
Vincristine
Etoposide
Cisplatin
Methotrexate
Carboplatin
Irinotecan
Topotecan
Docetaxel

Placlitaxel

These drugs are used in different combinations.

Some of the side effects of these chemotherapeutic agents have been outlined earlier under the treatment of breast cancer. The side effects of Vincristine include double vision, drooping eyelids, headache, jaw pain, tingling of the finger and toes with numbness (peripheral neuropathy), and constipation.

Some of the side effects of Cisplatin include nausea; vomiting; numbness of feet, fingers, and toes; blurry vision; possible kidney damage; and bone marrow suppression, resulting in pancytopenia.

Some of the side effects of Etoposide (VP 16) include bone marrow depression with low white blood cells, low red blood cells, low platelets; sores in the mouth; numbness in feet, fingers, and toes with tingling; loss of hair; nausea; vomiting; and alopecia.

To decrease the incidence of nausea and vomiting, different anti-emetic medications, such as Zofran or Kytril, in combination with Ativan, Benadryl, and Decadron, can be used.

Colorectal Cancer:

In 2013, there were 142,820 cases of colorectal cancer in the U.S. and 50,830 People died of this cancer during that year. In 2013, 1.24 million people in the world had colorectal cancer in the world and 608,000 people in the world because of colorectal cancer. Colorectal is the third leading cause of cancer deaths in the world in 2013.

In 2009, 16,520 blacks were diagnosed with colorectal cancer and 7,120 blacks died during that year. Blacks have in the U.S. had a 20% higher incidence of colorectal cancer and a 45% higher death rate compared to whites. Source: Journal of the National Medical Association Vol, 103, NO. 8. August 2011

Minorities in general have higher incidence of colorectal cancer and have higher rates of colorectal cancer deaths than do whites.

Risk factors for colorectal cancer include:

Genetic predisposition (family history of colon cancer)

History of prostate cancer
History of ovarian cancer
History of breast cancer
Physical inactivity
Obesity
Increase consumption of processed meat
Exposure to pesticide
Increase consumption of red meat
Colorectal polyps
Inflammatory bowel disease
Familial polyposis etc;

Colorectal cancer is a curable disease when diagnosed early and surgically removed. Common symptoms and signs of colorectal cancer:

1. Blood in the stools
2. Constipation
3. Diarrhea
4. Abdominal pain
5. Weight loss
6. Poor appetite
7. Hemorrhoids
8. Sudden development of inguinal hernia in a person in the cancer-age group (40 years old and older)
9. Anemia
10. Passing pencil-size stool
11. A combination of these signs and symptoms

How to diagnose colorectal cancer

To diagnose colorectal cancer, a complete history, and physical examination needs to be carried out. As part of this examination, a digital rectal examination needs to be done and the stool tested for occult blood. Sometimes, a person goes to the physician and states that he or she sees blood in the stool or on the toilet paper. Sometimes, a person might say that he or she has had hemorrhoids for a long time and suddenly the hemorrhoids have come out and are now bleeding. At times, a person in his or her 40s, or older, might come to see the doctor and reports that he or she has just developed an inguinal hernia with no known precipitating reason.

In all these instances, a complete lower bowel evaluation needs to be done to make sure that these signs and symptoms are not due to colon cancer. The stool needs to be tested for occult blood, unless gross blood is seen. It is important that the person being tested stays away from taking aspirin or NSAIDS for 7-10 days in the case of aspirin, and in the case of NSAIDS 12 to 24 hours.

It is also important that the person does not eat red meat for three days prior to testing the stool for blood. The person must not take Vitamin C in pill form for one week before having his or her stool the tested for occult blood. In addition, the person must not eat horseradish for several days before testing the stool for blood. Aspirin and NSAIDS will cause the stool hemoccult test to be positive because of the irritating effects on the lining of the stomach.

Red meat will cause the stool to be positive for blood because red meat has blood in it. Vitamin C causes the hemoccult test of the stool to be falsely negative for occult blood because Vitamin C is a reducing agent and the chemical reaction that is used in the test is an oxidation reaction.

So, adding a reducing agent to an oxidation reaction neutralizes the reaction, rendering it falsely negative. Eating horseradish can cause a person's stool to become black when it is exposed to the solution that is used to test the stool for blood. Taking Pepto-Bismol also causes the stool to become black, confusing it with bleeding from the stomach.

The tests most effective in evaluation of colorectal cancer consist of:

1. Digital rectal examination
2. Testing of the stool using the hemoccult test
3. Checking the serum ferritin
4. Checking the red cell distribution width (RDW) during a complete blood count
5. Testing for the soluble serum transferrin receptor level. (If elevated, it proves that the patient has iron deficiency anemia. This test is better than bone marrow iron stain test, the serum ferritin and the RDW.)
6. Barium enema
7. Colonoscopy
8. Flexible sigmoidoscopy
9. Rigid sigmoidoscopy
10. Virtual colonoscopy

According to the recent literature, flexible sigmoidoscopy is said to be as effective as colonoscopy detect cancer of the colon. Barium enema is an x-ray test during which the bowel is cleansed with cathartics, barium is put in the bowel from the rectum using a tube, and then x-rays are used to visualize the bowel, looking for abnormalities, such as cancerous growth.

There are several limitations with the barium enema. Among the limitations:

1. Retained stool in the bowel.
2. Barium enema is not able to diagnose colorectal if the cancer is located between 15 and 30 cm in the lower bowel from the entrance of the anus. This is so because the tube that is used to put the barium in the colon occupies that space, making it impossible to visualize a cancer that may be located in that space. Cancer is best discovered in that area by sigmoidoscopy or colonoscopy. In addition, another limitation of the barium enema is that if a mass or polyp is found it cannot be biopsied.

Colonoscopy is the best way to evaluate the colon because not only can the gastroenterologist see the entire lower bowel, but he or she can also biopsy any lesion or polyp that is there. Once a biopsy is taken from either a polyp or mass, the specimen is sent to the pathology laboratory for histological evaluation.

Colorectal cancer begins to develop at around age forty in blacks. In addition, blacks seem to produce more polyps and lager polyps than do whites. Blacks have more right-sided cancer of the colon, and right-sided colon cancer can be missed during colonoscopy than do left-sided colon cancer.

The followings are examples of colon cancer seen during colonoscopy.

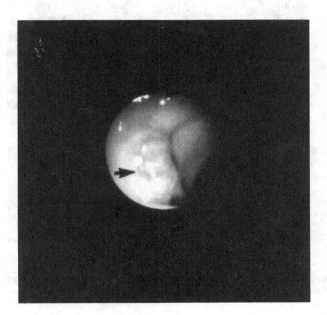

Figure 5.8 Colon cancer: sessile lesion of the colon (arrow)

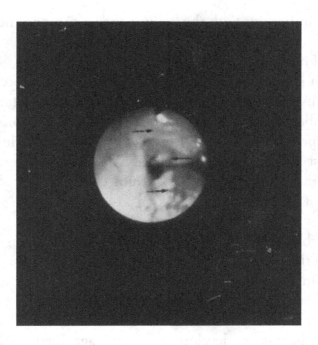

Figure 5.9-Large obstructing colon cancer with bleeding (arrows.

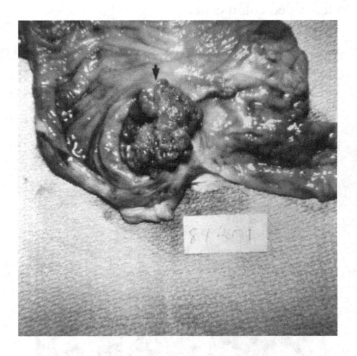

Figure5.10-Carcinoma in papillary adenoma of cecum (arrow).

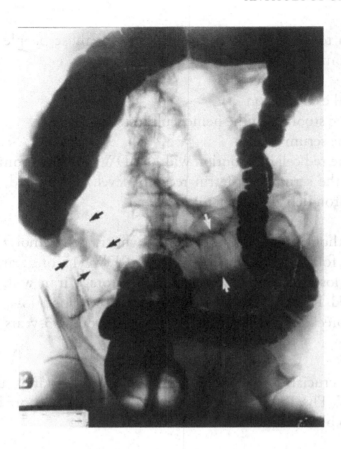

Figure 5.11*-*Barium enema: Apple core lesion of the cecum (white arrows) with small bowel obstruction (white arrows).

If the pathology report comes back that the polyp or polyps removed is or are negative for cancer, then in about two years the individual should have another colonoscopic examination. Some people have the propensity to develop polyps in their colon. It takes about 3-5 years for a precancerous polyp to develop into cancer. Some individuals who form a lot of polyps need surveillance colonoscopy every year for 2-3 years so that a polyp that has the potential to become cancerous can be removed before it becomes cancer. If the colonoscopy is negative, it can be repeated in 5 years.

The FDA has recently approved Celebrex to be used in people who have the propensity to form polyps in their colon. Celebrex, a Cox 2 inhibitor is used to treat arthritis. The enzyme cyclooxygenase is needed to mediate inflammation inside the colon and inflammation is a key component in the formation of colorectal polyps.

Using aspirin, NSAIDs and COX2 like Celebrex block the development of inflammation, thereby decreases polyps' formation.

It is very important to test frequently the stool of people who have the hereditary predisposition to colon cancer for blood, frequently using the hemoccult. It is also very

113

important to begin to do surveillance colonoscopy for those people starting at age 35 and to clinically monitor them by doing:

1. Digital rectal examination
2. Testing of the stool using the hemoccult test
3. Checking the serum ferritin
4. Checking the red cell distribution width (RDW) during a complete blood count
5. Testing for the serum transferrin receptor level. (If elevated, it proves that the patient has iron deficiency amenia.)

In a person without hemoglobinopathy, or who is not hemolyzing, and does not have either B12 or folate deficiency, has elevated RDW (15 or greater), that means he or she is probably losing blood slowly and losing storage iron with it. In the routine setting, the elevated RDW is the earliest sign of slow blood loss. This occurs from the time that the precancerous polyp starts oozing blood, 2-3 years before real cancer develops.

Therefore, it is crucial that the treating physician understands and knows how to interpret the RDW. The RDW is given as part of the CBC report by most reporting laboratories that do blood counts.

The third very important test that indicates blood loss and iron loss is the serum ferritin. The ferritin is the storage iron that humans have in their bone marrow, muscles, liver, spleen, the reticuloendothelial system, the brain, and other tissues in the body. A normal-size woman has 2.5 grams of iron in her body with 1.5 grams in the red cells and about 1 gram in the store, as ferritin. A normal size man has 3.5 grams of iron in his body. Each milliliter of blood has 0.5 mg of iron in it, it is easy to calculate how much iron an individual has lost when he or she becomes anemic by working backwards, and calculating how much her serum ferritin is.

One unit of blood, which is 500 cc, has 250 mg of iron in it. The normal serum ferritin in women is 10-291 ug/L and the normal serum ferritin in a man is 22-322 ug/L. The serum ferritin is a range and as such it takes several years of slow and chronic bleeding from whatever source to deplete the ferritin down. It is also important and crucial to understand that an individual must deplete his or her serum ferritin totally before he or she starts using the iron in the circulation.

When a person is bleeding occultly, iron is being lost slowly and in stages.
The first stage of iron lost is called, pre-latent or iron deficient erythropoiesis.
The second stage of iron lost is called latent or iron deficient state.
The third stage is called late latent stage or frank iron deficiency anemia.

In pre-latent stage of iron deficiency, the hematocrit is normal, the level of serum ferritin is starting to go down, and the RDW is high. In the latent stage of iron deficiency, the hematocrit is low normal, the level of serum ferritin has fallen lower, and the RDW is high. In the late latent stage of iron deficiency, the serum ferritin is low, the hematocrit is low, the RDW is high and mean corpuscular volume or MCV is low, and the reticulocyte count is low. In late latent stage of iron deficiency, frank iron deficiency anemia exists.

Understanding how iron is lost in occult gastro-intestinal bleeding, and, using this information to think back when evaluating patient at high risk or no obvious risk for colon cancer can help physicians to resect pre-cancerous polyps and in so doing prevents many people from dying from colon cancer.

When a person is bleeding slowly and chronically as is the case in cancer of the large bowel, rectum, small bowel, esophagus and stomach the first iron that is being lost is the iron in the store (the ferritin). Knowing that to be the case then, once it is noted that the range of the serum ferritin is starting to go down (being depleted) it is the crucial time to start evaluating the gastrointestinal tract to look for the reason or reasons for the blood loss.

In other words, if an evaluation is undertaken at this juncture, a resectable and curable precancerous polyp can be removed and cancer of the gastrointestinal tract, no matter where it is located, can be cured, in particular, if the cancer is located in the large bowel. The only cancer that may be difficult to cure surgically even if discovered and resected early is cancer of the esophagus.

If a woman is still menstruating regularly, the status of her iron kinetic is much more difficult to evaluate to determine the source or sources of her iron deficiency state.

If a mass is found during colonoscopy and biopsied and the pathology shows cancer, then a metastatic evaluation is carried out to determine if the cancer has or has not spread, before deciding to go ahead with surgical resection of the mass. The metastatic evaluation for colon cancer includes:

1. Complete blood count
2. Liver function tests such as SGOT, SGPT, alkaline phosphatase, LDH
3. CEA (carcinoembryogenic antigen)
4. Abdominal CT to look at the liver and the retroperitoneal area, etc., or abdominal sonogram
5. Chest x-ray or CT scan of the chest and bone scan
6. PET scan

If all these tests are normal, then the assumption can be made that the cancer has not spread to these organs; the patient can be scheduled for surgical resection of the cancerous mass.

The resected polypoid mass is sent to the pathology lab department for gross and histological evaluations. To know the extent of the spread of the colon cancer, a system of staging called Duke's staging is adhered to: Duke's A, Duke's B, Duke's C, and Duke's D.

or
Stage 1
Stage 2
Stage 3
Stage 4

Duke's A is when the cancer penetrates into the wall of the bowel but not through it. Duke's B is when the cancer penetrates through the wall of the bowel. Duke's C is when the cancer penetrates through the wall of the bowel and spreads to the surrounding lymph nodes. There exists more refinement of the Duke's staging, which defines Duke's B, B2, Duke's C and Duke's C2. Duke's D is widespread distant metastasis.

The Duke's staging of colon cancer is very important in that it dictates the type of treatment modalities that are provided for the patient with colon cancer. It is also important in outlining the prognosis of the individual who has colon cancer.

Duke's A and B colon cancer are surgically curable cancers. Duke's B2 oftentimes requires surgical resection with 6 months of adjuvant 5FU. Duke's C colon cancer is less likely to be surgically curable.

After surgical resection, the best adjuvant chemotherapeutic treatment for Duke's C colon cancer is Levamisole 150 mg every 8 hours for 3 days every 3 weeks with 5FU 450 mg/m2 weeks for 52 weeks.

At times surgical resection may be necessary in Duke's D lesion if a large cancer mass is found and is deemed to be potentially about to obstruct the colon. To avoid this problem, the surgeon then may decide to resect the cancer mass.

Otherwise, the treatment of Duke's D 5FU 500 mg/m2 IV bolus, Camptosar 125 mg /m2 IV over 90 minutes and Leucovorin 20 mg/m2 IV bolus on day 1, 8, 15 and 22 and 1 week off every month for 1 year.

Another frequently used regimen to treat Duke's or Stage 4 colon cancer is Oxaliplatin on Day 1, 85 mg/m2 IV over 2 hours, Leucovorin 200 mg/m2 over 2 hours IV, 5FU 400 mg/ m2 IV bolus and 5FU 600 mg/m2 as a continuous infusion over 22 hours. On day 2 Leucovorin 200 mg/ m2 IV over 2 hours 5FU 400 mg/m2 IV bolus, and 5FU 600 mg/m2 as a continuous infusion over 22 hours. This is repeated every 2 weeks. There have been good results seen using both these two regimens. Adding Avastin to different chemotherapeutic protocol has been effective at times. However, Avastin is a very expensive drug.

Other drugs used in cancer of the colon include:

1. Oxaliplatin
2. Irinotecan
3. Bevacizumab
4. Capecitabine
5. Cetuximab
6. Cisplatinum, 5FU, Mitomycin C for rectal cancer
7. Avastin
8. Radiation therapy is also used to treat cancer of the rectum either before or after.

Surgical removal of isolated liver mass from colon cancer has been done and is said to be at times successful.

Megace is at times added to the 5FU to increase the appetite of the patient with colon cancer and it helps with weight gain. Megace can cause clots to develop in the legs with serious clinical consequences. Oxandrin is also used to improve appetite in people with advanced colon cancer. The side effects are similar to Megace. Marinol is also quite effective in improving some cancer patient's appetite.

Another form of cancer that oftentimes develops in the large bowel is carcinoid tumor. The preoperative evaluation is the same, except that if the treating physician suspects carcinoid tumor, then serum serotonin or a 24-hour urine for (5HIAA) 5 hydroxyindoleacetic acid can be obtained as a baseline and to help firm up the diagnosis. These tests are helpful in the subsequent management of the patient with carcinoid tumor.

Non-Hodgkin's lymphoma of the large bowel does occur. The treatment approach is the same. First, surgical resection followed either by radiation therapy or by chemotherapy, depending on the histology and the extent of disease found at surgery.

Colorectal cancer is curable when found early. Therefore, yearly rectal examination and testing of the stool for blood once or twice per year and doing a complete blood count with RDW, serum ferritin and the serum-transferring receptors level together, can prevent colon cancer from ever killing anyone. It is very important for physicians to use the soluble serum transferrin level when evaluating black patients who may be suffering from sickle cell disease/ other abnomal hemoglobins that cause them to very high serum Ferritin/ RDW/ low MCV and yet may be bleeding from their GI track from pre-cancerous polyps or GI cancer.

If the treating physician does these tests and follow up on the results, pre-cancerous/ cancerous lesions of the colon, rectum, small bowel, and stomach and esophagus can be discovered early and treated appropriately.

Cancer of the esophagus:

In 2013, 32,430 people were diagnosed with cancer of the esophagus in the U.S. and 482,300 people were diagnosed with cancer of the esophagus in the world. 15.210 people died of esophagus cancer in the U.S. in 2013, and 406,800 people died from cancer of the esophagus in the world. Cancer of the esophagus is the eigth leading cause of cancer deaths in the world.

Cancer of the esophagus is 50% more common in blacks compared to whites. Esophageal cancer is always diagnosed when it has already in an advanced stage.

Alcohol abuse and tobacco smoking are risk factors in the development of cancer of the esophagus.

Other risks include:

> Barrett's esophagus
> Achlasia
> Plummmer-Vinson syndrome
> Celiac disease
> Consumption of too red meat
> HPV infection of the throat from HPV types 16 and 18
> Lye strictures of the esophagus etc;

The symptoms and signs of esophageal cancer include:

1. Difficulty swallowing
2. Upper stomach pain
3. Chest pain
4. Anemia
5. Weight loss etc;

The best ways to evaluate cancer of esophagus are:

CT
MRI
Esophagram
Endoscopy
Esophageal biopsy
CBC
Serum ferritin
CEA
Chemistry profile

Treatments of cancer of the esophagus include:

1. Surgical resection
2. Radiation therapy
3. Chemotherapy such as:
4. 5FU, Cisplatin
       Or
5. Epirubicin
6. Cisplatin
7. 5FU
       Or
8. Epirubicin
9. Oxaliplatin
10. Capecitabine
       Or
11. Irinotecan
12. Cisplatin
       Or
13. Vinorelbine

The 5 year survival for cancer of the esophagus is 11% for blacks and 18% for whites.

Cancer of the stomach:

In 2013, 21,600 people in the U.S. were diagnosed with cancer of the stomach and 750,000 in the world were diagnosed with canceer of the stomach in 2013 in the world and 736,000 people died of stomach in the world in 2013. Cancer of the stomach is causes the second most common cancer deaths in the world. Cancer of the stomach is most common in Japan and Scandinavia.

Cancer of the stomach is 2-3 times more common in blacks as compared to whites and the death rates are similarly higher for blacks as compared to whites. In addition, H pylori infection of the stomach can cause lymphoma in certain percentage of individuals.

Risk factors for stomach cancer include:

Genetic
Environmental
Smoked fish
Pickles
Processed foods
H pylori infection
Smoking
Alcohol abuse
Obesity etc;

Symptoms and signs of stomach cancer include:

1. Recurrent indigestion
2. Hyperacidity/Heart burn
3. Nausea and vomiting
4. Diarrhea and constipation
5. Bloating
6. Upper stomach pain
7. Weight loss
8. Anemia
9. Poor appetite
10. Fatigue
11. Vomiting blood etc
12. Black tarry stools etc;

The best ways to evaluate cancer of the stomach include:

1. Endoscopic examination with biopsy when necessary
2. Upper GI series
3. H. Pylori examination
4. CBC
5. Serum ferritin
6. Stool hemoccult
7. CEA etc;

Treatments of stomach cancer include:

1. Surgical resection
2. Chemotherapy drugs such as
3. Epirubicin
4. Cisplatin
5. 5FU
   or
6. Docetaxel
7. Cisplatin
8. 5FU in combination
   or
9. Epirubicin
10. Oxaliplatin
11. Capecitabine in combination
    or
12. Irinotecan
13. Cisplatin in combination

Cancer of the small bowel:

In 2013, 8,810 people in the U.S. were diagnosed with cancer of the small bowel and 1,170 people died from cancer of the small bowel in 2013 in the U.S. Cancer of the small intestine is a very rare form of cancer worldwide.

Cancer of the small intestine is more common in blacks as compared to whites. In 2005, 3.9 black males and 2.1 white males per 100,000 had cancer of the small intestine and 2.7 black females and 1.7 white females per 100,000 had cancer of the small intestine.

The death rate for cancer of the small intestine is higher in blacks as compared to whites. In 2005, 0.7 black males and 0.4 white males per 100,000 died of cancer of the small intestine and 0.5 black females and 0.3 white females died of cancer of the small intestine. Source: Surveillance, Epidemiology, and End Results (SEER) Program, 17 SEER Registries 200-2005.Division of cancer control and Population Sciences, National Cancer Institute, 2008

Risk factors for cancer of the small bowel include:

Crohn's disease
Intestinal polyposis
Celiac disease

AIDS

Puetz-Jegher's syndrome

Symptoms and signs of small bowel cancer include:

1. Abdominal pain
2. Bloating
3. Palpable abdominal mass
4. Weight loss
5. Blood in the stools
6. Iron deficiency anemia
7. Constipation
8. Small bowel obstruction etc;

The best ways to evaluate cancer of the small bowel include:

1. Complete history and physical examination
2. Abdominal CT scan
3. Capsule scoping of the small
4. CBC
5. Serum ferritin
6. CEA
7. Small bowel biopsy

The best treatments for cancer of the small bowel include:

1. Surgical resection
2. Chemotherapy such as
3. Docetaxel
4. Cisplatin
5. 5FU
> or
6. 5FU
7. Cisplatin
> or
8. Epirubicin
9. Oxaliplatin
10. Capecitabine
> or
11. Irinotecan
12. Cisplatin

The mother cells that give rise to the stomach and the small bowel are the same, as a result, chemotherapy drugs in the treatment of stomach and small bowel cancer are the same. Chemotherapy for stomach and small bowel cancer are not very effective.

Cancer of the Liver and intrahepatic bile duct:

In 2013, 692,000 people in the world had cancer of the liver. Cancer of the liver is the fourth most common cancer in the world. Each year 749,000 people die worldwide from hepatocellular carcinoma/cancer of the liver.

Liver cancer cancer is the fifth most common cancer in men and the seventh in women." Source: New England journal of medicine 365; 12 September 22, 2011 in the U.S.

In 2013, 30,640 people in the U.S. had cancer of the liver and 21,620 people died of cancer of the liver.

Cancer of the liver and intrahepatic bile duct is more common in blacks and othr minorities as compared to whites. In 2005, 13.2 black males and 8.2 white males per 100, 000 had cancer of the liver Intrahepatic duct in the U.S. and 4.0 black females and 2.9 white females per 100,000 had cancer of the liver intrahepatic duct.

In 2010, 6,316 whites, 3,022 Asians, 2,230, Hispanics and 1,397 had liver cancer.
The median survival for liver cancer was 15 months for Asians, 10 months for whites, Hispanics, and 8 months for blacks.

The death rates for cancer of liver intrahepatic duct are higher in blacks as compared to whites. In 2005, 10.3 black males and 6.7 white males per 100,000 and 3.9 black females and 2.9 white females died of cancer of the liver intrahepatic duct cancer in the U.S.

Risk factors for cancer of the liver include:

1. Hepatitis B
2. Hepatitis C
3. Alcohlism
4. Hemochromatosis
5. Alflatoxin B1
6. Cirrhosis
7. Anabolic steroid
8. Diabetes mellitus
9. Obesity

10. Alcohol abuse
11. Exposure to industrial toxins
12. Liver fluke
13. Vinyl chloride exposure
14. Arsenic exposure
15. Thorium dioxide exposure
16. Wilson's disease

The best ways to evaluate cancer of the liver include:

1. Complete history and physical examination
2. Abdominal ultrasound
3. Abdominal CT scan
4. CT guided liver biopsy
5. Alpha fetoprotein
6. CEA
7. CBC
8. SMA20
9. PT and INR
10. PTT
11. Cytology of abdominal fluid
12. Cell count of abdominal fluid
13. Gram stain of abdominal fluid
14. Culture of abdominal fluid
15. Protein and glucose analysis of abdominal fluid
16. Chest xray
17. Serum ferritin
18. C282Y in white patients
19. Serum hepcidin level
20. Serum ferroportin level

Signs and symptoms of cancer of the liver:

1. General weakness
2. Lassitude
3. Tiredness
4. Weight loss
5. Tiredness
6. Headache
7. Nausea/Vomiting
8. Needle marks from drug addicts
9. Alcoholism
10. Cirrhosis of the liver

11. Jaundice
12. Itching
13. Enlargement of the liver
14. Enlargement of the spleen
15. Portal hypertension
16. Esophageal varices
17. vomiting blood /Hematemesis
18. Ascites
19. Abdominal mass
20. Hemorrhoid
21. Rectal bleeding
22. Anemia
23. Possible positive hepatitis B or C
24. Possible HIV/AIDS
25. Iron overload
26. Leukopenia
27. Thrombocytopenia
28. Coagulopathy (high PT and PTT)
29. Dessiminated intravascular coagulopathy (DIC)
30. Abnormal liver function tests
31. Tissue confirmation of cancer of the liver
32. High serum ferritin
33. Hemolytic anemia
34. Iron deficiency anemia
35. Anemia of inflammatory diseases
36. Gynecomastia in men
37. Testicular atrophy
38. Plantar erythema
39. Spider angiomata
40. Recurrent vaginal bleeding
41. Secondary polycytemia

Treatments of liver cancer include:

Surgical resection
Radiation therapy
Chemotherapy treatment is not very effective in primary cancer of the liver (Hepatoma)
Some of the drugs in use to treat cancer of the liver include:
Doxorubicin
Cisplatinum
Capecitabine
Liver transplant as treatment modality is commonly carried out.

Blacks and other minorities are 36% less likely than whites to receive liver transplant.

Cancer of the gall bladder

In 2013, 10,310 men and women were diagnosed with cancer of the gall bladder in the U.S. and 3,230 people died of cancer of the bladder in the U.S. during that period.

Worldwide 38,309 people had cancer of the gall bladder in 2013 and the 5 years survival is only 20 percent. Sources: ACS Facts and Figures 2013 and WHO.

Risks for gallbladder cancer include:

Female sex
Obesity
Gall stones
Family history
Genetic (In the U.S. gallbladder cancer is most common in Native Americans)

Signs and symptoms of cancer of the gallbladder include:

Weight loss
Abdominal pain
Abdominal bloating
Chest pain
Appetite loss
Nauea
Vomiting
Yellowness of eyes
Yelloness of skin (jaundice)
Itching etc;

Evaluations of cancer of the gallbladder include:
History and physical examination
Abdominal ultrasound
Abdominal CAT scan with contrast by mouth and with IV contrast
Chest Xray
CBC
Complete chemistry profile
CEA
GGTP
PT/INR
PTT

Urinalysis
Gastrointestinal consult
Surgery consult

Treaments of gallbladder cancer include:
Surgical removal of the gallbladder
Radiationtherapy

Chemotherapy drugs to treat gallbladder cancer include:
5FU
Cisplatinum
Oxaliplatin
Gemzar
Xoleda
These chemotherapy drugs are frequently used in combination.

Cancer of the Pancreas:

In 2013, 45,220 people were diagnosed with cancer of the pancreas in the U.S. and 38,460 men women died of this cancer in 2013. Worldwide 250,000 people have pancreatic cancer every year and more than 250,000 people die yearly from pancreatic cancer.

The incidence of cancer of pancreas and the death rates of cancer pancreas are both higher in blacks and other minorities than in whites. In 2008, 17.1 black males and 14.8 black females per 100,000 had cancer of the pancreas and 10.7 white females and 13.5 white males per 100,000 had cancer of the pancreas in the U.S.

In 2007, 15.4 black males and 12.2 white males per 100,000 died of cancer of the pancreas and 12.4 black females and 9.1 white females per 100,000 died of cancer of the pancreas.

Signs and symptoms of cancer of the pancreas usually occur when it is too late to do much to save the patient. If the cancer is located near the head of the pancreas, it might cause the common bile duct to become obstructed, causing the patient to become jaundiced with no pain.

However, if the cancer is located at either the body or the tail of the pancreas, jaundice may occur due to metastasis to the liver.

Therefore, early development of jaundice due to cancer of the head of the pancreas may in some instances lead to the person seeking medical help. This could result in a positive outcome because of early surgical intervention. Left-sided, mid-abdominal pain in association with weight loss and poor appetite may also be signs of and symptoms of cancer of the pancreas.

Signs and symptoms of cancer of the pancreas include:

> Weight lost
> Poor appetite
> Abdominal pain
> Fever
> Jaundice
> Itching
> Nausea
> Vomiting
> Elevated liver function tests
> CEA
> Elevated CA19-9
> Anemia
> Palpable left sided mid abdominal mass

Risks for cancer of the pancreas include:

1. Tobacco smoking
2. Chronic pancreatitis
3. Diabetes mellitus
4. High fat diet
5. Cirrhosis of the liver.
6. Alcoholism
7. Obesity
8. Genetic predisposition
9. Eating too much red meat etc;

The best ways to diagnose cancer of the pancreas include:

1. Taking a good history
2. Physical Examination
3. Abdominal sonogram
4. Abdominal CT scan

5. Abdominal MRI
6. ERCP
7. PET scan
8. CT guided biopsy

During the ERCP or endoscopic ERCP if a mass is present, it can be seen and material can be obtained for diagnosis. In addition, a stent can be placed to relieve the obstruction of the common bile duct to relieve the jaundice, etc.

Cancer of the pancreas is very difficult to cure, but if found early, surgical resection is the preferred treatment but this cancer is hardly ever found early. There are many gastrointestinal procedures available to relieve the many symptoms and complications of pancreatic cancer but none is curable.

The most effective chemotherapeutic agents include:

Gemzar
Taxotere
Irinotecan
Oxaliplatin
Cisplatinum
Capecitabine
Tarceva
Afrinitor

These drugs are used in combination, but they are not curative most of the time and surgical removal and radiotherapy as modalities for pancreatic cancer have a role but they are not curative.

Other modalities of treatment in pancreatic cancer include:
Surgical resection
Radiation therapy

Cancer of the Brain

In 2013, 69,720 were diagnosed with cancer of the brain in the U.S. and 14,080 of them died of this cancer. The incidence of brain cancer is twice higher in whites as compared to blacks. However, the death rates for cancer of the brain is much higher for blacks and other minorities as compared to whites. This is so, because blacks and other minorities received inferior medical care for their brain cancer as compared to whites.

Worldwide 688,000 people have primary cancer of the brain and 175,000 people died of primary brain cancer in 2013. Sources: ACS, cancer facts and figures 2013 and WHO

Worldwide 170,000 brain metastsis occurred in 2013. Source: WHO

Symptoms and signs of brain cancer include:

1. Headache
2. Nausea
3. Vomiting
4. Blurry vision
5. Depression
6. Psychosis
7. Insomnia
8. Irritability
9. Weight loss
10. Dementia
11. Seizure
12. Weakness in arms
13. Weakness in legs
14. Difficulty talking
15. Difficulty with bowel function
16. Difficulty with urinary function etc;

Some of the most common brain cancers include:

1. Glioma
2. Astrocytoma
3. Meningioma
4. Acoustic neuroma
5. Oligodendroglioma
6. Glioblastoma multiforme
7. Medulloblastoma
8. Metastatic cancer to the brain etc;

Some of the most common cancer that can metastasize to brain includes

1. Lung cancer
2. Breast cancer
3. Colon cancer
4. Prostate cancer
5. Melanoma
6. Lymphomas

7. Leukemias
8. Head and neck cancer
9. Thyroid cancer
10. Cancer of the kidney
11. Sarcoma
12. Ovarian cancer
13. Cervical cancer
14. Uterine cancer
15. Testicular cancer etc;

The best ways to evaluate brain cancer include:

1. Complete history and physical examination
2. Brain CT Scan with IV contrast
3. Brain MRI with IV contrast
4. Brain biopsy
5. Chest x ray
6. CBC
7. SMA20
8. Possible lumbar puncture if metastatic cancer to the brain is suspected, using
9. a small fine needle
10. Cytology of spinal fluid
11. Glucose of spinal fluid
12. Protein of spinal fluid
13. Gram stain of spinal fluid
14. Cell count of Spinal fluid
15. Culture of spinal fluid

Treatments of brain cancer include:

1. Surgical resection
2. Radiation therapy
3. Chemotherapy such as:
4. Irinotecan
5. Carmustine
6. 6-Thioguanine
7. Procarbazine
8. Lomustine
9. Vicristine
10. Temozolomidine
11. 13-cis-Retinoic acid
12. BCNUetc;

Metastatic cancer to the brain is treated according to the primary tumor with chemotherapy plus radiation.

Cancer of the Cervix

In 2013, 12,340 women in the U.S. were diagnosed with cancer of the uterine cervix and 4,030 women died of uterine cervix during that period. Worldwide 500.000 new cases of cervical cancer are diagnosed every year and 275,000 women die every year from cervical cancer.

The incidence of cervical cancer is 50% higher in black and other minority women as compared to white women. Cervical cancer is diagnosed at a more advanced stage in black women as compared to white women. More black and other minority women die of cervical cancer than do white women.

Risk factors for cervical cancer include:

1. Having multiple sexual partners
2. Having sex with an uncircumcised man
3. Having sexual intercourse beginning at an early age
4. Having sexual intercourse with men who have many sexual partners
5. Using corrosive solutions such as vinegar and Lysol for vaginal douching
6. Exposing the cervix to human papiloma viruses types 16, 18, 31, 33, or 45, the virulent HPV types that can cause cervical cancer are 16, and 18. These two types of HPV are responsible for two third of cervical cancer.
7. Recurrent pelvic STD infections with Chlamydia, gonorrhea, trichomonas etc;
8. HIV/AIDS (women with HIV/AIDS have the propensity of developing a very invasive form of cervical cancer)

Some of the signs of cancer of the cervix include:

Abnormal vaginal bleeding
Severe pain during sexual intercourse
Bleeding after sexual intercourse
Recurrent and abnormal vaginal discharge
Persistent lower abdominal
Unusual severe abdominal pain during menstrual period
Recurrent breakthrough vaginal bleeding etc;

When adolescent girl starts having sexual intercourse at an early age, the cervical tissues are not yet matured enough to withstand the trauma associated with the act of sexual intercourse. Damages that occur to the cervical tissues during sexual intercourse exposing the cervical tissues to the possibility of developing dysplasia (abnormal cells) and the dysplasia can lead to cervical cancer as she grows up.

When the cervical tissues are exposed to the irritating effects of sexually transmitted diseases (STD), the irritation of the tissues causes dysplasia to occur which ultimately can lead to cervical cancer.

Exposing the cervical tissues to human papilloma virus (HPV) is highly associated with the development of cervical cancer. As outline above, many types of HPV are carcinogenic when they meet the cervical tissues.

Patients who are infected with the AIDS virus have a high propensity of development of invasive cancer of the uterine cervix. The uncircumcised penis carries under its foreskin, a thick, cheesy and malodorous secretion called smegma and this material, it is believed, can cause cervical cells to become abnormal /dysplastic when these cells are exposed to it recurrently, thus predisposing the cervix to the development of cervical cancer.

The labia minora and the clitoris of the female genitalia also produce smegma, but this smegma cannot reach the woman's cervix. Women, whose sexual partners are circumcised, such as Jewish women, have a lower incidence of cancer of the cervix.

Women who have sexual intercourse with men with large and uncircumcised penises have the highest incidence of cervical cancer because these penises can reach the uterine cervix during sexual intercourse depositing smegma on the cervix and causing physical trauma to the cervix. Smegma is known as a carcinogenic material.

Low socioeconomic status is associated with a higher incidence of cervical cancer due to a multitude of factors. One of the most important of these factors is the fact that poor women do not go as often to doctors for pap smears as do women whose socioeconomic status is higher. Usually, screening Pap smear begins at age 20 and continues yearly. High risk black women should have yearly Pap smear.

Starting at age 30, women who are at average risk who have 3 or more consecutive negative Pap smears may have Pap smears every three years. Starting at age 70, women who have 3 consecutive Pap smears consecutively and no abnormal Pap smear in 10 years, may stop having Pap smear. Exceptions can be made for individual women under certain clinical circumstances. Sexually active women ought to be tested for HPV, herpes, gonorrhea, Chlamydia, thrichomonas and HIV at the time of their Pap smears.

To diagnose cervical cancer, a cervical Pap smear needs to be done to look for abnormal cells that may be precancerous or cancerous. The Pap smear is very accurate when performed appropriately. The Pap smear is graded from Class I through Class

V. Class I is normal, Class II may be abnormal sometimes due to an inflammation or infection, etc.

If either an inflammation or infection is found, which causes a Class II Pap smear, it is recommended that the inflammation or the infection be treated and then the Pap smear repeated. If the Class II reverted to Class I after treatment, that is that. If on the other hand, the Class II persists, then further gynecological evaluation of the cervix is needed.

Table 7.1: Cytology Classification System

Bethesda System	*Dysplasia /CIN System*	*Papanicolaou System*
Within normal limits	Normal	Class I
Infections	Inflammatory atypia	Class II
Reactive changes		
Squamous cell abnormalities:		
Atypical squamous cells of undetermined significance	Squamous Atypia	Class IIR
Low-grade squamous intraepithelial lesion	HPV atypia	
	Mild dysplasia	CIN I
	Moderate dysplasia	CIN 2
High-grade squamous intraepithelial lesion	Severe dysplasia	Class III
	Carcinoma in situ	CIN 3
Invasive squamous carcinoma	Invasive squamous carcinoma Class V	Class IV

CIN. Cervical intraepithelial neoplasia HPV, human papilloma virus.
(Copied from Valiere Alcena, M.D., F.A.C.P., African-American Health Book)
Cervical cancer has four different stages from Stage 0 to Stage 4, with several subgroups in between.

Table 7.2: Cervical cancer staging FIGO
(International Federation of Gynecology and Obstetrics)

Stage	*Definition*
Stage 0	Carcinoma in situ, intraepithelial carcinoma; cases of Stage 0 should not be included in any therapeutic statistics for invasive carcinoma.

Stage I	The carcinoma is strictly confined to the cervix (extension to the corpus should be disregarded).
Stage IA	Invasive cancer identified microscopically. All gross lesions, even with superficial invasion, are stage IB cancers. Invasion is limited to measured stromal invasion with a maximum depth of 5 mm and no wider than 7 mm. (The depth of invasion should not be more than 5 mm taken from the base of the epithelium, either surface or glandular, from which it originates. Vascular space involvement, either venous or lymphatic, should not alter the staging.
Stage IA1	Measured invasion of stroma no greater than 3 mm in depth and no wider than 7 mm.
Stage IA2	Measured invasion of stroma greater than 3 mm and no greater than 5 mm in depth and no wider than 7 mm.
Stage IB	Clinical lesions confined to the cervix or preclinical lesions greater than IA.
Stage IB1	Clinical lesions no greater than 4 cm.
Stage IB1	Clinical lesions greater than 4 cm.
Stage II	The carcinoma has extended beyond the cervix, but has not extended onto the pelvic wall; the carcinoma involves the vagina, but not as far as the lower third.
Stage IIA	No obvious parametrial involvement.
Stage IIB	Obvious parametrial involvement.
Stage III	The carcinoma has extended beyond the pelvic wall; on rectal examination there is no cancer-free space between the tumor and the pelvic wall; the tumor involves the lower third of the vagina; all cases with a hydro-nephrosis of nonfunctioning kidney should be included, unless they are known to be due to other cause.
Stage IIIA	No extension unto the pelvic wall, but involvement of the lower third of the vagina.
Stage IIIB	Extension onto the pelvic wall or hydronephrosis or nonfunctioning kidney.
Stage IV	The carcinoma has extended beyond the true pelvic or has clinically involved the mucosa of the bladder or rectum.
Stage IVA	Spread of the growth to adjacent organs.
Stage IVB	Spread to distant organs.

(Adapted from International Federation of Gynecology and Obstetrics. Staging announcement: FIGO staging of gynecological cancers; cervical and vulva. Int J Gynecol 1995; 5:319.

As is the case with many other cancers, cervical cancer is found usually in a more advanced stage in black women than in white women. In white women, cervical cancer is found localized 90% of the time; but cervical cancer is found in a localized stage 70% of the time in black women. This is because black women usually do not seek treatment until their cancer is far more advanced than in white women. In all stages of cervical cancer, white women have a 67% 5-year survival rate. On the other hand, black women have a 59% 5-year survival rate.

This happens because minority women have Pap smears less frequently; so, their cervical cancers are detected in a more advanced stage, thus the lower 5-year survival rate of cervical cancer as seen in black and minority women, as compared to the 5-year survival rate in white women

Treatments of cervical cancer include:

Intraepithelial lesions are usually treated with superficial ablative techniques. If the cervical cancer is of the stage of micro-invasion and is less than 3 mm, stage IA1, it is treated with cone biopsy or what is referred to as extrafascial hysterectomy.

Stages of cervical cancer IA1, IB1, and IIA are usually treated with either radical hysterectomy or radiation therapy. Stages IB2 through IVA are usually treated with radiation therapy.

More advanced stages IIB, IIIB, IVB and IVA, etc., are treated with radiation therapy in association with chemotherapy and pain management. Chemotherapy for cervical cancer is not very effective.

The chemotherapeutic agents that are frequently used in advanced cervical cancer include:

Cisplatin
Bleomycin
Methotrexate
5FU
Isophamide

Cancer of the cervix is a curable disease when discovered early with Pap smear and appropriate gynecological treatments are provided.

The best treatments for cancer of the cervix are surgical removal of the cancer and radiation therapy. Combination chemotherapy using Cisplatinum, Methotrexate, 5FU and, Irinotecan and Leucovorin as adjuvant treatment after surgery is sometime effective in treating cervical cancer. Radiation therapy is also very effective as a treatment modality in cancer of the cervix.

Cancer of the Uterus:

In 2013, 49,560 women had cancer of the uterus and 8,190 women died of cancer of the uterus in the U.S. Worldwide there were 300,000 women endometrial cancer in 2013. In 2012, 74,000 women died from endometrial cancer in the world.

Overall, the incidence of uterine cancer is 40 % more common among whites females as compared to minority females, but minority females die of uterine cancer 60% more often. The reason for the higher death rate from uterine cancer in minority women is because minority women frequently ignore their symptoms and when they do go to their doctors, very often by the time they go to their doctors, their cancer is already too advanced to be cured.

The risk factors for uterine cancer include:

    Obesity
    Hypertension
    High level of estrogen in the blood
    Endometrial hyperplasia
    Nulliparity
    Early mernache
    Late menopause
    Ovarian cance
    Breast cancer
    Tomaxifen treatment
    Alcoholism
    Eating too much read meat
    Radiation to the pelvic area
    Genetic predisposition etc;

Symptoms and signs of cancer of the uterus:

    Abnormal menstrual periods
    Abnormal bleeding from the uterus
    Spotting in Postmenopausal women
    Vaginal bleeding in postmenopausal women
    Bleeding between menstrual periods in premenopausal women
    Abnormal vaginal discharge
    Crampy lower abdominal pain
    Recurrent bleeding after sexual intercourse
    Anemia etc;

Excess estrogen increases the incidence of cancer of the uterus because it affects the lining of the inside of the uterus (endometrial lining). The effect that estrogen has on the endometrial lining causes the uterus to develop a propensity to the development of uterine cancer. Because Tamoxifen has estrogenic effects, it affects the lining of the uterus negatively and thereby can increase the propensity of the uterine tissues to become cancerous in some women.

Women who have no children have an increased incidence of endometrial cancer because their uterus is constantly being stimulated with estrogen. Pregnancy allows the uterus to rest from estrogen for 7-9 months. These rest periods are important to allow the uterine tissues to get a period of time during which these tissues are free from strong estrogenic effects.

Early menarche is associated with increased incidence of uterine cancer because the uterine tissues have been exposed to estrogen for many years when, for example, a girl begins to menstruate at ages 8, 9, or 10. Similarly, late menopause is associated with increased incidence of uterine cancer because the longer a woman takes to stop menstruating, the longer her uterus is exposed to the effect of estrogen, thereby increasing the possibility of cancerous transformation of the uterine tissues.

Obesity increases the risk of cancer of the uterus because obesity increases the level cholesterol in the blood. Cholesterol is necessary for the production of all hormones in the body and the higher the concentration of cholesterol, the higher the level estrogen is going to be. The higher the concentration of estrogen the more the lining of the uterus will be stimulated and that increases the risk of uterus cancer.

1. Cancer of the Uterus/Endometrium is diagnosed by history, physical examination, and biopsy.
2. Pap smear
3. Endometrial Biopsy
4. Dilatation and curettage (D&C)
5. Hysteroscopic examination
6. Transvaginal ultrasound
7. Abdominal /Pelvic CT scan with contrast by mouth and IV Contrast
8. Abdominal/Pelvic MRI with IV contrast
9. CBC
10. Chemistry profile
11. CA125 serum level
12. Chest X-ray
13. Serum pregnancy test
14. PET scan
15. Colonoscopy
16. HE4 serum level

In addition the above outlined tests, PT/INR, PTT, Blood type and crossed matched and EKG and physical examination by an internist or Medical oncologist will be done to get the patient ready for surgery.

Once biopsy confirms that cancer of the endometrium exists, then the woman will be given the different treatment options. In addition, if it is decided that total hysterectomy is the main option, then an oncologycal gynecologist will be called in to evaluate the patient to perform the total hysterectomy. The surgical specimen will be sent to the pathology lab for staging.

Table 7.3: CLINICAL STAGE OF CARCINOMA OF THE ENDOMETRIUM
FIGO 2010 staging system (International Federation of Gynecology /Obstetrics)

1A Tumor confined to the uterus, no or< ½ myometrial invasion

1B Tumor confined to the uterus, > ½ myometrial invasion

II Cervical stromal invasion, but not beyond uterus

IIIA Tumor invades serosa or adnexa

IIIB Vaginal and/or parametrial involvement

IIIC 1 Pelvic node involvement

IIIC2 Para-aortic involvement

IVA Tumor invasion bladder and/or bowel mucosa

IVB Distant metastases including abdominal metastases and/or inguinal lymph nodes

Medical oncology
Management of Endometrial Cancer

Stage IA lesions of endometrial cancer (uterine cancer) are usually treated with total hysterectomy with bilateral salpingo-oophorectomy removal of the ovaries and the fallopian tubes. It is important to surgically remove the tubes and ovaries because the location of the cancer is such that it frequently spreads to the ovaries. The second reason is that most of the women who are affected by cancer of the uterus are postmenopausal.

Radiotherapy plays a major and significant role in the treatment of cancer of the uterus, in particular the stages that are not appropriate for surgical removal and yet not too advanced not to be treated.

The chemotherapeutic agents that are used in endometrial cancer include:

1. Cisplatin

2. Adriamycin
3. Cytoxan
4. Taxol
5. Carboplatin
6. Paclitaxel
7. Doxorubicin
8. Megestrol
9. Topotecan

These agents are used in different combinations.

Cancer of the uterus is a preventable and curable cancer if the proper preventative measures are taken and if the diagnosis is made early enough to prevent the cancer from becoming invasive. Early cancer of the uterus is curable most of the time with total abdominal hysterectomy. It is therefore important that women go to the gynecologist as soon as they notice unusual vaginal bleeding or spotting so that a thorough vaginal examination can be carried out and all necessary tests and biopsies can be done.

The best treatment for uterine cancer is hysterectomy, followed by radiation therapy. Advanced cases of uterine cancer after surgery and radiation are usually treated with either Tamoxifen or progestational hormones. If the hormonal treatment fails, then combination chemotherapy with Cytoxan, Adriamycin, and Cisplatin can be used.

Cancer of the Ovary:

In 2013, 22,240 women will be diagnosed with ovarian cancer in the U.S., 14,030 women will die of this cancer. Worldwide in 2013, 220,000 women are diagnosed annually with ovarian cancer and annually 140,000 women die from ovarian cancer in the world.

There two different cell types that cause ovarian cancer and there are the epithelial cell type and the germ cell type. The epithelial cell type is the most common cell type that causes ovarian cancer.

Ovarian cancer usually occurs in women 50-60 years of age or older. This cancer occurs most often in white women, Spanish women, black women, Native American women and Asian women in this order. It affects middle to upper class women more that poorer women. It also occurs more in developed countries as compared to developing counties.

Ovarian cancer is the fifth most common cancer in American women and the ninth most common cancer in women in the world and the number one cause of death among all genylogical cancers. While ovarian cancer is more common in white women, the death rates from ovarian is higher in black women and other minority women compared their white counterparts.

Risk factors for ovarian cancer include:
1. Being age 50 and older
2. Being white
3. Being of Ashkenazi ancestry
4. Having had breast cancer
5. Having BRCA1 and BRCA2 genes
6. Having had colorectal cancer
7. Having had cancer of the uterus
8. Childlessness
9. Infertility
10. Having history of mother, sister, grandmother, or maternal aunt wit cancer of the ovary etc;

Cancer of the ovary is very difficult to detect early, because the symptoms are very vague or nonexistent in the beginning. In early in ovarian cancer, there are often no signs or symptoms.

The symptoms and signs of ovarian cancer include:
Abnormal vaginal bleeding
Change in bowel habits
Bloating
Stomach upset
Gas
Crampy abdominal pain
Vomiting
Swelling of the abdomen
Abdominal pain

The best ways to diagnose cancer of the ovary include:

1. Pelvic examination
2. Abdominal examination
3. Pap smear
4. Pelvic sonogram/transvaginal ultrasound
5. Abdominal CAT and pelvic scan using contrast by mouth and IV
6. MRI of the abdomen
7. PET scan
8. CA125, which is a marker for cancer of the ovary. When this blood is elevated, it may mean that ovarian cancer is present.

9. HE4 serum level (human epididymis protein 4)
10. Colonoscopy

If an ovarian mass is documented by pelvic examination, pelvic sonogram, and abdominal CT scan, and ovarian cancer is suspected, then a laparoscopic examination can be carried out during which a biopsy can be taken for tissue evaluation. If nodes are seen, the interventional radiologist can do a biopsy under CT scan guidance to take tissue for histological studies. If the tissue taken is positive for cancer, then the gynecological oncologist can do a total hysterectomy with nodes dissection. The pathological specimen will be sent to the pathology laboratory to be studied by the pathologist and for histological staging.

Table 7.4: The most recent staging for ovarian cancer by FIGO/National cancer institute

Stage I:

Stage I ovarian cancer is limited to the ovaries.

Stage IA: Tumor limited to one ovary; capsule intact, no tumor on ovarian surface. No malignant cells in ascites or peritoneal washings.

Stage IB: Tumor limited to both ovaries; capsules intact, no tumor on ovarian surface. No malignant cells in ascites or peritoneal washings.

Stage IC: Tumor limited to one or both ovaries, with any of the following: capsule ruptured, tumor on ovarian surface, malignant cells in ascites or peritoneal washings.

The term, malignant ascites, is not classified. The presence of ascites does not affect staging unless malignant cells are present

Stage II:

Stage II ovarian cancer is tumor involving one or both ovaries with pelvic extension and/or implants.

Stage IIA: Extension and/or implants on the uterus and/or fallopian tubes. No malignant cells in ascites or peritoneal washings.

Stage IIB: Extension to and/or implants on other pelvic tissues. No malignant cells in ascites or peritoneal washings.

Stage IIC: Pelvic extension and/or implants (stage IIA or IIB) with malignant cells in ascites or peritoneal washings

Different criteria for allotting cases to stage IC and stage IIC have an impact on diagnosis. To assess this impact, of value would be to know if rupture of the capsule was (1) spontaneous or (2) caused by the surgeon; and, if the source of malignant cells detected was (1) peritoneal washings or (2) ascites.

Stage III:

Stage III ovarian cancer is tumor involving one or both ovaries with microscopically confirmed peritoneal implants outside the pelvis. Superficial liver metastasis equals stage III. Tumor is limited to the true pelvis but with histologically verified malignant extension to small bowel or omentum.

Stage IIIA: Microscopic peritoneal metastasis beyond pelvis (no macroscopic tumor).

Stage IIIB: Macroscopic peritoneal metastasis beyond pelvis 2 cm or less in greatest dimension.

Stage IIIC: Peritoneal metastasis beyond pelvis more than 2 cm in greatest dimension and/or regional lymph node metastasis.

Stage IV:

Stage IV ovarian cancer is tumor involving one or both ovaries with distant metastasis. If pleural effusion is present, positive cytologic test results must exist to designate a case to stage IV. Parenchymal liver metastasis equals stage IV.

Ovarian low malignant potential tumors almost never reach stage IV.

Radiation therapy plays a principal role in the treatment of early cancer of the ovary. In recent years, chemotherapy for ovarian cancer has been more effective. The most effective chemotherapeutic agents for epithelial cancer of the ovary used in combination are:

1. Cytoxan
2. Hexamethylmelamine
3. Doxorubicin
4. Cisplatin
5. Taxol
6. Paclitaxel

7. Carboplatin
8. Docetaxel
9. Topotecan
10. Liposomal
11. Doxorubicin
12. Gemcitabine
13. Capecitabine
14. Vinorelbine
15. Etoposide

Chemotherapeutic drugs in use to treat ovarian germ cell type in combination include:

1. Etoposide
2. Bleomycin
3. Cisplatin

The response rate in Stage II ovarian cancer when treated with platinum-based treatment is up to 50%. The 5-year survival for Stages III and IV ovarian cancer is about 20%, when treated with platinum-based treatment. The National Cancer Society has reported a 35% response rate with the combination of Taxol, Cisplatin, and Cytoxan in Stage II and IV ovarian cancer. Although cancer of the ovary is a very difficult cancer to treat, there has been excellent response to combination chemotherapy in recent years. The best treatment for cancer of the ovary is surgical resection of early/ stage 1 cancer of the ovary with adjuvant chemotherapy or radiation.

Cancer of the prostate:

In 2013, 238, 590 men had cancer of the prostate in the U.S. and 29, 720 men died of prospate cancer. Worldwide 899,000 men had prostate cancer and worldwide 238,000 men died of prostate cancer.

Prostate is much more common in black and other minority men compared to white men. Asians have a low incidence of prostate cancer. According to the American cancer society, "the average annual prostate cancer rate "between" 2001-2005 was 59% higher in black men than in white men". The death rate from prostate cancer is 2.4 times higher in black men than in white men according to the ACS. 5 of every 100 African American men are expected to die of prostate cancer.

In addition, prostate cancer occurs at an earlier age in black and other minority men than in white men.

Prostate cancer begins to occur at around age forty in black men and at around age 50 in white men. The two groups of black men in the world that have the highest rates of prostate cancer are African American men and black men from the Jamaica West Indies.

The incidence of prostate cancer in Jamaicans is 51.1 per 100,000.

Risks for prostate cancer in black men include:

Being African American
Age
High fat diet
Obesity
Caribbean born (specially Jamaicans)
Genetics
Recurrent prostate infection
Tobacco smoking
A difference in the activity of the gene PRDM9
Oncotype DX test evaluates which subgroup of prostate cancer is aggressive and more likely to spread and thus more deadly.

Symptoms of prostate cancer are divided in early symptoms and late symptoms.
Early symptoms of prostate cancer include:
Urge to urinate frequently
Difficulty to pass urine
Pain on urination etc;

Many men have early prostate cancer with no symptoms and their cancers are picked up during routine physical examinations. The symptoms of advanced prostate cancer include all the symptoms listed above plus:

Blood in the urine
Urinary retention
Lower abdominal pain
Urinary tract infection etc;

The ways to diagnose prostate cancer include:
Complete history
Complete physical examination
Digital rectal examination
Prostatic specific antigen (PSA)
Ultrasound of the prostate
Biopsy of the prostate

The PSA is crucial in establishing the diagnosis of prostate cancer. In prostate cancer the PSA is elevated. In obese men, the PSA may be abnormally lower because the higher blood volume the obesity creates. This fact must be taken into consideration when evaluating obese men for prostate cancer. This is particularly important in evaluating Black, Hispanics and Native American men because of the high percentage of obesity that exists in these groups of men.

Another important and indispensable part of the evaluation of prostate cancer is the digital rectal examination. During the digital rectal examination, the physician can tell if the prostate gland is enlarged, and if so, how enlarged. In addition, the physician can tell if the gland is nodular or if the gland is tender etc; there have been times when the PSA was normal and a cancerous nodule was palpated.

The medical conditions that cause an elevated PSA include:
Prostate cancer
Benign prostatic hypertrophy (BPH)
Prostatitis
Urinary tract infection
Rectal examination
Ejaculation

The different types of PSA are:
Total PSA
Free PSA
PSA velocity
Aged-adjusted PSA

The normal PSA is 0-4ng/ml

The prostate ultrasound is mandatory in the evaluation prostate cancer. During this test, suspicious calcification and other abnormalities can be seen. However, the prostate biopsy is the definitive procedure that can tell for sure if cancer exists in the prostate gland. This biopsy is carried out in urologist office under the guidance of ultrasound. The biopsy is done using a special needle that is inserted inside the rectum. The ultrasound guides the urologist to the different parts of the prostate gland to biopsy. The tissue is sent to the pathology laboratory for the pathologist to prepare and evaluate under the microscope. Waiting for the result of the prostate biopsy can be nerve racking for men.

Once the biopsy is done and the pathology result is back showing cancer in the prostate. The next step is for the urologist to meet with the patient and his wife, or girl friend or other love interest to discuss the treatment options.
The key point in this discussion is the stage of the cancer.

The most common staging system in use in the U.S. is:

"T stages (primary tumor)
N stages (Regional Lymph Nodes)
M stages (Distant Metastasis)
T stages (primary tumor)

In the T stages, the cancer is localized in the prostate gland surrounding areas.
Clinical:

TX—Primary tumor cannot be assessed
T0—No evidence of primary tumor
T1—Cannot detect tumor with imaging tests
T1a—Less than 5 percent of the prostate is affected by the tumor
T1b—More than 5 percent of the prostate is affected by the tumor
T1c—Tumor identified by needle biopsy, PSA elevated
T2—Tumor confined within prostate
T2a—Tumor affects one-half of one lobe or less
T2b—Tumor affects more than one-half of one lobe but not both lobes
T2c—Tumor affects both lobes
T3—Tumor extends through the prostate capsule
T3a—Tumor extends beyond the prostate capsule
T3b—Tumor invades seminal vesicle(s)
T4—Tumor is fixed or invades surrounding areas, such as the bladder neck,
External sphincter, rectum, levator muscle, and/or pelvic wall

Pathological staging:

pT2—Tumor confined to the prostate
pT2a—Tumor affects one-half of one lobe or less
pT2b—Tumor affects more than one-half of one lobe but not both lobes
pTc—Tumor affects both lobes
pT3—Tumor extends beyond the prostate
pT3b—Tumor invades seminal vesicle (s)
pT4—Tumor invades the bladder, rectum

N stages (Regional Lymph Nodes)
A N0 stage indicates the cancer has not spread to the lymph nodes.
N1 indicates the cancer has spread to one or more pelvic nodes.

Clinical:
    NX-Regional lymph nodes were not assessed

    N0—Tumor has not spread to regional lymph nodes
    N1—Tumor has spread to regional nodes

Pathological:

    pNX-Regional lymph nodes were not assessed
    pN0—Regional lymph nodes not affected by tumor
    pN1—Regional lymph nodes affected by tumor

    M stages (Distant Metastasis)
    A M0 stages indicates the cancer has not metastasized beyond the local lymph nodes.
    While M1 indicates the cancer has metastasized to distant lymph nodes and/or to other organs.

    MX-Distant metastasis cannot be assessed
    M0-No distant metastasis
    M1-Distant metastasis
    M1a-Non-regional lymph nodes affected by tumor
    M1b-Bones affected by tumor
    M1c-Other sites affected by tumor with or without bone disease"
    Sources: National Cancer Institute/American Cancer Society.

Treatment options for prostate cancer include:
Stage 1
    Radical prostatectomy (Using conventional surgical technic or DA Vinci/Robotic surgical technic inimically invasive)
                or
    External beam radiation
                or
    Seeds implantation
                or
    Watchful waiting

    Stage II Prostate cancer

    Radical prostatectomy as stage I plus radiation
                or
    External beam radiation
                or

Seeds implantation

Chemotherapy

Stage III Prostate cancer include

Radical prostatectomy as per stage I
or
External beam radiation
or
Hormonal therapy
or
Chemotherapy

Stage IV Prostate cancer

External beam radiation

Hormonal therapy

Chemotherapy

The hormonal medications in use to treat prostate cancer include

Lupron
Casodex
Zoladex
Eulexin

The chemotherapy medications in use to treat prostate cancer include

Taxol
Etoposide
Estramustine
Doxorubicin
Mitoxantrone
These drugs are used in advanced metastatic prostate cancer.

All treatments used to treat prostate cancer have side effects,
Proastatectomy as a treatment modality while effective can cause serious side effects.
Among these side effects include
Bleeding
Urinary incontinence
Urinary tract infection

Sexual impotence

Hormonal treatment is an integral part of the overall treatments of prostate cancer. However, hormonal side effects of the medications can be significant. Among these Side effects include.
Hot flashes
Enlargement of the breasts
No sexual desire
Sexual impotence

Chemotherapy drugs play a major and significant role in the treatments in prostate cancer.
Among these side effects are:

Nausea
Vomiting
Low white blood cells
Low red blood cells
Low platelets
Sores in the mouth
Loss of hair
Diarrhea
General weakness
Numbness in feet etc;

Some of the medications in use to treat sexual impotence after prostatectomy, radiation, and seeds implantation include
Viagra
Cialis
Levitra

Radiation and Seeds implantation both play major roles in the treatment of prostate cancer.
Some of the side effects of radiation as a treatment modality for prostate cancer include
Nausea
Vomiting
Weakness
Low white blood cells
Low red blood cells
Low platelets
Sexual impotence
Radiation proctitis

Rectal bleeding due to radiation proctitis

Some of the side effects of seeds implantation as a treatment modality for prostate cancer

Include:

Nausea

Vomiting

General weakness

Sexual impotence etc;

Prostate cancer is a curable cancer if diagnosed early.

Men ought to seek medical evaluation for prostate health starting at age 35 year if they are African Americans or Jamaicans and all other black men ought to seek medical evaluation for prostate health beginning at age 40.

All men whose fathers have had or have prostate cancer should seek medical evaluation for prostate health at age 35. Caucasian, Asian, and men of other ethnic ancestries should seek medical evaluation for prostate health beginning at age 50.

Cancer head neck:

In 2013, 41,380 people in the U.S. were diagnosed with head and neck cancer and 7,890 people died of head and neck cancer in the U.S.

Worldwide there are 600,000 cases of head and cancer annually 320,000 people die from head and neck cancer.

Head and neck cancer is 50 percent more common blacks and other minorities as compared to whites. The death rates are higher among blacks and other minorities with head and neck cancer than they are in whites.

Risk factors for head and neck cancer include:

Tobacco smoking

Alcohol abuse

HPV infection

Genetic transmission

Radiation to neck area during childhood

Some signs and symptoms of head and neck cancer include:

1. A sore that bleeds often and easily and fails to heal
2. Persistent hoarseness
3. Palpable mass in the neck

4. Pain on swallowing
5. Difficulty swallowing
6. Persistent sore throat etc;

Methods in use to diagnose o head and neck cancer include:
History
Physical examination
Fiberoptic Laryngoscopic examination
Chest x ray
CT SCAN of the neck
MRI of the neck
Biopsy of any lesion seen under general anesthesia

The best treatment for head and neck cancers is radiation therapy given 5 days per week for 6 weeks together with Cis-Platinum 100mg/m2 given on day #1, day #22 and day# 43. The response rate for radiation and chemotherapy for stages 1, 2, and 3, head and neck cancers is in the range of 75% world wide. The response rate for surgical resection of head and neck cancers with adjuvant radiation/ chemotherapy parallels the response rate of radiation and chemotherapy without surgical resection. Frequently surgical resection of head and neck cancers requires the removal of the voice box with a permanent tracheostomy.

Other drugs used to treat head and neck cancer are:

1. Paclitaxel
2. Docetaxel
3. Carboplatin
4. Ifosfamide
5. Methotrexate

In evaluating the throat using the fiberoptic laryngoscope, it is mandatory that the physician doing the scoping passes the laryngoscope through both nasal passages so as not to miss cancer and other lesions that may be located in the upper right or upper left of the nasal anatomy.

Some of the side effects of chemotherapy medications used to treat head and neck cancer include:

Nausea
Vomiting
Diarrhea
Loss of appetite
Weight loss

Sores in the mouth
Sores in the throat
Pain on swallowing
Low white blood cells
Low red blood cells
Low platelets
Fever
Infection
Dehydration
Severe pain in the mouth and throat
Numbness in feet etc

Some of the side effects radiation treatment used to treat head and neck cancer include:

Nausea
Vomiting
General weakness
Sore in the mouth
Sore in the throat
Severe damage to the upper esophagus with esophagitis
Dehydration
Low white blood cells
Low red blood cells
Low platelets
Infection
Severe damage to the salivary glands
Severe zerostomia (dry mouth)
Damage to teeth and gums with marked long term tooth decays
Severe damage to the skin around the neck with hyperpigmentation
Long term tiredness etc

Cancer of the Urinary Bladder:

In 2013, 72,570 people were diagnosed with cancer of the urinary bladder in the U.S. and 15,210 people died of this cancer.

Worldwide in 2013, there were 382,500 people that were diagnosed with cancer of the urinary bladder and 187,000 people die of cancer of the urinary bladder annually.

In 2008, 21.6 black males and 40.6 white males per 100,000 had cancer of the urinary bladder in the U.S. and 9.8 white females and 7.6 black females per 100,000 had cancer of the urinary bldder. Over all cancer of the rinary bladder is more common in men than women and it usally develops between the ages of 50 to 70.

In 2007, 7.9 white males and 5.4 black males per 100,000 died of cancer of the urinary bladder in the U.S. and 2.2 white females and 2.7 black females per 100,000 died of cancer of the urinary bladder in the U.S.

Urinary bladder cancer is twice more common in whites than blacks and other minorities, but the death rate is higher in blacks and other minorities than whites. In addition, the death rate for this cancer is higher in women than men.

Some of the risk factors for urinary cancer include:

Smoking
Exposure to industrial dyes
Exposure to industrial rubbers
Exposure to industrial leathers
Schistosomiosis heamatobium infection
Genetic inheritance

Symptoms of urinary bladder cancer include:

Urinary frequency
Urinary incontinence
Recurrent urinary infection
Blood in the urine (gross)
Microscopic hematuria
Urinary retention
Low back pain
Abdominal pain
Hydronephrosis
Weight loss
Poor appetite etc

The way to evaluate patients for possible urinary bladder cancer include

1. History
2. Physical examination
3. Urinalysis
4. Urine cytology
5. Ultrasound of the urinary bladder
6. IVP
7. CT of the urinary bladder

8. Cystoscopy with biopsy of suspected lesions

Surgery is frequently in the diagnosis and treatments of urinary bladder cancer.

Drugs in use to treat bladder cancer are:

1. Methotrexate
2. Vinblastin
3. Doxorubicin
4. Cisplatinum
5. Gemcitabine
6. Isfosfamine
7. Mesna
8. Placlitaxel
9. Inmmunotherapy with BCG installation in the urinary bladder.
10. Photodynamic therapy

The chemotherapy drugs are used in different combinations.

Kidney Cancer & renal pelvis:

In 2013, 65,150 people were diagnosed with kidney and renal pelvis and 13,680 people died of these cancers in 2013.

In 20134, Worldwide in 2013, 208,500 cancers of the kidney/renal pelvis were diagnosed and each year more 102,000 people died of cancer of kidney/renal pelvis.

Cancer of the kidney is somewhat more common in blacks and other minorities than in whites.

In 2005, 21.3 black males and 10.1 black females per 100,000 were diagnosed with cancer of the kidney in the U.S. and 18.8 white males and 9.5 white females per 100,000 were diagnosed with cancer of the kidney.

During that same time, 6.1 black males and 2.7 black females per 100,000 died of cancer of the kidney and 6.2 white males and 2.8 white females per 100,000 died of cancer of the kidney.

Some of the risk factors for cancer of the kidney include:

1. Being a man
2. Smoking
3. Exposure to asbestos

4. Exposure to cadium
5. Genetic inheritance
6. Being black
7. Von Hipple-Lindau syndrome
8. Hypertension etc

Signs and symptoms of cancer of the kidney include:

Hematuria (gross)
Hematuria (microscopic)
Low back pain
Palpable flank mass in lower abdomen
Unexplained and recurrent fevers
Weight loss
Poor appetite
Fatigue
Anemia
Polycytemia (hypernephroma) etc

Evaluating patients for possible cancer of the kidney

1. History
2. Physical examination
3. Urinalysis
4. Urine cytology
5. Ultra sound of the kidney
6. CT of the kidneys
7. MRI
8. PET scan
9. Chest x-ray
10. CBC
11. Complete metabolic profile

Treatments of cancer of the kidney include:

Surgery to remove the cancerous kidney
Possible radiation therapy
Possible chemotherapy
Chemotherapy medications in used to treat cancer of the kidney include:
Interferon-alpha
Bevacizumab
Interleukin-2
Sunitinib

Sorafenib
Temsirolimus

Testicular cancer:

In 2013, 7,920 men were diagnosed with testicular cancer and 370 men died of testicular.

Worldwide in 2013, 36,000 are diagnosed with tescular cancer annually and 1 in 5000 men die of testicular.

Testicular cancer is much more common in white men than in black and other minority men. In 2005, 1.4 black men and 6.3 white men per 100,000 were diagnosed with testicular cancer.

Risks for testicular cancer include:

Undescended testis
Family history of testicular cancer
Congenital abnormalities of the getourinary tract

Signs and symptoms of testicular cancer include:

A painless lump of the testicle
Pain in the testicle
Pain in the groin
Lower abdominal pain
Low back pain

How is testicular cancer diagnosed?

Examination of the testicles
Ultrasound of the testicle
Abdominal CT scan
Alpha Feto protein
Beta HCG
LDH
Biopsy of the testicular mass
Chest x ray
PET scan

How is testicular cancer treated?

Surgical removal of the affected testis (Orchiectomy)

Radiation therapy and or chemotherapy
The chemotherapy medications in use to treat stage II testicular include
Bleomycin
Cisplatinum
Etoposide
These drugs are used in combination every 28 days

Drugs in use to treat advanced stage testicular cancer include:

Cisplatinum
Vinblastine
Ifosfamide
Mesna
Or
Cisplatinum
Paclitaxel
Ifosfamide
Mesna

It is extremely important for men to examine there testicle frequently.
Testicular cancer is extremely sensitive to both radiation therapy and chemotherapy with a very high cure rate.

Leukemias

In 2013, 48,610 individuals were diagnosed will leukemia in the U.S. and 23,720 people died leukemia in the U.S. Worldwide in 2013, 300,000 people had leukemia. Leukemia is less common in whites than in blacks and other minorities.

The incidence of leukemia is 19.2 per 100,000 and 6.5 per 100,000 in blacks. In 2010, 970 black males and 860 black females are expected to die of leukemia.
Source: ACS Facts and figures for African Americans 2009-2010

The different types of leukemias are:

1. Acute lymphocytic leukemia
2. Chronic lymphocytic leukemia (CLL represents 35% of all leukemias in the world) and annually 75,000 people in the die of CLL in the world.
3. Acute myelogenic leukemia
4. Chronic myelogenic leukemia
5. Monocystic leukemia

6. Myelodysplastic syndrome
7. Acute megakaryocytic leukemia
8. T-cell leukemia/lymphoma due to HTLVI and II.

The risks for leukemia include:

Down's syndrome,
AIDS,
Exposure to ionizing radiation
Exposure to chemicals like benzene and other toxic chemicals
Genetic etc

Evaluations of leukemia include:

History and physical examination
CBC with differential
Complete chemistry profile
Urinalysis
LDH
LAP
ESR
HIV/AIDS blood test
Bone marrow aspiration
Bone marrow biopsy
Cell surface marker studies
Cytogenetic studies
Abdominal CT with contrast by mouth
Chest Xray
Chest CT
EKG
Echocardiogram
Rest MUGA

Sings and symptoms of Leukemia include:

Fatigue
Weight loss
Easy bruising
Nose bleed
Frequent infections
Enlarged liver
Enlarged spleen
Anemia

Elevated white blood cells
Low platelets
Abnormal peripheral blood smear
Abnormal bone marrow aspiration and bone marrow biopsy
Abnormal differential cells count on blood smear
Cytogenetics studies of chromosomal
Abnormal BCR/ABL Gene, QN, PCR (in CML)
Elevated LDH
Low leukocyte alkaline phosphatase (LAP)
Lymphocytes cell surface marker studies (CD5, CD 19, CD 20, and CD 23)

Different types of leukemias are treated with different chemotherapeutic regimens and bone marrow transplantation.
Induction therapy:

Acute lymphocytic leukemia (ALL) is treated with
Daunorubicin 50 mg/m2 IV every 24 hours on day 1-3
Vincristine 2 mg IV on days 1, 8, 15, and 22
Prednisone 60 mg/m2 daily on days 1-28
L-Asparaginase 6,000 U/m2 on days 17-28
There are Consolidation protocol and maintenance protocol available to treat ALL.
CNS prophylaxis is
Cranial irradiation is given with 1,800 rad in 10 fractions over 12-14 days
Plus Methotrexate 12 mg intrathecally every week for 6 weeks
Newer medications in use to treat ALL are
Imatinib 600 mg by mouth every day
Or
Dastinib 70 mg by mouth twice per day
Or
Clofarabine 52mg/m2 IV for 5 days

Acute Myelogenous leukemia (AML) is treated with
Cytarabrine 100 mg/m2/day Iv continuous infusion days 1-7
Daunorubicin 45 mg/m2 IV days 1-7
Or
Cytabrine 100mg/m2/day IV continuous infusion days 1-7
Doxorubicin 12mg/m2 days 2, 4, 6, and 8
There are several more protocols and single agents available to treat AML

Chronic lymphocytic leukemia (CLL) is treated with
Cytoxan 400 mg/m2 days 1-5
Vincristine 1-4 mg/m2 IV day (maximum dose 2mg)
Prednisone 100mg/m2 by mouth days1-5

Or
Fludaradine 25 mg/m2 IV days 1-5
Retuxan 375 mg/m2 IV days 1, and 4on cycle 1 and on day 1 there after
Or
Fludarabine 25 mg/m2 IV days 1-3
Cytoxan 250 mg/m2 IV days 1-3
Or
Retuxan 375 mg/m2 IV every week for 4 weeks
There are several more protocols and single agents' drugs in use to treat CLL.

Chronic Myelogenous leukemia is treated with
Imatinib 400 mg/day by mouth or 600 mg/day
Dasatinib 70 mg twice per day
Imatimid 400mg daily plus peginterferon alfa-2a 90ug weekly is said to be superior to Imatimid alone

Acute Promyelocytic leukemia is treated with
All-trans-Reteinoic Acid 45mg mg/m2/day by mouth in 2 divided doses until remission
Idarubicin 12 mg/m2/day IV on days 1-5

Hairy cell Leukemia is treated with
Cladribine 0.09 mg/kg/day IV as a continuous infusion days 1-7
Pentostatin 4 mg/m2 IV day 1
Repeat every 14 days for 6 cycles.

Lymphoma:

In 2013, 79,030 individuals were diagnosed with lymphoma in the U.S., that included 69,740 non-Hodgkin lymphoma and 9.290 Hodgkin lymphoma and 20,200 people died of lymphoma in 2013 in the U.S.

Worldwide in 2013, there were 600,000 people in the world have lymphoma and every year 25,000 people die from Hodgkin lymphoma and 40,000 die every in the world fom Non-lymphoma.

The incidence of lymphoma is higher in Caucasians than in Blacks and other minorities. In 2005, 2.9 black males and 2.3 black females per 100,000 were diagnosed with Hodgkin lymphoma and in comparison, 3.3 white males and 2.7 white females per 100,000 were diagnosed with Hodgkin lymphoma. During that time, 18.4 black males and 12.2 black females per 100.000 were diagnosed with Non-Hodgkin lymphoma and in comparison, 24.3 white males and 17.1 white females per 100,000 were diagnosed with Non-Hodgkin lymphoma.

The death rates for lymphoma are higher in whites compared to blacks and other minorities. In 2005, 0.5 black males and 0.3 black females per 100,000 died of Hodgkin lymphoma as compared to 0.6 white males and 0.4 white females per 100,000 died of Hodgkin lymphoma. During that time, 6.4 black males and 4.2 black females per 100,000 died of Non-Hodgkin lymphoma as compared to 9.7 white males and 6.2 white females per 100,000 died of Non-Hodgkin lymphoma.

Risks for lymphoma Hodgkin/Non-Hodgkin include

History of Infectious mononucleosis
Epstein—Barr infection (50% of Hodgkin lymphoma is associated with Epstein-Barr infection)
HIV/AIDS infection
HLTV 1 infection (this infection is most commonly seen in the Caribbean, southern island of Japan, Northeastern South America, Central America, and New Guinea.
Non-acquired immunodeficiency disease
H pylori infection of the stomach
Being a male
Being highly educated
Exposure to chemical
Genetic inheritance etc

Some of the signs and symptoms of lymphoma include:

Fever
Night sweats
Loss of appetite
Weight loss
Enlarged lymph nodes
Diarrhea
Fever of unknown origin FUO
Enlarged spleen
Enlarged liver
Abdominal pain
Jaundice
Anemia etc

The best ways to evaluate a person for the possibility of lymphoma include:

A complete history and physical examination
Chest ray
Chest CT scan
Abdominal CT scan
MRI of the chest/abdomen
PET scan
CBC
Complete chemistry profile
LDH
ESR
Urinalysis
PT/PTT
Bone marrow aspiration
Bone marrow biopsy
Cytogenetic studies
Lymphocytes cell surface markers
Lymph node biopsy

The best treatments available to treat Hodgkin's disease as published in the literature are:

(ABVD)
Doxorubicin
Bleomycin
Vinblastine
Dacarbazine

(ChiVPP)
Chlorambucil
Vinblastine
Procarbazine
Prednisone

(Stanford V)
Doxorubicin
Vinblastine
Mechlorethamine
Vincristine
Bleomycin
Etoposide

(ASHAP)
Doxorubicin

Methylprednisone
Cisplatin
Cytarabine

(CHOP)
Cyclophosphamide
Doxorubicin
Vincristine
Prednisone

Some of drugs available to treat non-Hodgkin's lymphoma as published in the literature are:

(CHOP plus Rituximab)
Rituximab
Cyclophosphomide
Doxorubicin
Vincristine
Prednisone

(CHOP-14 every 2 weeks)
Cyclophosphomide
Doxorubicin
Vincristine
Prednisone

(CODOX-M)
Cyclophosphomide
Vincristine
Doxorubicin
Methotrexate
Leucovorin
GM-CSF

(IVAC)
Etoposide
Ifosfamide
Mesna
Cytarabine
Methotrexate
GM-CSF

(DHAP)

Dexamethasone
Cisplatin
Cytarabine

(EPOCH plus Rituximab)
Rituximab
Doxorubicin
Etoposide
Vincristine
Cyclophosphamide
Prednisone

Radiation therapy is a major treatment modality in the treatments of lymphomas.

Multiple Myeloma:

In 2013, 22,350 people were diagnosed with multiple myeloma in the U.S. and 10,710 people died of multiple myeloma in the U.S. in 2013.

Worldwide in 2013, more than 220,000 people have multiple myeloma and about 66,000 people die every year from multiple myeloma.

Multiple myeloma is more than twice as common in blacks and other minorities as compared to whites and the death rate for multiple myeloma is more than twice in blacks as compared to whites.

Risk factors for multiple myeloma include:

   Being a man (multiple myeloma is more common in men than women are)
   Being black and other minorities
   Being age 50 or older
   Obesity
   Hypertension
   History of monoclonal gammopathy of undetermined significance (MGUS), each
year
   1 percent of people with MGUS develop multiple myeloma
   Exposure to radiation, benzene and other industrial chemicals

Signs and symptoms of multiple myeloma include
   Low back pain
   Rib cage pain
   Weight loss

Bone pain anywhere in the body
Weakness
Fatigue
Anemia
Blurry vision
Fever
Bence Jones protein in the urine
Monclonal M protein in the blood
Abnormal protein electrophoresis
Elevated IGG, IGM, IGA, and IGD in the blood
Low IGG, IGM, IGA, and IGD in the blod (seen in light chain myeloma)
Lytic lesions on bone x-rays.
Abnormal plasma cells level in bone marrow aspiration/biopsy
Elevated BUN
Elevated serum creatinine
Elevated serum calcium
Elevated ESR
Elevated LDH
High total protein
Low total protein (seen in light myeloma)
High serum calcium
High serum free light chain
Elevated Beta-2-microglobulin
Low or high white blood cells
Low red blood cells
Low platelets
Recurrent pneumonia
Recurrent urinary track infection
Sepsis (people with multiple myeloma are immunosuppresed and as such get infected frequently with bacteria, fungi, or viruses)

The different stages of myeloma

Stage 1
    "No anemia (in other words, a normal red cell count)
    A normal level of blood calcium
    No bone damage or a solitary plasmacytoma
    Low levels abnormal antibodies (immunoglobulin) in your blood or urine

Stage 2 includes anyone who does not fit exactly into 1 or stage
    Therefore, you would be stage 2 if you had 2 areas of bone damage. You can also have stage 2A or 2B. As with stage 1, this depends on whether your kidneys have been damaged at all by the myeloma.

Stage 3
   This is if you have
   Anenia (low red cell count)
   High levels of calcium in your blood
   More than 3 sites of bone damage
   High levels of abnormal paraproteins in your blood or urine

Stage 3 is also divided into stages 3A an 3B, with those in 3B, having a high creatinine level in their blood, indicacating that they have some kidney damage from their myeloma."

Treatments of multiple myeloma include both radiation for local bone pain and chemotherapy. The drugs in use to treat multiple myeloma include

   Melphalan 8-10mg/m2 days 1-4 by mouth
   Predisone 60 mg/m2 days 1-4 by mouth
   Repeat cycle every 42 days
   Or
   Melphalan 0.25 mg/kg/days 1-4 by mouth
   Prednisone 2mg/kg//days 1-4 by mouth
   Thalidomide 100-400 mg daily by mouth
   Repeat cycle every 42 days
   Or
   Vincristine 0.4 mg/day IV as a continuous infusion days 1-4
   Doxorubicin 9 mg/m2/day IV as a continuous in fusion days 1-4
   Dexamethasone 40 mg by mouth days 1-4, 9-12, and 17-20

   Or Velcade 1.3mg/m2 on day 1, 4, 8 and 11 and Adriamycin 30mg/m2 on day 4 and
   Dexamethasone 40mg IV or by mouth on day 1-4, 9-11 and 17-20 repeat cycle every
   21 days
   Stem cells transplant is an option for suitable patients.
   There are numerous other protocols in use to treat multiple myeloma.
   Bone marrow transplant is being quite often to treat patients with multiple myeloma with varying degrees of success.

Melanoma

The most serious and malignant form of skin cancer is melanoma and in 2013, 76, 690 individuals were diagnosed with melanoma in the U.S. and 9,480 people died of this cancer in the U.S. in 2013.

Worldwide in 2013, 200,000 people were diagnosed with melanoma and 48,000 people died from melanoma in 2013. Melanoma is more common in whites than blacks and other minorities are.

Risks factors for the development of skin cancer include:

1. Ultraviolet rays (exposure to the sun)
2. Being of fair complexion
3. Exposure to arsenic compounds
4. Exposure to radium
5. Exposure to coal tar
6. Family history of skin cancer
7. History of multiple skin moles
8. BRAF gene carriers

Signs and symptoms of melanoma include:

A mole that a change in color, size, and bleeds over the trunk, legs, abdomen, chest, arms a large brownish spot with darker speckles over sun exposed areas of the body

A lesion with irregular border and portions that is red, white, blue, or black over sun Exposed areas of the body Dark/black lesions on palms, soles of feet, fingertips, toes, mucous membranes in Mouth, nose, anus, and, vagina etc;

Evaluations of melanoma include:

History and physical examination
Close examination of the skin by a Dermatologist
CBC
Complete chemistry profile
ESR
Urinalysis
V600E test (newly approved by the FDA)
V600K test (newly approved by the FDA)
Chest Xray
Chest CT
Abdominal CT
PET scan
Skin biopsy

Any all lesions of concern should be examined by a dermatologist and appropriate biopsies taken when necessary. The most effective treatments for melanoma are surgical resection with regional lymph node removal, radiation therapy, immunotherapy, and chemotherapy.

The chemotherapy drugs in use to treat malignant melanoma include:
Dacarbazide 220mg/m2 IV days 1-3
Carmustine 150 mg/m2 IV days 1
Cisplatinum 25 mg/m2 IV days 1-3
Or
Temozolomide 75 mg/m2/day by mouth for 6 weeks
Thalidomide 200-400 mg/m2/day by mouth for 6 weeks
Or
Interferon Alpha-2b 15 million IU/m2 IV days 1-5, 8-12, and 15-19 induction
Interferon Alpha-2b 10 million IU/m2 Sc 3 times weekly post induction
Dacarbazide 200 mg/m2 IV days 22-26
Repeat every 28 days
New drugs approved by the FDA to treat melanoma include:
Yervoy
Zelboraf
Tafinlar
Mekinist

Thyroid Cancer:

In 2013, 60,220 people were diagnosed with thyroid cancer in the U.S. and 1,850 people died of thyroid cancer in the U.S. in 2013. Worldwide in 2013, 213,000 people were diagnosed with thyroid cancer and 25,000 people died from thyroid cancer in 2013.

Thyroid cancer is almost twice more common in whites than blacks and other minorities and the death rates for thyroid cancer are almost twice in whites than in blacks and other minorities.

Risk factors for thyroid cancer include:
Exposure to high dose radiation
People who were treated with radiation to treat tonsils/adenoids as children many years ago
History of thyroid goiter
Family history of goiter
Genetic inheritance etc
Signs and symptoms of thyroid cancer include:
A lump in the neck
Hoarseness

Problem swallowing
Enlarged lymph nodes around the neck etc;

How to evaluate a person for possible thyroid cancer:
History and physical examination
T4 and TSH blood tests
Thyroid ultrasound
Thyroid scan
Fine needle aspiration of a cold thyroid nodule
Chest x-ray

Treatments of thyroid cancer include:
Surgery to remove the thyroid gland
Radioactive iodine treatment to kill any remaining cancer cells
Synthroid

This thyroid hormone is to replace the hormone which the thyroid can no longer produce, and to suppress the ability of the pituitary gland from making TSH. People, who have had their thyroid glands removed, must take synthroid for the rest of their lives.

Much progress has been made in the detection and treatment of cancer and many cancers are curable when detected and treated early. However, much more needs to be done to understand the genetic transmission of cancer, the way cancer cells grow in the human body, so that genetic engineering can be used to prevent the growth of cancer cells in the human body. Society must do more to stop people from being exposed to cancer-causing agents and other toxic materials. Many people must stop their self-destructive habits such as cigarette smoking, alcohol abuse, and eating too many fat-rich foods; they must exercise more to lose weight to decrease their incidence of cancer.

The incidence of cancer and the death rates from cancer are much higher in Blacks and other minorities than Whites are. Higher rates of unemployment, lower level of education, high rates of uninsured and racism against Blacks and other minorities all play a role in both the cancer rates and death rates being so much higher in Blacks and other minorities compared to Whites. Both government and the private sector must make available more money for cancer research and cancer treatments so that cancer can be eliminated once and for all.

Chapter 6
KIDNEY DISEASES

There are more than 26 million people with kidney diseases in the U.S. and About 20 million more people are at risk for developing kidney diseases in the U.S. Worldwide there are more than 141,503,782 people with kidney diseases:

"Country—# of People
China—35,336,295
India—28,976,185
USA—26,000,000 ☐☐
Indonesia—6,487,322
Brazil—5,008,633
Pakistan—4,331,076
Russia—3,916,941
Bangladesh—3,845,292
Japan—3,464,206
Mexico—2,855,518
Philippines—2,346,281
Germany—2,242,434
Egypt—2,070,841
Ethiopia—1,940,774
Turkey—1,874,319
Iran—1,836,484
France—1,643,894
United Kingdom—1,639,717
Congo Kinshasa—1,586,566
Italy—1,579,504
South Korea—1,312,241
"South Africa—1,209,259
☐☐☐☐ Updated

Blacks and other minorities are at higher risk of developing kidney diseases and diseases of the urinary tract/bladder than whites and other ethnic groups.

Among the problems that can affect people and their urinary bladders are:

1. Urinary retention
2. Hematuria (bleeding from the urinary bladder and kidney)

3. Urinary tract infection
4. Cancer of the urinary bladder
5. Cancer of the kidney
6. Urinary incontinence
7. Prostate cancer
8. Sikle cell disease etc;

The most common causes of urinary retention include:

1. Diabetes mellitus
2. Stroke
3. Multiple sclerosis
4. Cancer of the bladder with bleeding and too much clots
5. Cancer of the kidney with bleeding and too much clots
6. Sickle cell disease with papillary necrosis, bleeding and too much clots
7. Urinary tract infection
8. Spinal cord injury
9. Benign prostatic hypertrophy
10. Prostate cancer

The most common causes of hematuria include:

1. Kidney stone
2. Urinary tract infection
3. Cancer of urinary bladder
4. Cancer of the kidney
5. Hemophilia
6. Von Willebran disease
7. Aspirin ingestion
8. Sickle cell anemia or sickle cell trait
9. Low platelets
10. Dessiminated intravascular coagulopathy (DIC) etc;

The most common causes of urinary tract infection include:

1. Diabetes mellitus
2. Stroke
3. Insertion of Foley catheter in the bladder
4. Old age with poor toileting
5. Multiple sclerosis
6. Cancer of the urinary bladder
7. Kidney stones with hydronephrosis
8. Cancer of the urether with hydronephrosis

9. Sexual intercourse (women)
10. Frequent baths
11. Tampon use
12. BPH etc;

The most common causes of cancer of the urinary bladder include:

1. Genetic predisposition
2. Exposure to different dyes at work
3. Tobacco smoking
4. Schistosoma haematobium etc;

The best ways to evaluate hematuria include:

1. Renal ultra sound
2. Bladder ultra sound
3. CT scan of the kidney
4. CT scan of the bladder
5. MRI of the kidey/bladder
6. Urine cytology
7. Urinalysis
8. Urine culture
9. Hemoglobin electrophoresis
10. Ova and parasite
11. Serum antibody screen for Schistosoma haematobium
12. Cystoscopy etc;

Diseases of the kidney that frequently affect include:

1. Infections UTI
2. Acute Pyelonephritis
3. Chronic Pyelonephritis
4. Hypertension
5. Diabetes mellitus
6. Hyperlipidemia
7. Kidney stone
8. Cancer of the kidney
9. Lupus (SLE)
10. Glomerulonephritis
11. Nephrotic syndrome
12. Papillary necrosis
13. HIV/AIDS
14. Thrombotic Thrombocytopenic Purpura (TTP)

15. Immune Thrombocytopenia (ITP)
16. Hemolytic uremic syndrome
17. Grastroenteritis
18. Polycystic kidney disease
19. Dehydration
20. Drug reaction
21. Azotemia-prerenal
22. Uremia (ESRD) etc;

Urinary tract infection is divided into lower tract urinary tract infection and upper tract urinary tract infection.

The most common symptoms of lower tract urinary tract infection include:

1. Urinary frequency
2. Burning on urination
3. Urinary hesitancy
4. Nocturia
5. Urinary retention
6. Gross hematuria
7. Microscopic hematuria
8. Fever
9. Chills
10. Head ache
11. Lower abdominal pain
12. General weakness
13. Tiredness etc.

The most common symptoms of upper tract urinary tract infection include:
all the above, plus flank pain, nausea and vomiting.

The best ways to evaluate UTI both lower tract UTI and upper tract UTI are:

1. Take good history from the patient
2. Do a complete physical examination
3. Do a urinalysis
4. Do a urine culture
5. Do 2 sets of blood culture
6. Do a complete CBC
7. Do SMA 20 chemistry profile
8. Renal ultra sound

If the person has UTI and is not febrile, he or she can be treated as an outpatient.

If he or she is febrile, he or she should be admitted to the hospital for in hospital treatments. The most common bacteria responsible for UTI in blacks are gram negative enteric Bacteria such as E coli, Klebsiella, Pseudomonas, Proteus, Enterobacter, and gram positive bacteria such as Enterococcus, Staphphylococcus aureus ect;

The antibiotics that are available to treat UTI include:

1. Ampicillin
2. Keflex
3. Kefzol
4. Cipro
5. Levaquin
6. Ceftazidime
7. Cetriaxone
8. Bactrim DS
9. Gentamicin
10. Tobramycin
11. Vancomycin
12. Zosyn
13. Nitrofurantoin etc;

Upper tract UTI is also called pyelonephrytis and must be treated with IV antibiotic for 14-21 days. Lower tract UTI in people who are febrile can be treated with antibiotic IV for 7-10 days if the blood cultures are negative. Sepsis due to UTI must be treated for 14-21 days with IV antibiotics.

Lower UTI in people who are afebrile can be treated with antibiotic by mouth for 3-4 days for first UTI or 7-10 days in those who have history of recurrent UTI.

Either people who have recurrent UTI lower tract or upper tract must be evaluated by an urologist to find out the reason for the frequent UTI. As part of the urological evaluation, the following tests must be done.

1. Urinalysis and culture
2. Ultrasound of the bladder
3. Ultrasound of the Kidneys
4. CT scan of the kidneys and bladder with contrast
5. CT scan of the kidneys without contrast looking for kidney stones
6. Cystoscopy
7. Urinary cylology
8. Hemoglobin electrophoresis

Sexually active women frequently have UTI which is associated with sexual intercourse. The way to prevent post coital UTI is for women to empty their bladder immediately after intercourse to prevent any bacteria that may have enter into the bladder during intercourse to be urinated thereby decreasing the incidence of UTI.

Women who frequently develop UTI after sexual intercourse are often given a Bactrim tablet or Nitrofurantoin tablet to take immediately after intercourse to suppress bacterial growth by of preventing UTI. Other things that increase the risk of UTI in women are the use of Tampon and taking frequent baths. Any who has frequent UTI should see a urologist for evaluation.

Kidney stones are quite common and this condition is quite painful. The most common stones are calcium oxalate and calcium phosphate. Calcium stones are most commonly seen.

The most common causes of kidney stones are:

1. Hyperuricosuria
2. Primary hyperparathyroidism
3. Intestinal hyperoxaluria
4. Hereditary hyperoxaluria
5. Hyperuricosuria
6. Gout
7. Lymphoma
8. Lymphocytic leukemia
9. Dehydration

The most common symptoms of kidney stones are:

1. Severe and excruciating lower back pain
2. Hematuria,(gross or microscopic)
3. Nusea
4. Vomiting

The best ways to evaluate people for kidney stones are:

1. Take a good history
2. Do a complete physical examination
3. Do a urinalysis to look for blood
4. Do a flat plate of the abdomen x-ray to look for a stone
5. Do a CT of the abdomen without contrast looking for a stone (Kidney stone protocol)
6. Strain the urine to look for stones

7. Do an SMA 20 chemistry profile
8. Do a serum uric acid
9. Do a CBC looking leukocytosis, lymphocytosis, elevated neutrophyls, elevated lymphocytes, blasts, or red blood cells (polycythemia)

The best treatments available to treat kidney stones are:

1. Pain killer medication
2. Allopurinol
3. Thiazide diuretic
4. Diet
5. Surgical removal of kidney stones
6. External Shock Wave Lithotripsy (ESWL)

Hematuria can occur in individuals who have abnormal coagulation problems such as

1. Hemophilia A and B
2. Factor V deficiency
3. Factor VII deficiency
4. Factor X deficiency
5. Factor XI deficiency
6. Von Willebran disease
7. Disseminated intravascular coagulopathy (DIC)
8. Thrombocytopenia (low platelet) due infection, PPT, ITP, Cirrhosis of the liver
9. Aspirin/ nonsteroidal anti-inflammatory drugs.
10. Sickle cell trait and sickle cell anemia (the reason for the hematuria in sickle cell disease is papillary necrosis of the kidney)

Hypertension is the number one disease in blacks in the United States. Three out of every four black adults aged 55 and older are hypertensive and 1 out of every five white adults are hypertensive. However, since hypertension is the number one disease in blacks, it is safe to say that three out of every four blacks aged 55 and older are at risk for kidney disease. The incidence of end-stage renal disease (ESRD) leading to renal failure is higher in blacks than in whites.

The reason that hypertension causes ESRD that ultimately results in the need for dialysis is that the kidneys have many vital structures within them that are essential for proper functions. Among those structures are the glomeruli, which are indispensable in the proper functioning of the kidneys. The elevated blood pressure causes plaques to develop inside the small vessels that carry blood and oxygen to the kidneys and the glomeruli within them.

Ordinarily, the inside of the blood vessels is smooth, and blood passes through them freely. When the blood pressure is high, as the blood passes through those vessels, the high pressure causes these vessels to lose their smoothness. The high pressure therefore damages the first layer of the vessels within the kidneys, resulting in plaque depositions.

The deposition of plaques in turn causes the narrowing of these vessels. The narrowing of the small vessels that is necessary to carry blood and oxygen to the glomeruli of the kidneys results in ischemia of the tissues of the kidney, resulting in the deaths of the glomeruli. The deaths of these glomeruli and other vital structures result ultimately in end-stage renal disease.

Blacks, Hispanics, and other people with the slightest trace of immediate African heritage fall within the category of people with low rennin by genetic predisposition. Asians also have low renin level in their blood for an entirely different genetic reason. Low-renin hypertension is referred to as high-volume hypertension.

However, as the kidneys fail, the renin level rises, resulting in greater elevation of the blood pressure, causing even more damage to the kidneys. Therefore, blacks who are hypertensive are at high risk of developing kidney disease from years of uncontrolled or poorly controlled blood pressure. Diabetes mellitus also causes kidney disease that can lead to ESRD.

In order to determine if the kidneys are sick and are about to fail from long years of being affected by hypertension or diabetes, the physician needs to do a history and physical examination and several blood tests, urine tests and radiological evaluation of the kidneys.

During the history and physical examination, the physician can determine how high the blood pressure is and whether the patient has evidence of hypertensive retinopathy (inside the eyes is the only place a physician can see a naked blood vessel in the human body without cutting the patient).

By examining the vessels inside the eyes, the physician can tell if the damage has occurred in the vessels because of longstanding and either untreated or poorly treated hypertension and the degree of damage. The kidneys are referred to as end organs as are the eyes, heart and brain, and if any of these end organs are damaged by the chronic effect of hypertension, then the examining physician can have a very good idea as to how long the blood pressure has been uncontrolled.

Further, the physician, by taking a history and examining the patient, he or she can tell whether the patient has entered into the uremic stage.

The best way to evaluate the kidneys for chronic kidney disease is to measure the glomerular filtration rate (GFR) and the amount of albumin in the urine.

Chronic renal disease has 5 stages, 1-5.

Stage 1.is GFR 90 ml/minute/1.73m2

Stage 2. is GFR 60-89ml/minute/1.73m2

Stage 3. is GFR 30-59ml/minute/1.73m2

Stage 4 is GFR 15-29ml/minute/1.73m2

Stage 5. Is GFR less than 15ml/minute/1.73m2?

Alternatively, urine can be collected for 24 hours to evaluate creatinine clearance and protein.

In uremia, a patient may have sweet breath, may have flaky salty material over his or her skin, or the patient may have swollen abdomen, swollen legs, the patient may be confused, the patient may have seizures, etc. On laboratory examination of the urine of the patient whose kidneys are failing chronically, the urine may be un-concentrated with a very low specific gravity. Normal specific gravity is about 1.010-1.025. A chronically sick kidney can only concentrate the urine to about 1.002-1.005. The specific gravity is the measure of the ability of the kidneys to concentrate urine. The sicker the kidneys are, the lower the specific gravity.

A chronically sick kidney from hypertension filters out plenty of protein. So by testing the urine during a routine urinalysis for proteins, the physician can be alerted as to how sick the kidneys are.

On microscopic examination of the urinary sediment, certain cellular materials such as certain types of casts can be seen.

By examining the electrolyte, like sodium, in the urine of a patient with failing kidneys, the physician can tell whether the kidneys are failing acutely, a condition called acute tubular necrosis due to some sort of acute event such as heart attack with a drop in the blood, sepsis with shock, acute and heavy bleeding with hypotension. Slow rogressive chronic disease such as hypertension or diabetes with damage to the kidneys canc also cause the kidneys to fail. The urinary sodium is easy to do. One needs only to get a few milliliters of urine from the patient and send it to the lab for urinary sodium testing.

In acute failure of the kidneys (acute renal failure), the urinary sodium is low. In chronic renal failure (the kidneys that have been failing for a long time), the urine sodium is high. This quick and easy test is of paramount importance in the treatment approach of a patient who shows up in the emergency room or the doctor's office with unexplained evidence of renal failure.

When the kidneys are failing acutely, they hold sodium in order to hold on to water to maintain the blood pressure to preserve the body and keep it alive.

On the other hand, chronic failing kidneys have lost their ability to hold on to sodium a long time ago, due to chronic damage that has occurred in the kidneys as a result of the insults of high blood pressure or diabetes to the kidneys; as a result, a large quantity of sodium is allowed to pass in the urine. Knowing this simple but crucial fact allows the physician to know how to approach both the acute and chronic medical management of the patient with failing kidneys.

Another indispensable crucial test that is done in every patient with failing kidneys who can pass urine is the 24-hour creatinine clearance. This test allows the physician to know the ability of the kidneys to function. It allows the physician to know how much function is left in the kidneys. The normal range of creatinine clearance in is 125 milliliters per minute down to about 75 milliliters per minute; and as a person gets older, these numbers decrease accordingly.

In order to do this test, the serum creatinine must be measured and a complete collection of all urine passed by the patient in 24 hours must be obtained and placed in a plastic bottle and sent to the laboratory to be tested. This urine must be kept refrigerated.

The next series of tests that are essential in evaluating the status of the kidneys are
Serum sodium
Potassium
Chloride
Bicarbonate
Creatinine
CBC

The reason why these tests are so important is that when the kidney is failing, it is unable to filter waste materials from the bloodstream properly, allowing these substances to accumulate in the body, and a reflection of this problem manifests itself with a rise in the BUN and serum creatinine first.

Then as the kidney failure progresses, the serum potassium rises while the serum bicarbonate decreases, resulting in a serious condition called hyperkalemic acidosis. Serum potassium of 6 or greater is a medical emergency that must be dealt with immediately because the high serum potassium can trigger cardiac arrhythmias, which can cause the death of the affected person with kidney failure.

Other serum chemistry tests that are important in evaluating a patient with kidney failure include the serum calcium, the serum phosphatase, the serum bilirubin, the LDH (lactic dehydrogenase), the CPK (creatinine phosphokinase), the total protein, and the serum albumin.

What role does an abnormality of each of these blood chemistry tests and CBC play in the evaluation of a patient with kidney failure? The blood tests to obtain in evaluating the kidney failure in patients include:

Serum sodium
Serum potassium
Serum bicarbonate
Serum chloride
Serum BUN
Serum creatinine
Serum phosphate
Serum calcium
Serum bilirubin
Serum protein
Serum albumin
Serum LDH
Serum CPK
CBC with differential

High serum sodium of 150-160, means that the kidney probably failed because of loss of volume (fluid) due to dehydration. Moreover, that rehydrating the patient with hypo-osmolar fluid such as water by mouth or water and sugar (D5W) intravenously, will normalize the sodium, and depending on how long the dehydration state existed, the kidney function will probably return to normal.

High serum potassium is quite a bit more complex and complicated than that because there are other conditions that can cause the serum potassium to be high that has nothing to do with renal failure. Assuming that the high potassium is due to kidney failure, then this occurs because the kidneys are unable to get rid of the breakdown products of proteins, which contain potassium plus potassium ingested as foods or beverages.

This also occurs because of electrolyte abnormalities of different types that cause the kidneys either to reabsorb too much potassium or to be unable to excrete enough potassium to maintain good potassium tolerance. The potassium accumulates in the blood, risking severe cardiac arrhythmias with potential lethal consequences if not brought down with either medications or dialysis.

Low serum bicarbonate known as acidosis, though important, is less crucial because the human body is made to tolerate acidosis much better than alkalosis the reverse of acidosis meaning the serum bicarbonate is high.

When the serum bicarbonate is high, low potassium result, which is as serious as high potassium in causing cardiac arrhythmias that, can lead to sudden death. Medications and/or dialysis can correct acidosis and high potassium.

The high serum BUN is a reflection of the inability of the kidneys to function well enough to get rid of the breakdown products of proteins. High BUN and creatinine are some of the indices of kidney failure. Even though high BUN and creatinine are important indices of renal failure, by themselves, they do not represent a threat to the life of a patient. However, when the BUN and creatinine are high, the potassium is at the critical level of 6.5 or greater. If the phosphate is high, the serum calcium is low, the creatinine clearance is 10 ml per minute or less, and the patient looks and feels sick, then the time has arrived for dialysis to start.

High phosphatase is a very important abnormality that must be corrected quickly because as the phosphatase goes up, the serum calcium goes down and the low serum calcium is potentially deadly because low calcium can cause cardiac arrhythmias, seizures, tetany with muscle cramps and twitching. Examining the blood for possible elevation of both total and indirect bilirubins is important because in acute and severe hemolysis, the kidney can acutely fail due to the clogging effect of debris from red blood cells, damaging the tubules of the kidneys.

Testing the blood for serum albumin is very important in renal failure because as the kidneys fail they allow protein to pass into the urine, reducing the serum albumin. This, in turn, causes fluid to pass into the extravascular compartment of the body, resulting in swelling of the abdomen and lower extremities, etc. This set of problems is referred to as "nephrotic syndrome." In nephrotic syndrome, the patient passes three (3) grams of protein or greater in the urine over a 24-hour period.

Testing the blood for total protein is very important because there are conditions such as multiple myeloma and other types of plasma cell dyscrasias in which the total protein is elevated and when protein is elevated, many bad things can happen, including a condition called hyperviscosity syndrome. If viscosity syndrome develops, the patient may experience blurred vision, dizziness, unsteady gait, memory loss, etc.
The acute treatment for hyperviscosity syndrome is plasma pheresis.

In multiple myeloma, renal failure occurs because light chain proteins filter out of the kidneys, resulting in severe damage to the kidney tubules, which causes renal insufficiency or renal failure to develop. There is a form of myeloma called light chain myeloma in which the total protein is typically low and this is so because the light chains are passing out in the urine in large quantities and not accumulating in the blood to be reflected as elevated total protein.

As the light chain proteins pass through the kidneys' tubules, the light chain proteins damage the kidneys.

In fact, light chain myeloma is more frequently associated with renal failure than multiple myeloma. Multiple myeloma is much more common in black and Hispanics than in whites and other racial groups. Therefore, it stands to reason that more balcks and Hispanics suffer from myeloma kidney than do whites are.

It is very important to test the blood for lactic dehydrogenase (LDH). For example, an elevated LDH may be seen in a patient who has an occult cancer that no one knows about yet. Sometimes many routine blood tests and the physical examination are normal but the LDH, BUN and serum creative are elevated. This could be a case of lymphoma, because in lymphoma and other cancers, the cancer cells grow via the anaerobic pathway, meaning that these cells grow in the absence of oxygen.

When cells grow in the absence of oxygen, lactic acid is produced as the product of the anaerobic pathway and lactic acid leads to lactic dehydrogenase (LDH). Therefore, a unilateral elevation of LDH in association with acute renal failure can mean one of several things:

1. Acute lymphoma with rapid cancer cell turnover, resulting in large breakdown products of protein making it difficult for the kidneys to filter them out in the urine, and the result is acute renal failure.
2. When the LHD is unilaterally high, it could be acute hemolysis due to hemolytic anemia or any other number of medical problems that can cause red blood cells to hemolyze.

Once hemolysis occurs, the by-products of the red cells will clog up the kidney tubules, which can result in acute renal failure. Blacks and Hispanics as well have the propensity to hemolyze because of sickle cell disease, thalassemia and sickle thalassemia, etc., and if these hemolytic episodes are not handled in a proper clinical way, acute renal failure can be one of the results. Some women of Greek and Italian ethnic background also have the propensity to have hemolitic diseases such as the beta thalassemia.

Elevation of serum creatinine phosphokinase (CPK) can be very important in the development of acute renal failure. There are many medical conditions that cause the CPK to be elevated so high as to be threatening to the health of the kidneys.

Among these conditions are rhabdomyolysis, caused by severe muscle trauma, severe seizure with muscle damage, muscle trauma because of a long march with trauma to the feet. Trauma to muscle because of marathon bongo drum beating with hands; all these conditions and more can cause damage to the skeletal muscles, resulting in acute damage to the tubules of the kidneys, which, if not treated properly, can cause kidney failure.

Therefore, when a patient presents with unexplained acute failure, testing the serum for elevation of CPK is an important thing to do. Any one of the statin anti-cholesterol medications can, at times, cause muscle breakdown, which if not recognized and properly treated, can lead to acute renal failure.

Doing a complete blood count in a patient who presents with acute renal failure is extremely important. Three parts of the CBC that a physician caring for a patient with acute renal failure must be concerned with:

1. The white blood cell count (WBC)
2. The platelet count
3. The hematocrit

A WBC of greater than 100,000 with lymphocytosis represents evidence of lymphoproliferative disorder out of control. The rapid cell turnover that occurs in this condition results in the production of a large amount of purine, a protein breakdown product that can clog the kidney tubules, resulting in acute renal failure.

If the platelet count is found to be very low, less than 40,000-50,000, in association with acute renal failure, that could mean several things. Low platelets, low hematocrit and acute renal failure could be seen in DIC, TTP, sepsis, Evan's syndrome as seen in SLE, leukemia or lymphoma, red cell transfusion reaction, AIDS, etc. Low hematocrit and acute renal failure could mean acute hemolysis with debris from the break-up of red cells clogging the kidney tubules, resulting in acute renal failure such as what occurs in thrombotic thrombocytopenia purpura (TTP). 1, 200 individuals in the U.S. develop TTP every year.

TTP causes renal failure because it is a small vessels disease that causes platelets to aggregate forming clots inside small vessels inside the kidneys preventing and oxygen to go to the kidneys. Abnormality in the activity of ADAMTS13 enzyme is responsible for hereditary TTP by its adverse effects on Von Willebrand factor.

Acquired TTP can occur because of

1. Cancer
2. Pregnancy
3. HIV/AIDS
4. Infection
5. Lupus
6. Some chemotherapy

7. Ticlopidine
8. Plavix
9. Cyclosporine A
10. Birth control pills and other estrogenic hormones etc;

TTP affects other organs beside the kidney, It also affects:

1. The Skin
2. The blood system
3. The brain
4. The heart

Symptoms and signs of TTP include:

1. Bleeding
2. Purpura (bleeding in the skin)
3. Thrombocytopenia (low platelets)
4. Anemia
5. Kidney failure
6. Stroke
7. Coma
8. Seizure
9. Cardiac arrhythmia ect;

The best ways to evaluate kidney failure due to TTP are:

1. Complete history physical examination
2. CBC
3. SMA20
4. Urinalysis
5. CPK
6. LDH
7. PT& INR
8. PPT
9. Glomerular filtration rate (GFR)
10. Plasma fibrinogen
11. Peripheral blood smear
12. Urinary sodium
13. Renal ultra sound
14. Chest x ray
15. EKG
16. Brain CT Scan with no contrast
17. Brain MRI with no contrast

18. EEG

The best treatments available to treat TTP associated kidney failure are:
Infusion of fresh frozen plasma, plasmapheresis, and aspirin by mouth or in suppository form if a patient is too sick to take it by mouth may be given.

Even though a patient may be bleeding because the platelet count is low, Aspirin is needed to disaggregate platelet on the one hand and to prevent further platelet aggregations on the other hand.

Dialysis is used to remove wastes from the body if the kidneys failed. Both acquired and hereditary TTP can have recurrent flare up 30-60 of the times necessitating treatments. The disease that is similar to TTP that can cause the kidney to fail is hemolytic uremic syndrome (HUS).

HUS is similar to TTP in that platelets aggregate inside small vessels in the body preventing blood and oxygen to freely flow to different organs in the body. The result are low platelets and hemolytic anemia. Hemolytic anemia occurs because as red blood cells try to pass through the vessels that are occluded with platelets and clots inside the small vessels, they get damaged resulting in microangiopathic hemolytic anemia.

The mechanism of platelets aggregation and clot formation occur in HUS because a substance such as endotoxin damages the inside small blood vessels, allowing platelets to get trapped which starts the platelets aggregation and clot forming process.
The most common cause of HUS is food poisoning (acute gastroenteritis) secondary to E.Coli OH157:H7 which occurs as result of contaminated hamburgers or other meat products. Other things that can cause HUS include:

1. Pneumonia cause by Steptococcus pneumonia bacteria
2. Ticlid
3. Quinine
4. AIDS etc;

Symptoms of HUS include:

1. Fever
2. Abdominal pain
3. Nausea
4. Vomiting
5. Diarrhea (sometimes blood)
6. Weakness
7. The best ways to evaluate HUS include:
8. Complete history and physical examination

9. CBC
10. Microscopic examination of peripheral blood smear, looking for schistocytes and helmet cells, if present, this establishes the diagnosis of HUS. Blood smear of patients with TTP,
11. Does not have schistocytes and helmet cells.
12. Reticulocytes count
13. Direct comb's test
14. SMA20
15. LDH
16. Urinalysis
17. Urine culture
18. Stools culture
19. Blood culture
20. Sputum culture and gram stain of sputum if there is a productive cough
21. Chest x ray
22. EKG
23. Abdominal ultrasound
24. Renal ultrasound

The following abnormalities are usually found in HUS:

1. Microangiopathic hemolytic anemia
2. Thrombocytopenia (low platelet count)
3. High reticulocyte count
4. High LDH
5. High indirect bilirubin
6. High alkaline phosphatase
7. High BUN
8. High serum creatinine
9. Low serum potassium (when the patient is vomiting and having diarrhea)
10. High serum potassium (when the kidneys failed)
11. High serum sodium
12. High serum bicarbonate (C02) (when the patient is vomiting and having diarrhea)
13. Low serum bicarbonate (C02) (when the kidneys failed)
14. Abnormal urinalysis with both protein and red blood cells found in the urine.
15. Sometimes anuria and kidney failure.

The treatments of HUS include:

IV fluid
Electrolyte replacement
Anti-fever medication (specifically (Tylenol by either mouth or suppository)

IV antibiotic to cover for both E. Coli OH157:H7 and for possible Streptococcus
Pneumonia
Folic acid
Anti—nausea medication
Anti—diarrhea medication
Pain medication
Plasmapherisis
Blood transfusion when the hemoglobin drops to less than 7 grams
Dialysis if renal failure develops.

In the pediatric age group, HUS is self limiting and supportive care with IV fluid and electrolyte replacement may be all the treatments that are necessary.

an other significant differentiating point between HUS and TTP, beside the angiopathic hemolytic anemia is the fact; in HUS the brain is never affected.

To prevent the devastation of the kidneys that leads to kidney failure, hypertensive and diabetic women have to decrease the salt and simple carbohydrate in their diets by half. Rather than eating an average of 7-8 grams of sodium per day, they ought to eat 3-4 grams of sodium per day. The decrease in sodium will decrease high blood pressure in women, which in turn will decrease their incidence of kidney failure.

Another common cause of kidney disease in Blacks, Hispanics and many other ethnic groups is sickle cell anemia. Sickle cell anemia damages the kidneys, because of both the occlusive and its inflammatory nature. Blood and oxygen flow to the glomeruli of the kidneys are both impaired, resulting ultimately in a significant percentage of people suffering with sickle cell disease developing end-stage renal failure requiring dialysis. Sickle cell trait often causes papillary necrosis, causing bleeding from the kidney, often the right kidney.

When hypertension, diabetes mellitus and sickle cell disease exist in same person, the incidence of kidney failure increases. Blood pressure of 130/80 is normal in a person not suffering from sickle cell disease, but in someone with sickle cell anemia, this is hypertension.

1. The most effective treatments for renal failure are a low-salt and low-protein diet.
2. When the renal function deteriorates to the point that the BUN and the creatinine are excessively high, along with high serum potassium, high phosphatase, low calcium and a very low creatinine clearance combined with evidence of uremia, dialysis becomes necessary.

Two types of dialysis are in routine use:

1. Peritoneal dialysis
2. Hemodialysis.

In the U.S. more than 500,000 people undergo dialysis yearly and wordwide about 2 million people receive dialysis on a regular basis.

More than 50,000 people died of kidney disease every year in the U.S. and worldwide 57 million people die yearly from kidney disease. The annual cost of kidney disease in the U.S. is 60 billion dollars.

Different clinical situations along with the patient's preference will help to determine which type of dialysis will be used to treat the individual patient with end-stage renal failure. Kidney transplant is an available option for some patients, if a match can be found.

"*

Country/Region	Extrapolated Incidence	Population Estimated Used
Kidney transplant in <u>North America</u> (Extrapolated Statistics)		
USA	16,551	314,831,647 (2012)
Canada	1,832	32,507,874
Mexico	5,915	104,959,594
Kidney transplant in Central America (Extrapolated Statistics)		
Belize	15	272,945
Guatemala	804	14,280,596
Nicaragua	302	5,359,759
Kidney transplant in Caribbean (Extrapolated Statistics)		
Puerto Rico	219	3,897,960
Kidney transplant in <u>South America</u> (Extrapolated Statistics)		
Brazil	10,376	184,101,109
Chile	891	15,823,957
Colombia	2,384	42,310,775
Paraguay	348	6,191,368
Peru	1,552	27,544,305
Venezuela	1,410	25,017,387
Kidney transplant in Northern Europe (Extrapolated Statistics)		
Denmark	305	5,413,392
Finland	293	5,214,512
Iceland	16	293,966
Sweden	506	8,986,400
Kidney transplant in Western Europe (Extrapolated Statistics)		
Britain (<u>United Kingdom</u>)	3,397	60,270,708 for UK
Belgium	583	10,348,276
France	3,405	60,424,213
Ireland	223	3,969,558
Luxembourg	26	462,690
Monaco	1	32,270
Netherlands (Holland)	919	16,318,199
United Kingdom	3,397	60,270,708
Wales	164	2,918,000
Kidney transplant in Central Europe (Extrapolated Statistics)		
Austria	460	8,174,762
Czech Republic	70	1,0246,178
Germany	4,645	82,424,609

Hungary	565	10,032,375
Liechtenstein	1	33,436
Poland	2,177	38,626,349
Slovakia	305	5,423,567
Slovenia	113	2,011,473
Switzerland	419	7,450,867
Kidney transplant in Eastern Europe (Extrapolated Statistics)		
Belarus	581	10,310,520
Estonia	75	1,341,664
Latvia	129	2,306,306
Lithuania	203	3,607,899
Russia	8,114	143,974,059
Ukraine	2,690	47,732,079
Kidney transplant in the Southwestern Europe (Extrapolated Statistics)		
Azerbaijan	443	7,868,385
Portugal	593	10,524,145
Spain	2,270	40,280,780
Georgia	264	4,693,892
Kidney transplant in the Southern Europe (Extrapolated Statistics)		
Italy	3,272	58,057,477
Greece	600	10,647,529
Kidney transplant in the Southeastern Europe (Extrapolated Statistics)		
Albania	199	3,544,808
Bosnia and Herzegovina	22	407,608
Bulgaria	423	7,517,973
Croatia	253	4,496,869
Macedonia	114	2,040,085
Romania	1,260	22,355,551
Serbia and Montenegro	610	10,825,900
Kidney transplant in Northern Asia (Extrapolated Statistics)		
Mongolia	155	2,751,314
Kidney transplant in Central Asia (Extrapolated Statistics)		
Kazakhstan	853	15,143,704
Tajikistan	395	7,011,556
Uzbekistan	1,488	26,410,416
Kidney transplant in Eastern Asia (Extrapolated Statistics)		

China	73,208	1,298,847,624
Hong Kong s.a.r.	386	6,855,125
Japan	7,176	127,333,002
Macau s.a.r.	25	445,286
North Korea	1,279	22,697,553
South Korea	2,718	48,233,760
Taiwan	1,282	22,749,838
Kidney transplant in Southwestern Asia (Extrapolated Statistics)		
Turkey	3,883	68,893,918
Kidney transplant in Southern Asia (Extrapolated Statistics)		
Afghanistan	1,607	28,513,677
Bangladesh	7,966	141,340,476
Bhutan	123	2,185,569
India	60,031	1,065,070,607
Pakistan	8,972	159,196,336
Sri Lanka	1,121	19,905,165
Kidney transplant in Southeastern Asia (Extrapolated Statistics)		
East Timor	57	1,019,252
Indonesia	13,440	238,452,952
Laos	342	6,068,117
Malaysia	1,325	23,522,482
Philippines	4,860	86,241,697
Singapore	245	4,353,893
Thailand	3,656	64,865,523
Vietnam	4,659	82,662,800
Kidney transplant in the Middle East (Extrapolated Statistics)		
Gaza strip	74	1,324,991
Iran	3,804	67,503,205
Iraq	1,430	25,374,691
Israel	349	6,199,008
Jordan	316	5,611,202
Kuwait	127	2,257,549
Lebanon	212	3,777,218
Saudi Arabia	1,453	25,795,938
Syria	1,015	18,016,874
United Arab Emirates	142	2,523,915
West Bank	130	2,311,204
Yemen	1,128	20,024,867

Kidney transplant in Northern Africa (Extrapolated Statistics)		
Egypt	4,290	76,117,421
Libya	317	5,631,585
Sudan	2,206	39,148,162
Kidney transplant in Western Africa (Extrapolated Statistics)		
Congo Brazzaville	168	2,998,040
Ghana	1,169	20,757,032
Liberia	191	3,390,635
Niger	640	11,360,538
Nigeria	1,000	12,5750,356
Senegal	611	10,852,147
Sierra leone	331	5,883,889
Kidney transplant in Central Africa (Extrapolated Statistics)		
Central African Republic	210	3,742,482
Chad	537	9,538,544
Congo kinshasa	3,286	58,317,030
Rwanda	464	8,238,673
Kidney transplant in Eastern Africa (Extrapolated Statistics)		
Ethiopia	4,020	71,336,571
Kenya	1,859	32,982,109
Somalia	468	8,304,601
Tanzania	2,033	36,070,799
Uganda	1,487	26,390,258
Kidney transplant in Southern Africa (Extrapolated Statistics)		
Angola	618	10,978,552
Botswana	92	1,639,231
South Africa	2,505	44,448,470
Swaziland	65	1,169,241
Zambia	621	11,025,690
Zimbabwe	206	1,2671,860
Kidney transplant in Oceania (Extrapolated Statistics)		
Australia	1,122	19,913,144
New Zealand	225	3,993,817
Papua New Guinea	305	5,420,280

"

*—Modified and updated

Total number of kidney transplants 329,182 was based on when the population was 6 billion.

In July 13, 2013 the population was 7,097,800,000

Chapter 7

GENITAL AND URINARY TRACT DISEASES IN MEN

Sexually transmitted diseases (STD) show much higher rates among some racial or ethnic minority groups than among whites". The rates of STDs are higher among black and other minorities than whites in the U.S. Source: CDC

Every year there are 19 millions new STDs in the U.S. There are 65 million individuals living with curable sexually transmitted diseases in the U.S.

Worldwide there were 499 million cases of STDs in 2013. Source: WHO

The most common STDs in the world and that also affect men are

Gonorrhea
Chlamydia
Syphilis
Trichomoniasis
Chancroid
Genital herpes
Genital warts
Hepatitis B
Hepatitis C
HIV/AIDS
HPV

The most common STDs in the U.S. in 2009 were:

Gonorrhea 301,174, 99.1 per 100,000
Chlamydia 1,244,180, 409.2 per 100,000
Syphilis 13,997, 4.6 per 100,000

"Blacks accounted for 71% of all gonorrhea cases in 2009. The gonorrhea rate among blacks was 20 times higher than whites". Source: CDC.

In 2007, the rates of syphilis were 28.2% in black males and 5.7% in white males in the U.S. The rates of Chlamydia were 8 times higher in blacks than whites, 1,398.7

cases per 100, 000 and 162.3 cases per 100,000. The rates of Gonorrhea were 662.9 cases per 100.000 among blacks and 19.1 cases per 100,000 among whites.

Genital herpes is a very common sexually transmitted disease. 68 million individuals are infected with Herpes Viruses I and II in the United States of America and about 1 million people become infected every year with these Herpes Viruses. Herpes Simplex Type II causes about 90 percent of genital herpes infections and Herpes Simplex Type I causes about 10 percent. 1 in 6 people in the U.S is infected with Genital Herpes. Genital herpes is most often transmitted during sexual intercourse or during oral sex with an infected partner.

It is possible for a man to transmit the herpes infection from a buttock or lip lesion; for example, from touching the infected area with his bare hand, then touch his genital area. Within 3 to 7 days after exposure, the first symptoms of genital herpes infection appear. The first symptoms are a burning or tingling pain or paresthesia in the perineal area. Genital herpes is 2 times higher African Americans than among whites. The incidence genital herpes is quite high among African American men and 40% of African American adults are infected with genital herpes. Source: CDC

The next thing that may happen is the development of a crop of small, water filled lesions, which are quite itchy. Sometimes, the affected man may feel a low-grade feverish feeling. The pain in the penis area may be quite severe with extreme tenderness on touching. Once the lesions break open, the area affected becomes more painful.

Lymph node enlargement in the inguinal area is common and often these lymph nodes can are tender and painful. In men who have AIDS, these herpetic lesions can accelerate in a severe and disabling manner all the way to the perianal area requiring hospitalization for intravenous medications and intramuscular pain medications to help ease the pain in these types of herpes infected men.

A man infected with herpes simplex may be able to infect a sexual partner during intercourse, even though he has no open herpetic sores. This occurs because of micro-tissue abresions that normally take place during sexual intercourse, allowing for men's or women's blood to enter into his or her sexual partner, resulting in the transmission of the herpes virus.

The incidence of genital herpes is quite high in males and herpes infection of the genital spares no ethnic groups and socioeconomic status. Any man who is sexually active can become infected with the herpes virus and this is particularly so if she has sexual intercourse without the use of a condom.

The diagnosis of herpes infection of the genital area can be made by culture taken from the infected areas or by rupturing the vesicles and culturing the fluid within them with clean culturette, place the culturette in a special herpes liquid medium in a tube, and send the tube to the microbiology lab for processing.

Sraping the ulcerated area on a clean slide and send it to the lab for a Zanck stain can also use to diagnose herpes. The culturing of the herpes infection is much more specific and definite evidence of the presence of the herpes infection if the culture is positive. Herpes infections tend to recur in the same area repeatedly. Stressful situations tend to cause the herpetic lesions to come back.

Some of the stresses that can cause the recurrence of herpes infections are the common cold, and stress associated with taking examinations in schools, work related stress, indigestion, etc. These stressful situations increase the level of adrenalin which has a lowing effect on the immune system allowing the dormant herpes infection to wake up and proliferate, causing the recurrence of the disease.

Treatment of Herpes Infection

If the genital herpes infection is more diffused and the patient is immunosuppressed the treatment is intravenous acyclovir. If the herpes infection is localized, the treatment is acyclovir by mouth or if the infection is localized and mild, acyclovir cream will help to relieve the symptoms but medication by mouth is needed, in addition. The question is how long to treat. Primarily, Genital herpes should be treated with acyclovir 200 mg by mouth, 5 times a day for 10 days or Valtrex 1000 mg by mouth, 2 times per day for 10 days.

Teatment for recurrent genital herpes is Valtrex 500 mg by mouth, 2 times per day for 5 days or acyclovir 400 mg by mouth, 3 times per day or Famvir 250 mg by mouth, 2 times per day for 5 days. The treatment for suppression of chronic genital herpes is Famvir 250 mg by mouth, 2 times per day or Valtrex 500 mg by mouth daily or acyclovir 400 mg 2 times per day.

This virus is very difficult to treat because it is slow growing, has a thick capsule, has the ability to hide for a very long time in the human body, and flares up on and off causing miseries for those who are infected. Therefore, the treatment for recurrent flare up of herpes infection may be for life.

Some of the most common signs and symptoms of STDs in men include:

Urethral discharge
Burning on urination
Genital ulcer
Swelling in the scrotum

Swelling in the inguinal area (bubo)

Lower abdominal pain

Fever etc;

Gnorrheal infection can become systemic and present with fever, chills, swollen and painful joints. When fluid is removed from a swollen joint, the fluid must be sent to the laboratory for cells count, gram stain, culture, protein, glucose, and LDH.

If the protein is high, the glucose is low, the cells count shows high white cells, and the differential count shows a high segmented polys, and Gram stain shows gram negative diplococci, this is indication of systemic gonorrheal infection with septic arthritis.

How to Diagnose Gonorrhea / Chlamydia in men

Urethral discharge is taken from the meatus of the penis, place on in a culture medium, and send to the microbiology laboratory for culture and gram stain and DNA probe. Some times, men have no symptoms of urethritis, are carrying chronic Gonorrhea/Chlamydia, and are able to transfer these infections in their ejaculate during sexual intercourse. The approach to treatment of Gonorrheal and chlamydial infections in men is guided by the clinical presentation.

How to treat Suspected or uncomplicated Gonorrhea/ Chlamydia in the office / outpatient Clinic:

The treatment is Ceftriaxone 250 mg IM in one dose with Doxycycline 100 mg 2 x per day for 14 days and. Alternatively, the patient can be treated with Floxin 400 mg by mouth twice per day, or Zithromax 500mg 2 tablets taken by mouth at the same time if Chlamydia is the suspected infection. If Gonorrhea is the suspected infection, then the same regimen can be used, except that the dose of Zithromax must be 3 grams by mouth taken at the same time.

Ceftriaxone is the best medication available to treat uncomplicated or suspected Gonorrhea intramuscularly in the office or in the clinic. Ceftriaxone, however, will not treat chlamydia and since it is oftentimes impossible to tell Gonorrhea from chlamydia, it is wise to treat for both by adding Doxycycline, Floxin, or Zithromax. These three medications are efficacious against Chlamydia. Floxin and Zithromax are both effective against both Gonorrhea and Chlamydia. Gonorrheal infection can be very complicated.

It is critical to tap the joint fluid and send it to the lab for gram stain, cell count, and culture. Treatment of Gonorrheal arthritis must be started immediately to prevent the destruction of the affected joint or joints.

In-Hospital Treatment of Gonorrhea

Ceftriaxone—2 grams IV every 12 hours

Doxycycline—100 mg p.o. or IV every 12 hours until the culture result is back from the laboratory.

Alternatively, Clindamycin—900 mg IV every 8 hours in addition to Gentamycin—2 mg/KG IM or IV and once the patient is improved then add Doxycycline—100 mg by mouth every 12 hours to complete a 14-day course.

Patients who cannot tolerate Doxycycline or who are allergic to Penicillin can be treated with Norfloxin 400 mg IV every 12 hours.

Once the culture result and sensitivity are back from the laboratory, then specific antibiotics can be used to treat the infection.

Prevention of Gonorrhea or Chlamydia Infection

1. Teenagers and older men ought not to be engaging in frivolous and irresponsible sexual intercourse.
2. They ought to strive to remain monogamous.
3. If they cannot abstain from sexual intercourse, then they must insist that their sexual partners use a condom during sexual intercourse. The use of a good condom not only prevents STD but also prevents unplanned or unwanted pregnancies.

The incidence of STD amongst working and middle class men in the United States and around the world is no less than it is amongst men of poorer socioeconomic status.

The incidence of STD in general is higher amongst young men from adolescence to adulthood because they frequently are less responsible about their sexual behavior.

There are 19 million new cases of STD (not including AIDS) reported annually in the United States according to a recent report by the Institute of Medicine. One-fourth of these cases are among teenagers according to that report. 22 percent of people above the age of 15 are carrying the herpes infection. It costs taxpayers $16.4 billion per year to treat STD in the United States. By the 11th grade, 70 percent of teenagers have had sexual intercourse and 40 percent of them have had four or more sexual partners.

In Chlamydia urethratis a few days after having sexual intercourse with an infected woman, the man will feel a burning sensation inside his penis. Around the same time, the man will see a slightly yellow to clear discharge coming out of his penis. At times there may be pain in the groin with low grade fever and burning on urination.

There are 2.8 million cases of Chlamydia annually in the U.S. As such, Chlamydia is the most commonly reported bacterial STD in the United States (According to the CDC). "Chlamydia rates in African Americans are eight times higher than in white Americans".

Chlomydia trachomatis is the most nationally reported STD in the US. In 2006, 1,031,000 cases of Chlamydia were reported by health departments in different localities in the U.S. Men become infected with Chlamydia through unprotected sexual intercourse. Men pass the infection to men in their ejaculates causing a mucopurulent endocervical discharge.

Some of the acute and chronic urethral complications of Gonorrhea and Chlamydia infections include:

1. Prostatitis
2. Epididymitis
3. Uretrhal stricture

Acute prostatitis in young sexually active men occurs usually because of Gonorrhea or Chlamydia infection. In older men, benign prostatic hypertrophy (BPH) is usually the cause of prostatitis. Chronic prostatitis is very difficult to treat because the prostate gland sits inside a very thick capsule which makes it very difficult for antibiotic to penetrate to kill the bacteria causing the infection. Frequently, a urologist has to massage the prostate gland in order to get the thick and mucoid material out of the prostate gland. Acute prostatitis can cause fever, chills, lower abdominal pain, pain in the groin, burning on urination and urinary frequency, malaise, vomiting, constipation, urinary retention etc;

Chronic prostatitis can cause many of the above symptoms on a recurrent basis plus, a dull lower abdominal pain, pain in the perianal area and discharge from the penis.

Evaluations of prostatitis include:

1. Taking a good history from the patient
2. Physical examination
3. Digital rectal examination of the prostate gland

It is not a good idea to massage the prostate gland in acute prostatitis because; this might lead to the spread of the infection into the blood stream leading to septicemia. If the patient has chills and high fever, this means that the infection has already spread into the blood stream and sepsis exists. In the setting of sepsis, urine and blood cultures must be taken and the patient needs in hospital treatment with IV antibiotic.

The preferred antibiotics in the setting of acute prostatitis with sepsis are
1. Ceftriaxone 2 grams IV every 12 hours plus Doxycycline 100mg twice per day by mouth for 7 days or Levaquin 750mg IV every 24 hours plus Doxycycline 100mg twice per for 7 days or Zithromax 500mg IV daily for 2 days followed by 500mg by mouth to complete a 10 day course of treatment. These combinations of antibiotics provide treatment for both Gonorrhea and Chlamydia.

For treatment of acute prostatitis with no fever, the choices of antibiotics are

1. Zithromax 500mg by mouth daily for 2 weeks or
2. Levaquin 250mg by mouth for 10 days
3. Floxin 400mg by mouth twice per day for 28 days or
4. Cipro 500mg by mouth for 2 weeks

Chronic prostatitis is treated with the same antibiotics as above, but the duration of treatment time is longer based on the clinical circumstances.

Epididymitis is acute and painful infection of the epididymis a tube located inside the testicle. Epididymitis is usually caused by STDs like Chlamydia and Gonorrhea in men between the ages of 20 to 40 years old. It causes swelling and redness of the affected testicle resulting in excruciating pain, some time associated with fever and chills. E. Coli can also cause epididymitis as well.

The diagnosis is made usually by the history, physical examination and if necessary ultrasound of the affected testicle. Treatments include antibiotics such as Levaquin, Floxin, Zitrhomax, Doxycycline, or Ceftriaxone, pain medication, Tylenol for fever, and bed rest. Any man with epididymitis needs to see a urologist.

Uretrhal stricture occurs because recurrent infection inside the urethra due to STDs such as Chlamydia or Gonorrhea. Trauma and viral infection can sometimes cause urethral stricture as well.

Symptoms of urethral stricture include:

Dribbling on urination
Intermittent urination
Incomplete empting of the bladder
Deflection of urination
Lack of urinary force
Frequent micturation

Some of the complications of urethral stricture include:
Urinary retention

> Urinary tract infection
> Inguinal hernia
> Hemorrhoids
> Rectal prolapse from straining
> Bilateral hydronephrosis

> The diagnosis is made by urethroscopy and urethrography
> Urethral stricture is treated by frequent dilatation or by bougies

Syphilis Infection

Syphilis has historically been one of the most common STDs to afflict mankind and has been in the new world since 1494 when Columbus and his men came to America. Syphilis is caused by the spirochete Treponema Pallidum.

"In the year 2008-2009 the number primary, early latent, late, late latent and congenital syphilis was 44,828 cases in the U.S. according to the CDC".

Worldwide hundred of millions of people are infected with syphilis and about 1.5 million pregnant women in the world are infected with syphilis resulting hundred of thousands of still birth and many thousands of congenital syphilis every year. Source: WHO

Syphilis is usually transmitted sexually, or from mother to baby. Once the organism is deposited into the human tissue it takes anywhere from 14 to 21 days for primary syphilis to develop.

In men, the parts of their genitalia first affected by early syphilis are the labia, fourchette or cervix. "During 2008-2009, the rate of primary syphilis increased in all racial and ethnic groups except non-Hispanic whites and Hispanics". The rate increased 11.6% among non-Hispanic blacks and non-Hispanic whites." CDC

In 2009, the rate primary syphilis was higher among non-Hispanic black men compare to white men. CDC-STD Surveillance. 2009

The first manifestation of primary syphilis is a chancre, which is often a painless sore. The chancre or syphilitic ulcer may be seen in the mouth, lips, arms, rectum, nipples, naval (belly button), etc. If left untreated, by 4 to 8 weeks the chancre would heal spontaneously. Untreated syphilis spreads via the lymphatic system to disseminate throughout the body to cause secondary syphilis.

The first manifestation of secondary syphilis is usually a rash over the body. The rash can occur in the palms of the hands and sometimes under the feet. The rash is often scaly, smooth and it may be itchy. This type of rash may resemble other rashes and may be difficult to distinguish just by looking at it. Because secondary syphilis is a systemic disease, it can cause sore throat, headache, fever, weight loss with aches and pains. There may be large glands in the neck, under the arms and elsewhere in the body.

After going through the primary and secondary stage in about 12 weeks, if syphilis remains untreated, then it enters into the latent stage. Many men may have symptoms and signs of primary and secondary syphilis without recognizing them. In about 2 years time if syphilis remains untreated, it enters into the tertiary stage. Tertiary syphilis is an advanced stage of syphilis, which can affect the heart, the liver, the brain, and other vital organs.

The chronic involvement of vital organs with untreated syphilis is guaranteed to cause death of individuals infected with it. Syphilis can cause a person to become paralyzed and can cause a person to develop seizures and even insanity due to changes in the brain.

Three outrageous, shameful, disgraceful, and inhuman and illegal experiments were done the past that allow for an understanding of chronic and devastating effects of untreated syphilis on the human body.

The first study was the Oslo study, which took place between 1891 and 1951. It included 2000 patients diagnosed clinically. The dark field test and Wasserman test were not yet in existence. Penicillin had not yet been discovered either so there was no effective way to treat these patients.

That study amply demonstrated the devastating effects of untreated syphilis on all parts of the human body, in particular, the brain, the aorta, the skeletal system, etc.

The second study was the infamous **Tuskegee study**, which took place from 1932-1974 in Tuskegee, Alabama under the control of the **United States Public Health Service.**

The shameful reason given for **this cruel, inhumane, barbaric, and racist study** was to find the effects of untreated syphilis on the human body. There were no scientific justifications for this study in view of the fact that the Oslo study had already shown all the bad things that untreated syphilis did to the human body.

From 1932 to 1974, under the leadership of the United States Public Health Service, 431 (Negro men) black men were injected with live syphilis organisms for the sole purpose of seeing what effects syphilis would have on their bodies. These

men did not sign consent for participating in the study. They did not know that they were being injected with live syphilis organisms.

The third study came to light in 2010 when a report came out showing that some of the same American scientists involved in the infamous Tuskegee study also carried out an experiment in Guatemala, injecting syphilis in 696 men and women Guatemalan prisoners, people with mental illness, and prostitutes. The experiments were carried out to test the effects of penicillin on STDs during 1946 to 1948. This discovery was made by a Wellesley College medical historian.

The U.S. Secretary of State Hillary Rodham Clinton and the Secretary of Health and Human Services Kathleen Sebelius apologized to the Guatemalan Government and the Guatemalan people for the actions of these American Scientists. Tax payer's money through the National Institute of Health financed the Guatemalan syphilis study.

The present U.S. Government under the direction of President Obam has ordered an investigation to be carried out by a Presidential Commission and the Institute of Medicine to find out what happened in the Guatemalan syphilis experiment.

In the history of the world, many events have taken place to catalogue men's cruelty towards each other: **Slavery, the Holocaust, the Rwanda Massacre, and the Tuskegee Study** and the Guatemalan syphilis experiment are a few such examples. In the Tuskegee Study, 431 men were sacrificed for nothing other than racism and bigotry, while the U.S. government, organized medicine, some black and white physicians, some white and black hospital administrators and society, at large, stood by silently. **How shameful and how disgusting?**

The first manifestation of primary syphilis is a chancre, which is often a painless sore. The chancre or syphilitic ulcer may be seen in the mouth, lips, arms, rectum, nipples, naval (belly button), etc. If left untreated, by 4 to 8 weeks the chancre would heal spontaneously.

Untreated syphilis spreads via the lymphatic system to disseminate throughout the body to cause secondary syphilis.

The first manifestation of secondary syphilis is usually a rash over the body. The rash can occur in the palms of the hands and sometimes under the feet. The rash is often scaly, smooth and it may be itchy. This type of rash may resemble other rashes and may be difficult to distinguish just by looking at it. Because secondary syphilis is a systemic disease, it can cause sore throat, headache, fever, weight loss with aches and pains. There may be large glands in the neck, under the arms and elsewhere in the body.

The physician has to be suspicious enough to order a blood test for syphilis. A scraping from the rash can be studied via dark field technique, which might show the spirochetes treponoma pallidum wiggling around under the microscope. Similarly, "scraping material" taken from the chancre seen in primary syphilis when placed on a glass slide, and covered with a cover slip and placed under the microscope will show the spirochetes, as well.

Other things that secondary syphilis may cause include arthritis, hepatitis, condyloma, uveitis, iritis, otitis, CVA, kidney problems such as glomerulo nephritis, hepatitis, weight loss, poor appetite, memory loss, seizure, meningitis, myocarditis, heart block, cardiac arrhythmias, heart failure, kidney failure etc.

After going through the primary and secondary stage in about 12 weeks, if syphilis remains untreated, then it enters into the latent stage. Many men may have symptoms and signs of primary and secondary syphilis without recognizing them.

In about 2 years time if syphilis remains untreated, it enters into the tertiary stage.
Tertiary syphilis is an advanced stage of syphilis, which can affect the heart, the liver, the brain, and other vital organs including neuro-syphilis. The chronic involvement of vital organs with untreated syphilis is guaranteed to cause death of individuals infected with it. Syphilis can cause a person to become paralyzed and can cause a person to develop seizures and even insanity due to changes in the brain.

How to Diagnose Syphilis

The tests that are presently in use to diagnose Syphilis are:

1. Dark field examination of material taken from a chancre.
2. VDRL (Venereal Disease Control Research Laboratory) or RPR
3. FTA-ABS (Fluorescent Treponema Antibody Absorption)

How Is A Dark Field Examination Done?

Material is taken from a chancre. It is placed on a glass slide. After prepping, a cover slip is placed on the specimen and placed under the microscope. The microscope is darkened in a special fashion to allow for proper visualization. A positive dark field is when spirochetes are seen wiggling around and around.

Seeing spirochetes under the microscope does necessarily means that a person has syphilis, because Yaws and Pinta also are diseases caused by spirochetes as well. They cannot be differentiated from the spirochete that causes syphilis morphologically. A positive VDRL in fact does not necessarily mean that a person has syphilis. There are many medical conditions in medicine that can cause false positive VDRL. Both Yaws and Pinta can cause a positive VDRL and yet the patients may not have syphilis.

How to Differentiate a False Positive VDRL/RPR from a Truly Positive VDRL/RPR

The test to do to differentiate a false positive VDRL/RPR is the FTA-ABS test. This test is always positive when a person has syphilis, because it is specific for the antigen produced by triponoma pallidum, which is the spirochete responsible for causing syphilis.

Treatment for the Different Stages of Syphilis

1. Primary syphilis—chancre stage (not allergic to penicillin) 1.2 million units of Benzathine penicillin in each buttock, IM.
2. Secondary syphilis—(not allergic to penicillin)—1.2 million units of Benzathine penicillin in each buttock IM weekly times three weeks in sequence.
3. Latent syphilis (not allergic to penicillin)—1.2 million units of Benzathine in each buttock IM weekly times three weeks in sequence.
4. Tertiary syphilis—(not allergic to penicillin)—1.2 million units of Benzathine penicillin in each buttock IM weekly times three weeks in sequence.
5. Neuro syphilis—(if not allergic to penicillin)—spinal tap ought to be done; send CSF for VDRL and FTA-ABS testing. If positive, admit patient to the hospital and treat with 12 to 24 million units per day of aqueous penicillin G IV for ten days or 600,000 units daily of procaine penicillin IM daily for 14 days. Either the IV or the IM treatment can be carried out on an outpatient basis.

Any man who is HIV positive, VDRL, and FTA positive must be assumed to have neurosyphilis. A spinal tap must be done and the CSF study for syphilis. It does not matter, in fact, whether the CSF is positive or not. Any HIV positive individual with positive VDRL and positive FTA-ABS must be treated in the same way as some one with documented neuro-syphilis as just outlined above, and additional weekly doses of Benzathine penicillin IM must be given for three weeks.

If a man is allergic to penicillin and has early stages of syphilis, the treatment of choice is Erythromycin or Tetracycline 500 mg by mouth, four times a day for 15 days. For more advanced stages of syphilis, including neuro—syphilis, the treatment of choice is Erythromycin or Tetracycline 500 mg by mouth four times a day for 30 days.

Other STDs and genital infections in men and how to treat them

Chancroid is an STD, which is caused by a bacterial organism called Haemophilus Ducrey. Among the signs and symptoms that occur 3 to 5 days after a man has sexual intercourse with an infected man are: pain and tenderness in the vulvae, ulcer formation in the area with a foul smelling odor, large inguinal nodes on both sides of the groin, which are quite tender and painful with subsequent formation of buboes. The diagnosis is made by gram stain, culture, or biopsy of a bubo or necrotic tissue from the vulvae. Treatment is usually Erythromycin 500 mg by mouth 4 times per day for 7 days or Ceftriaxone 250 mg intramuscularly one time.

Lympho-Granuloma Venereum (LGV) is an STD, which is caused by Chlamydia trachomatis serotype L1, L2, and L3 one week to 4 weeks after unprotected sexual intercourse with an infected man. Symptoms such as fever and headache may develop along with painless ulcer in groin areas. The infection frequently spreads via the lymphatic system into the anus and rectum resulting in ulcers, fistulas, and abscesses can develop. If left untreated, rectal stenosis can occur. The diagnosis is made by complement fixation and serologic antibody test to Chlamydia, so called Frei test. Treatment is Tetracycline or Erythromycin 500 mg 4 times a day for 3 weeks or Doxycycline 100 mg BID for 3 weeks.

Granuloma Inguinale is an STD that is caused by the bacterial organism Donovania granulomatosis. Small papules develop around the penis and groin, usually 1 to 12 weeks after sexual intercourse occurs with an infected man. These papules quickly develop into ulcers, which spread to the anus. Typically, if left untreated, fibrosis and scarring develop along with keloid and the development of elephantiasis due to destruction of the lymphatic system in the general pelvic area.

To make the diagnosis, tissue from the infected ulcers is stained with either Giemsa or Wright stain and examined under the microscope. Under the microscope Donovan bodies can be seen, confirming the diagnosis. Treatment is usually with Tetracycline 500 4 times per day for 3 weeks.

Condyloma acuminata, or venereal warts, is an extremely contagious STD, which is transmitted by skin-to-skin contact during sexual intercourse with an infected sexual partner. Venereal wart infection is frequently associated with other STDs such as Trichomonas etc. The organism that is responsible for venereal warts is human papilloma virus. These lesions proliferate more in men who are diabetic, or are immuno-suppressed.

Venereal warts can involve the penis and perianal area. The lesions can appear in a cauliflower formation. They frequently bleed and can be very difficult to treat.

The usual treatments include applications of Aldara cream, 25% trichloroacetic acid, salicylic acid in Collodion, or podophyllin resin, weekly to the warts. Sometimes, laser treatments, electro surgery, or cryosurgery with liquid nitrogen is used to remove the warts.

Molluscum contagiosum is an STD whose cause is a contagious virus which affects the vulva and perineal areas. It is quite contagious and is transmitted by skin contact. The treatment is electrosurgery.

Both Hepatitis C and Hepatitis B are primarily blood borne infections frequently transmitted by needle stick or blood products transfusions. These viruses can be found in both vaginal secretions and semen as such, can be transmitted sexually during sexual intercourse. About 10% of the U.S. of the adult's population may be undetected with hepatitis B. There is a vaccine for Hepatitis B, which is given in a 3-stage manner.

Worldwide 170 million people have chronic hepatitis C. Every year 4 million people are infected wity hepatitis C every year and 350,000 people die annually of hepatitis C. 2 billion people have hepatitis B infection. Worldwide thare are 360 million new hepatitis B in fection annually and 1.2 million People die every year from hepatitis B.

Four million People in the U.S. are infected with hepatitis C and about 5 10,000 people die every year from hepatitis C. There is no vaccine available for Hepatitis C yet. When Hepatitis C seriously affects the liver and the Hepatitis C viral load is high, and the liver biopsy shows high grade inflammation but no cirrhosis.

Alpha interferon injection is used three times per week, in conjunction with Ribavirin daily by mouth, both for 48 weeks, to treat the disease with good success, reducing the risk of liver failure and liver cancer. Ten thousands people die every year in the U.S. because of complications from hepatic C. Pegylated form of Alpha Interferon is now available for once per week use to treat Hepatitis C. Recently the FDA approved 2 new drugs to treat hepatitis C and there are telaprevir and boceprevir.

According to the most recent literature, **Hepatitis A** can also be transmitting via blood products transfusion and therefore via sexual intercourse as well.

Three methods exist to prevent STDs.

1. Prevention by using the method of sexual abstinence. This method is unrealistic.
2. Engaging in protected sexual intercourse by using a condom is a proven way to
3. Prevent most STDs. (like Chlamydia, Gonorrhea, Trichomonas, and Syphilis) or to 4. Provide some protection against STDs like HIV, HSV, Hepatitis B Hepatitis C, and H PV.

5. Curative treatments are available for almost all STD.
6. The prominent exceptions are AIDS and HSV for which there is no cure.

Treatments warts of the penis include:

Podofilox
Ttrichoroacetic acid
Imiquimod
Freezing with liquid nitrogen
Electrocautery
Surgical removal
Laser surgery

Many men are not circumcised either because of religious beliefs or because of cultural preferences. According to the WHO, 70% of men in the world are not circumcised.

While it is said by some that the penile foreskin adds to increased sensation to women during sexual intercourse, but it is a medical fact that the penile foreskin can cause many problems to men.

Uncercuncised men for example are proned to develop balanitis, phimosis, and paraphimosis to name a few. The foreskin of the penis also produces a waxy and rancid smelly material called smegma, which is suspected but not proven to cause cells of the cervix to become dysplastic when the cervical tissues are exposed to it.

Everything is relative, because proper hygiene would clearly make the transference of smegma from man to woman less likely. For further discussion about other urological problems in men, see chapter on prostate below.

Men who have genital and urinary tract health problems or concerns should seek advice from urologists.

Chapter 8
PROSTATE AND BLADDER DISEASES

In 2013, 238,590 men in the U.S. were diagnosed with prostate cancer and 29,720 men died of prostate cancer during that time. The incidence of prostate cancer in black American men and black men from the island Jamaica West Indies is more than twice that of other black men, white men and men of other ethnic groups.

Worldwide in 2013, 890,000 men were diagnosed with prostate cancer and 238,000 men died of prostate cancer.

What is the prostate gland?

The prostate gland is a gland the size of two walnuts that seat on either side of the neck of the urinary bladder.

What is the function of the prostate gland?

The Prostate gland secrete a liquid that helps to liquefy semen that is ejaculated by men during sexual intercourse, which allows the sperm to swim easier towards female eggs. That is the only useful function that the prostate is known to have.

The prostate gland can cause many miseries for men. In fact, all men, if live long enough will have one form of prostate problem or another.

The different problems that men are likely to suffer from with their prostate glands include:

1. Acute prostatitis (acute infection of the prostate gland)
2. Chronic prostatitis (chronic infection of the prostate)
3. Benign prostatic hypertrophy (enlargement of the prostate gland without the presence of cancer)
4. Urinary retention
5. Hematuria (blood in the urine)
6. Urinary track infection
7. Pyelonephritis
8. Sepsis
9. Prostate cancer

Which men who should worry about the development of prostate cancer?

All men have a high probability of developing prostate cancer but the incidence of prostate cancer is higher in black men than it is in men of other ethnic background.

For example, the incidence of prostate cancer is 2-3 times higher in Black American men than their white counterparts. Black American men and Jamaican men have the highest percentage of prostate cancer among all black men in the world and among men in general.

Risk factors for postate cancer include:

1. Heredity, that is if a man's father has prostate cancer; if his brother has prostate, colon, or breast cancer; if his uncle has prostate, colon, or breast cancer; if his mother has breast, colon, or ovarian cancer; if his aunt has breast, colon, or ovarian cancer. There is a 10% genetic crossover between prostate cancer, colon cancer, and ovarian cancer. In a certain mother is capable of transferring the gene for prostate cancer to her son. Once there is a cluster of cancer in the immediate family, any member of that immediate family has a higher likelihood of developing cancer of one kind or another, more so that the general population.
2. Obesity is associated of development of prostate cancer because the obese men have too much fat in their bodies, and therefore are able to use the cholesterol ring associated with fat to overproduce the male hormone-Androgen. The male hormone a man produces, the more he is able to stimulate the prostate gland, and the more the prostate gland is stimulated by the male hormone, the higher the incidence of developing prostate cancer.
3. Eating fat-reach diets—Eating too much fat leads to the production of too much male hormone-Androgen, which in turn results in over-stimulation of the prostate gland, resulting in a higher incidence of prostate cancer.
4. Frontal baldness is associated with a high incidence of prostate cancer, inparticular frontal baldness.
5. Several genes have been identified that predispose Black men and other men to a higher incidence of prostate cancer. Among these genes are TMPRSS2:ETS gene fusion in prostate cancer and the RAF genesetc;
6. It is believed that the fact that African-American men and Jamaican men eat a diet that is very rich in fat and that is why the incidence of prostate cancer is the highest in these two groups men than other black men and other men in the world. I was the first person to have made that observation in 1994 in my first book "The Status of Health of Blacks in the United States—a Prescription for Improvement", published by Kendle Hunt Publishing Company. The medical community has now recognized this as scientific fact.

At what age should black men begin to have themselves medically evaluated for prostate cancer?

Prostate cancer usually appears in black men at age 40. However, there are few cases known to have occurred as early as age 35. Prostate cancer usually appears in white males and males of other ethnicities at age 50, there are few cases known to have occurred as early as age 45 in them as well. 1 in 5 African American will be diagnosed with prostate cancer in their life times and prostate cancer is the second leading cause of cancer deaths in African American men.

What are the early symptoms of prostate cancer?

Usually there are no early symptoms.

What are the late symptoms of prostate cancer?

1. Blood in the urine.
2. Burning in urination.
3. Urinary frequency.
4. Hesitancy in urination.
5. Poor urinary stream.
6. Nocturia (getting up too many times at night to urinate).
7. Urinary retention.
8. Weakness.
9. Bone pain.
10. Constipation.
11. Paralysis from the waist down, due to spinal cord compression by the prostate cancer.

How can a man find out if he has prostate cancer?

To find out if a man has prostate cancer he must go to the doctor to have:

1. A digital rectal examination.
2. He must have a blood test done to examine the Prostatic Specific Antigen (PSA).

The rectal exam allows the physician to palpate the prostate gland to determine whether it is smooth, hard, or has a nodule, or whether the gland is 1+, 2+, 3+, or 4+ in size; 1+ being the smallest, 4+ being the largest.

The PSA is a blood test when elevated can mean that the man has prostate cancer. The normal PSA value is from 0 to 4.0 but is age-variable. In older men, PSA above four may not necessarily mean that prostate cancer is present. The normal value for PSA is set at a lower level for obese men than men of normal sizes. The more obese a man, the more diluted the concentration of the PSA is in his blood stream, because his blood volume is higher. For example, a PSA of 2.0 in an obese man may in fact be 5.0.

The PSA may be high in:

1. Acute prostatitis.
2. Chronic recurrent prostatitis.
3. Benign prostatic hypertrophy.
4. Post coital (a day after sexual intercourse).
5. Prostate cancer.

It is important to understand that a man may have a PSA of 1 and still has prostate cancer if he has a prostate nodule that is palpated during the rectal examination. In the same vain, a man may have a PSA of 1 in one year, and the next consecutive year the PSA is doubled to 2.0: that may indicate the presence of prostate cancer in that gland because of the doubling of the PSA value that occurs so rapidly.

It is also very important that close attention is paid to the difference that occurs in the PSA reading from year to year. If the PSA let us say was 1.8 in 1 year and the following year the PSA becomes 2.7, this is a PSA reflection of 0.9. This very important and may indicate the presence of cancer in the prostate gland. The accepted PSA Reflection is 0.7.

It is not unusual, for a man to present to the doctor with a high PSA and it is due to infection of the prostate or an enlargement of the prostate and not cancer.

By the age of 35, it is a good idea for Black men to begin the process of having yearly digital rectal examination and yearly PSA done. This is even more important if prostate cancer is known to exist in his immediate family.

How to evaluate an asymptomatic elevated PSA?

The first thing to do is to refer the man to a urologist. The urologist will take a history from him, examine him, and most likely do one or two things:

1. Depending on history he/she may choose to treat the man with an appropriate antibiotic.

2. After the completion of the course of the antibiotic, the urologist will likely repeat the PSA.
3. If the PSA returns to normal, he/she may decide to observe the patient.
4. If the PSA fails to return to normal, or did not change at all after the antibiotic treatment, the urologist is likely to recommend a prostate biopsy.
5. Alternatively, the urologist may decide to immediately recommend a prostate biopsy.
6. If the PSA velocity is greater than 0.7 form the previous year's PSA, that also calls for a prostate biopsy to done.

How is the prostate biopsy done?

The night before the biopsy, as well as the morning before the biopsy, the patient is given an antibiotic named Cipro to take. That prevents infections from developing. Then a special needle is used trough the rectum using sonographic technique as a guide and prostate tissue is taken from several parts of the prostate gland and placed in formalin and sent to the pathology laboratory for microscopic evaluation by a pathologist.

1. What if the prostate biopsy comes back indicting that cancer is present in the prostate *gland?*

2. What then must the man do?

The first thing is that the urologist is going to arrange for a meeting between the man and his wife, girl friend or significant other.

This meeting is extremely important because the man is going to hear this most unpleasant of all news in that he has prostate cancer. Any news telling anyone he/she has cancer is devastating to say the least, but telling a man that he has prostate cancer, and that his sexuality and life are both on the line is a matter of extraordinary emotional importance. For that reason, the man needs to have present during the discussion that is going to take place the one person that he trusts the most to help him handle the news of the moment.

Paramount in the discussion of the discovery of prostate cancer is what is the stage of the cancer? This is important because the stage of the cancer dictates what treatment alternatives the urologist can offer to the affected man.

A short synopsis of the staging system use to evaluate needle biopsy of the prostate is the Gleason stage system. The Gleason stages system rages from Gleason 1 to Gleason

10. The lower the Gleason stage, the more localized the cancer is and the better the prognosis. Conversely, the higher the Gleason stage, the more advanced the cancer is and the poorer the prognosis.

A Gleason stage up to 7 in most situations may lend itself to surgical intervention as a modality of treatment. A Gleason greater than 7 is less likely to be cured by surgery alone as a modality. A more detailed and thorough staging of prostate cancer is usually given after a pathological examination of the surgical specimen.

What are the different treatment modalities available to treat prostate cancer?

1. Nerve spearing—Radical prostatectomy for early stage prostate cancer.
2. Nerve-spearing Robatic prostatectomy
3. Radiation therapy.
4. Seeds placement.
5. Hormonal treatments for advanced prostate cancer.
6. Chemotherapy for metastatic prostate cancer.

Each one of these treatment modalities has their upsides and downsides.

The nerve spearing radical prostatectomy is offered as a curative treatment for early prostate cancer. It is a very extensive form of treatment during which the network of tubes within which sperm is produced is removed because frequently cancer cells are found hidden there. The nerves that are necessary to help a man to have an erection are evaluated and spared as best as possible to enable to have an erection some time in the future after surgery. Multiple nodes are removed and sent to the pathology lab to be evaluated for presence or absence of cancer. The valve that seats at the neck of the bladder is sacrificed to be sure that no cancer remains in that area.

Consequently the alternate valve which all men have and have never used before, is now used to attach the urether to enable the man to urinate once the Foley Catheter is removed several weeks postoperatively. The reason why it takes several weeks before the Foley Catheter can be removed is that it takes that long for the new valve to get accustom to function as a valve.

Radiation therapy is an excellent non-invasive modality to treat prostate cancer in men who for one reason or another are not good candidate for radical prostatectomy or their cancer's stage is not clinically appropriate for surgery.

The down side with radiation therapy for prostate cancer is that it is not always curative and it can cause proctitis, rectal bleeding and it can in significant percentage of cases cause erectile dysfunction.

Seeds Placement is superb alternative treatment for early prostate cancer for men who do not want surgery or who for medical reasons of one kind or another cannot have surgery. It too can cause erectile dysfunction in certain percentage of men.

In some men who have advanced prostate cancer seed placement can also be used as good treatment modality. In men, whose prostate gland is too large, hormone such as Leupron can be given intramuscularly to shrink the size of the prostate to allow for easier placement of the seeds. The seeds are radioactive materials that are placed inside the prostate gland to kill the cancer cells.

Hormonal treatments that commonly used to treat prostate cancer are:

1. Leupron (antitestosterone)
2. Flutamide (total Androgen Blockage)
3. Casodex
4. Zytiga

These hormones block the production of the male hormone from the prostate gland. By blocking the production of Androgen from the prostate gland, the growth of cancer cells are slowed down and the level of PSA in the blood decreases. Androgen is needed for prostate cancer cells to grow.

The side effects of Hormonal treatments for prostate are:

1. Erectal dysfunction
2. Gynecomastia (large breasts)
3. Feeling warm all the time (Hot flashes)
4. Sweating a lot

The most effective Chemotherapy presently to treat metastatic prostate cancer is TAXOL intravenously.

Another common problem that causes miseries for men is benign prostatic hypertrophy (BPH). BPH occurs when the prostate gland becomes enlarged and the enlargement impedes the free flow of urine. This results in frequent urination and sometime difficulty in urination.

The symptoms of BPH include:
Urinary frequency

Urinary urgency
Hesitancy on urination
Dribbling
Waking up at night multiple times to urinate
Weak urine stream
Leaking of urine
Burning on urination
Urinary tract infection
The diagnosis of BPH is established by the
History
Digital examination
Renal ultrasound
Cystoscopy

Treatments of BPH include:
Flomax 0.4mg by mouth daily
Avodart 0.5 mg by mouth daily
Terazosin 1mg, 2mg, 5mg, 10mg by mouth daily
Proscar 5mg by mouth daily

Minimally invasive procedures to treat BPH in use are"
Transurethral needle ablation
Transurethral microwave
High-intensity focused ultrasound

Surgical treatments to treat BPH include:
Transurethral surgery (TURP)
Laser surgery
Interstitial laser coagulation
Photoselective Vaporization"

The most common causes of urinary retention in men are:

1. Benign Prostatic Hypertrophy
2. Prostate cancer
3. Diabetes mellitus
4. Stroke
5. Multiple sclerosis etc;
6. Cancer of the bladder with bleeding and too much clots
7. Cancer of the kidney with bleeding and too much clots
8. Sickle cell disease with papillary necrosis, bleeding, and too much clots
9. Urinary tract infection

10. Spinal cord injury

The most common causes of urinary tract infection in men are:

1. Benign prostatic hypertrophy
2. Diabetes mellitus
3. Stroke
4. Insertion of foley catheter in the bladder
5. Old age with poor toileting
6. Multiple sclerosis
7. Cancer of the urinary bladder
8. Kidney stones
9. Cancer of the urether etc;

It is important that men understand the importance of having a digital rectal examination done every year from age 35 onward which can save their lives. It is equally important that white males and men of other ethnic background do the same by age 40. It is important that men understand that having a PSA blood test every year from age 35-40 onward can save their lives.

In particular, Black American men, Jamican men, other Black men and men in general, must be urged to modify their diet by removing the excessive amount of red meat, pork, fried foods, and replacing them with non-shellfishes fish, poultry, fruits, vegetables, beans, olive oil cooking oil and low simple carbohydrate foods, corn meal. In general, exercise along with a good diet program will help to decrease their total body fat and decrease their incidence of prostate cancer. All men no matter their racial make up ought to follow the advice of their physicians to decrease their incidence of prostate cancer.

A common problem that many men are suffer from is Erectil dysfunction (ED)
Some of the causes of ED include:
Diabetes mellitus
Hypertension
Atherosclerosis
Cerebrovascular accident
Multiple sclerosis
Radical Prostatectomy
Seed implantation into the prostate gland (in certain percentage of patients)
Radiation therapy to the prostate gland (in certain percentage of patients)
Low testosterone
Depression and other psychiatric disorders
Medication side effects etc;

The most effective medications available to treat **ERECTIL DYSFUNCTION** include:

Viagra

Cialis

Levitra

Injection of prostaglandin into the Penis

Muse

Penal implant

Viagra and the other similar medications work to bring about penal erection by releasing Nitric Oxide in the penis, which relaxes smooth muscle, and dilating the blood vessels that carry blood to the Penis. These two things bring about erection in men in this setting. Men can have a multitude of problems affecting their urinary bladders:

Among the problems that can affect men and their urinary bladders are:

1. Urinary retention
2. Hematuria (bleeding from the bladder)
3. Urinary tract infection
4. Cancer of the urinary bladder etc.

The most common causes of hematuria in men are:

1. Prostate cancer
2. Kidney stone
3. Urinary tract infection
4. Cancer of urinary bladder
5. Cancer of the kidney
6. Benign prostatic hypertrophy
7. Hemophilia
8. Von Willebran disease
9. Aspirin ingestion
10. Sickle cell anemia
11. Thrombocytopenia
12. Thrombotic thrombocytopenic purpura (TTP)
13. Desseminated intravascular coagulopathy (DIC)

The most common causes of cancer of the urinary bladder are:

1. Genetic predisposition
2. Exposure to different dyes at work
3. Tobacco smoking
4. Schistosoma haematobium etc;

The best ways to evaluate hematuria are:

1. Renal ultra sound
2. Bladder ultra sound
3. CT scan of the kidney
4. CT scan of the bladder
5. MRI of the bladder
6. MRI of the kidney
7. Urine cytology
8. Urinalysis
9. Urine culture
10. PSA
11. Hemoglobin electrophoresis
12. Ova and parasite
13. Serum antibody screen for Schistosoma haematobium
14. Cystoscopy etc;

Diseases of the kidney frequently affect men.
Among the diseases that can affect men's kidneys are:

1. Infections (UTI, Pyelonephritis
2. Kidney
3. Cancer of the kidney
4. End stage kidney disease
5. Glomerulonephritis
6. Nephrotic syndrome
7. Papillary necrosis
8. Polycystic kidney disease
9. Azotemia
10. Uremia etc;

The most common causes of urinary tract infection in are BPH, insertion of a foley catheter, kidney stones, sickle cell disease, aberrant urinary tract, prostate cancer, diabetes mellitus, stroke etc;

Urinary tract infection is divided into lower tract urinary tract infection and upper tract urinary tract infection.

The most common symptoms of lower tract urinary tract infection are

1. Urinary frequency
2. Burning on urination

3. Urinary hesitancy
4. Nocturia
5. Urinary retention
6. Gross hematuria
7. Microscopic hematuria
8. Fever
9. Chills
10. Head ache
11. Lower abdominal pain
12. General weakness
13. Tiredness etc.

The most common symptoms of upper tract urinary tract infection are:

all the above, plus flank pain, nausea and vomiting.

The best ways to evaluate UTI both lower tract UTI and upper tract UTI are:

1. Take good history from the patient
2. Do a complete physical examination
3. Do a urinalysis
4. Do a urine culture
5. Do 2 sets of blood culture
6. Do a complete CBC
7. Do SMA 20 chemistry profile
8. Renal ultrasound

If the man who has UTI and is not febrile, he can be treated as an outpatient.
If his febrile, he should be admitted to the hospital for in hospital treatments.

The most common bacteria responsible for UTI in men are gram negative enteric bacteria.
Some of the most common antibiotics available to treat UTI are:

Ampicillin
Keflex
Kefzol
Cipro
Levaquin
Ceftazidime
Cetriaxone
Bactrim DS
Gentamicin

Doripenem
Imipenem etc;

Upper tract UTI is also called pyelonephrytis and must be treated with IV antibiotic for 21 days. Lower tract UTI in men who are febrile can be treated with antibiotic IV for 10 days if the blood cultures are negative.

Lower UTI in men who are afebrile can be treated with antibiotic by mouth for 10 days. Levaquin by mouth is as effective as Levaquin IV.

Men who have UTI in lower either tract or upper tract must be evaluated by a urologist to find out the reason for the UTI. As part of the urological evaluation, the following tests must be done.

1. Ultrasound of the prostate
2. Ultrasound of the bladder
3. Ultrasound of the Kidneys
4. CT scan of the kidneys and bladder with contrast
5. CT scan of the kidneys without contrast looking for kidney stones
6. Urinary cylology
7. Serum PSA (after the UTI is treated)
8. Hemoglobin electrophoresis
9. Cystoscopy etc;

Men also frequently suffer from prostatitis.

In most sexually active younger men, prostatitis is usually due to exposure to either gonorrhea or Chlamydia during sexual intercourse. In the majority of older men, prostatitis is usually due to BPH or bldder infection. However, recent reports in the literature have documented significant increase in the incidence of STDs in elderly men.

The symptoms of prostatitis include:

Fever
Chills
Lower abdominal pain
Pain down the testicles
Low back pain
Pain in the groin
Dysuria
Frequent urination
Nausea
Vomiting

Head ache

Evaluations of prostatitis include:

Taking a good history

Physical examination

Urinalysis

Urine culture

Urethral culture for gonorrhea and Chlamydia

RPR

HIV blood test

Prostate ultrasound

It is not always a prudent idea for the prostate gland to be palpated by a physician when the gland is acutely infected. Doing so, may spread the infection in the blood stream causing sepsis.

The microorganisms that are frequently associated with the development of prostatitis include:

E.coli

Klebsiella

Proteus

Gonorrhea

Chlanydia

The medications in use to treat acute prostatitis include:

Levaquin

Cipro

Zythromax

Doxycycline

Teracycline

Floxin

Prostate infection can be very difficult to eradicate. The prostate gland sits inside a very thick capsule which is very difficult for antibiotics to penetrate. Because of that, the infection frequently becomes chronic.

The symptoms of chronic prostatitis include:

Recurrent lower abdominal pain

Chronic and recurrent pain in the groin

Dysuria

Frequent urination

Fever—when there is an acute flare up

Chills when there is an acute flare up

Evaluation of chronic prostatitis include

History

Physical examination

Palpation of the prostate gland

Urinalysis

Urine culture

Urethral culture for gonorrhea and Chlamydia

RPR

HIV blood test

Prostate ultra sound

Treatments of chronic prostatitis include:

Massage of the prostate gland by a Urologist to remove the thick and pussy material from the prostate gland

Levaquin for 4 weeks by mouth

Cipro for 4 weeks by mouth

Zythromax by mouth for 4 weeks

Doxycycline by mouth for 4 weeks

Floxin by mouth for 4 weeks

Kidney stones are quite common in men and this condition is quite painful.

The most common stones are calcium oxalate and calcium phosphate.

Calcium stones are most commonly seen in men.

The most common causes of kidney stones are:

Hyperuricosuria

Primary hyperparathyroidism

Intestinal hyperoxaluria

Hereditary hyperoxaluria

Hyperuricosuria

Gout

Lymphoma

Lymphocytic leukemia

Dehydration

The most common symptoms of kidney stones are:

Severe and excruciating lower back pain

Hematuria, (gross or microscopic)

The best ways to evaluate men for kidney stones are:

Take a good history

Do a complete physical examination
Do a urinalysis to look for blood
Do a flat plate of the abdomen x-ray to look for a stone
Do a CT of the abdomen without contrast looking for a stone
Strain the urine to look for stones
Do a SMA 20 chemistry profile
Do a serum uric acid
Do a CBC looking lymphocytosis (elevated lymphocytes count)

The best treatments available to treat kidney stones are:

Pain killer medication (Analgesic)
Allopurinol
Thiazide diuretic
Diet
Surgical removal of kidney stones
External Shock Wave Lithotripsy (ESWL)

Hematuria can occur in individuals who have abnormal coagulation problems such as

Hemophilia A and B
Factor V deficiency
Factor VII deficiency
Factor X deficiency
Factor XI deficiency
Von Willebran disease
Dessiminated intravascular coagulopathy (DIC)

Hamaturia can also occur because of platelet abnormalities such as

Thrombocytopenia (low platelet)
Thombopathy (qualitative platelet Abnormaqlity)

Hematuria can also occur because ingestion of aspirin and nonsteroidal anti-inflammatory drugs. Heparin, Lovenox, Pradaxa, Xarelto and Coumadin etc; can also cause hematuria. Another common cause of hematuria in men is sickle cell trait and sickle cell anemia. The reason for the hematuria in sickle cell disease is papillary necrosis of the kidney. Kidney stones, cancer of the kidney, cancer of the bladder and urinary tract infection are some of the frequent causes of hematuria.

All individuals with hematuria ought to be evaluated by a urologist.

Chapter 9
GYNECOLOGICAL
AND OBSTETRICAL DISEASES

AMONG THE MOST TROUBLESOME GYNECOLOGICAL problems affecting women are sexually transmitted diseases (STD). "CDC surveillance data shows a much higher rate of reported STDs among some racial or ethnic minority groups than among whites".

According to a report published by the CDC in February 14, 2013 there are 19.7 million cases of STDs annually in the U.S. and it costs $16 billion per year to treat these STDs." People between the ages of 15 to 24 accounts for half of the 19.7 million new infections in the U.S. annually." "HPV is the most common STD in all age groups and accounts for 14 million of all new infections."

"Curable sexually transmitted diseases cost $742 million, with Chlamydia, as the most common and most expensive." "Comparatively, HIV infects 41,000 people year in the U.S., but the life long treatment can cost $ 300,000 per person."

Worldwide there are 340 million new cases of syphilis, gonorrhea, Chlamydia and trichomoniasis in men and women ages 15-49 annually. Source: WHO

As outlined in chapter 7 above, the most common STDs in the world are:

> Human pappilomavirus
> Gonorrhea
> Chlamydia
> Syphilis
> Trichomoniasis
> Chancroid
> Genital herpes
> Genital warts
> Hepatitis B
> Hepatitis C
> HIV/AIDS

Every year there are 19 millions new STD's in the U.S. There are 65 million individuals living with curable sexually transmitted diseases in the U.S. By age 25, 1 out 4 people Americans will have an STD. According to recent reports every year there are about 1 billion unprotected sexual acts in the U.S. Every year, there are 750,000 unwanted teenage pregnancies in the U.S.

According to a recent report by the CDC, one in four young women is infected with at least one STD. 48% African American teenaged girls have an STD compared to 20% of white teenaged girls. All together, 3.2 million young women in the U.S. are infected with STD.

Fifty per cent of African American teenaged girls' ages 14-19 are infected with HPV, genital herpes or trichomonas. The most common STD's found in these teenage girls were HPV18% and Chlamydia 4%.

According to a recent report, a study carried out in Africa and published in March, 2008 Issue of Infectious Disease News, women who had sexual intercourse with Circumcised men, had a 12.5% decrease in genitourinary tract infections, such as trichomonas and bacterial vaginosis. The black women in the study did experience a decrease in HIV/AIDS when they had sexual intercourse with circumcised men.

The most STD's that infect black women are:

1. Genital herpes
2. Chlamydia
2. Gonorrhea
3. Syphilis
4. HIV/AIDS
5. Human papilloma virus (HPV)
6. Bacterial vaginosis
7. Trichomonas vaginitis
8. Vaginal candidiasis
9. Pelvic inflammatory disease (PID)
10. Venereal warts
11. Lymphogranuloma venerum
12. Chancroid
13. Granuloma inguinale
14. Condylomata acuminata
15. Molluscum contagiosum
16. Pelvic inflammatory disease (PID)
17. Tubo-ovarian abscess
18. Toxic shock syndrome

The 2009 incidence of the most common STDs in the U.S. are:

Gonorrhea 301,174, 99.1 per 100,000

Chlamydia 1,244,180, 409.2 per 100,000
Syphilis 13,997, 4.6 per 100,000
"Blacks accounted for 71% of all gonorrhea cases in 2009. The gonorrhea rate among blacks is 20 times higher than whites". Source: CDC.

One in four women is infected with genital herpes and according to CDC and half of African American women are infected with genital herpes simplex. 24 million people are infected with HPV in the U.S. 6.7 per 100,000 are African American women are infected with HPV and 2.5 white women per 100,000 are infected with HPV. Eighty per cent of sexually active American women by the age of 50 are infected with HPV.

Genital herpes is a very common sexually transmitted disease. 68 million individuals are infected with Herpes Viruses I and II in the United States of America and about 1 million people become infected every year with these Herpes Viruses. Herpes Simplex Type II causes about 90 percent of genital herpes infections and Herpes Simplex Type I causes about 10 percent. Genital herpes is most often transmitted during sexual intercourse or during oral sex with an infected partner.

It is possible for a woman to transmit the herpes infection from a buttock or lip lesion; for example, from touching the infected area with her bare hand, then touch her genital area. Women also could carry herpes infection which they got during birth from infected mothers. Within 3 to 7 days after exposure, the first symptoms of genital herpes infection appear. The first symptoms are a burning or tingling pain or paresthesia in the perineal area.

The next thing that may happen is the development of a crop of small, water filled lesions, which are quite itchy. Sometimes, the affected woman may feel a low-grade feverish feeling. The pain in the vulvar area may be quite severe with extreme tenderness on touching. Once the lesions break open, the area affected becomes more painful. Passing urine is painful if the area of the external meatus is infected (the opening where the urine comes out). Urinary retention can occur.

Lymph node enlargement in the inguinal area is common and often these lymph nodes can are tender and painful. In women who have AIDS, these herpetic lesions can accelerate in a severe and disabling manner all the way to the perianal area requiring hospitalization for intravenous medications and intramuscular pain medications to help ease the pain in these types of herpes infected women. A woman infected with herpes simplex may be able to infect a sexual partner during intercourse, even though she has no open herpetic sores.

The incidence of genital herpes is quite high in females and herpes infection of the genital spares no ethnic groups and socioeconomic status. Any woman who is sexually active can become infected with the herpes virus and this is particularly so if she has sexual intercourse without the use of a condom.

On examination, the physician is likely to see small vesicles over the labia majora, labia minora, the skin of the perineal area and the vulva. The cervix may be infected with the Herpes Virus and yet she may feel no pain because the cervical tissues may not manifest pain. She may have a mucous discharge as a part of a vaginitis associated with a herpes infection.

The diagnosis of herpes infection of the genital area can be made by culture taken from the infected areas or by rupturing the vesicles and culturing the fluid within them with clean culturette, place the culturette in a special herpes liquid medium in a tube, and send the tube to the microbiology lab for processing.

Scraping the ulcerated area on a clean slide and send it to the lab for a Zanck stain can also use to diagnose herpes. The culturing of the herpes infection is much more specific and definite evidence of the presence of the herpes infection if the culture is positive. Herpes infections tend to recur in the same area repeatedly. Stressful situations tend to cause the herpetic lesions to come back. Some of the stresses that can cause the recurrence of herpes infections are the common cold, menstruation, and stress associated with taking school examinations, work related stress, indigestion, etc.

These stressful situations increase the level of adrenalin which has a lowing effect on the immune system allowing the dormant herpes infection to wake up and proliferate, causing the recurrence of the disease.

Another very serious problem associated with genital herpes infection is when a woman is pregnant and has herpes infection of the genitalia at the same time. Women who are infected with genital herpes while pregnant can have spontaneous abortion or have premature babies. About 50-60 percent of babies born to women who have active genital herpes infection are infected themselves.

When a woman is infected with active herpes infection during pregnancy it is necessary that she is delivered by cesarean section to prevent the infant's mucous membrane from coming in contact with the infected birth canal of the mother, thereby preventing the infant from developing problems such as blindness, etc. Infants born to herpes simplex infected mothers can start having problems 3 to 4 days after birth and up to 60 percent of these infected babies die during the neonatal period. About 40 to 50 percent of those who survive can develop problems such as mental retardation, microcephaly, microphthalmos, and seizures.

Treatment of Herpes Infection

If the genital herpes infection is more diffused and the patient is immunosuppressed the treatment is intravenous acyclovir. If the herpes infection is localized, the treatment is acyclovir by mouth or if the infection is localized and mild, acyclovir cream will help to relieve the symptoms but medication by mouth is needed, in addition. The question is how long to treat. Primarily, Genital herpes should be treated with acyclovir 200 mg by mouth, 5 times a day for 10 days or Valtrex 1000 mg by mouth, 2 times per day for 10 days.

Treatment for recurrent genital herpes is Valtrex 500 mg by mouth, 2 times per day for 5 days or acyclovir 400 mg by mouth, 3 times per day or Famvir 250 mg by mouth, 2 times per day for 5 days. The treatment for suppression of chronic genital herpes is Famvir 250 mg by mouth, 2 times per day or Valtrex 500 mg by mouth daily or acyclovir 400 mg 2 times per day.

This virus is very difficult to treat because it is slow growing, has a thick capsule, has the ability to hide for a very long time in the human body, and flares up on and off causing miseries for those who are infected. Therefore, the treatment for recurrent flare up of herpes infection may be for life.

In 1996, 330 million cases of sexually transmitted diseases were reported worldwide. The rate of Gonorrhea rose by 9% during the period 1997-1999 (CDC) and there were 130 cases of Gonorrhea per 100,000 cases in women in 1999. Gonorrheal infection is more prevalent in younger women who are frequently more promiscuous starting from adolescents and teens who usually have multiple sexual partners. The bacterium responsible for causing the Gonorrheal infection is gram negative intracellular diplococcus (Neisseria Gonorrhea).

Gonorrhea is second most commonly reported STD health departments in different localities in the US. In 2006, 358,000 cases of gonorrhea were reported. Women, who are infected with Gonorrhea, become infected during sexual intercourse with men who are infected with Gonorrhea. Once infected, several things can happen to a woman. Five days to a week after being exposed, the woman may notice a foul smelling vaginal discharge with pain and irritation in the vaginal area.

If she does not seek medical care right away, the symptoms get worse as the infection travels upwards into her tubes causing an acute inflammation to occur. The infection also gets into the cervix and body of the uterus infecting these organs.

The infection may get into the ovaries resulting in tubo-ovarian infection, which can lead to the formation of tubo-ovarian abscesses. At this point the woman has what is called acute pelvic inflammatory disease (PID) secondary to Gonorrhea. The

Gonorrhea infection can go beyond the confines of the gynecological organs into the blood stream causing gonococcal septicemia or into different joints causing acute gonococcal arthritis of different degrees with the potential for destroying the affected joints if not treated promptly and effectively.

Sometimes because of failure to treat the acute infection the gynecologically infected organs stick to each other, causing adhesions to occur which can wrap around the bowels and sometimes around the liver on the right side of the abdomen. Pain in this area of the abdomen causing what is referred to as Fitz-Hugh-Curtis Syndrome with violin-like adhesive bands pulling on the liver capsule. Until these bands of adhesions are surgically lysed, pain in the right part of the abdomen persists, confusing the clinical picture.

How to Diagnose Gonorrhea in Women

The first thing to do is to take a good history as to the woman's sexual habits and her symptoms. It is important to find out when the woman's last menstrual period was because during a woman's menstrual period, the tissues in the gynecological organs are swollen, making it easier for both a freshly acquired infection to spread or a chronic infection to flare up causing acute gonococcal symptoms with severe pelvic pain.

The next thing to do is a good pelvic examination looking for a foul smelling vaginal discharge, cervical tenderness, tenderness of the neck of the cervix and the uterus, right or left lower abdominal tenderness with super pubic tenderness sometimes with rebound tenderness. The next most important thing to do is to send a special gonococcal test of the vaginal discharge to the bacteriology laboratory to try to determine if the gonococcal organism is causing the infection. This same specimen taken from the vagina can also be tested for Chlamydia.

Part of the vaginal discharge can be placed on a clean glass slide and smeared. Once the slide is dried, it can be stained with gram stain. The gram stained slide can be examined under the microscope. A number of things can be seen on that smear, including evidence of a purulent infection if many white blood cells are seen. Many different bacteria, both gram negative and gram positive, will be seen. There lies the problem with doing a gram stain on a specimen of discharge taken from the vagina.

There are many gram positives bacteria and gram-negative bacteria, which inhabit the vagina as their normal habitats. In particular, the gram-negatives bacteria that cause Gonorrhea looks exactly like other gram-negative bacteria that are found normally in the vagina. It is therefore almost useless to do a gram stain on a vaginal discharge when trying to make a diagnosis of Gonorrhea in a woman, unless gram negative intracellular diplococci are seen.

Once the pelvic examination is completed and appropriate specimens are sent to the different laboratories for testing, treatment for Gonorrhea can begin. It is important to realize that sexually transmitted diseases rarely present as one infection. Because of that, blood must be sent to the lab to test for syphilis, (VDRL), and for HIV (with consent). Vaginal secretion wet mount ought to be done and examine under the microscope to look for Trichomonas. A urinalysis can also be done, looking for Trichomonas in the sediment under the microscope. Vaginal and cervical swabs must be taken to culture for Herpes Simplex Numbers I, II, and specimen sent to test for HPV.

The approach to treatment of Gonorrheal and chlamydial infections in women is guided by the clinical presentation.

How to treat Suspected or uncomplicated Gonorrhea/ Chlamydia in the office / outpatient Clinic:

The treatment is Ceftriaxone 250 mg IM in one dose with Doxycycline 100mg two times per day for 14 days and Flagyl 250 mg by mouth twice per day for 4 days. Alternatively, the patient can be treated with Floxin 400 mg by mouth twice per day and Flagyl 500 mg 2 times per day for 14 days. Or Zithromax 500mg 2 tablets taken by mouth at the same time if Chlamydia is the suspected infection and Flagyl 250mg twice per day for 7 days to cover for Thrichomonas. If Gonorrhea is the suspected infection, then the same regimen can be used, except that the dose of Zithromax must be 3 grams by mouth taken at the same time.

Ceftriaxone is the best medication available to treat uncomplicated or suspected Gonorrhea intramuscularly in the office or in the clinic. Ceftriaxone, however, will not treat chlamydia and since it is oftentimes impossible to tell Gonorrhea from chlamydia, it is wise to treat for both by adding Doxycycline, Floxin or Zithromax. These three medications are efficacious against Chlamydia. Floxin and Zithromax are both effective against both Gonorrhea and Chlamydia.

The rational for using Flagyl by mouth, in the office or clinic, along with these other medications is because Trichomonas is frequently found along with the other infections. It makes sense to treat for it empirically. Flagyl is also very effective in treating bacterial vaginosis secondary to local anaerobic bacteria that inhabit in the vagina as they natural habitat

For women who are allergic to Penicillin who therefore cannot be treated with Ceftriaxone, the regimen containing Floxin or Zithromax can be used. For women who either had asymptomatic Gonorrhea or Chlamydia or become pregnant or for pregnant women who become exposed sexually to Gonorrhea or Chlamydia while pregnant, these women must be treated properly to prevent spontaneous abortion in the first trimester. There is higher incidence of pre-term labor in pregnant women who are infected with Gonorrhea or Chlamydia.

If a woman is infected with uncomplicated Gonorrhea and is pregnant, and is not allergic to Penicillin, the treatment of choice is Ceftriaxone 250 mg IM, one dose, and Erythromycin 250 mg 4 times per day for one week to cover for possible chlamydia infection. Spectinomycin can be used instead of Ceftriaxone in a pregnant Penicillin-allergic woman who is infected with uncomplicated Gonorrhea.

Tetracycline cannot be used in pregnancy in particular in the first trimester.
It will stain the teeth of the fetus. Nowadays, tetracycline is rarely used to treat Gonorrhea because the organism is frequently resistant to it.

If the fetus becomes infected with Gonorrhea the possibility of spontaneous abortion or stillbirth is quite high. If a woman who is infected with Gonorrhea becomes pregnant and is left untreated, close to 50 percent of the time the fetus being delivered by the woman will be infected during delivery. The fetus may develop sepsis, infection of the eyes, the scalp, arthritis, etc., secondary to Gonorrhea and the newborn baby will require intravenous antibiotics to treat him or her for the disease.

Gonorrheal infection can be very complicated and can cause acute pelvic inflammatory disease (PID). Second, it can cause acute inflammation of the tubes resulting in acute salpingitis. Third, the organism can migrate into the ovaries causing tubo-ovarian abscess. Fourth, the infection can involve the uterus causing endometrial inflammation. Fifth, the infection can leave the confines of the gynecological organs and spread into the blood stream causing sepsis. Once in the blood, it can involve many other organs in the body causing severe complications. Sixth, it can cause septic arthritis with pain, swelling of a joint or multiple joints is one of the most severe presentations of Gonorrheal infection in sexually active women.

It is critical to tap the joint fluid and send it to the lab for gram stain, cell count, and culture, glucose, and protein. Treatment of Gonorrheal arthritis must be started immediately to prevent the destruction of the affected joint or joints.

Lower abdominal pain, fever, cervical tenderness on pelvic examination with foul smelling vaginal discharge along with adnexal tenderness, high WBC, suggest the strong possibility of PID with possible tubo-ovarian abscess.

The different conditions that can cause abdominal pain in a woman of childbearing age include:

1. Acute appendicitis

2. Ectopic pregnancy
3. Urinary tract infection
4. Ruptured ovarian cyst
5. Acute diverticulitis is much less likely in this Age group, but can occur
6. Cancer of the large bowel is less likely in this age group, but can occur.
7. If she is diabetic, is therefore, prone to early vascular disease, she can have ischemic bowel.
8. If she has Polycythemia Vera or Essential Thrombocytopenia, she can have acute splenic vein thrombosis causing the abdominal pain.
9. Or if she suffers with inflammatory bowel disease, either ulcerative colitis or Krohn's disease in the affected part of the bowel causing severe lower abdominal pain.
10. If she takes birth control pills and has congenital antithrombin 3 deficiency, factor V Leiden deficiency, protein C or protein S deficiency, anticardiolipin antibody, elevated lipoprotein-a etc. she may become hypercoagulable and as a result, she may develop thrombosis of her intra abdominal vasculature which can cause severe lower abdominal pain, etc.
11. For the reasons just mentioned above, she may also develop pain in her lower leg because of Deep Vein Thrombophlebitis
12. She may also develop chest pain with shortness of breath because of pulmonary embolism associated with one of the thrombophilias outlined above.

When acute pelvic infection is suspected, the gynecologist can tap the cul-de-sac to remove fluid for culture if the pelvic sonogram shows the presence of fluid in the cul-de-sac. A serum pregnancy test can be done quickly to rule out the presence of pregnancy.

Pelvic sonogram, transvaginal or transabdominal sonogram can be done easily, even in a very sick woman; if she is too sick to drink fluid to fill her bladder then, a Foley catheter can be placed in her bladder and normal saline can be used to fill the bladder to permit the pelvic sonogram to be done.

Evaluation of the pelvic sonogram allows for evaluation of the uterus, the fallopian tubes, the ovaries, etc. It is also very useful to do a CT of the abdomen, which allows for complementary intrapelvic evaluation. The transvaginal ultrasound, may allow for better visualization of the intra pelvic structures.

Once these different tests have been done, then it is up to the treating gynecologist to decide whether to carry out laparoscopic examination to diagnose disease of the ovaries, the uterus, the fallopian tubes, etc., in the evaluation of pelvic and abdominal pain. It is also up to the gynecologist to decide whether the acutely sick woman needs a laparotomy to determine the reason for the pelvic and lower abdominal symptoms.

Once an acute intravaginal, intrapelvic, or systemic gynecological infection is either strongly suspected or confirmed, then in hospital intravenous antibiotics ought to be started immediately to treat the infection.

In-Hospital Treatment of Gonorrhea

1. Ceftriaxone—2 grams IV every 12 hours
2. Doxycycline—100 mg p.o. or IV every 12 hours until the culture result is back from the laboratory.
3. Alternatively, Clindamycin—900 mg IV every 8 hours in addition to Gentamycin—2 mg/KG IM or IV and once the patient is improved then add Doxycycline—100 mg by mouth every 12 hours to complete a 14-day course. Add Flagyl 500 mg every 6 hours during the acute phase of the infection to cover for not only possible accompanying Trichomonas infection but also anaerobic organisms that may be playing a role in the infectious process.
4. Patients who cannot tolerate Doxycycline or who are allergic to Penicillin can be treated with Norfloxin 400 mg IV every 12 hours.

Once the culture result and sensitivity are back from the laboratory, then specific antibiotics can be used to treat the infection.

Out patient treatments for gonorrhea include

1. Ceftriaxone 1 gram IM
2. Zetrhromax 500mg 2 tablets by mouth x 1

Prevention of Gonorrhea or Chlamydia Infection

1. Teenage girls and older women ought not to be engaging in frivolous and irresponsible sexual intercourse.
2. They ought to strive to remain monogamous.
3. If they cannot abstain from sexual intercourse, then they must insist that their sexual partners use a condom during sexual intercourse. The use of a good condom not only prevents STD but also prevents unplanned or unwanted pregnancies which are frequently unwanted.

The high incidence of Gonorrhea reported amongst "third world" women from developing countries as compared to women in the United States is due in part to the poorer socioeconomic status of women along with the higher incidence of drug abuse, which leads to risky behavior and or social aberrations. When people are high on drugs they inevitably become irresponsible, carefree and careless and the result is unprotected sexual intercourse and frequently with multiple sexual partners.

The incidence of STD amongst working and middle class women in the United States is no less than it is amongst women of poorer socioeconomic status. The incidence of STD in general is higher amongst young women from adolescence to adulthood because they frequently are less responsible about their sexual behavior.

There are 19 million new cases of STD (not including AIDS) reported annually in the United States according to a recent report by the Institute of Medicine. One-fourth of these cases are among teenagers according to that report. 22 percent of people above the age of 15 are carrying the herpes infection. It costs taxpayers $16.4 billion per year to treat STD in the United States. By the 11th grade, 70 percent of teenagers have had sexual intercourse and 40 percent of them have had four or more sexual partners.

Chlamydia Infection

There are 2.8 million cases of Chlamydia annually in the U.S. As such, Chlamydia is the most commonly reported bacterial STD in the United States (According to the CDC).

"Chlamydia rates in African Americans are eight times higher than in white Americans".

Chlamydia trachomatis is the most nationally reported STD in the US. In 2006, 1,031,000 cases of Chlamydia were reported by health departments in different localities in the U.S. Women become infected with Chlamydia through unprotected sexual intercourse and can infect their baby unborn babies. Men pass the infection to women in their ejaculates causing a mucopurulent endocervical discharge. The infection then can work its way up the woman's genital tract, infecting the uterus and the fallopian tubes. PID can result, causing chronic pelvic pain. Ectopic pregnancies and infertility occur frequently because of untreated chlamydia infection.

Women who are at risk Chlamydia should have a pelvic examination, and their vaginal cervical discharge should be tested for Chlamydia by culture, DNA probe, enzyme immunoassay (EIA) or nucleic acid amplification testing (NAAT).

Treatment can be started with Doxycycline 100 mg 2 times per day for 7 days or Floxin 300 mg 2 times per day for 7 days or Azithromycin 1 gram by mouth for 1 day or Erythromycin 500 mg by mouth 4 times per day for 7 days. If a woman is pregnant, she can be treated with Erythromycin 250 mg by mouth 4 times per day for 14 days or Azithromycin 1 gram by mouth for 1 day can be given. Similar to Gonorrhea,

Chlamydia infections are very often accompanied by one or two other STDs so the clinical thing to do is to test for Gonorrhea, draw blood for VDRL (syphilis test) and HIV, then treat for Gonorrhea, Chlamydia and Trichomonas until proven otherwise.

Treatment of Suspected Uncomplicated Chlaymdia Infection

1. Doxycycline 100 mg by mouth 2 times per day for 7 days.

or

2. Floxin 800 mg once by mouth with Ceftriaxone 250 mg IM and Flagyl 250 mg 4 times by mouth per day for 4 days.

or

3. Zithromax 1 gram by mouth

Complicated documented Chlamydia infection with acute pelvic infection can be treated with Doxycycline 100 mg ID q 12 hours IV for 7 days until symptoms improve then switched to by mouth for 10-14 days or Floxin 400 mg by ID q 12 hours IV for 7 days then for 10 to 14 days. or Zithromax 1 gram IV first day then 500mg IV for a total of 10 days.

Syphilis Infection

Syphilis has historically been one of the most common STDs to afflict mankind and has been in the new world since 1494 when Columbus and his men came to America. Syphilis is caused by the spirochete Treponema Pallidum.

"In the year 2008-2009 number primary, early latent, late, late latent and congenital syphilis was 44,828 cases in the U.S. according to the CDC".

Syphilis is usually transmitted sexually, or from mother to baby. Once the organism is deposited into the human tissue it takes anywhere from 14 to 21 days for primary syphilis to develop. In women, the parts of their genitalia first affected by early syphilis are the labia, fourchette, or cervix. "During 2008-2009, the rate of primary syphilis increased in all racial and ethnic groups except non-Hispanic whites and Hispanics". The rate increased 11.6% among non-Hispanic blacks and non-Hispanic whites." CDC

In 2009, the rate primary syphilis was higher among non-Hispanic black women compare to white women. CDC-STD Surveillance. 2009

The first study was the Oslo study, which took place between 1891 and 1951. It included 2000 patients diagnosed clinically. The dark field test and Wasserman test were not yet in existence. Penicillin had not yet been discovered either so there was no effective way to treat these patients.

That study amply demonstrated the devastating effects of untreated syphilis on all parts of the human body, in particular, the brain, the aorta, the skeletal system, etc.

The second study is the infamous **Tuskegee study**, which took place from 1932-1974 in Tuskegee, Alabama under the control of the **United States Public Health Service**

The shameful reason given for **this cruel, inhumane, barbaric, and racist study** was to find the effects of untreated syphilis on the human body. There were no scientific justifications for this study in view of the fact that the Oslo study had already shown what untreated syphilis could do to the human body. (As described in chapter 8)

From 1932 to 1974, under the leadership of the United States Public Health Service, 431 (Negro men) black men were injected with live syphilis organisms for the sole purpose of seeing what effects syphilis would have on their bodies. These men did not sign consent for participating in the study. They did not know that they were being injected with live syphilis organisms.

In 2010, a report came out showing that some of the same American scientists involved in the infamous Tuskegee study also carried out experiment in Guatemala injecting syphilis in 696 men and women Guatemalan prisoners, people with mental illness, and prostitutes. The experiments were carried out to test the effects of penicillin on STDs during 1946 to 1948. This discovery was made by a Wellesley College medical historian. The U.S. Secretary of State Hillary Rodham Clinton and the Secretary of Health and Human Services Kathleen Sebelius apologized to the Guatemalan Government and the Guatemalan people for the actions of these American Scientists. Tax payer's money through the National Institute of Health financed the Guatemalan syphilis study.

The present U.S Government has ordered an investigation to be carried out by a Presidential Commission and the Institute of Medicine to find out what happened in the Guatemalan syphilis experiment. (As described in chapter 8)

In the history of the world, many events have taken place to catalogue men's cruelty towards each other: **Slavery, the Holocaust, the Rwanda Massacre, and the Tuskegee Study** and the Guatemalan syphilis experiment are a few such examples. In the Tuskegee Study, 431 men were sacrificed for nothing other than racism and bigotry, while the U.S. government, organized medicine, some black and white physicians, some white and black hospital administrators and society, at large, stood by silently. **How shameful and how disgusting?** (as described in chapter 8)

Treatment for the Different Stages of Syphilis in women

1. Primary syphilis—chancre stage (not allergic to penicillin) 1.2 million units of Benzathine penicillin in each buttock, IM.
2. Secondary syphilis—(not allergic to penicillin)—1.2 million units of Benzathine penicillin in each buttock IM weekly times three weeks in sequence.
3. Latent syphilis (not allergic to penicillin)—1.2 million units of Benzathine in each buttock IM weekly times three weeks in sequence.
4. Tertiary syphilis—(not allergic to penicillin)—1.2 million units of Benzathine penicillin in each buttock IM weekly times three weeks in sequence.
5. Neuro syphilis—(if not allergic to penicillin)—spinal tap ought to be done; send CSF for VDRL and FTA-ABS testing. If positive, admit patient to the hospital and treat with 12 to 24 million units per day of aqueous penicillin G IV for ten days or 600,000 units daily of procaine penicillin IM daily for 14 days. Either the IV or the IM treatment can be carried out on an outpatient basis.

Any woman who is HIV positive, VDRL, and FTA positive must be assumed to have neurosyphilis. A spinal tap must be done and the CSF study for syphilis. It does not matter, in fact, whether the CSF is positive or not. Any HIV positive individual with positive VDRL and positive FTA-ABS must be treated in the same way as some one with documented neuro-syphilis as just outlined above, and additional weekly doses of Benzathine penicillin IM must be given for three weeks.

If a woman is allergic to penicillin and has early stages of syphilis, the treatment of choice is Erythromycin or Tetracycline 500 mg by mouth, four times a day for 15 days. For more advanced stages of syphilis, including neuro—syphilis, the treatment of choice is Erythromycin or Tetracycline 500 mg by mouth four times a day for 30 days.

It is very important to do follow-up VDRL after treating a person for syphilis. Every three months a repeat VDRL ought to be done to show that the VDRL titer is going down. Sometimes, the VDRL remains high even though adequate treatment was given. This situation can be quite confusing because a person can get re-infected with syphilis. It's hard to tell sometimes whether a person has become reinfected or not. An increasing VDRL titer after treatment may mean that re-infection may have taken place.

It is crucial that pregnant women are not treated with Tetracycline in the first trimester of pregnancy. Tetracycline will interfere with the calcification of bones and stains the teeth of the fetus / baby.

Other vaginal infections and STDs include
mucopurulent cervicitis
lympho-granuloma Venarum (LGV)
granuloma inguinale,
Candidiasis vulva-vaginitis
bacterial vaginosis
condylomata accumulate
molluscum contagiosum
chancroid
and toxic shock syndrome.

Causes Of Other STD and Vaginal Infections and How to Treat Them

Chancroid is an STD, which is caused by a bacterial organism called Haemophilus Ducrey. Among the signs and symptoms that occur 3 to 5 days after a woman has sexual intercourse with an infected man are: pain and tenderness in the vulvae, ulcer formation in the area with a foul smelling odor, large inguinal nodes on both sides of the groin, which are quite tender and painful with subsequent formation of buboes. The diagnosis is made by gram stain, culture, or biopsy of a bubo or necrotic tissue from the vulvae. Treatment is usually Erythromycin 500 mg by mouth 4 times per day for 7 days or Ceftriaxone 250 mg intramuscularly one time.

Mucopurulent cervicitis, bacterial vaginosis are STD caused by bacterial organisms, such as Gardnerella Vaginales, bacteroides, and Pepto cocci. Common symptoms are foul smelling vaginal discharge, and burning and itching in the vaginal area. The diagnosis of bacterial vaginosis is made by looking at a wet mount of vaginal discharge under the microscope showing the characteristic so called clue cells, checking the vaginal PH, a positive Whif test etc.

The usual treatment is Flagyl 500 mg 2 times per day for 7 days and Ampicillin 500 mg 4 times per day for 7 days, or Tetracycline 500 mg 4 times per day for 7 days. It is imperative that the woman's sexual partner gets treated, as well, to prevent re-infection when he next has unprotected sexual intercourse with her. Most recently, the CDC is recommending a single 2000mg of Flagyl to treat trichomonas in women and their sexual partners.

Candida vulvo-vaginitis is a yeast/fungal infection of the vulva and vaginal areas of the female reproductive organs and is one of the most common infections that a woman has to cope with. There are several predisposing conditions that create the setting, allowing for the development of this infection. Among these predisposing conditions are:

1. Diabetes mellitus
2. Antibiotic use
3. The use of birth control pills
4. Pregnancy
5. Frequent vaginal douching with corrosive anti-bacterial solution

A fungus called Candida albican causes vaginal candidiasis. Diabetes mellitus is highly associated with candida vulva-vaginitis, because the fungus grows best in the presence of sugar. If a woman is diabetic and her blood sugar is too high, her vaginal secretions also have too much sugar, thus favoring the growth of Candida albicans, causing vaginal infection. In fact, frequently, the first indication that may be woman is diabetic is when, suddenly, she begins having recurrent fungal vaginal infections.

How does antibiotic use cause fungal vaginitis (yeast infections as it is commonly referred to by women who have it)? Many different types of bacteria plus Candida albican live in the vagina as their normal habitats in harmony in a proper balance for the health of the vaginal environment. When a woman is treated with antibiotics of any kind, for any reason, it is believed that many of the bacteria in the vagina are decreased in number by the effect of the antibiotic on them. When that happens, the balance between the bacterial flora and the fungal flora may be changed in favor of the fungus allowing for fungal overgrowth resulting in a fungal vaginitis (yeast infection).

On the other hand, corrosive vaginal douching, such as Lysol and Vinegar and other substances like that, can cause vaginitis because some of these substances can kill the fungus that lives in the vagina, resulting in an overgrowth of bacteria causing a bacterial vaginitis to develop.

The diagnosis of vaginal yeast infection is made by a KOH wet mount on a glass slide which is looked at under a microscope by the examining physician. The presence of hyphae and spores of the Candida albican confirm the diagnosis.

It is wrong and ill advised for any woman to assume that she has a yeast vaginal infection when she develops a vaginal discharge. Self-treatment using over-the-counter vaginal creams can be fraught with danger, because there are many serious diseases that can first manifest themselves as discharge from the vagina. Examples are STD, cervical cancer to name a few. It is always best for a woman who develops a vaginal discharge to seek the help of a physician for proper pelvic examination and proper tests to establish a proper diagnosis and treatment of the vaginal problem, whatever it might be. Many poor women frequently cannot afford the cost of going to a doctor and, as a result, these women tend to use a lot of self-treatment, using all sorts of home remedies to treat themselves. This practice must be discouraged.

Treatments of fungal vaginitis (yeast infections)

Vaginal yeast infection is usually treated with anti-fungal creams or suppositories, such as Monistat vaginal cream or suppositories at bedtime for seven days or Femstat vaginal cream, Gyne-Lotrimin, etc. Frequently, one dose of Diflucan 150 Mg is sufficient to treat an episode of fungal vaginitis.

Lympho-Granuloma Venereum (LGV) is an STD, which is caused by Chlamydia trachomatis serotype L1, L2 and L3 one week to 4 weeks after unprotected sexual intercourse with an infected man. Symptoms such as fever and headache may develop along with painless ulcer in the vulva and vaginal areas. The infection frequently spreads via the lymphatic system into the anus and rectum resulting in ulcers; recto-vaginal fistulas and abscesses can develop. If left untreated, rectal stenosis can occur. The diagnosis is made by complement fixation and serologic antibody test to Chlamydia, so called Frei test. Treatment is Tetracycline or Erythromycin 500 mg 4 times a day for 3 weeks or Doxycycline 100 mg BID for 3 weeks.

Granuloma Inguinale is an STD that is caused by the bacterial organism Donovania granulomatosis. Small papules develop around the vagina, usually 1 to 12 weeks after sexual intercourse occurs with an infected man. These papules quickly develop into ulcers, which spread to the anus, vagina, perineum, and cervix. Typically, if left untreated, fibrosis and scarring develop along with keloid formation in association with vaginal stenosis and the development of elephantiasis due to destruction of the lymphatic system in the general pelvic area.

To make the diagnosis, tissue from the infected ulcers is stained with either Giemsa or Wright stain and examined under the microscope. Under the microscope Donovan bodies can be seen, confirming the diagnosis. Treatment is usually with Tetracycline 500 4 times per day for 3 weeks.

Condyloma acuminata, or venereal warts, is an extremely contagious STD, which is transmitted by skin-to-skin contact during sexual intercourse with an infected sexual partner. Venereal wart infection is frequently associated with other STDs such as Trichomonas vaginitis infection or bacterial vaginosis, etc.

The organism that is responsible for venereal warts is human papilloma virus. These lesions proliferate more in women who are diabetic, on birth control pills, pregnant or are immuno-suppressed.

Venereal warts can involve the perivaginal area, the vulva, and the perianal area.

The lesions can appear in a cauliflower formation. They frequently bleed and can be very difficult to treat.

Pregnant women whose perivaginal and vulva area are infected with the venereal wart may have to undergo a cesarean section to prevent the baby from coming into contact with this most infectious virus. The usual treatments include applications of Aldara cream, 25% trichloroacetic acid, salicylic acid in Collodion, or podophyllin resin, weekly to the warts. Sometimes, laser treatments, electrosurgery, or cryosurgery with liquid nitrogen is used to remove the warts.

Molluscum contagiosum is an STD whose cause is a contagious virus which affects the vulva and perineal areas. It is quite contagious and is transmitted by skin contact. The treatment is electrosurgery.

Both Hepatitis C and Hepatitis B are primarily blood borne infections frequently transmitted by needle stick or blood products transfusions. These viruses are found in vaginal secretions and semen and therefore can be transmitted sexually during sexual intercourse.

There is a vaccine for Hepatitis B, which is given in a 3-stage manner. There is no vaccine available for Hepatitis C yet. When Hepatitis C seriously affects the liver and the Hepatitis C viral load is high, and the liver biopsy shows high grade inflammation but no cirrhosis. Alpha interferon injection is used three times per week, in conjunction with Ribavirin daily by mouth, both for 48 weeks, to treat the disease with good success, reducing the risk of liver failure and liver cancer. Ten thousands people die every year in the US because of complications from hepatic C. Pegylated form of Alpha Interferon is now available for once per week use to treat Hepatitis C. (see chapter 8)

According to the most recent literature, **Hepatitis A** can also be transmitting via blood products transfusion and therefore via sexual intercourse as well.

Another serious vaginal infection that women can be affected with is **toxic shock syndrome.** The most frequent cause of toxic shock syndrome is the use of certain vaginal tampons. The causative organism is a toxin from Staphylococcus. The usual symptoms can vary from flu-like to lower abdominal cramps with fever and excessive vaginal bleeding associated with sepsis. Once recognized, treatment with IV antibiotics against Staphylococci is effective and curative.

Three methods exist to deal with STDs.

1. Prevention by using the method of sexual abstinence. This method is unrealistic.
2. Engaging in protected sexual intercourse by using a condom is a proven way to
3. Prevent most STDs. (like Chlamydia, Gonorrhea, Trichomonas, and Syphilis) or to Provide some protection against STDs like HIV, HSV, Hepatitis B Hepatitis C,
4. and H P V.
5. Curative treatments are available for almost all STD. The prominent exceptions

6. are AIDS and HSV for which there is no cure.

Women of all ethnic groups are prone to a multitude of gynecological problems. When women are pregnant, more often than not, the pregnancies go on to excellent to excellent outcomes. However, for reasons that will be discussed later in the chapter, many things can go wrong with both expecting mothers and their infants changing pregnancy into a very serious medical situation with the potential for many possible catastrophes.

Pre-menstrual syndrome, known as PMS, is a complex of symptoms that occur 7 to 10 days before the onset of menstrual blood flow. PMS has been described since the time of Hippocrates. Symptoms of PMS are many and varied in different women. Some of the most common symptoms of PMS, according to the literature, are:

1. Irritability
2. Lack of concentration
3. Tiredness
4. Mood swings
5. Depression
6. Insomnia
7. Weight gain
8. Crying spells
9. Suicidal ideation among some women
10. Breast achiness or pain
11. Poor appetite
12. Decreased libido
13. Diarrhea or constipation

Many theories have been postulated regarding the causes of PMS. Among them are abnormal levels of different hormones such as Estrogen, Progesterone, cortisone, and androgens. Both too much and too little of these hormones are able to bring about the symptoms of PMS. Still more abnormalities, such as too much anti-diuretic hormone, deficiencies in the levels of vitamins A, B6, decreased levels of magnesium, melatonin, reactive hypoglycemia, abnormal menstrual stress, and psychosocial problems, all are believed to contribute to make PMS worse. Ovulation seems to play a major role in the causation of PMS. PMS does not occur before puberty nor does it occur after menopause, or in women who are prevented from ovulating.

The symptoms of PMS seem to be made better by ingestion of Vitamin B6, water pills, and birth control pills. Some women who suffer from PMS respond to hypnosis. Some women respond to dietary management such as low fat, low carbohydrates, decrease intake of tea and coffee and reduced caffeine ingestion. After a hysterectomy to treat problems such as uterine fibroids, etc., if the ovaries are removed, the symptoms of PMS seem to go away. The ingestion of NSAIDS non-steroidal anti-inflammatory drugs like Naproxen Advil, Motrin and birth control pills with progesterone seem to help. Using too much nerve calming pills or sleeping pills should be discouraged due to their addictive potential. However, medication such as Selective Serotonin Reuptake Inhibitors (SSRI) like Zoloft and Paxil seem to control the symptoms of PMS.

Another common syndrome that frequently afflicts women is **premenstrual dysphoric disorder (PMDD).** The different components of this disorder include

1. Depressed mood.
2. Anxiety or tension
3. Affective liability
4. Anger or irritability etc. Zoloft or Paxil seems to work very well in relieving these symptoms.

Dysmenorrhea is a common problem that plagues women the world over. There are primary and secondary Dysmenorrheas. Usually symptoms of Dysmenorrhea commence 6 to 12 months after a young girl starts to see her period (menarche). Some in the literature attribute the cause of dysmenorrhea to such things as uterine contractions. There is evidence that the level of prostaglandins is high, in particular PGF2 and PGE2. During the secretory phase of the menstrual cycle the level of prostaglandins seems highest. The interplay between prostaglandins and the general conditions of the uterus and interference of blood flow to it, resulting in cramping and pain and seem to be operating in primary Dysmenorrhea.

In some women, symptoms of Dysmenorrhea start as soon as the period begins and ends between 48 and 72 hours. The pain can be quite severe. It is located usually over the lower abdomen below the umbilicus, sometimes going around the lower back.

Some women actually pass out from the intensity of the pain and can't function for a day or two when they have their periods. Diarrhea, nausea, vomiting, headache and extreme fatigue are the frequent symptoms that some women experience during their menstrual period.

Secondary dysmenorrhea is associated with such conditions as chronic PID, endometriosis, uterine fibroids, intrauterine contraception device (IUD), etc.

The main treatments of primary dysmenorrhea include NSAIDS (nonsteroidal anti-inflammatory drugs), such as Motrin 600 mg four times per day, Naprosyn 250 mg three times per day, Anaprox 275 mg three times per day, Advil 2 tablets four times per day, Aleve 2 tablets three times per day or Aspirin 325 mg one tablet three times per day, etc.

These medications work by counteracting the effects of prostaglandins on the uterus thereby reducing uterine contractions. Women who suffer from congenital bleeding disorders, such as Hemophilia and Von Willebrand disease ought not to take any of the above-mentioned medications because they will make their bleeding problems worse. Women with peptic ulcer disease also ought not to take these medications because they will make their peptic ulcer worse and can cause gastrointestinal bleeding.

Women who only have mild symptoms of hyperacidity can take H2 blockers such as Axid, Tagamet, Pepcid or Zantac along with the NSAIDS to both ameliorate symptoms and to prevent ulcer formation. (Prilosec, Protonic, and Nexium will work fine to relieve the symptoms of hyperacidity as well). The best medication to prevent NSAIDS-induced ulcer is Cytotec 100 mcg 3 times per day, along with the ingestion of the NSAIDS.

Birth control pills also work to ease the symptoms of Dysmenorrhea. They do so by reducing menstrual blood flow and by inhibiting ovulation. Some women use both birth control pills and NSAIDS in order to get relief. Treatments for secondary dysmenorrhea are essentially based on treating the underlying causes such as treatments for endometriosis, uterine fibroids, PID, removing IUD, uterine polyps, uterine malformations, and cervical stenosis, etc.

Prescribing NSAIDS or birth control pills may at times be useful. Women are encouraged to see their gynecologists for help with dysmenorrhea problems. Fibroid tumors of the uterus are extremely common in women and can cause a long list of minor and major complications. About 70% percent of white women by the time they reach 50 years of age develop uterine fibroids and about 90% of black women by the time they reach age 50 develop fibroids. (Source: Ame. J. Obstet, Gynecology. 188 (1) 100-07, 2003) Fibroid tumors are about 3 to 4 times more common in Black and Hispanic women, than in their white counterparts.

The cause of uterine fibroids is not known. Fibroids develop from smooth muscles in the wall of the uterus. Estrogens and possibly progestins have a marked effect on the growth of uterine fibroids, facilitating their growth to very large sizes at times. Uterine fibroids are not seen before menarche and usually do not get larger after menopause. Women who take estrogen for menopausal symptoms or osteoporosis, etc. have an increased chance of having their fibroids increase in size, even though they are no longer menstruating.

It is speculative to say why Black and Hispanic women have such a high incidence of uterine fibroids. The fact that Blacks, in general, or anyone with any degree of Negroid genes in their being, tend to have a very high propensity to develop keloids (excessive connective tissue, collagen and scaring) when the skin is traumatized by cutting or abrasion. The constant shedding of the lining of the uterus from within and other traumatic events that the uterus must undergo by necessity makes the theory of "uterine keloids" as the basis for uterine fibroids quite tantalizing. Some White women have keloids too, but to a much lesser degree.

The symptoms of uterine fibroids include:

1. Abdominal mass causing lower abdominal pressure.
2. Lower back pain
3. Constipation
4. Urinary frequency
5. Abdominal pain
6. Pain on intercourse
7. Urinary retention
8. Vaginal bleeding between periods
9. Heavy and prolonged vaginal bleeding with clot formation.
10. Secondary iron deficiency anemia because of chronic vaginal blood loss.
11. Weakness and lassitude because of iron deficiency.
12. Panic attacks and depression occur in many of those women resulting from the fear associated with pain and other symptoms Associated with uterine fibroid and the prolonged blood loss. Uterine fibroid and its associated symptoms including the prolonged vaginal bleeding and bleeding in between menstrual Cycles interfere with a normal sex life between sexual partners.

About 11% of women with uterine fibroids who bleed excessively have Von Willebrand disease. (Source: Internal Medicine News Sept. 15, 2003.)
Uterine fibroids create a major problem for a woman's fertility. For one thing, there are a significant percentage of women whose infertility is attributed to uterine fibroids.

On the other hand, it is hypothesized that the very sizes of some uterine fibroids make it very hard for some women to carry a fetus to term because the large size of fibroids inside the uterus prevent fetuses from growing by being crowded out. The result may be spontaneous abortion, or preterm labor and premature delivery.

Frequently, however, the fibroids are multiple but small enough to allow for the growth of fetuses allowing pregnancies to go to completion. Occasionally, the uterine fibroids have to be removed via a procedure called a myomectomy leaving the uterus in place in order to allow the woman a chance to conceive and carry on a pregnancy to term.

There are women who are not in a position to get pregnant but prefer a myomectomy to a hysterectomy because these women want to keep their uterus. Black women views of womanhood are in large measure similar to the views of white women and women of other races, but there are some differences known mostly to the communities of black women.

One of the key differences is that many black women are reluctant to have hysterectomies because of the unsubstantiated notion that when a woman loses her womb she is no longer sexually desirable to her male sexual partner. It is not clear as to where this false notion originated, but it is pervasive in many communities where black women reside. Many these women spend a great deal of time discussing this topic in their doctor's offices.

Removing a woman's uterus for a legitimate medical reason does not diminish a woman's ability to function sexually. If a woman's ovaries are removed, the woman will undergo surgically induced menopause in the same way as if she had undergone menopause naturally.

As stated earlier, excessive vaginal blood loss is a common problem associated with uterine fibroids and results in iron deficiency anemia leading to weakness, lassitude, shortness of breath and an overall chronic unwell feeling.

Pelvic ultrasound is the best radiological test to diagnose uterine fibroids along with the pelvic examination. Sometimes fibroids can grow to very large sizes, presenting as an endocervical mass, which requires a more extensive evaluation to make sure that the woman is not suffering from cancer, such as sarcomas. Large uterine fibroids can be palpated as a large pelvic/ abdominal mass, which can cause abdominal pain, nausea, vomiting, constipation, bloating, poor appetite, urinary incontinence and urinary tract infections, etc.

Evaluation consists of abdominal CT scan, pelvic ultrasound, CBC, blood chemistries (SMAC), ESR, and Ca125. Sometimes even a barium enema is carried out along with the physical examination. If there is nothing other than uterine fibroid, then the woman is referred to a gynecologist.

The usual treatments for uterine fibroids in women of childbearing age who wish to have children are myomectomy or embolization. Sometimes, D&C is done to rule out other causes of the vaginal bleeding. Some time; Lupron is given intramuscularly or other medical treatment is given to decrease the size of uterine fibroids and/or to reduce bleeding.

For women 40 years or older who are no longer interested in having children or in preserving their uterus, hysterectomy, is the usual method of treatment.

Symptoms of menopause can be treated in a variety of established ways. The development of osteoporosis because of removal of the ovaries is possible but women of immediate African ancestry have a very low incidence of osteoporosis as a fact of hereditary. However, many black women have low vitamin D which can cause osteoporosis. (see chapter on osteoporosis).

Much more information regarding uterine fibroids and their treatments exist and each individual woman ought to consult her gynecologist when she faces problems relating to uterine fibroids.

Endometriosis

Endometriosis is a gynecological problem that causes a lot of problems for women the world over. Black women appear to have a higher incidence of endometriosis than white women. Endometriosis tends to affect women when they reach 30 years of age in most instances and seems to decrease when these women reach menopause. Sometimes adolescent girls suffer with endometriosis as well. This is often discovered when these girls are having difficult menstrual periods and severe dysmenorrhea.

Endometriosis results from endometrial glands overgrowths outside the endometrial cavity. These growths can occur in nearby areas like the urinary tract, the gastrointestinal tract, ovaries, part of the uterine cervix and the cul de sac, the sigmoid colon, and the appendix, etc.

Some of the symptoms of endometriosis include lower abdominal pain, dyspareunia and dysmenorrhea, etc. Infertility is a common problem in women who suffer with endometriosis. The gynecologist usually makes the diagnosis and various modalities of treatment exist to deal with this serious condition. Surgical resection of the lesions (endometriomata) and hormones are the treatments frequently used.

The reader is encouraged to consult with her gynecologist for a more thorough explanation of this most serious condition.

Among the diseases that afflict women is cancer of their reproductive organs. The most common cancers seen in the reproductive organs of women are:

1. Cervical cancer
2. Uterine cancer
3. Ovarian cancer

Uterine cancer is more common in black women than in white women. The reasons are many, but chief among them is the fact that most black women are more obese than do white women. Obesity is highly associated with uterine cancer. The reason why obesity increases the incidence of uterine cancer is because fat cells can convert to estrogen, by some adrenal hormones. The higher the level of estrogen in a woman's blood, the more the lining of the uterus gets stimulated which, in turn, can lead to uterine cancer. Estrogen, therefore, is suspected to be the number one culprit in the cause of uterine cancer.

Other predisposing factors in the causation of uterine cancer are Hypertension, gallbladder disease, diabetes mellitus, and estrogen treatment. Oral contraceptives and pregnancy seem to protect against uterine cancer. Pregnancy protects against uterine cancer, because when a woman is pregnant, her uterus is protected by very high progesterone level for 7-9 months. So the more pregnancies a woman has, the less her chances of developing uterine cancer and conversely the fewer the pregnancies a woman has, the greater her chances of developing cancer of the uterus.

Irregular and or excessive vaginal bleeding is one of the most common signs seen in uterine cancer. Endometrial biopsy or D and C is test used to diagnose endometrial cancer. Any woman who is experiencing irregular or excessive vaginal bleeding ought to see the gynecologist for a pelvic examination, Pap smear and, possibly an endometrial biopsy. It is always abnormal for a woman to bleed in between her menstrual cycle.

If the endometrial biopsy is positive for cancer, the usual practice is for the affected woman to be staged, often to undergo a total hysterectomy, and to be treated by adjuvant post-op treatment with either chemotherapy and/or radiation therapy which, may be needed for advanced cancers.

According to the American Cancer Society, 43,470 women in the year 2010 were diagnosed with uterine cancer and 7,970 of these women died of uterine cancer that year.

In 2009, 3,780 black women were diagnosed with uterine cancer in the U.S. and 1,240 of these women died of uterine cancer. Women over age 50 are more prone to develop uterine cancer. Weight loss and pelvic pain may be symptoms of uterine cancer. A greater percentage of black women die of uterine cancer than white women. One of the main reasons for this disparity is the fact that many black women do not go as frequently

The consequence of this lack of gynecological evaluation is cancer of the uterus is usually discovered in a more advanced stage in most black women than in their white counterparts, making it much more difficult to cure this sub-group of women of their uterine cancer, which is highly curable if detected and treated early.

In 1998, the five-year survival rate for early uterine cancer was 96%, the relative survival rates for uterine cancer for white females exceeded that of black women by fifteen percent, which is very telling and unacceptably too high.

The second most common cancer of the female reproductive organs is cancer of the ovary. According to the American Cancer Society, 21,880 new cases of ovarian cancer were diagnosed in the United States in the year 2010 and 1,850 women died of ovarian cancer in the year 2010. In 2009, 1,330 black women died of ovarian cancer in the U.S.

What makes ovarian cancer difficult to diagnose is the fact that there are no early symptoms that a woman can detect. The earliest symptom is usually swelling of the abdomen due to fluid in the abdomen.

The other presenting symptoms are abdominal pain, nausea and vomiting, all of which are late signs and often mean intestinal obstruction because of metastatic cancer wrapping itself around the bowel.

The tests and radiological examinations in use to diagnose ovarian cancer inclue:

Pelvic examination
Transvaginal ultrasound
CT scan of the pelvis with oral and IV contrast
Abdominal CT scan with contrast
MRI of the pelvis with IV contrast
Ca125.

Transvaginal ultrasound is a useful test to screen for ovarian lesions. A group of women was screened using Transvaginal Ultrasound, it had a sensitivity of 81%, a specificity of 98.9%, and the positive predictive value was 94%, while the negative predictive value was 99.97%. ***Source: Oncology News International, May 2000, Vol. 9 No. 5.*** The best way to diagnose ovarian cancer or any other cancer is tissue diagnosis on an excisional biopsy specimen.

The known risk factors for ovarian cancer are genetic predisposition. The cancer gene mutation or trait is transmitted in an autosomal dominant fashion with variable penetrance. Women with one first degree relative with ovarian cancer have two to four times the risk of developing ovarian cancer. Not having any children is a predisposing factor for ovarian cancer. Conversely, having two to three pregnancies to term decreases the incidence of ovarian cancer.

Too much fat in the diet increases the incidence of ovarian cancer. Many black women eat a fat rich diet, which plays a role in their increased incidence of ovarian cancer. Taking birth control pills seems to decrease the incidence of ovarian cancer by 30 to 60%. and so does a prior tubal sterilization or hysterectomy.

Black women have twice the incidence of ovarian cancer as compared to white women. Symptoms of ovarian cancer are very nonspecific making it very difficult to diagnose. Evidence from recent literature shows the extent of the problem, when it comes to the examination of the female pelvis. Bimanual pelvic/abdominal examination missed 36 percent of fibroids and 70 percent of abnormalities in the adnexa (a part of the pelvis) of women. (*Source: American Journal of Obstetrics and Gynecology, 1996; 175: 1189-1194*)

This is an alarming finding because with managed care companies (HMO) reluctant to pay for tests, who will pay for screening pelvic ultrasound to detect early ovarian cancer so it can be treated early in the hope of curing the affected woman?

As stated above, about one to 10 percent of ovarian cancer runs in families. Single women, nuns and women who have never had children have a higher incidence of ovarian cancer. Birth control pills seem to decrease the incidence of ovarian cancer. This occurs apparently because birth control pills suppress ovulation and interferes with ovarian functions.

The Ca125 blood test, may be elevated in some postmenopausal women with ovarian cancer and transvaginal ultrasound may help to diagnose ovarian cancer early enough to save the lives of women who have ovarian cancer.

The usual approach to the treatment of ovarian cancer is total hysterectomy with removal of the ovaries and the fallopian tubes and the uterus, with resection of surrounding nodes, omentum and adjuvant treatment with chemotherapy, radiation therapy, or a combination of both. The five-year survival for ovarian cancer was 44 percent for white women in 1991, as compared to 38 percent for black women a difference of 6 percent.

Cervical cancer is the third most common cancer of the female reproductive organs. Unlike ovarian and uterine cancers, cervical cancer is seen most frequently in younger women. There are multitudes of factors that predispose women to cervical cancer. Among these risk factors are:

1. Sexual intercourse at an early age. The reason for this risk is that the cervical tissues are not mature enough to withstand the trauma and irritating effects of sexual intercourse and exposure to some oncogenes which cause some of the young cells in the cervix of these young women to become dysplastic and which starts the malignant processes in the cervix of these women.
2. Multiple sexual partners are another predisposing factor to the development of cervical cancer. The more men a woman has sexual intercourse with, the more irritations and oncogenes the woman's cervix is exposed to. The more traumas

the cervix suffers during sexual intercourse and the more frequent exposure to high risk HPV, the more dysplastic the cervical tissue can become.

The best tests to diagnose HPV are Pap smear and DNA probe.

There are many types of HPV viruses. Some HPV viruses are categorized as low risk for cervical cancer and some are categorized as high risk. The low risk HPV is types 6, 11, 40. 42. 43, 44, 54,61,72,73, and 81. HPV types 6 and 11 are most commonly associated with genital warts. The high risk HPV for cervical cancer is 16, 18, 31, 33, 39, 45, 51, 52, 56, 58, 59, 68, and 82. HPV # 16 is the most common HPV type that is associated with
cervical cancer.

According to the CDC, 15% of the U.S. population is infected with HPV. Altogether, 20 million people in the U.S. are infected with HPV. Every year, 6.2 million people get infected with HPV, making it the most common STD in the U.S.

The most effective treatments for pre-malignant cervical lesion caused by HPV include:

1. Surgical removal
2. Cryotherapy
3. Laser surgery
4. Electrocautery

Treatments of genital warts include:

1. Podofilox
2. Ttrichoroacetic acid
3. Imiquimod
4. Freezing with liquid nitrogen
5. Electrocautery
6. Surgical removal
7. Laser surgery
8. Veregen ointment (recently approved by the FDA)

To prevent HPV a vaccine has been approved by the FDA. Gardisil is anti HPV vaccine approved for used against types 6, 11, 16, and 18 in females ages 9-26.
Worldwide, cervical cancer affects 470,000 women and 233,000 deaths yearly.

In addition, there is the issue of male hygiene which is most important because the more unclean a man is the more irritating materials he is likely to bring into contact with a woman's cervix. Probable irritants that can be brought into contact with a woman's cervix are such things like bacteria, viruses, fungi, and smegma from under the man's penis or foreskin.

Cervical changes, whether brought about by infections or chemicals contained in solutions used by women during douching, may result in predisposing to the development of cancer of the cervix.

Many black men are not circumcised either because of religious beliefs or because of cultural preferences. According to the WHO, 70% of men in the world are not circumcised. While it is said by some that the penile foreskin adds to increased sensation to women during sexual intercourse, but it is a medical fact that the penile foreskin can cause many problems to women.

Uncercuncised men for example are proned to phimosis, paraphimosis, and balanitis, to name a few. The foreskin of the penis may also produce a waxy and rancid smelling material called smegma, which is suspected but not proven to cause cells of the cervix to become dysplastic when the cervical tissues are exposed to it.

It is further speculated, that Jewish women have a lower incidence of cervical cancer in part because Jewish men are circumcised and are therefore unlikely to transfer smegma to their female partner's cervix. Conversely, it is also speculated that black women have a higher incidence of cervical cancer, in part, because many black men are not circumcised and therefore are more likely to transmit smegma to their female sexual partner's cervixes.

Everything is relative, because proper hygiene would clearly make the transference of smegma from any man to any woman less likely. The woman's vagina also produces smegma but it is located in the labia minora and cannot get to her cervix.

Multiple sexual partners and, starting intercourse at an early age, recurrent and chronic infections are much more important factors in the causation of cervical cancer than any other possibilities. Human Papilloma virus (HPV) plays the central role in the causation of cervical cancer.

Women infected with the HIV/AIDS are prone to develop an invasive and aggressive form of cervical cancer and the causative factor is believed to be human Papilloma virus. Black women in the U.S. are particularly affected by this problem because of the higher incidence of HIV/AIDS infection prevalent in African American women.

According to recent literature, women in the United States spent $250 million dollars per year on over the counter medications to treat fungal vaginal infections, $120 million dollars per year on vaginal douching products and about $50 million dollars per year on vaginal deodorants. All this adds up to $420 million dollars per year on over the counter products to self treat vaginal symptoms. The most effective treatment available to treat fungal vaginitis is Diflucan (fluconazole) 150 mg per day by mouth; one dose. There are several anti fungal vaginal creams on the market; many of them can be bought without a prescription.

Cervical cancer is easily diagnosed by doing a Pap test (Papanicolaou) the procedure is carried out by placing a speculum inside the woman's vagina while she is on the gynecological examining table with her feet properly placed in the stirrups. With good visualization, using a bright lamp, the examining physician is able to fully see the cervix, and using a small wooden spatula, or a cytobrush, multiple specimens are taken from different parts of the cervix and placed on a clear glass slide marked "cervix" or in liquid based container for thin layer preparation.

Slides are quickly sprayed with a fixative solution, labeled with the patient's name and the appropriate identification, and sent to the cytology laboratory to be prepared for microscopic examination by a trained cytologist/pathologist. Sample for liquid based cytology are labeled and send to the lab in the jars. (see chapter on cancer)

The Pap smear used to be classified as follows:

Class 1 Normal
Class II Inflammatory Atypia
Class III Dysplasia
Class IV Carcinoma in situ
Class V Invasive carcinoma

Over the past decade, a uniform system of terminology has gradually been developed leading to the Bethesda Guidelines endorsed by the American Cancer Society and the American College of Obstetric Gynecology When to start doing Pap smear?

3 Years after first penile intravaginal sexual intercourse. No later than age 21.

How often to do Pap smear?

Every 2 years, if using liquid based cytology—until age
Every 3 years, after age 30, if 3 consecutive technically satisfactory PAP/HPV screens were normal.
Annually if immunosuppressed (HIV+, after transplants,) DES+, HR-HPV+

When to stop doing Pap smear?

After total abdominal hysterectomy or total vaginal hysterectomy for benign disease without history of previous CIN or immunosupprssion.

After age 70, or if 3 consecutive technically satisfactory Pap screens were normal in the previous 10 years. Continue annual screening Pap smear for immunosuppressed, DES + and HPV+ women. (see chapter on cancer)

False positive Pap smears on glass slides used to be about 20 percent. This finding is troubling, but if a colposcopic biopsy is done, the true diagnosis can be made. Recently the recommendation for Pap smear has been changed and women are therefore encouraged to seek advice from their gynecologists to help them decide when they need to get their pap smear.

The colposcope is a type of microscope with low magnification, which is used by a gynecologist to visualize a woman's cervix looking for abnormalities of different types while at the same time taking biopsies of the suspected tissues looking for cancer. At times, a camera may be attached to the colposcope to allow pictures to be taken of tissues of the cervix, which can be re-photographed later as a way of checking up on the cervix.

Laparoscopic examination is used frequently to examine the pelvis to evaluate different abnormalities felt on pelvic examination, or seen on transvaginal ultrasound and CT scan of the pelvis. A small incision is made around the umbilicus to introduce the instrument so that the gynecologist can carry out different procedures in a minimally invasive way.

Early noninvasive lesion of the cervix has no symptoms. Vaginal bleeding is the most frequent symptom of invasive carcinoma of the cervix. The bleeding may occur after:

1. Sexual intercourse
2. Excessive and prolonged menstrual bleeding
3. Bleeding between periods
4. Sometimes post-menopausal bleeding in some women only has a purulent vaginal discharge. Some have a mucoid or serous vaginal discharge, as their only symptoms are complaint.
5. Most cancers of the cervix are of the squamous cell type about (90-95 percent,) the rest are adeno carcinoma or adeno squamous carcinoma.

Different Stages of Cancer of the Cervix

Stage O	Carcinoma in Situ
Stage I	Carcinoma Confined to the Cervix
Stage IA	Micro-invasive
Stage Ia1	Minimal microscopically evident stromal invasion
Stage Ia2	Lesions detected microscopically that can be measured
Stage IB	Lesions of greater than Stage Ia2 usually bulky cervix
Stage II	Carcinoma Extends in the Cervix but not Extended to the Pelvic Wall
Stage III	Carcinoma Extended to the pelvic Wall
Stage IV	Carcinoma Extended Into the Pelvic Wall, Clinically Involving the Mucosa of the Bladder or Rectum
Stage IVa	Spread of the Cancer to Adjacent Organs
Stage IVb	Spread of the Cancer to Distant Organs

(Modified from the International Federation of Gynecology and Obstetrics)

As part of the clinical staging of cervical cancer, certain blood and x-ray tests need to be done:

1. Chest x-ray
2. Skeletal x-rays
3. Intravenous pyelography to make sure that the ureters are not involved with cancer or CT with contrast.
4. Sigmoidoscopic examination to make sure that cancer has not invaded the lower bowel.
5. CT scan of the abdomen and pelvis with contrast looking for possible metastasis
6. MRI of the pelvis with contrast
7. CBC looking for anemia
8. SMA20 looking for abnormal liver function and abnormal kidney function. Abnormal liver function tests in this setting means liver metastasis. Abnormal kidney function tests, such as high BUN and creatinine, may mean that the ureters have been invaded with cervical cancer obstructing them and causing the rise in BUN and creatinine.

Cryosurgery, laser, electrocoagulation, Loop electro diathermy excision, and cervical cone biopsy are used to treat early cervical cancer. (Intraepithelial neoplasia or dysplasia) Hysterectomy is used to treat invasive cervical cancer.

Radiation therapy is an effective treatment modality for some advanced stages of cervical cancer; specifically Stages IIIa, IIIb and IVa Stave IVb, sometimes are treated with radiation for palliation of vaginal bleeding.

Chemotherapy is used for palliation in cervical cancer because their effectiveness is limited.

Cancer of the cervix is a curable disease if diagnosed early and treated early. (See chapter 7 on Cancer). According to the American cancer Society, in the year 2007, 11,150 women developed cancer of the cervix and 3,670 of these women will die of cervical cancer during that same period.

One of the most common and potentially deadly conditions that affect pregnant women is toxemia of pregnancy. Toxemia of pregnancy is a rather complex syndrome with multiple categories and varied levels, which occur to different degrees and differing severity.

Even mild toxemia of pregnancy can be a threat to the life of both mother and unborn fetus and because of this; the syndrome must be recognized and treated quickly to avoid catastrophic results.

According to the most recent literature, it is believed that pre-eclampsia begins early in pregnancy and it has 3 distinct sequential phases. In phase one; there is incomplete invasion of the trophoblast into the endometrium, which is probably due to maladaptive immune response in the pregnant mother, leading to inadequate formation of the placenta. This process then causes the development of the second phase during which, there is a decrease in the levels of angiogenic growth factor, resulting in increased level of placental debris in the mother's blood, resulting in placental ischemia. The third phase causes the full pre-eeclamsia syndrome. All three phases must be necessary for there to clinical pre-eclamsia/eclamsia to exist. (see below)

The American College of Obstetrics and Gynecology classifies hypertensive disorder in pregnancy this way:

1. Pre-eclampsia/eclampsia (hypertension peculiar to pregnancy)
2. Chronic hypertension (of whatever cause)
3. Chronic hypertension with superimposed pre-eclampsia
4. Late or transient hypertension

Toxemia of pregnancy is divided in several categories, as just stated. The first part is pre-eclampsia. Mild pre-eclampsia occurs most frequently in young women during their first pregnancies. Usually it occurs in the third trimester of pregnancy. The medical criteria that must be met to think a pregnant woman has pre-eclampsia is blood pressure 140/90 to 160/110, urinary protein greater than 500mg for 24 hours, mild edema of hands or face.

Patients with sickle cell anemia usually have low blood pressure 100-60 to110-70 so a blood pressure of 130/70 in a patient with sickle cell anemia or sickle cell trait may represent hypertension and in the setting of pregnancy may be associated with pre-eclampsia and therefore may need to be treated with medication.

Severe pre-eclampsia occurs when the blood pressure is greater than 160/110; urinary protein is greater than 500mg for 24 hours or 3 to 4+ along with edema of hands or face. In addition, the woman may become oliguric (putting less than 400 cc of urine in a 24 hours period), headache, blurry vision, and altered consciousness, cyanosis, or pulmonary edema, pain in the upper abdomen, liver function test abnormality, and thrombocytopenia. A special problem of hypertension associated with pregnancy is eclampsia. Eclampsia includes all of the above problems seen in pre-eclampsia in addition to grand mal seizure.

Diseases that predispose a pregnant woman to pre-eclampsia and eclampsia are:
Hypertension, acute or chronic pyelonephritis, collagen vascular diseases, systemic lupus erythematosus, obesity, diabetes mellitus, high blood cholesterol elevated triglyceride level etc. Sequelae of pre-eclampsia and eclampsia include persistent or chronic hypertension.

There is another syndrome called HELLP syndrome seen in pre-eclampsia, which is hemolysis, elevated liver enzymes and low platelet count. It is seen usually in women who have had preexisting hypertension, previous pre-eclamptic pregnancies, who are 25 years or older and whose pregnancy is less than thirty weeks. The woman may or may not be hypertensive; HELLP Syndrome is now regarded as a form of severe pre-eclampsia.

What causes pre-eclampsia-eclampsia? No one knows what causes pre-eclampsia-eclampsia. Several theories have been mentioned but no definitive proofs have been put forth to explain the different things that happen in pre-eclampsia/ eclampsia. The two most written-about and talked-about theories are the prostaglandin theory, which states that in hypertensive pregnancies the level of PGI2 or prostacyclin is low, while the level of thromboxane A2 is elevated this situation causes peripheral vascular resistance and causes platelets to become activated. The other theory states that pre-eclampsia and eclampsia are the result of utero-placental ischemia.

According to this theory, utero-placental ischemia causes production of vasoconstrictive substances, which lead to the development of a substance called aldosterone this, in turn, causes salt retention and water retention with elevation of blood pressure. Recently, it has been discovered that there exists placental tissue damage, which cause the release of placental products, (Cytokines, (TNF, IL VEGF) which cause vascular and tissue damage.

This complex of problems leads to poor function of the placenta, which may be the reason for the development of pre-eclampsia. These abnormalities were found in some non-pregnant women 3 years after their last pregnancies which were complicated by pre-eclampsia. These abnormalities were reversed using antioxidant such as Vitamin C.

Treatment of pre-eclampsia-/eclampsia is quite complex and the obstetricians are in control of directing that treatment with frequent help from the internists. The treatment includes diet management with weight control, decreased salt intake, treatment of high blood pressure, and frequent urinalysis to detect proteinuria and measuring serum uric acid, BUN, Creatinine, Platelets, and LFT.

Some anti-hypertensive medications that are used in pre-eclampsia / eclampsia are:

1. Apresoline by mouth or IV
2. Aldomet /Labetalol by mouth or IV
3. Diazoxide IV
4. Minipres by mouth
5. in hypertensive crisis, Nitroprusside IV
6. IM or IV Magnesium sulfate is used for prevention of seizures etc.

Another frequent complication of pregnancy is **gestational diabetes.** About 1-3 percent of pregnant women develop gestational diabetes. The screening for gestational diabetes usually begins between the 24th and 28th week of pregnancy. Screening for diabetes in pregnancy follows these guidelines:

1 hour after giving the woman 50 grams of glucose to drink, the blood sugar should be less than 135mg/d. If this glucose challenge test is positive, a 3 hour oral glucose tolerance test is performed.

The Oral Glucose Tolerance Test:

The three-hour glucose tolerance test is used to diagnose diabetes mellitus.

A fasting pregnant woman is given 100 grams of glucose in liquid form to drink to do the test. Blood is drawn at specific intervals to test the level of glucose. An example of a normal 3-hour glucose tolerance test is fasting blood glucose 105, 1 hour after drinking the glucose solution 190; 2 hours, 165; 3 hours, 145. The ideal blood glucose in a pregnant woman is 60-100 fasting. If the fasting blood sugar is 105 or greater, then the woman is started on a strict diet of measured calories and carbohydrates to maintain the glucose level at the normal range and the woman is encouraged to increase her physical activity as initial steps.

Here is a long list of problems, which can occur during the pregnancies of diabetic women. The pregnant diabetic woman can develop:

1. Pre-eclampsia
2. Eclampsia
3. Hyperglycemia
4. Diabetic ketoacidosis
5. Diabetic coma

The fetus of a diabetic mother can be very large (macrosomia) resulting in a difficult and possibly traumatic delivery. The fetus may suffer from immature or underdeveloped organs such as the lungs, the liver, the brain, and pituitary gland. Congenital abnormalities are more common in a baby born to a diabetic mother, than to a non non-diabetic.

Some of the more common congenital abnormalities are:

1. Cardiac abnormalities
2. Neural tube defects
3. Spina bifida

Intrauterine death is also more common in these women.
If diet and exercise are not enough, then insulin is started to control the blood sugar.

The obstetrician uses a specific insulin formula to calculate the amount of insulin the woman needs to control her blood sugar. Most oral hypoglycemic agents are contraindicated during pregnancy because they cross the placenta and can cause malformation in the fetus. It is crucial that very strict normal blood sugar control is maintained throughout pregnancy to prevent the development of any problems in either the mother or the fetus.

According to the literature, twenty percent of Black women who had gestational diabetes will go on to become diabetic within 10 years post delivery and 10 percent of white women who had gestational diabetes will develop diabetes mellitus within 10 years post delivery.

Several autoimmune diseases that may get worse during pregnancy and some of them can first develop during pregnancy. Some of these diseases include:

1. Rheumatoid arthritis
2. Systemic lupus erythematosus (SLE)
3. Idiopathic thrombocytopenic purpura (ITP)
4. Thrombotic Thrombocytopenic Purpura (TTP)

5. Graves disease
6. Myasthenia gravis

Only three of these conditions will be discussed, because they are the most commonly seen in pregnancy.

1. **Rheumatoid arthritis** is an autoimmune disease, which causes inflammation of the joints causing severe pain and frequently destroying these joints. It can also involve many other organs. It affects mostly people between the ages of 20-60 but, at times, affects children and it can flare up during pregnancy. Many medications that can be used to treat the symptoms of rheumatoid arthritis but most of these medications cannot be used during pregnancy. Salicylates, which are the main ingredient in aspirin, do cross the placenta, which means that side effects such as fetal bleeding, altered renal function, oligohydramnios, premature closure of the ductus venosus can occur.

   In addition, the woman might bleed excessively at the time of delivery. So caution must be used in these circumstances. NSAIDS are very good to treat arthritis but again with caution, because their side effects might present problems similar to those of aspirin for both the fetus and neonate. Steroid can be used during pregnancy and is a very effective medication to treat rheumatoid arthritis. It is best to avoid medications of any kind during pregnancy except in special circumstances, which may be individualized.

2. **Systemic lupus erythematosus** (SLE) is an autoimmune disease which is more common in woman. SLE is seen quite frequently in women of color and it is 3 times more common in black women than among white females. Between the years 1979 to 1998 the death rate from SLE in black women in the age range 45 to 64 rose to about 70%. Women of childbearing age get affected more with SLE. SLE affects all organs in the human body and frequently flares up can cause a multitude of serious medical complications with possible deadly consequences. During pregnancy, SLE flares up may endanger both the life of the mother and the fetus. Therefore, it is risky for any woman with active, uncontrolled SLE to get pregnant.

3. **Idiopathic thrombocytopenic purpura** is an autoimmune disease frequently seen in pregnancy. When ITP is seen in pregnancy, both the welfare of the mother and fetus has to be weighed and carefully monitored. Fetal hemorrhage is the most frequent problem seen.

Corticosteroid is the treatment of choice if petechiae and bleeding are present, or severe thrombocytopenia occurs. Neonatal bleeding is not frequent if the platelet count is 50,000 or greater. When delivery is nearing and if cervical dilatation allows it, fetal platelets count can be obtained by fetal scalp sampling. If the platelet count is less than 50,000, cesarean section ought to be done to prevent brain hemorrhage in the fetus because of passage through the birth canal. On the other hand, if the platelet count is 50,000 or greater, vaginal delivery can be allowed to go on. Several more bleeding problems exist that can occur in pregnant women, but will not be discussed here.

Menopause is a well known condition that affects women the world over. Women reach natural menopause when they stop menstruating Most women are born with about 450,000 eggs (ova) in each ovary and by the time a girl starts to menstruate (menarche), (which usually starts between the ages of 9 and 14), she is left with about 200.000 eggs. She continues to lose thousands of eggs as she releases (ovulates) one egg per menstrual cycle every month until she reaches her menopause.

Different women stop menstruating at different ages past 40 years of age. Some women stop menstruating at age 45 and some women stop at age 55, etc. When a woman reaches natural menopause, she no longer ovulates cyclically.

Hormones, which the pituitary gland produces (pituitary gonadotrophins); control the function of the ovaries to produce estrogen and progesterone. Both of these hormones dictate what goes on in a woman's menstrual cycle. As a woman gets older, the ability for the ovaries to produce these hormones lessens and lack of estrogen in her blood stream is believed to cause her to begin to experience the symptoms of menopause.

The symptoms of menopause include hot flashes, sweating, dizziness, heart palpitation, insomnia, tiredness, lethargy, depression, and crying spells, head ache, etc. As a woman gets older she may begin to experience dryness of the vagina with dryness of the urethral meatus resulting in symptoms, which resemble bladder infection. Frequently, some women experience pain during sexual intercourse, which causes them to avoid having sex with their husbands or boy friends, resulting sometime in serious discord.

Black women as a rule are more obese than white women and obesity may contribute to lessen the symptoms of menopause in obese women. Post-menopausal obese women have plenty of fat from which to produce estrogen under the influence of their adrenal glands. Fat cells are able to transform the adrenal precursors of estrogen into estrogen.

All hormones in the human body need cholesterol from fats to form that first chemical ring (the cholesterol ring) in the formation of hormones such as estrogen, etc. So when a woman's ovaries become atrophied because of menopause and are no longer able to produce estrogen, estrogen must be provided exogenously in different forms to satisfy the body's need of estrogen.

Estrogen containing hormones have been documented to be associated with an increase risk some serious medical problems such as:

1. Coronary heart disease and heart attacks
2. Breast cancer
3. Stroke
4. Deep vein Thrombophlebitis (clot in the legs)
5. Pulmonary embolism (clot in the lungs) etc.
6. Cancer of the Uterus

According to recent literature, using menopausal hormone (estrogen or progestins) to treat symptoms of menopause is considered unsafe for women. Estrogen and/or progestins use in menopausal women is associated with increase breast cancer, ovarian cancer, coronary artery heart disease, stroke, deep vein thrombophlebitis, and pulmonary embolism and increase death rates.

One of the most serious problems associated with the menopausal state is osteoporosis (brittle bones). Osteoporosis causes bone breakages, resulting in severe pain in the spine, hips and wrists, etc. As a fact of genetic inheritance, women of color suffer less from osteoporosis than do white women. It is not altogether clear why Blacks suffer less from osteoporosis than whites do. Women of all races suffer equally from age related osteoporosis. (See chapter on Osteoporosis.)

The negative aspects of increased estrogen production in obese women are that obese women have a higher incidence of both breast cancer and cancer of the uterus. The higher the level of estrogen in a woman's blood stream, the stronger her bone structure, but the higher her risks of her developing both breast cancer and uterine cancer. This is so because the high estrogen level over-stimulates tissues in the breasts and uterus thereby increasing their risks of developing cancer much more easily. According to some studies,

Post-menopausal women who are treated with estrogen for more than 10 years have a high probability of developing fatal cancer of the ovaries up to 29 years after the estrogen treatment was discontinued. *(Source: JAMA, March 21, 2001, Vol. 285, No. 11)*

The mechanisms through which some of complications of menopausal hormone treatment can occur are well known. When a woman takes estrogens, there are substances in her body called anti-thrombin III, protein C and proteins S, which are necessary in the proper levels to keep the blood properly thinned. When the levels of these coagulation substances are low, the blood becomes too thick resulting in its slow motion inside the blood vessels and the usual result is clot formation, leading to DVT in the extremities.

Clot from DVT can break off and cause pulmonary embolism (clots in the lungs), strokes and clots to other vessels such as the vessels in the kidneys, around the heart and inside the abdomen, etc., resulting in lethal consequences.

Women who have OB/GYN health problems or concerns should seek advice from OB/GYN physicians.

Chapter 10
GASTROINTESTINAL DISEASES

DISEASES OF THE GASTROINTESTINAL TRACT are among the most common diseases that people suffer from.

More than 1 billion people in the world have no access to health care. 36 million people die every year in the world because of noncomunicable diseases such as:

CVD
Cancer
Diabetes
Chronic lung diseases etc;
All together, 56 million people die every year in the world because of diseases of on kind or another including gastrointestinal diseases. WHO

The most frequent GI symptoms that people go to see the doctor for consist of:

1. Heartburn
2. Bitter taste in the mouth
3. Indigestion
4. Bloating
5. Gaseousness
6. Increased flatus
7. Nausea
8. Vomiting
9. Loss of appetite
10. Easy filling of the stomach when eating (dysphagia)
11. Pain on swallowing food
12. Pain in the stomach area
13. Pain in the abdomen
14. Recurrent diarrhea
15. Rectal bleeding
16. Pain on defecation
17. Hemorrhoids
18. Burning pain in the chest
19. Hematemesis (vomiting blood) etc,

The reasons for these symptoms include:

1. Hiatal hernia
2. Reflux esophagitis
3. Slow motility of the esophagus
4. Esophagitis due to fungal infection of the esophagus
5. Cancer of the esophagus, etc.
6. Gastroesophageal reflux disease (GERD)
7. Duodonal ulcer
8. Cancer of the stomach
9. Crohn's disease
10. Gastric ulcer
11. Mallory Weiss tears
12. Esophgeal varices
13. Ulcerative colitis

"There are two different types of hiatal hernia: the sliding type and the paraesophageal type" Both types cause significant symptoms such as heartburn, regurgitation, and bitter taste in the mouth, and chest pain. In hiatal hernia, acid backs up toward the throat, causing the symptoms just outlined. As the acid bathes the part of the esophagus that dips into the stomach, the symptoms develop. Bleeding due to hiatal hernia occurs frequently because of erosion that the acid causes in the wall of the part of the esophagus affected by the acid.

More bleeding occurs in para esophageal hernia than in sliding hernia. The reason why more bleeding occurs in para esophageal hernia than in the sliding type is because in the para esophageal type of hiatal hernia, the part of the esophagus that is involved is stuck in one place. In the sliding type of hiatal hernia the affected part slides up and down into the area containing the acid, exposing the esophageal tissues much less to acid and thus reducing the incidence of bleeding.

Chronic coughing and throat irritation are frequent symptoms of GERD.

Another important and serious condition that affects the esophagus is achalasia. People who have AIDS frequently suffer with esophagitis due to fungal infection, viral infection such as cytomegalovirus, or herpes viral infection resulting in severe pain on swallowing.

The incidence of smoking and alcohol abuse is quite high among blacks and, as a result, their incidence of cancer of the esophagus is higher than among blacks who do not drink alcohol and do not smoke tobacco.

One of the most common complaints that the physician sees in his or her office is stomach pain. The reasons for the stomach complaints are many and wide-ranging in characteristics. A frequent contributor to stomach problems is the ingestion of contaminated foods resulting in indigestion and/or acute gastroenteritis with nausea and vomiting.

Another common reason for acute gastroenteritis is viral infection affecting the stomach, resulting in stomach pain, stomach cramps, nausea, vomiting, and fever. Because most blacks are poorer than their white counterparts are, they eat foods that are of a lower quality and frequently these foods become contaminated resulting in infectious gastroenteritis from bacteria such as Staphylococci bacteria, E. Coli, Salmonella, Shigella, Campylobacter, etc.

Another common and frequent complaint of the stomach problems in blacks is stomach pain due to ulcers. The reason why stomach ulcers are so much more common in blacks as compared to whites is that blacks face racial discrimination every day. As a person faces racial bigotry, the person first becomes intensely angry, followed with intense fear. Both anger and fear cause the stomach to produce an excessive amount of acid and the increased level of acid in the stomach causes a burning pain, indigestion, and, eventually, ulcer of the stomach. In order to cope with the daily pressure and stress of racial discrimination, blacks frequently resort to alcohol abuse and cigarette and other tobacco smoking, both of which, via different mechanisms, can cause severe stomach problems including peptic ulcers.

Smoking cigarettes places a large amount of nicotine in the bloodstream, causing marked acid secretion, which increases symptoms of peptic dysfunction and increases the incidence of peptic ulcer disease. Therefore, people who smoke have more ulcers of the stomach.

Peptic dysfunction is one of the common symptoms of alcohol abuse. Some of these symptoms include nausea, vomiting, retching, stomach pain, gastritis, hematemesis (vomiting of blood), and Mallory-Weiss, as a result of forceful and persistent vomiting due to the adverse effects of alcohol on the stomach and the junction into the stomach. (Mallory-Weiss tear is a tear that occurs at the junction where the esaphogus enters into the stomach—Gastro-Esaphogeal Junction, this tear can occur as a result of forceful and prolonged vomiting/wretching from any cause, but it is seen most frequently in alcoholics.)

A Mallory-Weiss tear causes severe upper gastrointestinal bleeding, occurring because of forceful vomiting and retching, resulting in a tear at the junction where the esophagus meets the stomach. Mallory-Weiss tears occur most frequently in alcoholics.

One of the most serious upper gastrointestinal complications of chronic alcohol abuse is esophageal varices. Varices are small superficial blood vessels that develop on the surface of the esophagus because of portal hypertension, which is the result of occlusion of the small vessels within the liver. The occlusions of these vessels cause the spleen to become enlarged, which in turn causes the development of portal hypertension. Because the esophageal varices are superficial, they bleed easily, frequently and profusely. It is almost impossible to stop the bleeding from esophageal varices.

All the different treatments that have been tried have very little effectiveness. Bleeding from gastritis is an extremely common occurrence. Alcohol is quite irritating to the lining of the stomach, and because of this irritation, bleeding occurs. This bleeding can be quite profuse at times.

Attached to the lower part of the stomach and to the beginning of the large bowel is the organ called the small intestine.

The most common abnormalities that affect the small intestine are:

1. Malabsorption.
2. Inflammatory bowel disease (Crohn's disease).
3. Cancer of the small bowel.
4. Aterial-venous (AV) malformation
5. Lymphoma of the small intestine
6. Cancer of the small intestine
7. Bacterial infection of the small intestine
8. Viral infection of the small intestine
9. AIDS of the small intestine
10. Tuberculosis of the small intestine
11. Scleroderma of the small intestine
12. Parasitic infestation of the small intestine
13. Chronic pancreatitis etc;

Many other conditions affect the small intestine.
Malabsorption can occur because of
Tropical sprue
Non-tropical sprue
Gluten enteropathy
Scleroderma
Chronic pancreatitis
AIDS etc;

Patients suffering from these conditions, frequently develop severe diarrhea with massive loss of fluid, minerals, electrolytes, and vitamins. Malabsorption results in general weakness, overall worsening the patient's condition.

Sprue—tropical type, the cause of which is not known but is probably due to some form of microorganism, which releases a toxin into the small bowel, resulting in malabsorption of iron, folic acid, vitamin B12 and a multitude of minerals and electrolytes. Weight loss, anorexia, diarrhea, and anemia are some consequences of tropical sprue.

Nontropical sprue is another abnormality of the small bowel. This form of sprue is due to intolerance to gluten, which is a protein found in wheat and its products. It is believed that this form of sprue is inherited via a dominant gene of incomplete penetrance. The result of this type of sprue is diarrhea, malabsorption, weight loss, and anorexia.

One of the common symptoms of small bowel disease is pain around the umbilicus. Another frequent symptom of small bowel disease is diarrhea. Still another common symptom of small bowel disease is rectal bleeding. The rectal bleeding can be due to angiodysplasia or AVM, ischemic colitis, Crohn's disease, Meckel's diverticulum, polyps and cancer, etc. The lower part of the small bowel is attached to the large bowel and the large bowel is afflicted with the most devastating disease of the gastrointestinal tract, namely cancer.

In the year 2009, 16,890 blacks were diagnosed with colon rectal cancer in the United States and 7,120 blacks died of colon rectal cancer. Another common cause of colon-rectal bleeding is polyps of the colon. Polyps of the colon can bleed, but can also give rise to cancer of the colon. Still another frequent cause of colon and rectal bleeding is diverticulosis of the colon.

Diverticular disease of the colon is more common in the blacks who live in developed countries as compared to the blacks who live in the third world. Blacks who live in the third world have more meager diets that contain more roughage, more fibers, and less fat, which allow for more regular and more bulky bowel movements. The lack of roughage, and the lack of fibers and too much fat lead to constipation, which is associated with increase in the incidence of diverticular disease of the colon and colon cancer.

Diverticular bleeding is most often painless. Painful diverticular bleeding may be associated with diverticulitis. Diverticulitis is a condition that results from an infected diverticulum. Diverticulum is an outpouching from the inside wall of the bowel. Every now and then erosion occurs in these diverticuli due to actions of the stool on them. The result is acute diverticulitis, which causes abdominal pain, fever, chills, and malaise. Diverticulitis is a very serious condition, which can cause abscesses and sometimes perforation of the large bowel, resulting in peritonitis and death of the affected person if left untreated.

Another frequent cause of bleeding from the lower GI tract is AVM. Bleeding associated with AVM (arteriovenous malformation) is not only common but, at times, very difficult to diagnose and even more difficult to treat. Ulcerative colitis and Crohn's disease are common in blacks and the most common problems associated with these conditions are anemia and rectal bleeding.

Ischemic colitis is seen in elderly individuals who suffer from diabetes mellitus and arteriosclerotic disease and is associated with rectal bleeding and abdominal pain, fever chills, and elevated white blood cell count. Bloody diarrhea is seen frequently in AIDS patients because of enterocolitis due to fungi, viruses, bacteria, protozoa and parasites. Enterocolitis is a serious problem in anyone who is afflicted by it, but it is particularly devastating in AIDS patients because of their already weakened condition.

Constipation is a common problem and one of the reasons women frequently seeks medical advice. Constipation can be due to many different things. Poor dietary habits can lead to constipation. A diet deficient in roughage, fiber, and bulk can cause constipation. An underlying condition such as hypothyroidism can cause constipation. Taking medications such as calcium channel blockers to treat hypertension or to treat angina pectoris can cause constipation because the calcium channel blocker relaxes the smooth muscle of the colon, preventing contraction of smooth muscles, which is necessary for the colon to excrete its contents, namely the stool.

Taking too many laxatives is a frequent cause of constipation. When an individual uses laxatives too frequently, the colon becomes lazy, and loses its ability to contract properly and will not work without help to excrete stool. This condition is called cathartic colon. The treatment for this is to retrain the person as to the proper bowel habits to help him or her to refrain from using cathartics to bring about a bowel movement.

Constipation must always be brought to the attention of the physician because frequently constipation can be the first sign noticed in cancer of the large bowel.

The same can be said of diarrhea as it is related to cancer of the colon. Any significant changes of bowel habits ought to be brought to the attention of a physician because major pathologies can be the reason of the change in bowel habits.

Another frequent ailment is hemorrhoids. Hemorrhoids are found on the very end of the lower GI tract, namely the anus. Hemorrhoids have many causes, but the most frequent ones consist of:

1. Straining at stool due to impatience
2. Constipation causing a person to strain at stool
3. Obesity resulting in too much pressure being placed on the anal area
4. Too much weight gain during pregnancy resulting in too much pressure on the anal area

5. Occupational hazards such as driving long distances over long periods of time
6. Standing for long periods of time over many years
7. Obstructive colonic polyps or cancer of the colon resulting in straining at stool.

If a person suddenly protrudes a hemorrhoid while at the same time passing pencil-thin stool, that usually means there is something obstructing the normal passage of the stool resulting in acute protrusion of a hemorrhoid and that person needs immediate medical attention to evaluate the large bowel by colonoscopic examination to seek out the problem. One of the frequent symptoms associated with the anal area is bleeding. Bleeding from the rectum is always serious and must always be evaluated medically.

It is necessary to bring it to the attention of a physician anytime blood is seen coming from the rectum. Self-diagnosis of rectal bleeding, assumed to be due to hemorrhoids, leads frequently to the missing of early diagnosis of colon and rectal cancer.

Blacks and other minorities and in particular black and minoritithy women have a tendency to be bashful to seek medical help when they see blood in their stools. This is a most dangerous habit, which can cause a person to delay the diagnosing of serious problems such as colon or rectal cancer.

In addition to hemorrhoids, there are other conditions that can cause bleeding in the part of the perirectal area; among these conditions are anal fissures and inflammation-associated colitis, both of which can cause rectal bleeding.

How to evaluate gastrointestinal complaints

The first thing a physician must do is to take a careful history. The next step is to carry out a careful physical examination. Having done these two things, the doctor should next try medications along with diet modifications. Depending on the severity of the symptoms and /or the physical findings, intervention by way of blood tests, x-ray tests, or endoscopy/colonoscopy/sigmoidoscopy/examinations might be carried out in an attempt to establish a diagnosis. If the patient's complaint is inability to swallow liquid or solid foods, then a CBC, SMA 20 chemistry profile, and serum ferritin are the necessary and appropriate blood tests to do.

Doing an upper GI series, with an esaphogram, or doing an endoscopy of the upper GI tract is the appropriate and necessary x-ray or endoscopic examination. These examinations are capable of discovering all abnormalities that cause symptoms and diseases of the upper and lower GI tracts.

If a patient's complaint is pain in the stomach, heartburn, hyperacidity, vomiting blood or bleeding from the stomach, then doing a CBC, serum ferritin, upper GI series, endoscopic examination, and abdominal sonogram are sufficient to discover most of the problems associated with the upper GI tract, the gall bladder and the pancreas.

Frequently, an abdominal CT scan is needed to help evaluate the pancreas to be certain pancreatic cancer is not causing the patient's abdominal pain. Abdominal sonogram is the choice test to diagnose stones in the gall bladder, while the abdominal CT is good to evaluate cancer of the gall bladder and the liver.

To evaluate the small intestine, one needs to do an upper GI series with a small bowel follow-through. It is not routine to do endoscopic examination of the small bowel. To evaluate the large intestine, one can do a barium enema, which is putting barium in the intestine through the rectum into a rubber tube, and once the barium is in the large bowel then x-ray pictures are taken in different positions. They are gastroenterologists who are trained to scope the small intestine. In addition, a special capsule study can be done to evaluate the small intestine.

An instrument called a sigmoidoscope can be used to look inside the lower bowel. There are two different types of sigmoidoscopes, a rigid one, and a flexible one. The rigid scope can be passed up to 30 cm, and the flexible scope can be passed up to 60 cm. Different complaints and different circumstances dictate which procedure is done.

There is an instrument called a colonoscope, which is a long, flexible, and hollow instrument that allows the gastroenterologist to examine the entire large bowel, looking for abnormalities. Biopsies can be taken during these procedures and lesions such as polyps can be removed entirely, and cancerous mass can be biopsied.

According to the recent literature, flexible sigmoidoscopic examination missed up to 34% of cancer of the colon. Therefore, since the bowel preparation is the same for both colonoscopy and flexible sigmoidoscopy, it is preferable to do a colonoscopy instead of flexible sigmoidoscopy. When necessary, an anoscope can be used to look inside the rectum to evaluate local problems in that part of the bowel.

How can people prevent the development of some of these gastrointestinal ailments?

Starting with the esophagus, people will decrease their incidence of esophageal cancer by stopping cigarette smoking and alcohol abuse. Both of these bad habits cause a predisposition to the development of cancer of the esophagus. Esophageal varices are associated, most frequently, with alcohol abuse and alcoholic liver disease.

If people would abstain from alcohol abuse, their incidence of alcohol-associated esophageal problems would likely disappear.

Hiatal hernia is a frequent problem and it can be quite troublesome, at times resulting in heartburn and sometimes in iron deficiency anemia because of slow but chronic bleeding from the hiatal hernia. People can help themselves by losing weight and in so doing they can either prevent and/ or decrease the incidence of hiatal hernia. About 51% of blacks in the United States are obese/overweight, and 80% of black women are obese/overweight. Obesity plays a significant role in the development of hiatal hernia and the worsening of its symptoms.

Symptoms associated with diseases of the stomach are more common in black and other minorities as compared to whites and the reasons are many.

To start with, the foods that most black and other minorities like to eat have too much fat, salt, and spices in them. When the combination of a diet of fatty, salty, and spicy foods, cigarette smoking, and alcohol abuse are considered and added to the day-to-day stress that poor minorty people have to deal with, it is easy to see why the incidence of stomach ailments of all sorts is so much higher in them than in whites.

According to the recent literature, a microorganism lives in the stomach of many individuals who have chronic peptic ulcer disease of the stomach. This organism is called Helicobacter pylori. H. pylori is said to play a major role in the causation of peptic ulcer. It is also said that if left untreated this organism can ultimately cause cancer (lymphoma) of the stomach to occur. To diagnose this infection, gastric material is taken from the stomach and tested for the presence of the organism.

A blood test is also available for the presence of H. pylori antibody. The CLO test can also be done by getting a sample of gastric juice and adding a chemical solution to it. If the solution turns yellow to orange color, the test is positive. There is also a breath test available to test for the presence of H pylori as well. A stool test is also available to diagnose H pylori.

Obesity is very highly connected with gallstones formation and gall bladder diseases. Further, many Blacks and other minorities suffer with hemolytic diseases such as sickle cell anemia and sickle thalassemia and thalassemias that predispose them to gall bladder stone disease. Minorities who suffer from these hemolytic anemias produce a substance called indirect bilirubin, which is a pigment that comes from the breakdown products of the hemolyzed red cells. The bilirubin pigment forms bilirubin stones in the gall bladder.

However, most of the gallstones seen in obese people are cholesterol stones. Symptoms of gall bladder stones, which include nausea, vomiting, right-sided abdominal pain which can at times be referred to the left side of the upper abdomen, can easily be confused with diseases of the stomach such as peptic ulcer or hiatal hernia with reflux. Symptoms of gall bladder disease can also be confused with diseases of the pancreas. Both acute and chronic pancreatitis can have symptoms that are similar to gall bladder disease. Frequently, a person would present to the doctor with jaundice and no pain.

Then the question becomes is it due to gallstones occluding the common bile duct, resulting in backing up of bile into the bloodstream, or is it due to a tumor (usually cancer at the head of the pancreas pressing on the common bile duct), causing the jaundice to occur. This condition is called painless jaundice.

Many other serious conditions that can affect the gall bladder, such as ascending cholangeitis, cancer of the gall bladder, gangrene of the gall bladder, etc. Another common cause of abdominal pain is disease of the pancreas. In women, the most common disease of the pancreas is acute pancreatitis. Gallstones are the second most common cause of pancreatitis. Gall bladder and gallstones diseases are quite high in incidence in American Indians and Eskimos.

Gallstones cause pancreatitis by blocking some of the tubes that carry enzymes out of the pancreas, resulting in back flow of enzymes into the pancreas, and causing inflammation of the pancreas. This pancreatitic inflammation starts the process of acute pancreatitis.

The most common reason why people suffer from pancreatitis is alcoholism, although the incidence of alcohol abuse is high in whites than it is in blacks and other minorities. Alcohol is very toxic to the pancreas, resulting in acute inflammation causing acute pancreatitis. Acute pancreatitis causes abdominal pain, nausea, vomiting, fever, dehydration, electrolyte imbalance and high serum or urine amylase.

When pancreatitis occurs along with other tissue damage, resulting in chronic pancreatitis, pseudocyst of the pancreas and pancreatic abscess can also occur. The symptoms of chronic pancreatitis include the symptoms outlined in acute pancreatitis, plus severe diarrhea, malabsorption, weight loss, and diabetes mellitus, etc.

The reason why malabsorption and diarrhea occur in chronic pancreatitis is that the pancreas, having been destroyed by the effect of alcohol, is not able to produce the different enzymes that are necessary for proper digestion of foods. In particular, fatty foods cannot be digested, resulting in oily diarrhea. The reason that diabetes mellitus occurs in chronic pancreatitis is that the cells that produce insulin are located in the pancreas, and once the pancreas is destroyed then insulin cannot be made. The result is high blood sugar in the blood and all of its consequences.

Many more conditions affect the small bowel and large bowel that can cause pain, and among them are ulcerative colitis and Crohn's disease. Some of the first signs are rectal bleeding, cramps, diarrhea, pain, iron deficiency anemia, etc. No one knows what causes Crohn's disease and ulcerative colitis. To diagnose inflammatory bowel diseases, both barium studies and colonoscopic examinations are used.

To diagnose inflammatory bowel of the small bowel, barium study is needed. Diagnosis of inflammatory bowel disease of the large intestine can be made by both barium studies and colonoscopic examinations. In inflammatory bowel disease, the inner surface of the bowel is swollen and inflamed and bleeds easily.

The cause or causes of these changes are not known in spite of many years of research. In addition to abdominal pain, diarrhea, and rectal bleeding, there is an increased incidence of colorectal cancer in people suffering with inflammatory bowel disease.

How to evaluate diseases of the gastrointestinal tract

The beginning of the GI tract is the mouth, and the best way to evaluate the mouth is by the naked eye. To evaluate the throat, sometimes an instrument like the laryngoscope may be used.

To evaluate the esophagus, either barium swallows followed by x-ray or endoscopy can be used.

To evaluate the stomach, the best two ways are upper GI series with barium swallow or endoscopic examination, during which the different parts of the stomach can be directly visualized and, when necessary, biopsies can be done. It is important to understand that if a gastric ulcer is detected during the upper GI series, then endoscopic examination must be carried out so that it can be biopsied to rule out cancer. Gastric ulcers have a high propensity to be cancerous and must always be biopsied when discovered. There are multitudes of other abnormalities that can be found in the upper GI tract during the endoscopic examination.

The best way available to evaluate the small bowel is using barium swallow with small bowel follow-through. Some of the diseases found in the small bowel are Crohn's disease, cancer, malabsorption, Meckel's diverticulum, arteriovenous malformation, polyps, cancer etc.

To evaluate the large bowel (colon or intestine), barium enema, colonoscopy, rigid or flexible sigmoidoscopic examination is used. Using these examinations, the physician can evaluate the entire large bowel from the anus up to the area where the large bowel is joined with the small bowel. Conditions such as cancer, polyps, diverticulosis, ulcerative colitis, ischemic colitis, arteriovenous malformations, hemorrhoids, anal fissures, etc., can be discovered and, when necessary, biopsies can be taken to determine the true nature of some of these diseases, to allow for appropriate treatments," whether surgical or medical treatments".

How to best treat the different diseases of the gastrointestinal tract

One of the common complaints that bring patients to the physician's office is heartburn. Heartburn is due to hiatal hernia with reflux esophagitis. Women suffer a lot from this condition because of the fact that a large percentage of women are obese and obesity has a close association with hiatal hernia and heartburn. The best treatments consist of:

1. Weight loss
2. Low-fat diet
3. Decrease of caffeine intake
4. Decrease of alcohol consumption
5. Sleeping with head of the bed up, or placing 2-3 pillows under one's head when sleeping, to prevent the free flow of acid to reflux up towards the throat
6. Reglan 10 mg, 15 minutes before meals, three times a day and at bedtime.
7. H2 blockers like Zantac, Axid, Pepcid, Tagamet etc
8. Protein pump inhibitors (PPI's) like Nexium, Prilosec, Prevacid, Protonic, and AcipHex

Regland works to propel the foods down the stomach with more ease, preventing too much acid production. When food sits in the stomach too long, too much acid is produced. It backs up toward the upper chest, causing hyperacidity, heartburn, and bad taste in the mouth, bad breath and, frequently, severe chest pain simulating cardiac chest pain and, at times, a chronic cough. Whenever the stomach detects food it sends a signal to the lining of the stomach where the acid-producing cells are located to secrete more acid to digest the food.

The idea then is to help move the food along so that less acid is produced, thereby decreasing the symptoms of heartburn. H² blockers such as Tagamet, Axid, Zantac, and Pepcid are used also in hiatal hernia with reflux with very good success because these medications block the production of excess acid, preventing the formation of ulcerations around the esophagogastric junction, thereby decreasing the symptoms of heartburn. Protein pump inhibitors such as Prilosec, Prevacid, Nexium and Protonic, AcipHex are also very effective in medical management of GERD (gastroesophageal reflux disease).

There is no definite surgical procedure available to repair hiatal hernia in common use, though there have been some recent claims being made that hiatal hernia can be repaired using laser. However, GERD is being treated laparoscopically using a wraparound surgical technique that seems to be enjoying some degree of success.

Antacids such as Mylanta, Maalox, Rolaids, etc. are also helpful in relieving symptoms of heartburn and hyperacidity associated with hiatal hernia with reflux.

The most common disease of the stomach is ulcer. Other diseases of the stomach that are frequently seen are cancer, lymphoma, gastritis associated with aspirin ingestion or alcohol abuse and H. Pylori infection, etc.

The best treatment available to treat stomach ulcers is the H2 blockers, such as Tagamet, Axid, Zantac, Pepcid and more powerful acid blockers, namely protein pump inhibitors like Prilosec, Prevacid, Nexium, Protonix, AcipHex etc. These medications are commonly used for two months to treat ulcers that are proven by upper GI series or endoscopic examination. After two months, a repeat upper GI series or endoscopic examination is done. If the ulcer is healed, then based on symptoms, the physician may choose whether to continue treatment for a few more weeks or not.

If the ulcer is only partially healed, then treatment with H2 blockers can continue for two more months. If the last two months of treatment trial of the ulcer still fails to heal it fully or not at all, then at this point a biopsy via endoscopic examination becomes mandatory to rule out cancer. It is now accepted practice to test for H. pylori at the time of endoscopic examination, using gastric tissue via biopsy to test for the presence or absence of this microorganism. (see above for a discussion regarding other tests available to diagnose H pylori)

H. pylori is believed to play a major role in the causation of peptic ulcer disease and malignancy of the stomach, such as lymphoma, as stated above. H. pylori is the most common nosocomial infection in the world.

About 50% of the world population is infected with H. pylori. About 75% of the population of New York City it is said carries the H. pylori organism in their stomach because of migration of people from different parts of the world who live there. Countrywide in the U.S., the incidence of H. pylori is 30%. Chronic peptic ulcer disease is associated with H. pylori, the latter being tagged as a causative reason for the development of the ulcer.

There are several protocols available to treat H. pylori but Prevpac is a frequently used one. It is used for either 10 days or 14 days. H. pylori get into the body through the" oral /fecal" route. It is important to understand that diagnosing peptic ulcer using the upper GI series is only 65%-70% accurate, while diagnosing peptic ulcer using endoscopy is about 95%-100% accurate.

Surgical treatment is still used for treating ulcers of the stomach under specific circumstances. When an ulcer of the stomach fails to stop bleeding in spite of all medical treatments and in particular when the patient who is bleeding receives too much blood; a gastrectomy is usually carried out to stop the bleeding and save the patient's life. Another situation that requires gastrectomy is when a biopsy of the stomach reveals the presence of cancer, a gastrectomy is usually undertaken to remove the cancerous part of the stomach. More often than not, other treatments such as chemotherapy and/or radiotherapy are used as additional treatments when cancer of the stomach is surgically removed.

The small intestine is frequently affected by Crohn's disease, and the most frequent treatment for Crohn's disease is steroids with Azulfidine steroid enemas with added folic acid to prevent the folic acid deficiency that the Azulfidine causes. Surgical resection of part of the small intestine is also frequently carried out as part of the treatment for small bowel Crohn's disease.

Another common disease of the small bowel is cancer. The cancer seen in the small bowel can vary from solid tumor like adenocarcinoma, lymphoma, carcinoid tumor, and different types of metastatic cancer to the small bowel. Another frequent disease of the small bowel is sprue, both tropical sprue and non-tropical sprue. The treatment of choice for tropical sprue is antibiotics such as Tetracycline and the treatment for non-tropical sprue is a gluten-free diet.

Many other serious medical problems can affect the small intestine such as arteriovenous malformation causing severe bleeding, Meckel's diverticulum with severe bleeding and severe malabsorption due to chronic pancreatitis and a multitude of other causes.

The different treatments for these different diseases of the small intestine are handled individually as each disease situation warrants.

The large bowel is the site for a multitude of diseases, some very serious and some less serious, but, nevertheless, many are afflicted by them. Some of the most frequent diseases and conditions of the colon include:

1. Diarrhea
2. Constipation
3. Diarrhea alternating with constipation

4. Abdominal cramps
5. Flatulence
6. Abdominal pain
7. Rectal bleeding
8. Ulcerative colitis
9. Crohn's disease of the colon
10. Diverticulosis
11. Diverticulitis
12. Bacterial overgrowth
13. Lactose intolerance
14. Acute infectious gastroenteritis
15. Parasitism
16. Ischemic colitis
17. Intestinal obstruction
18. Colon cancer
19. Rectal cancer
20. Rectal fissures
21. Hemorrhoids
22. Inguinal hernias
23. Familial polyposis
24. HIV/AIDS
25. Lymphoma
26. Blind loop syndrome etc;

Diarrhea occurs for a multitude of reasons in humans, resulting in serious discomfort and inconveniences. Cancer of the colon is frequently presented with diarrhea as an initial complaint. Sometimes the diarrhea occurs because there is a mass obstructing the colon but watery stool is able to pass around it, expressing itself as diarrhea. Sometimes diarrhea occurs because of other cancers such as carcinoid tumor, mucus-producing adenocarcinoma of the colon, etc. Diarrhea is frequently seen in people who are suffering from ulcerative colitis or Crohn's disease of the colon.

Diarrhea is seen in both acute and chronic pancreatitis. Diarrhea is frequently seen in individuals suffering from sprue. Diarrhea is seen frequently in people suffering from irritable bowel syndrome. Parasitic infestations such as giardiasis are frequently manifested with diarrhea and there are multitudes of other parasitic infestations which cause diarrhea. Many individuals abuse cathartics and come to the physician with a complaint of chronic diarrhea when in fact the diarrhea is self-afflicted.

Lactose intolerance is quite common in blacks. About 65% of blacks suffer from this condition and develop the disease to one degree or another at some point in their lives. In addition to abdominal cramps, flatulence, nausea, gaseousness, lactose intolerance causes diarrhea. There is an enzyme called lactase, which is produced by certain cells in the lining of the intestine, and the role of this enzyme is to break down lactose into glucose and galactose.

If a person lacks lactase completely or has a diminished quantity of this enzyme, when that person ingests dairy products such as milk, cheeses, butter, etc., he or she develops symptoms of lactose intolerance as just outlined. The ingested lactose becomes almost like a cathartic, resulting in bowel discomfort. Lactose intolerance is hereditary, but oftentimes it gets worse as a person gets older.

Avoiding dairy products is the mainstay of treatment. Some individuals with a mild to moderate form of this condition may benefit from taking a pill called LactAid or drinking milk containing LactAid. Blacks suffer from lactose intolerance in combination with lack sun of exposure, plus the fact the darker the skin, the harder it is for the sun's rays to penetrate and stimulate vitamin D production are the reasons why vitamin D deficiency is so high in blacks and other people with dark skin. (see the chapter on osteoporosis for a more detailed discussion about vitamin D deficiency).

AIDS is one of the most prevalent diseases that causes diarrhea. The causes of the diarrhea seen in AIDS patients are due to a multitude of different microbial, viral, fungal, and parasitic organisms, and in some cases cancer, such as rectal cancer or Kaposi's sarcoma, lymphoma can also cause rectal bleeding and diarrhea. CMV-associated enterocolitis is quite common in AIDS patients. Herpes simplex gastroenteritis with diarrhea is common in AIDS patients. Other well known microorgisms that can cause dirrhea in AIDS patients include Giardiasis, amoebiasis, candidiasis, cryptosporidium, isospora belli, salmonella, shigella, etc.

Lymphoma of the GI tract with diarrhea is reasonably common. Another common cause of diarrhea is acute infectious gastroenteritis with diarrhea due to contaminated foods. The foods, water, raw vegetables, poultry, and meats can become contaminated with fecal-associated bacteria including salmonella, shigella, E. coli, campylobacter (usually seen in red meat/ground meat), Listeria, typhoid, and cholera organisms etc. These foods also can become contaminated with staphylococci resulting in severe abdominal pain, nausea, vomiting, diarrhea, and fever, sometimes resulting in dehydration, electrolyte imbalance, rectal bleeding and, at times, death of the affected individuals.

Poorly cooked meats are a good source of E. coli contamination. In the case of staphylococcus food poisoning, the endotoxin that this organism produces is actually ingested by the individual being contaminated, resulting in symptoms 6-8 hours later.

This happens quickly because the bacterial organisms do not have to multiply in the intestine in order to produce the endotoxin that is produced by the staphylococcal organism. In other situations, the bacteria need time to multiply in the colon to bring about the symptoms. Therefore, a person may get sick 1 day, 1 ½ days, or 2 days later. Diarrhea is clearly a very common medical problem and must be dealt with seriously when it develops. Self-diagnosis can be very dangerous.

It is a good idea to let your physician know if you are troubled with diarrhea so that appropriate steps can be taken to evaluate the cause or causes of the diarrhea and the proper treatments can be prescribed. Viral gastroenteritis includes Rotavirus, Norwalk virus, enteroviruses, reoviruses etc.

Clostridium difficile is a very common cause of diarrhea in and out of the hospital. When it occurs inside the hospital, it is usually due to nosocomial transmission (from a person to another). When it occurs outside the hospital, it is most frequently due to exposure to antibiotics. Antibiotic exposure can cause it to occur inside the hospital as well. 1 out of 10 people with C. difficile die. Other causes of diarrhea include hyperthyroidism, irritable bowel syndrome, lactose intolerance, chronic pancreatitis, short loop syndrome, etc.

Constipation is an extremely common complaint. Constipation is found in all ethnic groups. Blacks living in the third world suffer less with constipation because their diets have more grains and roughage, resulting in more normal bowel movements. Constipation, as a condition, can be due to numerous things, and prominent among these are the following:

1. Stress
2. Poor eating habits
3. Hypothyroidism
4. Taking laxatives too often, resulting in a condition called cathartic colon—that is to say, the colon has lost its ability to contract properly because the individual is compulsively abusing laxatives to bring about daily bowel movements. It is not necessary to have a bowel movement every day. A bowel movement every other day is perfectly fine.
5. Constipation due to medications. Good examples of medications that can cause constipation are the calcium channel blockers. The very reason why these medications work to bring down blood pressure is by relaxing the smooth muscles within the vessel in the people taking them. The intestines have smooth muscles in them and once these smooth muscles are relaxed, the bowel is likely to lose its contractile force, resulting in constipation. Fortunately, these very important medications don't cause this problem in everybody who takes them.
6. Irritable bowel syndrome, a condition associated with spasm of the bowel is frequently associated with abdominal cramps and constipation.
7. The most feared condition sometimes seen in people who are constipated is cancer of the large bowel.

Cancer of the large bowel causes constipation by mechanically preventing stool from passing through the area where the cancer is, resulting in pencil-sized stools and straining during defecation.

Before prescribing treatments for any of these conditions, thorough evaluations must be carried out to be sure of the cause or causes of these symptoms. In the case of constipation, it most probably plays a major role in the causation of cancer of the large intestine. This happens because the foods and fluids we consume in the developed world contain a lot of cancer-causing materials. These materials are either outright carcinogens or cancer promoters.

Some of these cancer promoters are things produced by the human body itself. For instance, when a person eats a lot of fat containing foods such as red meat, the body via the biliary system produces a lot of bile acids in order to digest fats contained in these red meats. These bile acids are very harsh and irritating to the tissue of the large intestine. The long-term effects of the constant irritation of the tissues of the colon result in the development of colon cancer.

Constipation is bad, because not only is it uncomfortable, but it also can predispose the colon to the development of many serious medical conditions, and colon cancer is among them.

Abdominal cramps are a very common complaint and it can be due to things such as constipation, diverticulitis, lactose intolerance, irritable bowel syndrome, acute and chronic infections, parasitic infestation, ulcerative colitis, Crohn's disease, enterocolitis, acute and chronic pancreatitis, cancer of the stomach, cancer of the gall bladder, cancer of the pancreas, cancer of the colon, and stress, etc.

Flatulence is a condition that manifests itself by excessive passing of gas from the rectum. It is a normal biological function to pass gas from the rectum. The gas that is formed and expelled from the rectum is essentially methane. It is, however, abnormal when the gas a person passes is malodorous (smells bad) and when the frequency of passing gas is excessive and when the amount of gas one is passing is excessive. When a person passes large amounts of malodorous gas from the rectum too frequently, clearly this situation requires medical evaluation.

There are many conditions that affect the GI tract that can cause a person to produce too much and malodorous gas from the rectum, but the most common reasons are lactose intolerance and eating too much gas-producing foods such as green bananas, cabbage, peas, beans and dairy products when one is lactose intolerant.

Abdominal pain can be due to many things, including acute appendicitis, acute peritonitis due to conditions such as intra-abdominal abscess of different types, ischemic colitis, ulcerative colitis, cancer, peptic ulcer, perforated peptic ulcer, gall bladder disease, acute and chronic pancreatic diverticulitis, kidney stones.

Other common causes of abdominal pain are acute gastroenteritis due to viral, bacterial, fungal, and parasitic and protozoal infections. One of the severest and most common abdominal pains is due to menstruation.

Menstrual pain causes much distress in women of all ethnic groups. Black and Hispanic women have a higher incidence of uterine fibroids than white and Asian women do. Uterine fibroids worsen menstrual pain and bleeding.

Women with uterine fibroids suffer a lot from menstrual cramps, abdominal pain, and heavy and prolonged menstrual bleeding with passing of blood clots. The pain occurs during menstruation, in part, because of the effects of prostaglandin on the smooth muscle inside the uterus causing muscle contractions and pain.

Rectal bleeding is a frequent complaint for which people seek help from a doctor. Most people think they have hemorrhoids when they see blood in their stools. While hemorrhoids are frequently responsible for rectal bleeding, it is wrong to assume that if blood is coming from one's rectum, it must be due to hemorrhoids that are bleeding. Yes, hemorrhoids can bleed but so can rectal cancer, colon cancer, small bowel cancer, cancer of the stomach, colon polyps, diverticulosis of the colon, ischemic colitis, Meckel's diverticulum, angiodysplasia of the GI tract, and anal fissures, etc.

In fact, a person with no previous history of hemorrhoids who suddenly develops hemorrhoids either with or without bleeding would be wise to seek medical help because an obstructing polyp or cancer of the colon or rectum can cause that person to be straining during defecation, resulting in the development of hemorrhoids. That is not to say that every time someone develops a hemorrhoid he or she necessarily has colon or rectal cancer, but that possibility exists if the person is in the cancer age group of 45 years or older.

If a person bleeds from the rectum, regardless of age, he or she requires a lower gastrointestinal evaluation by colonoscopy to determine the cause. In point of fact, a person in the cancer age group with known hemorrhoids, which have been quiescent, that suddenly comes out and starts to bleed ought to also seek medical care to be certain that he or she does not have other reason or reasons to explain the sudden aggravation of the heretofore-quiescent hemorrhoids.

Blacks and other minorities seem to have a higher predilection to the development of hemorrhoids because they eat a poor diet with lots of fat, less grain, less vegetables and overall use less bulk, resulting in more constipation, which in turn leads to more hemorrhoids due to more straining during defecation. Another obvious reason that blacks have more hemorrhoids than do whites is that blacks tend to be more obese and obesity places a great deal of stress on the lower end of the GI tract, namely the anal area, resulting in hemorrhoids and their associated pain and bleeding symptoms.

Bleeding from the rectum is always abnormal and ought to be evaluated by a physician. The treatments for hemorrhoids are many and each person's case may be different from another person, because the cause or causes can differ. Conservative treatments, such as anal suppositories containing steroids, along with Sits baths or surgical removal of hemorrhoids, either the conventional way or with laser, are being used. Stool softeners, weight loss, and diet modifications are all approaches that can work for different people. It is best really to see your physician who can evaluate you and tailor a treatment program that is suitable for you.

Inflammatory bowel disease, which represents in the aggregate ulcerative colitis and Crohn's disease, are diseases of unknown cause, which cause different degrees of inflammations of the gastrointestinal tract, resulting in bleeding from the rectum, abdominal pain, and sometimes fever, weight loss, diarrhea, iron deficiency anemia, etc.

Sometimes, people suffering from inflammatory bowel disease can develop acute abdominal pain, megacolon, perforated viscous, intestinal obstruction, intestinal abscess, peritonitis, requiring emergency surgical intervention. Inflammatory bowel disease cuts across racial lines and oftentimes starts in the pediatric age group. Inflammatory bowel disease imposes a major burden on the individuals suffering from it and frequently these individuals develop significant psychological problems such as depression and the like.

No cure has been found for inflammatory bowel disease, but significant progress has been made with different forms of steroid medications either in pill form, intravenously, or in enema form. Medications such as Azulfidine as well as Asocal have made a big difference in the majority of people suffering from inflammatory bowel disease. There is a higher incidence of colon cancer in people suffering from inflammatory bowel disease. The reason is not altogether clear, but certainly the repeated inflammatory reactions and scarring that the bowel is exposed to for sure play a major role in the genesis of the development of bowel cancer in these individuals.

Polyps of the colon are quite common in modern society. It is believed that this is so because those who live in the modern world eat poorly. That is to say, people in the developed world eat poorly because they eat too much fats, carbohydrates and salt and not enough grains, roughage, and vegetables and fruits. Some of the vegetables and fruits that people eat in the developed world are contaminated with insecticides placed there by some food growers to prevent insects from destroying their crops, hence maximizing their profit margins at the expense of the consumers. It is believed that the interplay of all these factors plus genetic predisposition facilitates the development of colonic polyps, which in time three to five years may become cancerous. People in the third world develop only a fraction of the colon cancer that people in the modern world suffer from.

Blacks in Africa and other third world countries suffer only a fraction of the colon cancer that American Blacks and other minorities suffer from. Dietary habits have a lot to do with blacks' health problems. They eat too much red meat, too much bacon, too many eggs and too much fat and too little of grains, fruits and vegetables. The "soul food" tastes good but it's not healthy food.

The inability to pay for the healthy foods remains a serious problem among poor blacks, and this economic problem is getting worse instead of better. As the economic situation of black people in this country worsens, the health of blacks will continue to get worse. The incidence of colon cancer is going to get worse as black people's diet gets poorer in the United States and the poorer diet is a direct reflection of the poor economic status of blacks as compared to whites.

Another condition that predisposes to the development of colon cancer is familial polyposis. Familial polyposis is a hereditary condition that parents who carries this gene pass on to their children. The children who inherit this gene develop multiple polyps in their colons and, unfortunately, develop colon cancer arising from these polyps. Once a diagnosis of familial polyposis is established, surgical treatment is advised to remove the colon via total colostomy and prevent colonic cancer from developing.

Diverticulosis of the colon is another common condition seen in the developed world. This is related to the dietary habits of people who live in the developed world. A diet that is deficient in bulk and roughage predisposes to the development of diverticulosis. Diverticula are small outpouchings from the wall of the large bowel. Every so often, the walls of some of these diverticula erode resulting in vascular breakdown, which in turn results in bleeding.

Sometimes this bleeding can be severe and life threatening and the bleeding is usually painless and recurrent. Frequently, the only real treatment that is available is surgical removal of the part of the bowel that is bleeding in order to stop the bleeding when all other conservative treatments have failed.

Diverticulitis occurs when a diverticulum or many diverticula become infected. Sometimes diverticular abscesses can develop. Diverticulitis occurs because the outpouching membrane from the wall of the bowel is bathed with fecal materials and fecal materials contain many bacteria. When the membrane of the diverticulum becomes inflamed and infected, the result is the development of diverticulitis. The symptoms of diverticulitis are abdominal cramps and pain, usually in lower abdominal area, fever, chills; sometimes diarrhea with or without blood and increased white blood cell count (leukocytosis) can occur.

Treatments of diverticulitis include antibiotics by mouth with low-residue diet, for low-grade diverticulitis. For moderate-grade diverticulitis, patients should be admitted to the hospital and keep NPO (no foods by mouth); treatment is given through IV fluids and IV antibiotics. Patients with high-grade diverticulitis with possible diverticular abscesses also need to be hospitalized, keep NPO and treated with IV antibiotics.

Hyperalimentation may be given to sustain the patient off all foods. Sometimes, if peritonitis is deemed to exist because of perforation of the bowel resulting from diverticulitis, surgical resection of the affected part of the bowel may be necessary.

Bacterial overgrowth or blind-loop syndrome occurs when a situation exists that allows bacteria to grow in a part or parts of the bowel where a piece of bowel is left in a pouch-like manner due to surgical repair or due to multiple diverticula.

One of the consequences of blind loop syndrome is low B12 level and all its consequences. A good indication that blind loop syndrome may exist is a very high folic acid level in the blood in conjunction with a low serum B12 level. The approach to make this diagnosis is to try to correct the problem if possible, by treating the condition with antibiotics to eradicate the bacteria that are causing the overgrowth, and then replenish the B12 level with B12 injections.

The enzyme lactase is found in cells that are located in the walls of the intestine to facilitate breakdown of lactase into glucose and galactose; both are sugars found in milk. When the amount of lactase is too low or completely absent, this breakdown process (metabolism) is impaired. The result is abdominal cramps, bloating, nausea, flatulence, and, frequently, diarrhea.

In children, this is particularly troublesome because infants need the calcium and other nutrients that milk contains for proper growth. In infants the treatment is milk substitutes. In adults, the treatments include abstinence from milk and other dairy products or lactase containing milk or taking LactAid when eating or drinking dairy products.

Acute bacterial gastroenteritis can be very serious and sometimes fatal, as well as moderate-to-mild. This usually occurs because of eating contaminated foods, usually with fecal material from food handlers who don't wash their hands after using the bathroom. The fecal contamination can also occur in the plants where the meat or poultry products are prepared for shipping to supermarkets or a variety of other ways in the chain of events that the foods pass through before they get to the consumer's table.

Improperly cooked and contaminated foods in fast food places is a common situation that can result in acute staphylococcus or E. coli gastroenteritis or any number of other causative bacterial gastroenteritis. Microorganisms including E. coli, salmonella, shigella, staphylococcus, campylobacter, cholera, and viruses of different types can cause gastroenteritis. Salmonella or shigella gastroenteritis is a common form of gastrointestinal infection that can cause misery for travelers.

Acute infectious gastroenteritis causes fever, headache, nausea, abdominal pain, and vomiting, severe diarrhea, which can result in marked dehydration, bacteremia with sepsis and sometimes death if not treated in time and properly. When traveling abroad in certain countries, it is prudent to avoid drinking the water. Use only bottled water even to wash the mouth or to brush one's teeth. Do not eat raw or rare meat. Eat meat or fish that is well cooked. Eat only hard-boiled eggs. Do not eat uncooked vegetables of any kind.

Before leaving to go away, make sure you check with your physician to get you a supply of Cipro 750 mg tablets or 500 mg. to be taken one tablet twice per day in the event you get sick with diarrhea. Levaquin 500 mg once per day is just as effective to treat infectious gastroenteritis. Erythromycin 500 mg 4 times per day is the treatment of choice for infectious gastroenteritis that is caused by campylobacter.

Anti-diarrhea medications such as Lomotil, Imodium, and Kaopectate suspension are important to have on hand to treat the diarrhea. Compazine 10 mg tablets to be taken 3 times per day for nausea or vomiting or Zofran 4 mg once per day also are important to treat the symptoms of acute gastroenteritis. Pepto-Bismol taken one tablespoon 4 times per day helps to ease some of the crampy symptoms of acute gastroenteritis

Do not be alarmed if your stool becomes black when taking Pepto-Bismol, it is not blood; the bismuth in the Pepto-Bismol that becomes black because of bacterial actions on it. Tarry-black stool, called melena, smells distinctly like old blood, and is a terrible smell. Pepto-Bismol associated black stool smells like regular stool, except it is black. When not sure, check with your physician.

Frequently, acute infectious gastroenteritis requires treatment in the hospital with IV fluid, electrolyte replacement IV and IV antibiotics. The IV fluid must contain dextrose with sodium chloride of different concentrations. The purpose of the dextrose is to maintain the affected patients in an anabolic state to hasten recovery. In this setting, even a diabetic patient can be given dextrose with added regular insulin. More commonly, the affected patient can be treated at home with medications by mouth.

Acute gastroenteritis can also be due to viruses. Viral gastroenteritis is quite common and can be very severe if not treated promptly and properly and can lead to a multitude of complications such as electrolyte imbalance, cardiac arrhythmia, renal failure, and DIC, depending on different underlying chronic medical problems and the age of the individuals affected, and death can result.

Treatments of viral gastroenteritis are fluid IV or by mouth to prevent dehydration and electrolyte replacement by mouth by ways of soups, sodas, juices or IV. Antipyretics such as Advil and Tylenol are important to bring fevers down. Anti-diarrhea and anti-nausea medications such as just described are very important in dealing with these conditions.

Differentiating bacterial, viral, fungal, or parasitic gastroenteritis is left to the judgment and clinical experience of the examining physician. He or she can usually arrive at the proper diagnosis with a high degree of certainty.

Ischemic colitis usually occurs in the elderly with multiple medical problems such as diabetes mellitus, arteriosclerotic heart disease, etc. Ischemia colitis occurs when the blood flow to the affected bowel is impeded either because the patient's blood pressure falls for one reason or another, preventing blood to flow properly to perfuse the bowel. Lack of blood flow causes a segment of the bowel to become ischemic, resulting in abdominal pain. Sometimes, the circulation of blood is occluded by a clot that is thrown to that area from an embolus, usually from the heart, resulting in occlusion of blood causing ischemia of that part of the bowel, which means, if not diagnosed quickly, the affected bowel will die resulting in a multitude of complications with possible death as a final result.

Surgical resection is frequently carried out to treat ischemic colitis. Once ischemic colitis becomes a serious consideration in the differential diagnosis of abdominal pain in an elderly person who presents to the doctor with abdominal pain, a flat plate of the abdomen must be done. A sign called finger printing can sometimes be seen on that x-ray film and if seen, ischemic colitis is highly possibly present. However, even if that is seen or not seen, angiogram is necessary to confirm the presence of ischemic colitis. The most frequently used treatment of ischemia colitis is surgical resection of the ischemic bowel.

Intestinal obstruction is an extremely common medical problem, which brings patients to physicians complaining of nausea, vomiting, and abdominal pain, and feeling generally sick. The list of things that can cause both small and the large intestine to be obstructed is quite long. Things such as:

1. Adhesions resulting from previous abdominal surgical procedures
2. Fecal impaction

3. Tumor of different types
4. In the third world and to some degree in rural south of the United States, where parasitic infestations are common, certain parasites such as ascaris can cause obstruction of the bowel.

Many inflammatory conditions such as ulcerative colitis or Crohn's disease that can destroy and cause narrowing of the lumen of the bowel, causing fistula to develop, resulting in intestinal obstruction. At the other extreme, these inflammatory bowel diseases can at times present with a condition called megacolon, whereby the lumen of the bowel becomes markedly enlarged, representing a surgical emergency.

Megacolon is best diagnosed by obtaining a simple x-ray of the abdomen called flat plate of the abdomen. Many things or conditions that can cause the intestine to become mechanically obstructed or to lose its ability to contract, resulting in the backing up of intestinal contents, resulting in nausea, vomiting, abdominal pain, etc.

Colorectal cancers are common in all groups in the United States. These cancers are more common in minority women as compared to white women. This is due to many reasons, and prominent among these reasons are the fat-rich diet that many blacks eat and the fact that so many blacks are obese/over weight and the fact that blacks, as a rule, go less frequently to physicians to be examined. By the time a black person develops symptoms such as abdominal pain, nausea, vomiting, diarrhea, rectal bleeding because of colorectal cancer, often the cancer is already in an advanced stage.

If the person is lucky, the rectal bleeding might be due to a precancerous polyp or some other nonmalignant lesion.

Intestinal obstruction is treated with a Cantor tube that is passed through the nose into the bowel. This tube has a little bag at the end of it filled with mercury to pull it down into the bowel slowly, forcing the area of obstruction to open. Every day an x-ray of the abdomen is obtained to see the progress of the tube and to see if the obstruction has opened up.

The tube is attached to a machine called the Gomco machine to suction gastrointestinal contents, relieving the nausea, vomiting and abdominal pain. During this period, the patient is fed with intravenous fluid containing saline, glucose, and potassium chloride. Suctioning GI contents in this fashion causes the loss of a large amount of potassium chloride and it is crucial that potassium be replaced to prevent severe hypokalemia, which can cause serious cardiac complications.

Rectal fissures are lesions of the rectum, which represent cracks in the rectal tissue. They can bleed and are quite painful. Rectal fissures are treated with Sitz baths and different ointments made specifically for treating superficial rectal ailments.

Hemorrhoids are tissue protrusions that occur immediately inside the rectum (internal hemorrhoids) or immediately outside the rectum (external hemorrhoids). Hemorrhoids may at times be associated with obesity, causing undue pressure to the anal area, and pregnancy, resulting in weight gain and pressure to the anal area. Both pregnancy and obesity occur more frequently in black and other minority women than in white women. That is to say, black and other minority women, as a rule, have more children than white women and with each pregnancy the incidence of developing hemorrhoids increases. Many other factors are associated with hemorrhoids having nothing to do with obesity or pregnancies.

Conditions such as constipation commonly lead to the development of hemorrhoids. Colorectal cancer can at times result in the development of hemorrhoids or the aggravation of pre-existing hemorrhoids. If pre-existing hemorrhoids suddenly got worse, either by bleeding or by coming out, causing pain, this may be the result of an obstructing lesion above in the colon or the rectal area, causing straining at stooling. The high pressure generated during straining causes the development of hemorrhoids and the aggravation of pre-existing hemorrhoids.

It is therefore always necessary to pay close attention to the complaints of rectal bleeding or worsening of pre-existing hemorrhoids by undertaking a lower gastrointestinal evaluation by a skilled gastroenterologist to be certain that no underlying cancerous mass is causing the obstruction.

Inguinal hernia can be associated with colorectal cancer. An obstructing mass within the large bowel inevitably causes the person harboring the mass to generate a great deal of pressure in the muscle of the lower abdomen. This set of interactions can result in tearing of intra-abdominal muscle causing the development of inguinal hernia. It is therefore very important to investigate a woman who is in the cancer age group, age 45 and older, who spontaneously develops an inguinal hernia.

Any person who fits this profile ought to have a lower GI evaluation with either a barium enema or a colonoscopy before she undergoes an inguinal hernia repair.

Many gastrointestinal diseases are seen commonly in blacks; therefore it is crucial that blacks pay close attention to the multitude of factors outlined in this chapter to help them from falling victims of these diseases.

Chapter 11

SPRUE /GLUTEN ENTEROPATHY/ CELIAC DISEASE

Celiac disease is a genetically transmited-immune mediated disease that affects both children and adults. The worldwide incidence of celiac disease varies between one in 100 to one in 300 people or one per cent of the world population and it affects men, women, children and people of races. Source: WHO"

The disease is seen 1.5-2 times more often in women as compared to men. It is also seen more frequently in first degree relative (10 to15%), type 1 diabetes, (3 to 16%), Hashimotos's thyroiditis (5%), or other autoimmune diseases (including autoimmune liver diseases, sogren's syndrome, and IgA nephropathy), Down's syndrome (5%), Turner's syndrome (3%), and IgA deficiency (9%). Source NEJM367; 25 December 20, 2012

In the U.S. 3 million people suffer with celiac disease. Celiac disease/gluten enteropathy causes and an allergic like reaction to occur in the small bowel when predispose people eat wheat containing foods. The foods hat can cause the symptoms of celiac disease include wheat, rye and barely.

Signs and symptoms of celiac disease include
Abdominal cramps
Bloating
Diarrhea
Foul smelling stools
Fat rich stools
Stools containing undigested food particles
Lactose intolorance
Malabsorption
Low cholesterol level in the blood
Weakness
Weight loss
Iron deficiency anemia
Folic acid deficiency anemia
Vitamin B12 deficiency anemia
Vitamin D deficiency
Vitamin K deficiency
High Protombin/INR due to low vitamin K

Skin bruising due to low vitamin K
Increase bleeding due to low vitamin K
Osteoporosis
Peripheral neuropathy
Electrolytes deficiencies
Low serum magnesium level

High parathyroid hormone level due to both low vitamin D and low magnesium levels
Elevated liver function tests (AST, and ALT)
Muscle weakness
Muscle cramps
Numbness in extremities due to low serum B12
Poor memory due to low serum B12
Mesntral irregularity
Infertility
Growth retardation in children
Skin rash (dermatitis herpetiformis)
Sores in the mouth etc;

Other diseases associated with Sprue/ celiac disease include
Systemic Lupus (SLE)
Rheumatoid arthritis
Hypothyroid disease
Hyperthyroid disease
Ulcerative colitis
Chron's disease
Type 1 diabetes
Insulin dependent diabetes mellitus
Hashimoto's thyroiditis
See paragraph 2 above

Evaluations of Sprue/celiac disease include:
History and physical examination
Blood pressure
Pulse
Temperature
Respiratory rates
CBC
Complete metabolic profile
Blood culture
HIV/AIDS blood test
Lipid profile

T4 and TSH
Stool for ova and parasite
Stool culture
Stool Gram stain
Stool leukocytes
Stool for C. difficle toxin A and B
24 hour stools for fat
Serum B12
Serum Folate level
Serum Ferritin
Serum vitamin D25 level
Serum Magnesium level
Serum parathyroid hormone level
PT/INR
PTT
Serum IgA anti-tissue transglutaminase antibodies (tGTA) positive in Sprue/celiac disease
Serum anti-endomysium antibodies (EMA) positive in Sprue/celiac disease
ANA
Rheumatoid factor
ESR
Abdominal ultrasound
Abdominal CT scan
Endoscopic examination
Colonoscopy
Small bowel biopsy (abnormal small bowel villi are seen in people who have celiac disease).

Treatments of Sprue/Celiac disease include
Gluten free diet
No wheat
No rye
No barley
No grain
No cereal
No pasta
No breads
No crackers
No cakes
No pies
No Cookies
No oats
No mustard

No candy bars
No lunch meats
No ice cream
No salad dressings
No canned soups
No yogurt
No process foods that have wheat
No beers made with wheat
No milk
No cheese
Give Vitamin B12 IM monthly
Give folic acid 1 mg by mouth daily
Give vitamin D 2000 units by mouth daily
Give 1 gram calcium by mouth daily
Give Ferrous sulfate 325 mg by mouth 3 times per day
Give vitamin C 250 mg 3 times per day to allow for better absorption of iron
Eat potato, soy, rice, meat, fish, chickens, eggs, fruits, vegetables, beans, peas etc;

Chapter 12
TROPICAL SPRUE

Tropical sprue is disease that affects people who live in the tropic or people who frequently visit the tropic. The disease occurs because of bacteria that cause inflammation/swelling of the the wall of the small intestine.

Signs and symptoms of tropical srpue include:

Abdominal cramps
Abdominal pain
Diarrhea (foul smelling stools)
Steatorrhea (fat filled stools)
Stools with undigested foods
Fever
Weight loss
Fatigue
Weakness
Malnutrition
Anorexia
Menstrual irregularity
Infertility
Muscle cramps
Tingling in extremities
Numbness in extremities
Poor memory/dementia
Low vitamin B12
Low vitamin folic acid
Low vitamin D level
Low vitamin K level
Low vitamin a level
Low vitamin E level
Low serum magnesium level
Low serum phosphorus level
Electrolytes imbalance
Cardiac arrhythmia
Hypotension
Kidney disease
High serum parathyroid hormone level

Osteoporosis
Low serum Ferritin level
Abnormal villi of the small intestine on biopsy

Evaluations of tropical sprue include:

History
Physical examination
Blood pressure
Pulse
Respiratory rate
CBC
Complete metabolic profile
Lipid profile
T4 and TSH
B12 level
Serum Ferritin
Folate level
ANA
ESR
PT/INR
PTT
Rheumatoid factor
HIV/AIDS blood test
Vitamin D level
Serum magnesium
Serum phosphorus
Parathyroid hormone level
Blood culture
Stool culture
Ova and parasite
Stool leukocytes
Stool gram stain
Stool A and B C. difficile toxins
24 hour stools for fat
Abdominal ultrasound
Abdominal CT scan
Endoscopy
Colonoscopy
Small intestine scoping
Small intestine biopsy
Bone density

Treaments of tropical sprue include:

Tetracycline 250mg four times per day by mouth
Doxycycline 100mg twice per day
Bactrim DS one tablet twice per day
B12 1mg IM monthly for at least 1 year
Folic acid 1mg by mouth daily for at least 1 year
Ferrous sulfate 325mg three times per day till the hematocrit and the ferritin levels become normal
Replace vitamin D level by mouth
Replace magnesium by mouth or IV
Replace phosphorus by mouth or IV
Replace potassium by mouth or IV
One tablet of multivitamin dayly etc;

Chapter 13
DIARRHEAL DISEASES/ FOOD POISONING

Diarrheal diseases are very common and every year there are 5 billion episodes of diarrheal diseases worldwide. Every year 2 million people die from diarrheal diseases in the world and 1.5 million of these deaths occur in children under the ages of two years. In addition, a diarrheal disease is the number one cause of malnutrition of children in the world. Source: WHO

Every year there are 211 million cases of diarrheal diseases in the U.S. And 1 in 6 people in the U.S. get gastroenteritis every year. Source: CDC

Each year 76 million people get sick from food poisoning in the world and and food poisoning causes 1.8 million deaths per year. Every year 48 million people in the U.S. get sick from food poisoning and 325,000 are hospitalized from food poisoning. Every year food poisoning kills 5,000 peaople in the U.S. The medical Cost of food poisoning per year in the U.S. is $152 billion. : Sources CDC and WHO:

According to the CDC the most common sources of foodborne illnesses are leafy vegetables such as spinach, kale and lettuces 23% and dairy products 14% and they also found that dairy products were responsible for 16% of hospitalizations, leafy vetables 14% and poultry 12%. Other sources of food poisoning include poultry, meat, fish, shell fish, and contaminated water etc;

There are two types of diarrheal disease:

The noninflammatory and the inflammatory types, example of the noninflammatory type include Cholera and Giardia and example of inflammatory type include microbes like Shigella and Entamoeba histolytica.

Cholera and Giardia cause diarhhea by interfering with intestinal fluid absorption causing massive watery diarrhea, abdominal cramps, fever, and dehydration. Shigella, Entamoeba histolytica viruses, bacteria, cause diarrhea, abdominal pain, nausea, vomiting, and fever.

Diarrheal /food poisoning diseases are transmitted from person to person and via fecal contaminated foods to the oral route.

Risk factors for diarrheal/food posoning dieases include:

Residing in coutries where diarrheal diseases are prevalent
Traveling to countries where diarrheal diseases are prevelant
Residing in hospitals
Residing in nursing homes
Children in day care centers
Living in overcrowding houses
Having type O blood type
Eating contaminating foods
Drinking contaminated water
Eating contaminating fruits
Eating contaminating vegetables
Eating contaminating eggs
Eating contaminating hambuger meats
Eating contaminating meats
Eating contaminating chickens
Eating contaminating shell fish
Eating contaminating fish
Using bath rooms without washing one's hands
AIDS
Anal sex (HIV, Giardia, and Entomoeba histolytica can be transmitted via this route)
Eating in restaurents with unsanitary conditions
Traveling on cruise ships
Cancer
Radiation therapy
Chemotherapy
Non-acquired immunodeficiency diseases etc;

Bacterial organisms that can cuase diarrheal/food poisoning diseases include:

Staphylococcus aureus
Escherichia coli (E. coli O157:H7)
Shigella species
Campylobacter
Salmonella
Vibrio vulnificus
Yersinia
Listeria
Clostridium botulism
Clostridium perfringes
Clostridium difficile

Viruses that can cause diarrheal diseases include:
Adenovirus
Rotavirus Norvovirus
Calcivirus

Protozoa organisms that can cause diarrheal diseases include:

Entomoeba histolytica
Giardia lamblia
Cryptosporidium

Symptoms of diarrheal diseases include:

Nausea
Vomiting
Abdominal pain
Diarrhea
Bloody diarrhea
Fever
Sepsis
Weakness
Fatigue
Head ache
Joints pain
Muscle cramps
Thirst
Dehydration
Hypotension
Kidney failure
Confusion
Desseminated intravascular coagulopathy (DIC)
Anemia
Deaths in many cases.

Evaluations of diarrheal dieases include:

History and physical examination
Vital signs
Stool culture
Stool Gram stain
Stool leukocytes
Stool ova and parasites examination
Toxin and antigen assays of stool

"Xtag GPP (Gastrointestinal Pathogen Panel) stool test (this test was approved by the FDA in January 2013, it can detect 7 bacterial pathogens-Clostridium difficile toxin A and B, Campylobacter, E.coli O157,

E. coli Lt/ST, Salmonella, Shigella, and Shigella-like toxin producing E. coli stx 1/stx 2

2 viruses—N Rotavirus and Noroviruses, 2 parsites Cryptosporidium and Giardia"

CBC

Complete metabolic—chemistry profile

T4, T3, and TSH

Blood culture

RPR blood test

HIV blood test

Serum IgA (Giagia lambia diarrheal disease can be senn in people who have IgA deficiency)

Serum titer for entamoeba histolytica

EKG

Chest Xray

Abdominal CT scan

Individual microorganisms that cause grastroeneritis include:

Staphylococcus aureus
Campylobacter Jajuni
Clostridium botulinum
Clostrium perfringes
Shigella
E.coli
Salmonrlla
Salmonela typhi
Vibrio vulnificus
Cryposporidium
Entomoeba histolytica
Giardia lamblia
Listeria
Hepatitis A
Hepatitis E
Noroviruses
Rotavirus ect;

Chapter 14
STAPHYLOCOCCUS GASTROENTERITIS

Treatments of diarrheal diseases are different for different causative organisms.

The most frequent food born diarrheal infection is staphylococcus areus associated infection. Staphylococcus food infection is the result poorly refrigerated foods, in particular diary products containg foods such as milk, cheese, cream, ice cream, and other foods such as rice, grits, meats, chicken, fish that left outside too long. Staphylococcus is every where, on the hands, nostrils, mouth, the skin, kitchen counters etc;

Staphylococcus aureus develops the fastest because the bacterium produces an endotoxin in the food that is being infected. The person being infected actually swallows the already made endotoxin in the contaminated food making them sick in 1 to 6 hours. The endotoxin causes the swelling and inflammation in the colon that results in the symptoms complex that are responsible for the diarrheal disease manifested in staphylococcus aureus gastroenteritis/enterocolitis.

Outpatient treatments for staphylococcus aureus gastroenteritis include:

Compozine 10mg by mouth every 6 hours
or
Zofran 4 mg by mouth every 8 hours
Cipro 500 mg by mouth every 12 hours for 7 days
Lomotil or Emodium may be given to ease the diarrhea
Peptobismol 15cc 4 times per day as needed
Tylenol may be given for fever

If patient is unable to drink and eat, to avoid dehydration, the patient ought to be hospitalized.

Patients with staphylococcus aureus who present to the emergency room with high fever, chills, abdominal pain, vomiting, diarrhea should be admitted into the hospital. These patients need abdominal CT scan, Chest Xray, EKG, blood cultures stool culture, stool gram stain, stool leukocytes count, stool ova and parasites, CBC, Complete chemistry metabolic profile, Clostridium difficile toxin, Cipro 500mg IV every 12 hours or Cefriaxone 1 gram IV every 12 hours, Zofran 8 mg IV every 8 hours

Tylenol 650mg by mouth every 4 hours for fever, D5 normal saline, and 20MEQ of potassium at150cc per hour
Lacted Ringer's at 150cc per hour
Infectious disease and gastroenterology consults.

Chapter 15
E.COLI GASTROENTERITIS

Escherichia Coli O 157: H7 infection is a very common infection, humans get infe ted with it by coming in contact with it by eating foods contaminated with feces from human or animals like cows. It is most frequently transmitted by contaminated meat, chicken, unpasteurized milk, fruits, unpasteurized apple cider, vegetables such as lettuce, alfalfa sprouts, unpastericed juices, and contaminated water. The most virulent E. coli that causes intestinal infection is E. coli O157:H7. It gets people sick whitin 1-8 days.

The most frequent symptoms of E. coli gastroenteritis include:

Nausea
Vomiting
Abdominal cramps/pain
Bloody diarrhea
Fever
Weakness
Thtombocytopenia
Hemolytic anemia
Bruising of the skin due to low platelets
Hemolytic uremic syndrome
Sepsis
Dehydration
Kidney failure

Evaluations of E. coli gastroenteritis include:

Complete history and physical examination
Vital signs
Stool culture
Stool Gram stain
Stool leukocytes test
Stool ova and parasites
Stool for C. difficile toxin A and B
Xtag GPP stool test
Blood culture
CBC

Complete chemistry-metabolic profile
PT/INR
PTT
Reticulocyte count
Close review of peripheral blood smears
Serum LDH
HIV blood test
Urinalysis
Chest xray
EKG
24 hour urine creatinine clearance
24 hour urine protein
Glomerular filtration rate (GFR)
Renal ultrasound
Abdominal CT scan

Treatments of E.coli O157:H7 gastroenteritis include

Hospital admission
IV fluid with D5 Normal saline with 20MEQ of potassium at 150cc per hour
Lacted Ringer's 150cc per hours
Tylenol 650mg by mouth every 4 hours for fever
Antibiotics, aspritin, NSAID, and Lomotil ought to be avoided in gastroenteritis
due to O157:H7 as these might make the disease worst.
Traveler's diarrhea can be treated with Cipro 500mg by mouth twice per day for
1 week or Azithromycin 500mg by mouth for 1 week.

If Hemolytic uremic syndrome develops, a hematologist needs to take over the management of this proble. If kidney failure develops, a nephrologist needs to take over the management of the kidney failure. Dialysis can be carried out on people who require it.

The best way to prevent O157:H7 E. coli gastroenteritis is adhere to personal hygiene and cook foods to a temperature of 160 degrees and avoid eating contaminated foods.

When traveling to underdevelop countries, don't dring the water. Don't eat uncooked foods and avoid eating uncooked vegetables. In addition, it is a good idea to carry both Cipro, Zithromax, Compozine, or zofran with you to take at the first sign of symptoms.
Infectious disease and gastroenterology consultations.

Chapter 16
SHIGELLA GASTROENTERITIS

Shigella gastroenteritis is very serious infection. World wide 166 million people get infected with the shigella bacterium and 1 million people die from the infection. Source: WHO. In the U.S., 14, 000 people get infected with Shigella and 1 percent of those infected with Shigella die annually in developed countries like the U.S.

Shigella gastroenteritis occurs by fecal contamination from person to person and inparticular those living in crowded dwellings and food handlers. It is transmitted from contaminated sea foods, water and ready to eat food products. People become sick 24 to 48 hours after eating contaminated foods.

The symptoms of Shigella include:

Fever
Nausea
Vomiting
Watery diarrhea
Mucoid diarrhea
Bloody diarrhea
Abdominal cramps
Abdominal pain
Anorexia
Malaise
Dehydration etc;

Evaluations of Shigella gastroenteritis include:

History and Physical examination
Vital signs
Chest xray
Abdominal ultrasound
Abdominal CT scan
EKG
CBC
Complete chemistry-metabolic profile
Blood culture
Stool culture

Stool ova and parasites
Stool leukocytes
Stool Gram stain
Xtag GPP stool test
Blood HIV test
T4 and TSH

Treaments for Shigella gastroenteritis include

Water by mouth
Fruit juices
Diluted tea
No foods by mouth
Intravenous fluid with Normal saline with 20 MEQ of potassium per liter
Intravenous fluid with Normal saline and glucose with 20 MEQ of potassium per liter
Lacted Ringer's at 150cc per hour
After a few days of putting the stomach to rest start with bananas, rice, applesauce and toast
Zofran 4 mg by mouth every 4 hours for nausea and vomiting
Zofran 8 mg IV every 8 hours for nausea and vomiting
Reglan 10 by mouth every 6 hours as needed for nausea and vomiting
Compozine 10 mg by mouth every 6 hours as needed for nausea and vomiting
Cipro 500mg IV every 12 hours
or
Cipro 500mg by mouth every 12 hours
or

Ceftriaxone 1 gram IV every 12 hours
or
Azithromax 500mg by mouth every 12 hours
or
Azithromax 500mg IV every 12 hours
or
Bactrim DS 1 tablet twice per day
Infectious disease and gastroenterolgy consultations

Chapter 17
CAMPYLOBACTER GASTROENTERITIS

Campylobacter Jejuni food poisoning/diarrheal illness is the most common food born gastroenteritis in the world. 2.4 million People in world get sick every year from Campylobacter dirrheal illness/gastroenteritis. Source: WHO

In 2010, 845,000 individuals got sick from Campylobacter gastroenteritis in the U.S.
Source: CDC All together, there 17 different spices, and 6 subspices of Campylobacter bacteria but C. Jejuni is the one that causes diarrheal disease/ gastroenteritis in humans.

Campylobacter Jejuni is transmitted by eating contaminated chicken, meat, water and when cross contamination occurs with other foods. Campylobacter infection occurs usually as a result animal or human feces that come in contact with chicken, meat, water or unpasterized milk. More infants, children than adults and more men than women get infected by campylobacter.

Each year 124 People die from Campylobacter gastroenteritis/diarrheal illness. Worldwide most People who get sick from Campylobacter jenuni don't die from it except infants, children, and those who have HIV/AIDS.

Sources of Campylobacter infection include:

Poultry
Pig
Cattle
Sheep
Shelfish
Cats
Dogs
Pets
Ostriches

Campylobacter Jejuni is transmitted trhough poorly cooked chicken, meat, unpasterized milk, water, anal sex, and coming in contact with all the above things when there are contaminated, plus cross contamination in kitchens.

Symptoms of Campylobacter begins from 2-5 days and sometime up to 10 days from the time of comtamination.

The symptoms of Campylobacter include:

Nausea
Vomiting
Abdominal cramps
Abdominal pain
Diarrhea
Bloody diarrhea
Fever
Pain in joints
Weakness
Head ache
Dizziness etc;

Complications of Campylobacter infection include:

Septic arthritis of joints
Endocarditis
Guillan-Barre syndrome (about 1 in every 100 cases of Campylobacter diarrheal infection results in Guillan Barre with general paralysis. This usually occurs several weeks after the onset of the C. infection.
Sepsis
Hepatitis
Pancreatitis
Appendicitis
Cholecystitis
Urunary tract infection etc;

Evaluations of Campylobacter diarrheal/gastroenteritis infection include:

History and physical examination
Vital signs
Stool culture
Stool ova and parasites
Stool toxin A B for C. Difficile
Xtag GPP stool test
Stool leukocytes
CBC
Complete chemistry-metabolic profile
Urinalysis

Urine culture
Blood culture
Erythrocyte sedimentation rate
HIV blood test
Acute hepatitis A, B andC, profile
Abominal ultrasound
Abdominal CAT scan
Chest xray
EKG
Echocardiogram
IV fulid with Noral saline with 20 MEQ of potassium in each liter at 150cc per
or
IV D5 normal saline with 20 MEQ of potassium in each liter at 150cc per hour
or
Lacted Ringer's 150cc per hours

Zofran 8 mg IV every 8 hours for nausea and vomiting
or
Zofran 4 mg by mouth every 8 hours for nausea or vomiting
or
Compazine 10mg by mouth every 6 hours for nausea and vomiting
or
Regland 10 mg by mouth every 8 hoursn for nausea and vomiting

Peptobismol 1 table spoon every 6 hours as needed

The most frequent antibiotics in use to treat Campylobacter diarrheal/gastroenteritis
are:
Erythromycin 500 mg IV or by mouth every 6 hours for 10-14 days
or
Azythromycin 500mg IV or by mouth every 12 hours for 7-10 days

or
Tetrcycline 250mg by mouth every 6 hours for 10-14 days

If a person with Capylobacter diarrheal/gastroenteritis disease is septic, dehydrated with pancreatitis, hepatitis, cholecystitis, appendicitis, or Guilland Barre, he or she should be hospitalized for in hospital care.

The ways to prevent the transmission of Campylobacter include:

Wash hands with soap and water

Cook foods to tempeture to 167 F

Drink only pasteurized milk

Animal and poultry handlers should use gloves when touching and while working with them

Food handlers should wash their hands with soap and water should ware gloves when handling foods.

When traveling to underdeveloped countries dring only bottle water or boil water

Don't eat raw vegetables and fruits when traveling to areas where Campylobacter infection is prevalent

Don't let foods sit unrefrigerated for more than 2 hours

Wash hands always after using bath rooms etc;

Chapter 18
SAMONELLA GASTROENTERITIS

Salmonella is a very common cause of diarrheal disease/gastroenteritis.
    Worldwide 93.8 million cases of salmonella gastroenteritis are reported every year.
    The annual death rate due to Salmonella diarrheal disease is 155,000.

In the U.S. more than 1 million cases of Salmonella gastroenteritis were reported
In 2011, 20,000 cases resulted in hospitalization and 378 people died. Source: CDC

Salmonella can cause three different kinds diseases:

Gastroenteritis
Typhoid fever
Bacteremia/Sepsis

Risk factors for Salmonella infection include:
Eating contamineted raw meat
Eating or drinking raw eggs
Eating undercooked meat, eggs, poultry, eggs products and unpasteurized milk
Contaminated knives, cutting surfaces
Infected food handlers
Owners of birds or reptiles
Living group homes
Traveling to countries where poor sanitary conditions exist
AIDS
Unacquired immunodeficiency diseases
Chemotherapy treatment
Radiotherapy treatment
Sickle cell anemia
Long term steroid treatment
Bilogical medications
Anti-rejection medications during organ transplants

Symptoms of Salmonella Diarrheal disease/gastroenteritis include:

Symptoms of salmonella develop between 1-3 days after exposure
Nausea

Vomiting
Fever
Abdominal cramps/pain
Diarrhea
Chills
Headache
Muscle pain/myalgia
Blood in stool

Evaluations of Salmonella diarrheal disease/gastroenteritis include:

History and physical examination
Blood pressure
Pulse
Temperature
Respiratory rate
Stool culture
Stool Gram stain
Stool leukocytes
Stool ova and parasites
Stool toxin for Clostridium difficile
Xtag GPP stool test
CBC
Complete chemistry-metabolic profile
Blood culture
Urinalysis
RPR
HIV blood test
Hemoglobin electrophoresis
Malaria smear
Chest xray
Abdominal sonogram
Abdominal CT scan
Brain CT
Brain MRI
Lumbar puncure
Spinal fluid culture
Gram stain of spinal fluid
Spinal fluid glucose
Spinal fluid protein
EKG
Echocardiogram

Complications of salmonella gastroenteritis include:

> Dehydration
> Dry mouth
> Dry tongue
> Reduced urine output
> Joints swelling
> Joint pain
> Sepsis
> Septic arthrtis
> Endocarditis
> Osteomyelitis
> Meningitis
> Seizure
> Brain abscess etc;

Treaments of Salmonella diarrheal/gastroenteritis include:

> Usually symptoms resolve in five to seven days requiring no treatments at all
> Re-hydration with water by mouth to treat dehydration
> Intavenous fluid with normal saline with 20 MEQ of potassium per liter at 150cc per hour
> or
> Intravenous normal saline and glucose (D5W) with 20 MEQ of potassium per liter at 150cc per hour
> or
> Lacted Ringers 150cc per hour

> If the symptoms get worst, then antibiotics can be used to treat the infection.

Antibiotics in use to treat salmonella diarrheal disease/gastroenteritis include:

> Ampicillin 1 gram IV every 4 hours for 7-14 days
> or
> Ceftriaxone 1 gram IV every 12 hours for 7-14 days
> or
> Cipro 500mg IV or by mouth every 12 hours for 7-14 days
> or
> Bactrim DS 1 tablet every 12 hours for 7-14 days

> Peptobismol 1 table spoon every 6 hours by mouth
> Compozine 10 mg by mouth every 6 hours for nausea and vomiting

Zofran 4 mg by mouth every 8 hours for nausea and vomiting

Prevention of Salmonella diarrheal disease/gastroenteritis includes:
Wash hands after using bath rooms
Cook chicken, turkey, red meat, ground meat, eggs thoroughly up to a temperature to 167 degree F
Don't drink unpasteurized milk
Don't eat or dring raw eggs
Wash hands with soap and water after handling birds, reptiles
When traveling to developing countries don't dring water unless it is boiled and drink bottle water, don't eat uncooked vegetables, don't eat uncooked fruits
Avoid living in crowded housing etc;

Chapter 19
TYPHOID FEVER

Typhoid fever is caused by Salmonella serotype typhi. After infection occurred, it takes from 5 to 21 days for symptoms to appear. Typoid fever occurs because of contaminated food and water.

Worldwide 13 million people get typhoid fever every year and 500,000 people die every year. Each year about 400 people contracted typhoid fever in the U.S. These infections occur as a result U.S. Citizens traveling to developing countries.

The symptoms of typhoid fever include:

Head cahe
Sore throat
Cough
Diarreha or constipatation
Intestinal bleeding
Poor appetite
Abdominal pain
General aches and pain
Slow heart rate
Fever up to 104
Chills
Lethargy
Dehydration
Seizure in children

Evaluation of Typhoid fever include

History
Physical examination
Temperature
Pulse
Blood pressure
Respiration rate
Oxygen saturation
Stool culture
Stool Gram stain

Stool leukocytes
Stool ova and parasites
Stool toxin A and B for C. difficile
Xtag GPP stool test
CBC
Complete metabolic profile
Blood culture
Urinalysis
Urine culture
Chest xray
Abdominal CT scan
Echocardiogram
EKG

Treatments of typhoid fever include

Intravenous fluid with normal saline glucose and 20 MEQ of potassium at 150cc per hour

or

Nomal saline and 20 MEQ of potassium at 150cc per hour

or

Ringer's lactate at 150cc per hour

Ampicillin 1 gram IV every 4 hours or Ampicillin 500mg by mouth every 6 hours

or

Cipro 500mg IV or by mouth every 12 hours

or

Amoxicillin 500mg by mouth every 8 hours

or

Ceftriaxone 1 gram IV or IM every 12 hours

or

Bactrim DS 1 tablet by mouth every 12 hours

or

Gentamicin 1.5 mg/kg IV every 8 hours

Zofran 4 mg IV or by mouth every 8 hours for nausea or vomiting
Compozine 10mg every 6 hours for nausea or vomiting
Tylenol 650mg by mouth every 4 hours for fever or Ibuprofen 400-600mg every 6 hours Aspirin is not to be used in children to treat fever because it might cause Reye's syndrome.

Complications of Typhoid fever include:

Aspirin is contraindicated in typhoid fever because it might cause acute degranulation of mast cells resulting in hypotension and shock.

Bacteremia/Sepsis

Arthritis

Reiter's syndrome

The typhoid organism can remain in the gall bladder for a very long time while causing no immediate symptoms, while sheding salmonella taphi in the stool resulting in recurrent thyphoid fever infection in a carrier of salmonella typhi.

Chronic carriers of slamonella typhi can transmit the infection to people.

Chapter 20
LISTERIA GASTROENTERITIS

Listeria gastroenteritis develops whitin 9-48 hours afer eating lunch meats, hot dog, cheese, unpasteurized milk, eating unwashed eaw food products, and exposure to contaminated soil and water. It may take as long as 2 months before symptoms appear sometimes.

About 2.500 people in the U.S. get sick every from Listeria and about 500 people die every year from Listeria in the U.S.

Risk factors for Listeria infection include:

HIV/AIDS
Chemotherapy
Radiation therapy
Cancer
Alcoholism
Cirrhosis of the liver
Organ pransplants
Long term treatment with steroid
Biological medications
Pregnancy

Symptoms of Listeria gastroenteritis include:

Nausea
Diarrhea
Abdominal cramps
Abdominal pain
Fever
Muscle aches
When listeria enters into the blood it can cause
Sepsis
Meningitis
Headache
Stiff neck
Confusion
Seizure

During pregnancy symptoms of listeria infection include
Miscarriage
Still birth
Premature delivery
The infants may have irritability, fever, vomiting and may refuse feedings

Evaluation of listeria infection include:

History and physical examination
CBC
Complete chemistry profile
Blood culture
Urine culture
Lumbar puncture (brain CT or brain MRI should always be done before lumbar puncture)
CSF culture
Gram stain of CSF
Cells count of CSF
Protein lrvel of CSF
Glucose level of CSF
LDH of CSF
Stool culture
Stool Xtag GPP
Brain CT
Brain MRI etc;

Treatments of listeria infection include:

Zofran 4mg IV or by mouth every 8 hours for nausea or vomiting

Tylenol 650mg every 4 hours for fever

NSAIDs for fever

Aspirin 650mg every 6 hours for fever
Lomotil 1tab every 6 hours for diarrhea

Imodium A-D 2mg every 6 hours for diarrhea

Kaopectate II caplets 1 tab qid for diarrhea

Peptobismol 1 table spoon 4 times per day for diarrhea

Ampicillin 1 gram IV every 6 hours
>
> or

Amoxcicillin 500mg by mouth every 8 hours
>
> or

Bactrim DS 1 tab twice per day
>
> or

Levaquin 500mg IV every 24 hours
>
> or

Levaquin 500mg by mouth every 24 hours

D5 normal saline at 150cc per hour
>
> or

D5 ½ nomal saline at 150cc per hour

Ringer's lactate at 150cc per hour etc;

Prevention of listeria infection includes:

Wash hands with soap and water after using the bath room
Heat hot dogs, lunch meat, and deli meat well
Wash vegetables well before eating
Keep all foods well regfrigerated
When traveling to developing countries, dring only bottle water, do not eat uncooked vegetables, do not eat uncooked foods of any kind etc;

Other bacterial gastroenteritis includes:

Clostridium botilinum which causes gastroenteritis when people eat contaminated foods such as improperly home canned foods, salted fish, smoked fish, baked potatoes and foods that kept outside at warm temperature for long period of time.
Symptoms begin to develop between 12-72 hours.

Clostridium perfringens causes gastroenteritis when people eat contaminated foods such as meats, gravies and stews. Clostridium perfringes causes symptoms to appear between 8-16 hours after ingestion.

Vibrio vulnificus causes gastroenteritis when people eat contaminated raw oysters, poorly cooked muscles, clams and scallops. Symptoms begin between 1-7 days from ingesting these foods.

Chapter 21
GIARDIA LAMBLIA GASTROENTERITIS

Giadia lamblia gastroenteritis is a parasitic infection that is very common and causes about 22,000 people in the U.S. to get gastroenteritis every year and about 200 million people around the world to get gastroenteritis evry year.

The organism is transmitted via the fecal oral route primarily due to contamited foods and water.

Risk factors for getting from giardia lamblia include:

Eating raw food products
Drinking contaminated water
Infected food handlers
Residing in institutions
Residing in nursing homes
Day-care workrs
Traveling to developing countries
Failure to wash hands after using the bath room
Anal sex
HIV/AIDS
Non-acquired immunodeficiency diseases
Sickle cell anemia
Chemotherapy
Radio therapy
Long term steroid treatment
Biological medications
Organ transplants etc;
A-spleenic (people who have no spleen)
Pergnancy
Symptoms of giardiasis can begin to develop 1-2 weeks after exposure.

Signs and symptoms of giardia gastroenteritis include:

Nausea
Loss of appetite
Vomiting

Diarrhea watery or loose stool
Cramps in the stomach
Cramps in the abdomen
Bloating
Burping
Malabsoprtion
Vitamin B12 deficiency
Blood in the urine (hematuria)etc;

Evaluation of giardia gastroenteritis includes:

History and physical examination
CBC
Complete chemistry profile
Serum IGA (people with IgA deficiency are at high risk for giardiasis)
Stool for ova and parasites
The entero-test
ELISA blood test (this test can detect giardiasis up to 90%)
Bladder sonogram
Urinalysis
Urine culture
Urine cytology
Urology consultation
Hemoglobin electrophoresis
Medications to treat giardia gastroenteritis include:
Metronidazole (Flagyl)
Albendazole
Tinidazole
The course of treatment usally lasts for 5-10 days
Compozine
Kytril
Zofran
Lomotil
Immodium
Kaopectate
Peptobismol etc;

Chapter 22

CRYPTOSPORIDIUM GASTROENTERITIS

Every year there are 300,000 cases of cryptosporidium infection in the U.S. and worldwide there are 2.5 million cases of cryptosporidium gastroenteritis annually.
Worldwide there are 100,000 deaths annually from cryptosporidium.

Cryptosporidium infection occurs mainly in children and in people with HIV/AIDS.
When this infection occurs in healthy people, the infection is usally self limited.

Risk factors for cryptosporidium gastroenteritis include:

Child care workers
Children in day care centers
People who travel to developing countries
Swimers who drink contaminated water in pools or lakes
Parents of infected children
Anal sex
Oral to anal sex
Hickers who drink comtaminated water
Campers who drink contaminated water
Handlers of infected animals
Pregnancy
Chemotherapy treatments
Radio therapy treatment
Long term steroid use
Biological medications
HIV/AIDS
Non-acquired immunodeficiency diseases etc;

Signs and symptoms of cryptosporidium gastroenteritis include:

Nausea
Vomiting
Watery diarrhea

Dehydration
Abdominal cramps
Abdominal pain
Fever etc;

Evaluations of cryptosporidium gastroenteritis include:

History and physical examination
CBC
Complete chemistry profile
PT/INR, PTT
Urinalysis
Serum B12
Stool culture
Xtag GPP stool test
Stool for ova and parasites
Stool for white cells
Abdominal ultrasound
Small bowel biopsy
HIV/AIDS 1 and 2 blood test

Treatments of cryptosporidium include:

Nitazoxanide
Zithromax
Imodium A-D
Lomotil
D5 normal saline at 150cc per hour with 20 meq kcl
Lacted Ringer's at 150cc per
HAART for AIDS patients

Complications of cryptosporidium gastroenteritis include:

Dehydrtation
Weight loss
Acute cholecystitis (acute gall bladder infection)
Hepatitis
Acute pancreatitis
Infection of the small bowel
Headache
Joint pain

Fatigue
Dizzy spells
Pain in the eyes
Malabsorption
B12 deficiency
Deaths can occur in people with AIDS.

Chapter 23

ENTAMOEBA HISTOLYTICA GASTROENTERITIS

Worldwide 50 million people have entamoeba histolytica gastroenteritis every year and about 100,000 people die in the world every year from this infection.

Entamoeba histolytica is a parasitic organism that is transmited via the fecal oral route and is most common in developing countries. In the U.S. the prevalence E. histolytica is about 4% and most these cases are asymptomatic.

Risk factors for E. histolytica include:

Living in developing countries
Eating contaminated foods
Drinking contaminated water
HIV/AIDS
Anal sex
Anal/oral sex
Cancer
Long term use of steroid
Biological medications
Chemotherapy treatment
Radio therapy treatment
Non-acquired immunodeficiency diseases
Pregmancy
Children
Neonates
Malnutrition etc;

Signs and symptoms of entomoeba gastroenteritis include:

Nausea
Vomiting
Watery diarrhea
Bloody diarrhea
Rectal bleeding
Abdominal cramps
Abdominal pain

Fever
Weight loss
Anorexia etc;

Evaluations of E. histolytica include:

History and physical examination
CBC with differential
Complete chemistry profile
PT/INR, PTT
Stool for ova and parasites
Stool culture
Serologic testing
Plymerase chain reaction (PCR)
HIV/AIDS 1 and 2 blood tests
ESR
Chest xray
Abdominal sonogram
Andominal CAT Scan with contrast both by mouth and IV
Abdominal MRI with IV contrast
Infectious disease consultation
GI consultation
Surgical consultation etc;

Complications of Amebiasis include:

Toxic megacolon
Fulminant colitis
Necrotizing colitis
Rectovaginal fistula
Amebic liver abscess
Brain abscess
Seizure
Bowel perforation
GI bleeding
Peritonitis
Sepsis
Intusssception
Empyema
Anemia
Leukocytosis
Eosinophilia
Elevated liver function tests

Elevated ESR
DIC
Malabsoption
B12 deficiency etc;

Treatments of entomoeba gastroenteritis/amebiasis include:

Flagyl
Paromomycin
Tinidazole
Iodoquinol
Broad spectrum IV antibiotics as indicated

For peole who need to be admitted to the hospital, D5 and normal saline at 150cc per hour or

Lactated Ringer's at 150cc per hour
Zofran 4mg IV of by mouth every 8 hours
Compozine 10mg by mouth every 6 hours
Lomotil 1 tablet every 6 hours as needed for diarrhea
Imodium A-D 1 tablet every 6 hours as needed for diarrhea
Tylenol 325mg 2 tablets every 4 hours for fever.

Chapter 24
YERSINIA ENTEROCOLITICA

Yersinia enterocolitica is a Gram negative coccobacillus. It causes disease both in humans and animals such as cattle, der, birds and pigs. Most of these animals become asymptomatic carriers. Once the organism enters into the human body through the mouth, it replicates in the ileum and invades Peyer's patches. From there it dessiminates into the mesenteric lymph nodes resulting in enlarged lymph nodes.

The pain on the right side of the abdomen is frequently confused with appendicitis.
In immunosupressed individuals, the Yersinial organism can spread to the liver and spleen causing the development of abcesses.

Risk factors for Yersinia enterocolitica infection include:

Eating fecal contaminated foods
Eating raw pork
Eating undercooked pork
Eating chitterlings (pork intestine)
Drinking unpasteurized contaminated milk
Drinking contaminated water
Touching infected cattles, pigs and birds
Hemochromatosis

Symptoms of Yersinia enterocolitica include:

Nausea
Vomiting
Abdominal pain
Fever
Watery bloody diarrhea
Lymphadenopaty (enlarged nodes)
Joint pain
Skin rash (erythema nodosom) etc;

Evaluations of Yersinia enterocolitica include:

History and physical examination
Temperature

Blood pressure
Pulse
Repiratory rate
Oxygen Saturation
Stool culture
Stool leukocytes
Stool ova and parasites
Stool toxin
CBC
Complete metabolic-chemistry profile
Serum ferritin
Blood culture
HIV blood test
Erythrocyte sedimentation rate
ANA
Rheumatoid factor
PPD (TB test)
Abdominal CT scan
Abdominal sonogram
Chest x-ray
Gastroentorology consultation to a colonoscopy
Infectious disease consultation

Treatments of Yersinia enterocolitica include:

Intravenous fluid with Normal saline plus 20MEQ of potassium in each liter at 150cc per hour or
Normal saline with D5W plus 20 MEQ of potassium in each liter at 150cc per hour
or
Ringer's lactate at 150cc per hour
Zofran 4mg IV every 8 hours as needed for nausea and vomiting or Compozine 10mg every 6 hours as needed for nausea and vomiting
Ceftriaxone 1 gram IV every 12 hours or Levaquin 500mg IV or by mouth every 24 hours or Bactrim DS twice per day.

Prevention of Yersinia enterocolitica includes:
Wash hands with soap and water after using the bath room
Don't eat undercooked meat
Don't drink unpasteurized milk
Wash hands with soap and water after touching raw meat
Wash hands with soap and water after handling pigs, cattles, and birds
Refrain from eating chitterlings.

Chapter 25

CLOSTRIDIUM DIFFICILE DIARRHEAL DISEASE/GASTROENTERITIS

Clostridium difficile diarrheal disease/gastroenteritis is a very common infection that results from taking some antibiotics and nosocomially. In addition the infection can also develop when a person is exposed to individuals carrying the bacterium in their bowels.

Tree million C. difficile infections occur in hospitals every year in the U.S. and 20,000 C. difficile infections occur in community settings in the U.S. every year. 14,000 people die from C. difficile infection every year in the U.S.

Millions of people get infected with C. difficile around the world every year and many thousands of them die as a result of C. difficile diarrheal illness.

Many people both children and adults carry the C. difficile organism in their colon as carrirers and never get sick.

The facilitities where the C.difficile organism is found include:

Hospitals
Extended care facilities
Nursing homes
Nurseries
Community centers
Neighborhood health centers
Living in the communities (about 32% of community based C.Difficile infection had some contact with health care facilities in recent pass).

The materials that are frequently contaminated with C.difficile spores include:

Furnitures
Linens
Bedpans
Toilets seats
Floors
Hands
Telephones

Rings
Stethoscopes
Diaper pails etc;

The antibiotics that have been known to cause C. diffficile diarrheal disease/gastroenteritis and pseudomembrenous colitis include:

Clindamycin
Amoxicillin
Ampicillin
Cephalosporins/Keflex
Bactrim
Cipro
Penicillin
Erytrhomycin
Levaquin etc;

Other risk factors for C. difficile colitis include Ulcerative colitis and Crohn's disease with no exposure to antibiotics. HIV/AIDS, non-acquired immunodeficiency diseases, Cancer, Radiotherapy, and chemotherapy.

Symptoms of C. difficile diarrheal/gastroenteritis include:

Fever
Chills
Diarrhea
Constipation
Nausea
Loss of appetite
Weight loss
Abdominal cramps/pain
Dehydration
Electrolytes imbalance

Evaluations for C.difficile diarrhea include:

History and physical examination
Temperature
Blood pressure
Pulse
Repiratory rate
Oxygen Sturation
Stool for C. difficile toxin A an B

Stool culture
Xtag GPP stool test
Stool ova and parasites
Stool Gram stain
Stool leukocytes
Blood culture
CBC
Complete metabolic /chemistry profile
Urinalysis
Urine culture
Chest x-ray
Abdominal CT scan
EKG
Flexible sigmoidoscopy
Colonoscopy etc;

A negative A and B toxin for C. difficile does not rule out C. colitis therefore, it is necessary to sigmoidoscopy or colonoscopy to document colitis/pseudocolitis.

In addition, it is not necessary for some one to have diarrhea for the suspicion of C. difficile infection to be arisen. People can develop sepsis with high fever due C.difficile infection and be constipated. It is prudent always to check for C. difficile infection in anyone with unexplained fever in the hospital.

Treatments of C. difficile colitis include:

Stop the antibiotic causing the colitis

Intravenous fluid with Dextrose and normal saline plus potassium at 150cc per hour
or
Normal saline plus potassium at 150cc per hour

Ringer's lactate at 150cc per hour

Tylenol 325mg 2 tablets every 4 hours to keep temperature below 100

Flagyl 250mg four times per day by mouth for 14 days or 500mg three times per day by mouth for 14 days
or
Vancomycin 125mg four times per day by mouth for 14 days
or
Fidaxomicin is newly approved by the FDA to treat C. difficile colitis, it is more effective because it is bactericidal as compared to Flagyl and Vancomycin which are

bacteriostatic. Recurrence of C.difficile infection occurs less often in patients with non-NAP strains of C.dificile bacterium.

The dose of Fidaxomicin is 200mg twice per day by mouth for 10 days.
Fidaxomicin should be the antibiotic of first choice in C.difficile colitis.
Stool transplantation ("While the standard antibiotic treatment cured 27% of patients in the trial, fecal trnsnplants cured 94%") Source: Einstein connection; Issue 45, Jan 30,2013

Cpmplications of C. difficile colitis include:
Dhydration
Low blood pressure
Electrolytes imbalance
Kidney failure
Dessiminated intravascular coagulopathy
Megacolon
Perforation of the bowel
Peritonitis
Death

Prevention of C. difficile colitis includes:

Wear mask, gown, and gloves to the rooms of patients with C. colitis
Disinfection of stethoscpoes after examining patients with C. dificille colitis are mendatory
Wash hands with soap and water
Use antibiotics only when necessary
Retest stools of people recently treated for documented C. difficile for several months
Avoid using the same toilets with people being treated for C. difficile colitis or recently treated for C. difficile colitis
If at all possible avoid residing in adults home, nursing home and all other crowded residential facilities.

Chapter 26
VIRAL GASTROENTERITIS

Viral diarrheal disease/stomach flu is quite common.

The viruses that frequently cause diarrheal disease/Gaatroenteritis include:

Norvovirus (responsible for 50% to 70% of all gastroenteritis in adults and is the most common cause of gastroenteritis in the U.S.) Source CDC

Norvovirus (Norwalk virus)

Every year norvovirus cause 21 million cases of gastroenteritis in the U.S.
Every year norvovirus causes 70,000 hospitalizations and 500 deaths in the U.S.

Worldwide there are 90 million cases of norvovirus gastroenteritis every year resulting in 218,000 deaths annually.

Rotavirus

Worldwide 133 million people develop rotavirus gastroenteritis every year and in the U.S. there 3 million cases of rotavirus gastroenteritis. In the U.S. rotavirus causes 60,000 hospitalizations, resulting in 40 deaths.

Rotavirus gastroenteritis kills 1.3 million people in the world evry year. 500,000 of them are children.

Adenovirus
Calcivirus
Sapovirus

Viral gastroenteritis occurs through the oral fecal route, symptoms develop 1-3 days for Norvovirus and 1-3 days for Rotavirus.

Risk factors for viral diarrheal disease/gastroenteritis include:

Poor hand hygiene
Failure to wash hands with soap and water after using the bath room
Touching bath room door nobes after using the bath room
Living in the same house with a person who has stomach flu

Living in crowded living facilities
Young children
School children
Day care workers
Childern in day cares
Children living in developing countries
Adults living in developing countries
Being in the hospitals
Nursing homes residents
Dormitory residents
Being in cruise boats
Eating contaminated foods
Drinking contaminated water/fluids
Shaking hands
HIV/AIDS
Anal sex
Anal/ oral sex
Non-acquired immunodeficiency diseases
Cancer
Chemotherapy treatment
Radiothearapy treatment

Symptoms of viral gastroenteritis/stomach flu include:

Nausea
Vomiting
Abdominal cramps
Abdominal pain
Diarrhea
Fever
Chills
Headache
Muscles ache
Malaise
Weakness
Poor appetite
Dehydraion etc;

Evaluations of viral gastroenteritis/stomach flu include:

History and physical examination
Blood pressure
Pulse

Temperature
Respiratory rate
Oxygen saturation
CBC
Complete metabolic-chemistry profile
Urinalysis
Stool culture
Xtag GPP stool test
Stool for ova and parasite
Stool leukocytes
Stool Gram stain
Stool for C. difficile A and B toxin
Blood culture
Polymerase chain reaction (PCR) for individual viruses
Chest X-ray
Abdominal ultrasound
Abdominal CT scan may or may not be necessary

Treatments of viral gastroenteritis/stomach flu include:

Intravenous fluid with normal saline and glucose plus 20 MEQ of potassium at 150cc per hours
or

Half normal saline and glucose plus 20 MEQ of potassium at 150cc per hour
or
Ringer's lactate at 150cc per hour

Zofran 8mg IV every 8 hours for nausea and vomiting
or
Compozine 5 or 10 mg IM every 6 hours

Peptobismol 1 table spoon every 6 hours as needed for abdominal cramps

Complications of viral diarrheal disease/gastroenteritis include:
Dehydration
Electrolytes imbalance
Hypotension (low blood pressure)
Cardiac arrhythmias
Kidney failure
Disseminated intravascular coagulopathy
Deaths.

Chapter 27
CHOLERA

Cholera associated diarrheal disease/gastroenteritis affects 3-5 million people in the world every year and kills 100-120,000 every year.

In the U.S. about 10 cases of cholera are reported every year, half of these cases are acquired outside of the U.S. Deaths are rare from cholera in the U.S.

Source: WHO

More recently, 485,000 cases of cholera have been reported in Haiti and 6,700 deaths have been reported because of cholera. According to the U.N. the cholera in Haiti was brought to Haiti from peace keepers from Nepal.

Cholera Vibrio is a Gram negative bacterium that causes infection of the small bowel trough fecal contamination of foods and water. "The Cholera bacterium releases a potent toxin (CTX) which binds to the intestinal wall, where it interferes with the normal flow of sodium and chloride. This causes the body to secrete enormous amounts of water, leading to diarrhea and rapid loss of fluids and salts. "Two 2 subgroups of Vibrio cholera cause dirrheal disease and there are V. cholera O1 and O139. Vibrio cholera O1 causes the majority of cholera outbreaks in the world.

The majority of people infected with Vibrio Cholera don't get sick eventough, they can transmit the infection to other people. About 10-20 percent of those who become infected develop full blown cholera diarrheal disease/gastroenteritis.

Risks of Cholera diarrheal disease/gastroenteritis include:

Living slums where there are many people with no running water, no bathroom facilities and poor sanitary conditions
Living in overcrowded camps
Comsuption of fecal contaminated foods and water
Eating raw and uncooked shellfish
Raw fruits and vegetables
Surface water/well water
Contaminated grains
Travel to developing countries where Cholera epidemic is common
Reduced acid in the stomach (hypochlorhydria), The Cholera organism cnnot survive in an acidic enveroment)
Type O blood type

Evaluations of Cholera diarrheal disease/gastroenteritis include:

History and physical examination
Temperature
Blood pressure
Pulse
Respiratory rate
Oxygen Saturation
Stool culture
Stool Gram stain
Stool leukocytes
Stool ova and parasites
Stool toxin
Blood culture
CBC
Complete metabolic Chemistry profile
Urinalysis
T4 and TSH
HIV blood test
PT and INR
PTT
Chest Xray
Abdominal CT scan
Abdominal ultrasound
EKG
Internal medicine consultation
Infectious disease consultation
Gastroenterology consultation
Cadiology consultation
Nephrology consultation

The symptoms of Cholora diarrheal disease/gastroenteritis include:

Watery diarrhea
Nausea
Vomiting
Dehydration
Fever
Seizures
Muscle cramps
Lethargy
Exteme thirst
Sunken eyes

Low blood pressure
Low urine output
Electrolytes imbalance
Cardiac arrhythmia
Sock
Diseminated intravascular coagulopathy (DIC)

Complications of Cholera dirrhea disease/gastroenteritis include:

Hypoglycemia (low blood sugar)
Hypokacemia (low serum potassium)
Kidney failure etc;

Treatments of Cholera diarrheal disease/gastroenteritis include:

Salty water solution by mouth
Intravenous fluid with Normal Saline plus 20 MEQ of potassium chloride in each liter at 200cc per hour or
Intravenous fluid with Normal saline and glucose plus 20 MEQ of potassium in each liter at 200cc per hour or
Intavenous Ringer Lactate at 200cc per hour

Antibiotics in use to treat cholera include:

Doxycycline 300mg single dose adults
Tetracycline 500mg three times per day for 3 days a adults
Trimethoprim/sulfamethoxazole 160 mg adult
Azythromax 500mg adults
Tetracycline 12.5mg/kg three times per day children
Trimethoprim/sulfamethoxazole 5mg/gk children
Zythromax 250 mg children

Anti-emetics:

Zofran 4mg every 8 hours IV or by mouth as needed for nausea and vomiting
Compozine 10mg by mouth every 6 hours as needed for nausea and vomiting

Anti-pyretic s (anti—fever)

Tylenol 325mg 2 tablets every 4 hours for fever
Aspirin 325mg 2 tablets every 4 hours as needed for fever

Advil 1 tablet every 8 hours as needed

Motrin 400-600mg every 6-8 hours as needed

Don't use motrin, Advil or Aspirin if the kidney has failed or if there is bleeding.

Prevention of Cholera dirrheal disease/Gastroenteritis include:

Wash hands thourougly with water and soap after using the bath room

Drink unly bottled water

Don't drink water unless you boiled it yuorself

Don't eat uncooked fish of anykind

Don't eat shell fish

Eat foods that are completely cooked

Don't eat foods from street vendors.

Travlers to countries where Cholera epidemic is prevalent only if you absolutely must

Make sure your physician gives you prescriptions for Tetracycline, Doxycycline, Bactrim or Zythromax and Zofran to carry with you when you travel to developing countries where the incidence Cholera is high (Pregnant women should not take Tetracycline)

When there, follow all the suggestions above

When you return, even if you don't feel sick, see a physician to have your stool cultured for Cholera.

Chapter 28
CONSTIPATION

Constipation is very common medical condition. It affects 12% of people in the world and 2% of people in the U.S. Women and the elderly are more affected than other people are.

Conspitation occurs when the large bowel fails to contract to propel the fecal matter in a normal way to allow for its excretion through the rectum. Most people move their bowels every once per day, or 3-4 times per week, or twice per week. If a person spends 1 week or more without moving his or her bowel, he or she is constipated.

Signs and symptoms constipation include:

Straining during defecation
Passing hard stools
Incomplete evacuation of stools
Two or less bowel movement per week
Internal hemorrhoids
External hemorrhoids
Rectal bleeding
Rectal pain
Abdominal cramps
Abdominal pain
Bloading
Nausea
Vomiting
Iron deficiency anemia etc;

The risk factors for constipation include:

Eating non-bulky foods
Not drinking enough water
Eating to much fatty foods
Stress
Lack of exercise
Diabetes mellitus
Hypothyroidism
Depression

Pain medications
Irritable bowel syndrome
Pregnancy
Colon cancer
Anorexia nervosa

Bulimia
Stroke
Multiple sclerosis
Parkinson disease
Old age
Some calcium containing antacid
Nacrcotic pain medications

Evaluations of constipation inclue:

History
Physical examination
CBC
Complete metabolic profile
Hemoglobin A1c
Serum ferritin
T4 and TSH
Chest-ray
X-ray of the abdomen
Abdominal CT scan
Sigmoidoscopy
Colonoscopy
Virtual colonoscopy
Barium enema

Treaments of constipation include:

Milk of magnesia
Miralax
Colace
Ducolax tablets
Ducolax suppositories
Senokort
Metamucil
Citrucil
Benefiber
Sena-S

Unifiber
Phospho-soda
Cascara
Epson salt
Fleet enema
Oil retention enema
High colonic enema
Citrate of magnesia
Colyte
Castor oil etc;

Complications of Laxatives include:

Laxatives abuse
Cathartic colon
Electrolytes unbalanced
Cardiac arrhythmias
Vitamin K deficiency
Bleeding
Anemia etc;

Chapter 29
HEMORRHOIDS

Hemorrhoids are very common and about 50% of people in the world develop hemorrhoids by the time they reach age 50. There are two types of hemorrhoids. There is external hemorrhoid and external hemorrhoid. Hemorrhoids develop because of too much pressure on veins from the pelvis and rectal area.

Causes of hemorrhoids include

Constipation
Diarrhea
Pregnancy
Straining during bowel movement
Obesity/overweight
Anal intercourse
Diabetes mellitus
Hypothyroidism

Symptoms of hemorrhoids include:

Rectal bleeding
Discomfort in the anal area
Pain in the anal area
Itching in the anal area
Iritation in the anal area
Swelling in the anal area
A lump in the anal area
Leakage of stools etc;

Evaluations of hemorrhoids include:

History and physical examination
CBC
Complete metabolic profile
T4 and TSH
Anascope
Sigmoidoscopy
Colonoscopy

Treatments of hemorrhoids include:

    Anisol cream
    Anisol ointment
    Anisol suppositories
    Sizt bath
    Stool softeners

    Fiber rich foods
    Eating plenty of fruits
    Eating plenty of vegetables
    Eating plenty of grains
    Consumption of plenty of water
    Anti dirrheal medications to treat dirrhea
    Rubber band ligation
    Coagulation
    Hemorrhoidectomy
    Sclerotherapy (injection) etc;

Complications of hemorrhoids include:

    Iron deficiency anemia
    Thrombosed hemorrhoids
    Hemorrhoids may develop because of obstruction from rectal cancer as well as colon cancer.

It is never normal to bleed from the rectum therefore, anytime someone sees blood coming from the rectum, ought to be evaluated by a physician.

The development of hemorrhoids itself warrants a complete medical evaluation by physicians.

Chapter 30
DIVERTICULOSIS

Diverticulosis is a condition in which small pouches/sacs arise from the wall of the large intestine. These pouches/sacs develop more frequently in lower left part of the colon called the sigmoid. Each individual pouch/sac is called a diverticulum.

People who suffer from this condition is said to have diverticular disease.

Every now and again fecal materials cause erosion in the walls of diverticuli resulting in bleeding. Once an individual bleeds from diverticuli, he or she tends to have recurrent bouts of diverticular bleeding on and off.

Diverticular disease is more common in developed countries compared to underdeveloped countries. Diverticular disease begins to develop at age 40 and 50% of People residing in industrial countries have diverticulosis after age 60.

A diet poor in high fiber foods plays a major role in development of diverticulosis, hence the reason why diverticulosis is less common in the developing world where people eat a fiber rich diet and the reverse is true in the developed world where people eat a fiber poor diet.

Symptoms of diverticulosis include:

    Painless rectal bleeding
    Low red blood cells count (Anemia)
    Low blood pressure
    Shock
    Rapid heart rate etc;

    Evaluations of diverticular bleed include:
    History
    Physical examination
    Rectal examination
    Temperature
    Blood pressure
    Pulse
    Respiratory rate
    Oxygen saturation
    CBC

Complete metabolic profile
PT/INR, PTT
Chest x-ray
EKG
Bleeding scan
Colonoscopy
ABO blood typing and indirect coomb's screening

Treatments of diverticular bleed include:

Intavenous fluid with D5/normal saline at 150cc per hour
Nasal Oxygen at 2 liter per minute nasal canula
Transfuse with packed red blood cells if indicated for severe blood loss anemia.

Prevention of diverticulosis/diverticular bleed includes:

Red meat free diet
Low far diet
High fiber diet
Diet full of poultry, fish, vetables, fruits and grain
Diet free of seeds containing foods
Diet free of hot and spicy foods etc;

Chapter 31
DIVERTICULITIS

Diverticulitis develops when diverticuli pouches/sacks become infected because of stools entered inside them or otherwise cause them to become inflamed. 25% of people with diverticular disease develop diverticulitis.

Symptoms and signs of diverticulitis include:

Abdominal pain
Abdominal cramps
Fever
Chills
Nausea
Vomiting
Constiptation
Rapid heart rate
Rapid pulse rate
Elevated white blood cells (WBC)
Elevated ESR

Complications of diverticulitis include:

Diverticular abscess
Intestinal perforation
Peritonitis
Sepsis
Death

Evaluations of diverticulitis include:

History
Physical examination
Rectal examination
Stool hemoccult
Temperature
Pulse
Rspiratory rate
Oxygen saturation

CBC with differential
Complete metabolic chemistry profile
Serum amylase
Serum lipase
Urinalysis
Urine culture
Blood culture
Chest Xray
Abdominal sonogram
Abdominal / pelvis CT scan with contrast by mouth and IV
EKG
Surgical consultation
Gastrointestinal consultation
ABO blood typing
Type and screen

Treatments of diverticulitis include:

Intravenous fluid with D5/normal saline at 150cc per hour
Or
Normal saline IV at 150cc per hour

Nasal oxygen at 2 liter per minute nasal cannula

Transfuse with blood as needed for anemia

Ceftriaxone 1 gram IV every 12 hours, plus Flagyl 500mg IV every 6 hours
Or
Cipro 500mg IV every 12 hours, plus Flagyl 500mg IV every 6 hours
Or
Levaquin 500mg IV every 24 hours, plus Flagyl 500mg IV every 6 hours
Or
Unysin 3 Gram IV every 6 hours
Or
Zosyn 3.375 Gm IV every 6 hours

Prevention of diverticulitis includes:

Avoid eating popcorn
Avoid eating nuts
Avoid eating pumpkin
Avoid eating sunflower
Avoid eating Hot peppers

Avoid eating spicy foods
Avoid eating tomatoes
Avoid eating Zucchini
Avoid eating strawberries
Avoid eating raspberries
Avoid eating poppy seeds
Avoid eating cucumbers
Avoid eating red meat

When a person has diverticulosis/diverticulitis it is ok to eat
Bread
Beans
Whole grain
Cereal
Oat meal
Poultry
Fish
Shrims
Eggs
Seedless fruits
Seedless vegetables
Milk
Cheese

People who suffer from diverticulosis/diverticulitis ought to follow the advice of their physicians.

Chapter 32
ANEMIA

Anemia is common in all racial groups.

Hemoglobinopathies

1. Sickle cell disease
2. Beta-Thalassemia
3. Alpha-Thalassemia
4. Hemoglobin C C
5. Hemoglobin AC
6. Hemoglobin SC
7. Hemoglobin sickle thalassemia
8. Hemoglobin persistent of hemoglobin F
9. Hemoglobin D
10. Hemoglobin E
11. Hemoglobin Lepore

1. Autoimmune hemolytic anemia (warm types)
2. Cold agglutinin hemolytic anemia
3. Paroxysmal cold hemoglobinuria
3. Hereditary spherocytosis hemolytic anemia
4. Paroxysmal Nocturnal hemoglobinuria (PNH)
5. Drug-induced hemolytic anemia
6. G6PD associated hemolytic anemia
7. Cirrhosis of the liver (Hyperslpenism associated hemolytic anemia)
8. Thrombotic Thrombocytopenic Purpura (TTP) associated anemia
9. Disseminated intravascular coagulopathy (DIC) associated anemia
10. Blood transfusion reaction associated anemia etc;

HEMOGLOBIN F

Elevated Hemoglobin F can be seen in different abnormal hemoglobinopathies.
Sickle cell anemia
Beta-thalassemia
Hereditary persistence of fetal hemoglobin (HPFH)

Delta-beta-thalassemia etc;

In sickle cell anemia the level of hemoglobin F level varies.

In hereditary persistence of fetal hemoglobin is moderately elevated but, the hemoglobin A2 is normal and the MCV is also normal. The heterozygous and homozygous carriers are asymptomatic.

In Beta-thalassemia, there is a decrease in the synthesis of β **ch**ain, resulting in a normal hemoglobin F level and elevated A2 level and low MCV.

In Delta-beta thalassemia there is a reduction in the synthesis of both β and δ chain synthesis with elevated hemoglobin F, normal A2 and low MCV.

HEMOGLOBIN D

Hemoglobin D is an autosomal recessive variation of hemoglobin A that develops in the beta-blobin chain of hemoglobin A. Hemoglobin D develops because of a substitution of glutamic acid for glutamine at codon 121 of the β chain.

There are several varients of Hemoglobin D and there are Hb D Punjab (hemoglobin Los-Angelese, a substitution of glycine for glutamic acid at codon 121)
Hb Ibadan (a substitution of lysine for threonine at codon 7)
Hemoglobin D is seen most commonly in people from
India
Pakistan
Ireland
England
Australia
Holland
Iran
Turkey
China

Homozygous hemoblobin DD is rare and causes only mild symptoms with an enlarged spleen and a mild hemolytic anemia. Hemoglobin Beta thalassemia is a more severe form of hemoglobin D disease and causes moderate hemolytic anemia.

HEMOGLOBIN E

Hemoglobin E is a hereditary abnormality that occurs as result of a substitution of lysine for glutamic acid at position 26 of the Beta globin chain. This abnormality causes thalassemia to develop because of decrease in Beta globin chain.

Hemoglobin E thalassemia is seen most frequently in people from
Vietnam
Cambodia
Laos
Thailand
Filipino
China
India
Turkey
Homozygous hemoglobin E causes slpeenomegaly and hemolytic anemia.
Other hemoglobin E diseases include hemoglobin sickle/ E disease and hemoglobin E/ β.
Both these two types of hemoglobin E disease cause hemolytic anemia.

HEMOGLOBIN LEPORE

Hemoglobin Lepore occurs because of a cross over "between the delta and and beta globin loci." Hemoglobin Lepore has 2 normal alpha chains and 2 delta fusion chains.
Hemoglobin Lepore is commonly found in people from
Greek
Itali
Yugoslavia
Rumania
Turkey
Africa
Papua
India

Individuals who suffer with hemoglobin lepore have the same problems as those who have Beta-thalassemia and all its associated complications.

Other common types and causes of anemia include

1. Sickle cell disease
2. Beta—thalassemia
3. Alpha-thalassemia
4. Sickle cell C disease
5. Sickle-Beta thalassemia
6. Hemoglobin CC disease
7. Hemoglobin AC disease
8. Chronic diseases
9. Mixed collagen vascular diseases

10. Poverty
11. Malnutrition
12. Parasitic infestation
13. Multiple child births
14. Uterine fibroids
15. Lead poisoning
16. Iron deficiency
17. Vitamin B12 deficiency
18. Folic acid deficiency
19. Sickle cell trait
20. Kidney failure
21. Alcoholism
22. Itravenous Drug abuse
23. Hepatitis C
24. Hepatitis B
25. Cirrhosis of the liver
26. AIDS
27. Hemochromatosis
28. Lupus
29. Arthritis
30. Cancer
31. Sarcoidosis
32. Endocarditis etc;

Five percent of the world population carries the genes for sickle disease and thalassemia. Each year 300,000 babies are born with sickle cell disease in the world.

Two million five hundred thousands black Americans carry the gene for sikle cell anemia and have sickle trait and about 100.000 black Americans have sickle disease.

Anemia is more common in women than men are because more women suffer from iron deficiency. Iiron deficiency anemia is more common in women because ninety percent of black women 50 year and older have uterine fibroids and 70% of white women have uterine fibroids. Uterine fibroid causes heavy menstrual blood loss. Menstrual blood loss causes iron loss. The average menstrual blood loss is between 45 and 50 cc of blood per month, assuming normal gynecological functions.

The quantity of blood loss that occurs during abnormal menstrual bleeding cannot be measured because of clots that form during that abnormal process. In addition, the average blood loss for each delivery varies depending on a multitude of factors. In addition, during delivery of a natural childbirth, a women can lose anywhere from as little as 200 cc to as much as 600 cc of blood.

The period of bleeding can extend up to one to two weeks after delivery, depending on different circumstances. In a difficult delivery requiring an episiotomy or a cesarean section, the amount of blood lost has to be quantified based on many factors, not the least of which is how proficiently the procedure was done by the doctor and whether the haemostatic status of the woman in question was normal. Black and other minority women have more children than do white women. The average iron loss during each normal pregnancy is 750 mg, which is the equivalent of 3 units of blood.

Anemia is more common in certain racial groups than others because of the fact that some racial groups suffer more from conditions such as abnormal hemoglobin, poverty, parasitic infestation, AIDS etc;

Blacks
Greeks
Italians
Asians
South East Asians
Indians

Black women and other minority women are more afflicted with a condition called PICA than are white women. Women who suffer from PICA have iron deficiency anemia. Blacks are more likely to have hereditary types of anemia that are passed on to them from their parents and which they, in turn, pass on to their children. Blacks and other minorities have a high incidence of colorectal cancer, which is often associated with bleeding with resulting secondary anemia. In addition, many blacks and other minorities live in the deleloping world exposing them to parasitic infestation. Parasitic infestation causes blood loss from the colon resulting in iron deficiency anemia. Many individuals living in the deloped countries like the UK and the U.S. et; suffer from anemia because malnutrition resulting from poverty.

What is anemia?

Anemia is a condition in which the human body has low concentration of red blood cells.

Why is too little blood bad for the body?

Low concentration of red blood cells is bad for the body because red blood cells are needed to carry oxygen to all the organs in the body for proper body functioning.

When an individual is anemic, the different organs in the body are deprived of the proper amount of oxygen, resulting in the condition referred to as anoxia. An anoxic organ can become sick because of oxygen deficiency. Red blood cells contain a substance called hemoglobin. Hemoglobin has as its function to bind with oxygen in order to carry it to the different places in the human body where it is needed.

There exists an invisible man-conceived curve in the human body called the Oxygen Dissociation Curve. When the right amount of oxygen is present in the blood, this curve is well balanced in the middle and is shifted to the right to deliver oxygen to the tissues. When something happens that causes anemia to develop, the end result is that the red blood cells hold onto oxygen, and the curve is shifted to the left, resulting in the inability of the red cells to discharge their content of oxygen to the different tissues of the body, resulting in improper perfusion of the tissues with oxygen. The Oxygen Dissociation Curve is influenced by the pH of the blood.

What are some of the symptoms of anemia?

To answer this question one must know how long the person has been anemic and how severe the anemia is. A normal hemoglobin and hematocrit in a woman is 13.0-14.5 grams hemoglobin and normal hematocrit is 38% to 42% hematocrit. Normal hemoglobin in man is 14.0-16.0 grams and normal hematocrit is 45% 50%.

The more acute the blood loss, hemolysis or inability to produce red blood cells results in lower red blood cell count, which results in anemia and the less able an individual is to tolerate it. The younger the person who is losing blood is, the better he or she is able to tolerate the anemia. The older the person is who is acutely losing blood due to bleeding or hemolysis, the less well he or she is able to tolerate the anemia. Older people are more likely to have underlying medical problems, such as heart disease, kidney disease, hardening of the arteries in the brain, etc., making it easier for the anemia to complicate these already precarious conditions.

People who have had anemia for a long time are better able to tolerate their anemia because they have had enough time for their bodies to adjust to the effects of the anemia. In time, many of these chronically anemic people's vital organs, such as the heart, the brain, the kidneys and many other organs would be affected by the anemic state but it would happen gradually. The most common symptoms of anemia are weakness, malaise, headaches, shortness of breath, tiredness, irritability, depression, chest pain, menstrual irregularity, infertility, insomnia, etc.

What conditions must exist in the human body before anemia can occur?

1. A person must be bleeding or must have bled.
2. A person must be hemolyzing red blood cells (that is, breaking up red blood cells in the body).
3. A person's bone marrow must have stopped producing red blood cells because of bone marrow failure, or
4. The bone marrow cavity is replaced by other cells, such as cancer cells, etc., leaving little or no room for red blood cells to be made, or
5. The bone marrow may also be replaced by fibrous tissues such as occurs in a condition known as myelofibrosis. Any combination of the aforementioned conditions interplaying at the same time can result in anemia.

What are the physical signs of anemia?

The signs of anemia are many and frequently coincide with the type of anemia the person is suffering from.

If a person presents to the emergency room or to the doctor's office and is acutely bleeding, from the vagina, the rectum, or vomiting blood from an upper gastrointestinal tract or from the urinary tract, his or her pulse rate will be fast, his or her blood pressure might be low and he or she may be having pain. Severe and acute bleeding from any of these sites resulting in about 1800 cc of blood loss or more will likely cause a drop in the blood pressure.

Another frequent sign of acute blood loss anemia is rapid heart rate.
The reason for the rapid heart rate is that this is the heart's way of trying to make up the difference by increasing the cardiac output in an attempt to help deliver enough oxygen for proper body functions. If the anemia persists for many years, the heart may fail because of what is called high output heart failure.

Other physical signs of anemia include:

1. Paleness of the skin
2. Pale nail beds
3. Pale conjunctivae in the entire human body the only place where naked vessels can be seen is in the eyes. By looking at the conjunctivae (the white of the eye) the examining physician can see blood vessels with the naked eyes and can tell if these vessels are pale, indicating chronic blood loss.
4. In addition, if the patient is hemolyzing, different degrees of icterus (yellowishness) can be observed by the examining physician. There are many

other conditions having nothing to do with hemolytic anemia that can cause scleral icterus.

5. Rapid breathing

6. Flow heart murmurs, which is a function of the thinness of the blood as it passes through the heart valves.

●

What are the most common anemias?

The most common anemias include:

1. Iron deficiency anemia

2. The second most common anemia are anemia such as sickle cell anemia (SS), sickle cell C (SC), sickle cell thalassemia, homozygous hemoglobin C, Alpha thalassemia and Beta thalassemia.

3. Another common anemia seen more frequently is lead poisoning-associated anemia. These individuals get exposed to lead as youngsters, and never realizing that they had this problem, therefore, they sought no treatment and as adults, they continue to suffer with this anemia.

4. Still another common anemia seen in many poor people is nutritional deficiency anemia. Many poor people are forced by virtue of their impoverished conditions not able to eat nutritious foods because these foods are, for the most part, expensive. Moreover, this state of poor nutrition begins at an early age, as many poor young people go to school with no breakfast and eat only the food that is provided as part of the school lunch program. The quality and quantity of these foods vary from communities to community. In many instances, these foods are prototypes of fast foods, which are neither healthy nor nutritious. Frequently, a combination of these different anemias coexists in the people, making their anemic state much more difficult and complex to diagnose and treat. According to recent reports, 58 million American citizens live below the poverty line and 25% of blacks in the U.S. live below the poverty line. It has also been reported that some 14 million children in the U.S. go to bed at night hungry.

5. Alpha thalassemia is quite common in blacks—32% of blacks carries the Alpha thalassemia hemoglobin gene but only 2% develops anemia (Alpha thalassemia minor)

6. Beta thalassemia is quite common.

7. Sickle cell anemia is quite common in blacks and other people of color

8. Autoimmune hemolytic anemia is quite common and frequently seen in association with lupus (SLE).

9. Pernicious anemia is also common in blacks and seems to have a predilection for young black women.

10. Other B12 deficiency anemia is also common.

11. Folic acid deficiency anemia is common.

12. Anemia of acute blood loss is also common in blacks and can occur for a variety of reasons.
13. Another common anemia frequently seen in blacks is anemia of chronic disease or anemia of inflammatory diseases.
14. HIV/AIDS associated anemia is quite common.

Chapter 33
IRON DEFICIENCY ANEMIA

Women have iron deficiency anemia more often than men because of blood loss during menstruation, during childbirth, as a result of gastrointestinal bleeding from different diseases of the GI tract, Pica, and eating foods that are poor in iron. In addition, men and women have iron deficiency anemia because gastrointestinal bleeding from ulcer, cancer of the esophagus, esophageal varices, cancer of the small bowel, meckel diverticulum of the small bowel, colon cancer, hemorrhoids etc.

As of 2012, the world has over 7 billion people. Thirty percent of the world population suffers from hunger. Hunger and malnutrion play a major role in high incidence of anemia. More than 2 billion people in world have iron deficiency anemia. WHO

Eight hundred and sixty eight million people in the world suffer from hunger and malnutrition 2012 and Fifteen million children die every year because of hunger in the world. WHO

Fifty million people in the U.S. suffer fron hunger including 1 in 6 adults and 1 in 5 children and fity million Americans are getting food stamps. Source: USDA

People who migrated to the United States from regions of the world, such as South America, Latin America, Central America, the Caribbean, Africa and other tropical countries where the incidence of parasitic infestation is high are more likely to be infested with parasites.

The iron deficiency anemia is the of blood loss due to worms sucking blood from their intestines, resulting therefore in loss of blood in the stool. Parasitic infestation is a serious problem for black people, many of whom are surviving on a meager diet to begin with, while at the same time they are losing a significant percentage of their intake of nutrients to parasites that afford them no symbiosis in return. That is clearly an unfair deal.

What aggravate the situation even more is the fact that black women, be it in the U.S. or anywhere else in the world, and have a higher birth rate and pregnancies than do white women. The reasons that many black women have more children than white women are many and run the whole gamut of factors such as cultural preferences, religious beliefs, poverty, and lack of formal education, lack of professional status, and psychosocial and psycho-racial circumstances and economic reasons.

In third developing countries, black women have many children for several reasons:

1. The family needs many children to tend and take care of the farms.
2. Religious beliefs do not permit the use of birth control in many parts of the third world.
3. These women have many children as a way of pleasing the men, who equate having many children with an expression of their virility, masculinity, and sexual prowess and as an expression of their manhood in general. Many developed countries for religious reasons encourage women to have many children. In the U.S. many religious groups also encourage women to have many children.

Interestingly, the same feelings and expressions permeate the society of the Americas and the Caribbean Basin communities and other black communities in the world. Many black and Hispanic women in U.S. society hold to these same values and beliefs.

These practices are rooted in the African culture, and that culture has its traces well imprinted in the psyche of many of the black men and women who inhabit the Americas and other parts of the world. Whether they would choose to acknowledge these most truthful and important historical facts or not is a different story altogether.

Many people abuse alcohol to a significant degree and alcohol abuse is associated with many conditions that can cause iron deficiency anemia. For instance, alcohol abuse frequently causes gastritis. The blood that is lost because of gastritis can lead to iron deficiency anemia when the gastritis occurs recurrently, as is often the case.

Alcohol abuse frequency causes esophageal varices with recurrent bleeding, and this too can cause iron deficiency anemia. Alcohol abuse frequently causes damage to the liver resulting in alcoholic liver disease (cirrhosis of the liver), which can cause breakthrough vaginal bleeding in women and stomach ulcer, resulting in iron deficiency anemia. The incidence of colon cancer is quite high in blacks in the U.S. and in the world, and one of the most common signs of colon cancer is iron deficiency anemia.

Drinking tea with food in the stomach can cause a person not to be able to absorb iron that is contained in the food, making iron deficiency anemia worse. The reason why drinking too much tea can contribute to low iron level in the blood is because tea contains tannic acid, and tannic acid binds the iron that is in the food, preventing its absorption from the stomach. So people ought to be aware that drinking tea is okay but it is best to drink tea on an empty stomach.

How to evaluate iron deficiency anemia in women

The first thing to do in evaluating blacks with iron deficiency is measure the CBC, reticulocyte count, and serum ferritin. Iron deficiency as a disease has several stages
Stage 1 is called prelatent iron deficiency
Stage 2 is called latent iron deficiency state or iron deficient erythropoiesis
Stage 3 is frank iron deficiency anemia. Each millimeter of blood contains 0.5 mg of iron.

BLOOD SMEAR IN IRON DEFICIENCY ANEMIA

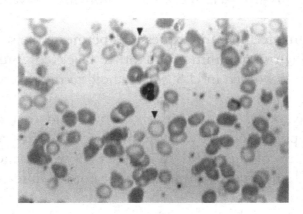

Figure 33.1-Peripheral blood smear showing hypochromic

It is said, according to the World Health Organization, that more than 2 billion people of the 7 billion people in the world suffer from iron deficiency anemia. Undoubtedly, most of these iron-deficient individuals are women because by nature most women must lose blood menstrually since menarche and it continues until they become menopausal. As childbearing mothers, by necessity, women also must lose iron through fetal iron usage during pregnancy. Many women also lose iron during childbirth and through breastfeeding. Breast milk contains iron, and as a mother feeds her infant she loses iron in the breast milk. Breastfeeding worldwide is more common in black women, and in poor women than in white women and upper-class women.

Iron deficiency is most probably much more common than the 2 billion reported by the World Health Organization for several reasons. Iron deficiency state is one of the leading diseases in the world in blacks. Iron deficiency state is defined as total body iron store depletion that leads ultimately to iron deficiency anemia. Long before iron deficiency anemia comes about, the loss of blood, and the iron it contains, had already begun.

The first iron a person loses when he or she is bleeding slowly is the iron from the store, as reflected by the serum ferritin. Iron is stored as ferritin in the bone marrow, the muscles, the spleen, the liver, and other tissues of the body, including the iron that is located in the cytochrome system of the brain, which is needed for proper uses of oxygen by the brain to make the brain function well to carry the daily activities.

When the iron stored is depleted, even before evidence of anemia appears, people whose iron store is absent feel tired all the time, can't concentrate well, yawn a lot, become irritable easily, and feel overall unwell. An average size adult man has 2 grams of iron as storage iron in his body and 1.5 grams of iron in his circulating blood as circulating iron for a total body iron of 3.5 grams.

The average size adult woman has 1 gram of iron in her iron store as storage iron, and 1.5 grams of iron in her circulation as circulating iron. 1 gram of iron is the equivalent of 4 units of blood, because each unit of blood contains 250 mg of iron. Once a person loses the entire iron store, as reflected by a serum ferritin of less than 10 to 15, and then he or she begins to use up the circulating iron for the production of red cells. As the level of the circulating iron decreases, iron deficiency anemia starts to set in, which gets worse and worse over time, resulting in low hematocrit, low MCV and low red cells per million and high RDW. At this juncture, he or she looks pale and feels very tired.

It is important for a treating physician to understand iron kinetics because it enables him or her to determine very early whether a person is slowly bleeding and losing iron. When an individual is bleeding slowly and occultly, the very first blood test to become abnormal is the RDW (red cells distribution width). The RDW becomes elevated when an individual begins to lose blood slowly. The RDW is elevated in all diseases that cause microcytosis, such as thalassemias, iron deficiency anemia, and macrocytic anemias such as B12 deficiency, folate deficiency, and hemolytic anemias.

The next blood test that becomes abnormal when a person is bleeding slowly and chronically is the serum ferritin. Ferritin is a phase 2 reacting protein and therefore can be falsely high in inflammation and infection. It is therefore prudent to always interpret the serum ferritin with this fact in mind. Serum ferritin ought to be looked at as a scale, in that if the level of ferritin is going down, that represents blood and iron loss and the patient must be evaluated accordingly.

In the case of cancer of the GI tract, the decreased level of serum ferritin can be detected very early, sometimes as much as four years prior to the person becoming anemic or prior to the person having any symptoms that might make him or her suspect that he or she may have colon cancer. It is, therefore, important to test the stool for occult blood, which is mixed with the rest of the stool, making it difficult for the eye to see. It takes 25 cc of blood in the gut to cause the stool hemoccult to become positive. The RDW comes with the CBC and, as just mentioned, is elevated in slow chronic bleeding. The serum ferritin test costs only about $56.00 in most clinical laboratories.

When it is interpreted properly, the serum ferritin can help to save thousands of black from dying as a result of GI cancer, because, by evaluating black folks early the doctor can remove the precancerous or cancerous lesion either endoscopically via biopsy or via colonoscopic biopsy or surgically.

A new test that is now clinically available called the soluble serum transferrin receptor level, which is much more sensitive to diagnosed iron deficiency anemia. This test is not affected by either infection or by inflammation. An elevated soluble serum ferritin level is firm evidence of iron deficiency anemia, even if the serum ferritin is normal or high. Iron is attached to the receptors in the transferrin protein to be carried to the early red blood cells in the bone marrow to produce new red blood cells. When there is no iron, these receptor sites remain unoccupied and, as such, their level is elevated, hence the value of this test.

Starting at age 40, Blacks and Hispanics ought to have a colonoscopy, because the incidence of colon cancer begins to develop at around that age in these groups. Blacks also have larger polyps and seem to have more right sided colon cancer than do whites. Right sided colon cancer ate missed more often during colonoscopy than left sided cancer.

Other conditions that can cause iron deficiency consist of:

1. Gastroesophageal reflux disease
2. Peptic ulcer
3. Chronic gastritis associated with ingestion of aspirin or nonsteroidal anti-inflammatory drugs or alcohol abuse
4. Diverticulosis
5. Inflammatory bowel diseases, such as ulcerative colitis, Crohn's disease
6. Bleeding esophageal varices
7. Heavy vaginal bleeding due to uterine fibroids, Von Willebrand's disease, etc.

Uterine fibroids are quite common in black women. By age 50, about 90% of black women have uterine fibroids (Source: American Journal of Obstetrics and Gynecology. 188(1) 100-07, 2003). Heavy vaginal bleeding is sometimes the result of Von Willebrand's disease in about 11% of women (Source: Internal Medicine News, September 15, 2003).

What can people do to prevent iron deficiency anemia and what are the best ways to treat it?

1. Since most blood and iron are lost during menstruation in women, women must be evaluated and treated for any dysfunctional vaginal bleeding that can be the result of uterine fibroids or other problems, as to minimize blood loss and iron loss with it. A simple bleeding test from the tip of a finger done of aspirin for two weeks and of NSAIDS for 12 hours can help to determine if a woman has Von Willebrand's disease or not. The normal bleeding time is up to 7 minutes. Von Willebrand's disease consists of qualitative platelet abnormalities which prevent platelets from aggregating properly, resulting in prolonged bleeding. A special Von Willebrand' disease complete profile test is available and very accurate to establish the diagnosis of Von Wllibebran's dieae.

2. Von Willebrand's disease is the most common bleeding abnormality in the world, affecting several million individuals to one degree or another. Making the diagnosis can in most instances be quite complicated, so when this diagnosis is being considered, it is a good idea to refer the black men and woman to a hematologist for both evaluation and treatment. Excessive vaginal bleeding, nose bleed, bleeding from the GI tract and urological tract and, penis etc, due to Von Willebrand's disease is treated with 20 micrograms of Desmopressin (DDAVP) in 50 cc of normal saline IV over half an hour.

3. Women who have Von Willebrand's disease and don't know they have it and they get treated with birth control pills or other hormones to control heavy menstrual flow. One of the reasons why sometimes that treatment works is precisely because they probably have Von Willebrand's disease and the estrogen in that hormone raises the Factor V111 Von Willebrand's factor which, transiently improve platelet functions, slowing down the bleeding.

4. Blacks and other people from third world countries and African-Americans who reside in the rural South of the U.S. must have their stool tested for parasites, which, if found, can be in part responsible for chronic blood loss due to parasites attaching themselves to the wall of the bowel, sucking up blood, resulting in iron deficiency. Blacks, who because of their living condition which place them at high risk for parasitic infestation. Those either lived in the third world before at one point in the past or in the rural South of the U.S. or who visited countries where they could have been infested with parasites, to have their stool checked by the parasitology laboratory for the possibility that parasitism may be partly responsible for their iron deficiency.

5. Another common problem that some women are afflicted with that causes iron deficiency anemia is a habitual condition called pica. There are different types of pica eating clay or other types of dirt, eating starch, or eating ice. In the United States, some women are afflicted with PICA and in particular those who reside in the South. Eating clay or starch binds iron as it goes to the stomach, preventing its absorption. PICA is a psychological problem that is developed

into a habit and it is very hard to stop. It is ingrained in part of the culture in certain parts of the black community, this has been going on for hundreds of years, and is very difficult to eradicate, but it must be dealt with because it adds to the degree of iron deficiency anemia that these women suffer from. When these women are pregnant, that's when the PICA habit seems to be most acute when they eat clay, starch, or ice.

6. Still another contributing factor to iron deficiency anemia is drinking tea with one's meal. It is a small contributing factor to iron deficiency, but it is one, nevertheless. Tea contains tannic acid, which binds iron in the stomach, preventing its absorption. The best way for a person to drink tea is on an empty stomach or three or four hours after eating iron-containing foods to allow the stomach a chance to absorb the iron.

If the iron deficiency anemia is severe, sometimes, blood transfusion is necessary. Otherwise, iron deficiency is best treated with iron tablets by mouth. There are several iron preparations on the market such as Ferrous Sulfate, Ferrous Gluconate, Ferrous Fumarate, and Slow Fe, Corvite Fe 150 1 tablet per day, Multigen plus Caplets 1 tablet per day, Multigen Caplets 1 tablet per day and Ferrex 28 1tablet daily.

For people who cannot tolerate iron because of nausea, diarrhea, and constipation or so severely iron deficient, Vonofer IV 100mg per day can be used.

In order to treat iron deficiency properly, patients must take one 325 mg tablet daily for one week with foods, then one tablet twice per day for one week, then one tablet three times per day. 180 mg of iron must be taken daily in order for 60 mg per day can be absorbed. Taking less iron than that, will not correct the anemia properly.

Chapter 34
SICKLE CELL ANEMIA

The genetic abnormalities that cause these different anemias are quite different and, as a result, the severity varies. The severest of these anemias is sickle cell anemia. About 8.0% of the Black-American population carries the sickle cell gene (sickle cell trait). This number is the same for Caribbean Blacks as well as Latinos and 300 million people worldwide have sickle cell trait.

Sickle disease affects million of people mostly in Africa, the Mediterranean and North America. Nigeria alone has about 4 million people with sickle cell disease.

A cardiologist from Chicago Dr James Bryan Herrick and his intern Dr Ernest E. Irons first discovered sickle cell disease, the clinical entity, in the U.S. in 1910. They made the discovery in a 20 year old black dental student named Walter Clement Noel studying dentistry in Chicago from the island of Grenada in the Caribbean. This biomolecular abnormality causes the red blood cell of the sickle cell patient to become sticky and deformed and develop into a half-moon or banana-shaped cell. The normal red cell is disc-shaped.

Only about 100, 000 Black-Americans actually have sickle cell anemia, the homozygous type (full-blown sickle cell disease) and 3,600,000 have sickle cell trait. At birth, 1:625 Black-American babies born are expected to develop sickle cell disease. Sickle cell disease has an important historical background. This research done in sickle cell anemia gave birth to the entire field of molecular biology and to a great extent modern science and modern medicine. Dr Linus Pauling made the discovery that the substitution of valine for glutamic acid in position 6 of the beta globulin chain is responsible for the basic abnormality that causes red blood cells to sickle in people who carry the sickle cell gene.

These abnormalities in the red cell membranes cause the red cells to develop a great deal of difficulty passing through small vessels to deliver oxygen to tissues of the heart, the brain, the kidneys, the liver, the bone, the eyes, the spleen, the skin, the muscle and the rest of the tissues of the body. The lack of oxygen delivery to these different organs is responsible for many of the problems associated with sickle cell disease.

Historically, the sickle cell gene can be traced to three main areas of Africa. The most prevalent sickle cell gene came from Benin near Nigeria in Central Africa. Another gene came from Senegal on the West Coast of Africa. The third gene came from the Bantu-speaking area of Central Africa. There are 4 million people with sickle cell disease in Nigeria. These genes are also known as 1. **BEN** for Benin 2. **CAR** for Central African Republic and **SEN** for Senrgal.

The same three genes can be found within North American Blacks and in the Caribbean. The African slaves who were brought here against their will to work the fields and to do forced labor brought these sickle cell genes to the North American continent during the slave trade. Over the close to 500 years since slavery started, the sickle cell gene has had ample time to penetrate the North American Black race, causing much devastation and leaving a lot of pain, suffering, despair and death in its wake. As early as 1670, there is evidence that clinical sickle cell disease existed in a Ghanaian family. Sickle cell disease does not only affect Blacks. Sickle cell disease affects some Indians, Italians, and Arabs, and the same percentage of Hispanics throughout the Americas are affected by sickle cell disease, as are Blacks, which is 8.5%.

Sickle cell disease is a preventable disease, if individuals who carry the gene for this deadly disease would learn the pros and cons of how the disease is inherited. If a woman who is not carrying the sickle cell trait gene marries with a man who is carrying the gene for sickle cell trait and they decide to have children, 50% of the children will be born without the sickle cell gene and 50% will carry it. If both individuals are carrying the sickle cell trait, 25% of their children will be born normal, 25% will be born with the full-blown sickle cell disease, and 50% will be born carrying the sickle cell trait.

If one of them has the full-blown sickle cell disease and the other is normal, 100% of the children will be born carrying the sickle cell trait. If one of these two individuals is carrying the sickle cell trait (AS) and one has the full-blown sickle cell disease (SS), 50% of the children will be born with the sickle cell trait (AS) and 50% will be born with the full-blown sickle cell disease (SS).

If both of these individuals have full-blown sickle cell disease (SS), 100% of their children will be born with full-blown sickle cell disease (SS). Once a person is carrying either the sickle cell trait (AS) or sickle cell disease (SS), many factors interplay to make that person sick and suffer from sickle cell disease.

What makes sickle cell as deadly as a disease is the inability of the hemoglobin S to carry oxygen to the different tissues and organs of the body for proper body functions. The basic effect of the hemoglobin molecule is the substitution of valine for glutamic acid in the beta globulin chain at position 6, as mentioned earlier, which causes sickle cell hemoglobin to gel where there is lack of oxygen.

This process is called polymerization. This basic abnormality is responsible for most of what is wrong in sickle cell disease. Because of polymerization, the red cells become stiff and sticky and therefore are unable to pass freely through small vessels such as venules, arterioles, capillaries and other medium-sized vessels, resulting in vascular occlusion. Vascular occlusion which occurs because of these sticky, misshaped, half-moon or banana-shaped red cells prevents red cells from delivering oxygen normally to tissues in the body of people who are affected by sickle cell disease.

White blood cells also contribute to the occlusive processes that occur in sickle cell disease. White cells secrete a series of adhesive proteins that result in an inflammatory reaction within the vessels of the sicklers. This inflammatory reaction participates in the vascular occlusion that occurs in painful sickle cell crisis. Platelets may also contribute to the vascular occlusion processes by secreting abnormal proteins within the vessels of the sicklers.

Sickle cell disease is a multi-system disease and, as such, affects every major and minor organ in the human body, starting with the skin, which is the largest organ in the human body. The lower extremities can develop ulcers due to skin breakdown. The brain of a sickle cell patient is damaged early and severely, resulting frequently in stroke at an early age, from 4 to 6 years old.

Blacks with sickle cell disease frequently present acutely with one or several of the following crises:

1. Painful sickle cell crisis
2. Hemolytic crisis
3. Hypoplastic crisis
4. Acute chest syndrome
5. A combination of all the aforementioned crises occurring in tandem
6. Splenic sequestration in sickle thalassemia or sickle cell C disease

Painful sickle cell crisis

Painful sickle cell crisis occurs because of occlusion of the small vessels in the body due to the misshaped, sticky red cells making it difficult for them to pass through these vessels to carry oxygen for proper perfusion of tissues. The lack of oxygen delivery to these tissues results in tissue anoxia. The anoxic tissues secrete kinins, mentioned earlier, which cause the burning pain in different parts of the body. This pain can at times be quite severe.

The basis of the painful sickle cell crisis is when the body of the sickle cell patient is under stress, such as infection, which raises the pulse rate, causing the need for more oxygen delivery to tissues to be more severe.

When that need cannot be met, that further aggravates the anoxia, causing a painful crisis to be triggered and made worse.

Another frequent predisposing factor in the development of painful crises is cold weather, which causes vasoconstriction, preventing oxygen delivery to tissues in sufficient amounts, causing ischemia to occur in these tissues, and the result is pain.

Most recently, new information has come out in the literature outlining some of the mechanisms responsible for the occlusive nature of sickle cell disease. The sickled red cells cause damage to the inner lining of blood vessels. The damaged inner lining of blood vessels produces a series of adhesion proteins. These adhesion proteins are said to play a major role in causing occlusion of red blood cells, resulting in painful sickle cell crises. It is believed that both white blood cells and platelets produce proteins that play a role in the vascular occlusive nature of sickle cell disease. (Ref.: American Society of Hematology Education Program Book, 1998).

Treatment of painful sickle cell crisis

The painful sickle cell crisis is best treated with pain medication such as Dilaudid IM or by mouth, morphine sulfate IM, IV or by mouth, Percocet, by mouth, Toradol by mouth or IM, and IV fluids. Some blacks with sickle cell disease, by virtue of the fact that they have an enlarged heart due to repeated assault to the heart by the sickle cell disease over a long period of time, may be in heart failure chronically, so giving them IV fluids may be detrimental.

It is important that people with sickle cell disease who come to the emergency room with painful crisis be evaluated thoroughly by physical examination and by chest x-ray to be certain that they do not have congestive heart failure before being given large amounts of fluid. Giving too much fluid to a sickler can throw the patient into pulmonary edema, which, if not understood quickly, can result in the death of the patient. Pain medication, oxygen, and transfusion of fresh blood are indicated in the treatment of patients with sickle cell disease who are in pain.

It must be clearly understood that the vast majority of patients with sickle cell disease who suffer with recurrent painful crises are, by necessity, addicted to the pain medications that they have been receiving over the years. In spite of this fact, however, these patients must be given ample amount of pain medication when they are in pain, for this is the only way to help them ease their suffering. If it can be determined that an infection triggers the painful crisis, then that infection must be treated with appropriate antibiotics to help alleviate the crisis.

Tests, such as chest x-ray, blood culture, urine cultures, etc. and CBC with reticulocytes count must be done before starting antibiotic treatment. Trying to treat a patient with painful sickle cell crisis with an underlying infection, without treating the infection, is just not going to work. The infection must be treated simultaneously, while the pain is being treated in order to handle the situation in its totality.

The most effective pain medication to treat sickle cell painful crisis is morphine sulfate. Demerol (meperidine) is frequently used to treat patients with painful sickle cell crisis, but it is a bad medication for this purpose. The reason that Meperidine (Demerol) is a bad pain medication to use in the treatment of painful sickle cell crisis is because Meperidine breaks down in the body into Normeperidine, which accumulates in the body because of its very long half-life.

Normeperidine has no significant pain-relieving effect. Normeperidine, however, causes insomnia, anxiety, agitation and seizure, all of which are very bad for people suffering with pain due to sickle cell disease. Morphine sulfate therefore is the recommended pain medication to treat sickle cell patients suffering with pain.

Hemolytic crisis

People with sickle cell disease hemolyze a certain percentage of their red blood cells at all times, and that is the nature of their disease. It is, however, not clear as to the reason or reasons why suddenly patients with this disease begin to hemolyze grossly. When individuals with sickle cell disease develop the hemolytic crisis, they drop their hematocrit abruptly, resulting in shortness of breath, joint pains, general weakness, and sometimes acute congestive heart failure.

The hemolysis can be so brisk, causing the patients to suddenly develop dark looking urine, then their eyes become as yellow as an orange, when, the day before, the situation was not like that at all, and they need to be quickly brought into the hospital and treated appropriately. Other evidence of the hemolytic crisis is a markedly elevated LDH, total and indirect bilirubin and elevated reticulocyte count.

Treatments of the hemolytic crisis

Once it is recognized that a patient is in acute hemolytic crisis, the patient must be admitted to the hospital and oxygen, nasally or by mask, administered along with fresh packed red blood cells. If the patient shows signs of congestive heart failure, Lasix IV must be given to prevent worsening of the CHF. Folic acid, either by mouth or by IV, must also be given to the patient.

Treatments of acute hemolytic crisis

People with sickle cell disease hemolyze their red blood cells all the time, which is part of the disease process. The half-life of their red blood cells is extremely short, maybe 10 to 20 days, as compared to 120 days in a normal person. However, under the stress of an infection or some other circumstances, some of them known, some of them unknown, these individuals can acutely begin to hemolyze, resulting in a rapid drop in their hematocrit.

When this happens, a number of things can develop such as acute shortness of breath, chest pain, drop in blood pressure with shock, and an acute heart attack can occur because of this severe drop in hematocrit. This occurs because of the inability of the heart to pump sufficient blood to carry oxygen to the myocardium.

Acute hemolytic crises must be discovered quickly and treated carefully with fresh packed red cells under the cover of IV Lasix or other loop diuretics to prevent acute pulmonary edema from occurring. In addition to a very low hematocrit, high bilirubin, high LDH, and high reticulocyte count also occur in acute hemolytic crisis.

In addition to replacing blood with fresh packed cells, a high dose of folic acid must also be given when the patient is acutely hemolyzing. The recommended dose of folic acid in patients with chronic hemolytic disease such as sickle cell is as much as 25 mg of folic acid per day and not the usual 1 mg per day of folic acid, which is given for nutritional deficiency. One milligram of folic acid is inadequate in people who are chronically hemolyzing.

Failure to understand this fact can result in the inability of the patient who is chronically hemolyzing to make sufficient red cells. As an individual hemolyzes, the body attempts to make new red cells to meet the demand created by the hemolytic state and uses all available folic acid to make new red cells. Everybody who is hemolyzing chronically is, by definition, folate deficient.

The need to give fresh packed red cells to chronically anemic patients has been mentioned earlier. This is a very important concept to understand because when a severely anemic patient needs a blood transfusion, the anemia can be made worse if she is transfused with old packed red cells that have been sitting in the blood bank for a long time. As blood sits in the blood bank, the level of 2-3 Diphosphoglycerate (2-3 DPG) constantly decreases.

Blood that is depleted in 2-3 DPG, when infused in an already anemic person, shifts the oxygen dissociation curve further to the left, making it much more difficult for that person to deliver oxygen to the tissues. What needs to be done do is to give fresh packed cells, less than a week old, so that a sufficient amount of 2-3 DPG can be delivered into the blood stream to shift the oxygen dissociation curve to the right, allowing for better delivery of oxygen to the tissues.

If a person has underlying ischemic myocardial disease, as is frequently the case in peple with sickle cell disease, then the ischemic myocardial disease can be made acutely worse, resulting in either worsening of underlying congestive heart failure. This can even lead to an acute heart attack or can cause serious cardiac arrhythmias to occur because of the worsening myocardial ischemia.

Hypoplastic crisis

The hypoplastic crisis usually occurs because of an infection that suppresses the bone marrow or because of folic acid deficiency or some other insult to the bone marrow that causes it to fail. Evidence that a patient has developed hypoplastic crisis is an acute drop in the hematocrit and a low reticulocyte count. Treatment of hypoplastic crisis includes oxygen, blood transfusion, folic acid administration, and treatment of any underling infection if any exists.

Acute chest syndrome

Acute chest syndrome is the most serious and potentially lethal of all the sickle cell crises. Next to painful crisis, acute chest syndrome is the second most common reason patients with sickle cell disease get admitted to hospitals, and acute chest syndrome is the cause of death in 25% of all deaths of sickle cell disease patients. Surgery is a major risk factor for the development of acute chest syndrome. Some 25% of patients with sickle cell disease who undergo elective surgery develop acute chest syndrome.

In acute chest syndrome the sickle cell patient usually presents with chest pain, tachycardia, fever, cough, shortness of breath, low oxygen saturation, high white blood cell count, high baseline hemoglobin, low platelet count, together with infiltrates on the chest x-ray.

The nature of the acute chest syndrome appears to be multifactorial and is associated with inflammatory cytokines causing vascular endothelium damage with fat embolism and pulmonary infarction. Secretory phospholipase A2 is an inflammatory substance that is produced in the lungs in ACS and liberates free fatty acids, which in turn cause acute pulmonary fat embolism to occur.

The level of secretory phospholipase A2 is quite high in the blood of patients with ACS and is elevated before the onset of ACS and when detected confirms the diagnosis of ACS. Infection plays a major role in ACS. In patients with ACS, when bronchoscoped, several different microorganisms were found. Included in the list of microorganisms were different bacteria and viruses. The most common bacteria found were Chlamydia pnuemoniae, Mycoplasma pneumoniae, respiratory syncytial virus, Parvovirus, Rhinovirus, etc.

Treatments of acute chest syndrome

1. Patients who are having pain should be given pain medication such as morphine sulfate to relieve their pain.
2. Oxygen must be given.
3. Incentive spirometry every 3-4 hours while awake is crucial to prevent atelectasis and eventual pneumonia.
4. Transfusion of fresh packed red blood cells must be given and if necessary exchange transfusion ought to be given.
5. Broad-spectrum IV antibiotics must be given because they are felt to play a major role both in genesis of ACS and in its complications.
6. Blood for secretory phospholipase A2 should be obtained and the level ought to be used to monitor the activity of the syndrome.
7. Daily chest X-ray is necessary to monitor lung infiltrates if there are any.
8. Frequent arterial blood gas is needed to monitor the lung functions of these patients.
9. It is very important to avoid giving too much IV fluid to patients with ACS so as to prevent the development of pulmonary edema and other complications such as adult respiratory distress syndrome (ARDS), etc.

Splenic sequestration

Splenic sequestration as a sickle crisis is seen most frequently in infants but can also be seen in adults who have either sickle C disease or sickle thalassemia.

The reason why patients with SC or sickle thalassemia can have this form of sickle crisis is because frequently they have spleens and these spleens are enlarged.

Therefore, when patients in this category present with acute left-sided mid-abdominal pain, splenic sequestration with impending rupture of the spleen must be considered and an abdominal CT scan and a surgical consult must be obtained immediately. Oftentimes, people who carry the sickle cell trait (AS) do not realize that the AS state carries its own list of medical problems. These problems include prominently:

1. Hematuria with occasional severe gross bleeding from the kidney because of papillary necrosis of the left kidney more often than the right kidney, as mentioned earlier.
2. Arthritis of the hips, knees, and spine.
3. Inability to concentrate the urine properly, although general kidney function is normal.
4. Anemia, more severe in menstruating women because of concomitant iron deficiency due to iron loss as part of the menstruation cycle. About 35% to 40%

of the red cells are sickle in AS trait as compared to 60% to 70% in people with SS disease.

5. Infraction of the spleen can occur in situations where ambient oxygen pressure is too low in people with sickle cell trait. But, people with sickle cell trait are able to tolerate simulated high altitude with no problem. People with the sickle cell trait have been engaging in strenuous physical activities, including professional sports, with no difficulty. Usual medical management with analgesics, iron by mouth, with IV fluids, blood transfusions, when necessary, and high-dose folic acid, up to 25 mg per day, are the mainstay in the everyday treatment of patients with sickle cell disease. The usual 1 mg dose of folic acid given daily is grossly inadequate as outlined earlier. Blacks who have sickle cell disease and are pregnant must take folic acid to improve their level of hemoglobin as well as to guard against neuro-tubular disease.

6. Recently, several reports have appeared in the medical literature outlining evidence of sudden cardiac arrest and deaths in young athletes with sickle cell trait during straineous atheletic activities.

Other acute complications of sickle cell disease include:

1. Gross hematuria due to papillary necrosis of the kidney
2. Acute chest syndrome
3. Pulmonary Embolism
4. Acute myocardial infarction (heart attack)
5. Congestive heart failure, which is due to the cardiomyopathy associated with the secondary hemochromatosis.
6. Acute gouty arthritis, due to the rapid red cell turnover associated with the chronic hemolytic state
7. Stroke
8. Acute multi-organ damaged syndrome
9. Sickle cell disease hemolytic transfusion reaction syndrome.

There are several more recently described complications of sickle cell disease, such as the effect of increased viscosity due to high hematocrit in a person with sickle cell anemia. A hematocrit of 30%-35% or higher interferes with oxygen delivery to the tissues, resulting in hypoxia and can be associated with thrombosis (clot formation). As part of this increased viscosity scenario another syndrome, called acute multi-organs damage syndrome, can occur. Because of the hypoxia associated with increased hematocrit, several organs can become damaged at the same time, resulting in an acute medical emergency. These are the most frequently damaged organs during this syndrome:

1. The kidneys causing hematuria (blood) in the urine, or the kidneys can fail (acute renal failure)

2. Necrosis of the liver can occur
3. The bone marrow may become necrotic, resulting in the propagation of fat emboli
4 Acute pancreatitis can occur
5. Acute stroke as well as acute myocardial infarction can occur.

To prevent the acute multi-organs damaged syndrome, the hematocrit of the sickle cell patients ought to be kept between 27%-29% (Ref: American Society of Hematology Education Program Book, Dec. 2000).

Still another serious complication of sickle cell disease is a hemolytic transfusion reaction that can occur in patients being transfused with red blood cells to treat anemia associated with sickle cell disease. This problem is called sickle cell transfusion reaction syndrome. Some of the indications that a patient with sickle cell may be experiencing sickle cell transfusion reaction syndrome include:

1. Worsening of the painful crisis while receiving blood transfusion
2. A marked drop in the patient's hematocrit and acute inability to make new red blood cells, as manifested with a low reticulocytes count
3. A rapid drop in the hematocrit after receiving blood transfusion (the hematocrit drops to a lower percentage than before the transfusion of red cells were given)
4. Subsequent transfusions of red blood cells may make the anemia worse and, at times, this situation can be severe enough to cost the affected woman her life. This problem must be recognized quickly and when and if it occurs, to avoid transfusing a patient who is suffering from this problem.

BLOOD SMEAR SHOWING SICKLE CELLS

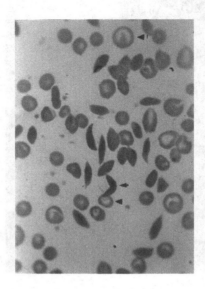

Figure 34.1-Arrow showing sickle cell (banana-shaped cell). Arrow head showing a target cell in a black person with sickle cell anemia, with thalassemia combined (sickle thalassemia).

Other types of anemias seen in blacks are folic acid deficiency, B-12 deficiency and autoimmune hemolytic anemia. Sickle cell disease frequently affects the bone and brain of individuals suffering from it.

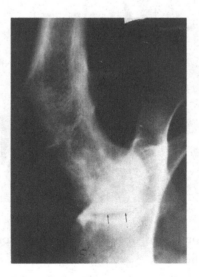

Figure 34.2-Arrows showing avascular necrosis (lack of blood flow to bone) of femoral head with flattening necrosis of head bone in a black person with sickle cell disease.

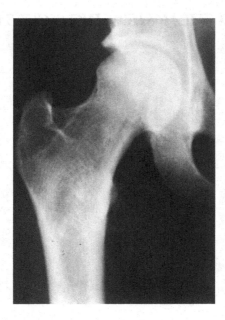

Figure 34.3-X-ray of a normal hip

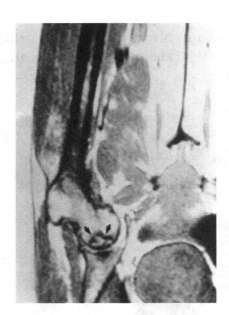

Figure 34.4-MRI of femoral head of hip of a black person with sickle cell disease. Arrows showing avascular necrosis.

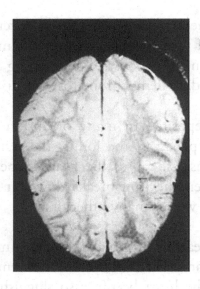

Figure 34.5- Arrows showing multiple infarcts (stroke) in the brain of a black person with sickle cell disease as documented by brain MRI.

The treatment of sickle cell hemolytic transfusion reaction is administration of corticosteroid intravenously. A rising reticulocytes count and hematocrit is an indication that the patient is getting better (Ref: American Society of Hematology Education Program Book, 2000).

The heart is always affected in a rather severe way in patients with sickle cell disease. The mechanism through which the heart gets affected in sickle cell disease is similar to all the other affected organs, through a vascular occlusive mechanism. The vessels carrying blood to the heart to deliver oxygen are of all different sizes.

The smaller they are, the easier it is for them to get occluded by the very nature of the sickle red cells. Sickled red cells just cannot pass through these small vessels easily, and there lies the basis of the ischemia that occurs in the muscle of the heart in women suffering with sickle cell disease. The ischemia causes the release of substances called kinins, which are chemicals that tissues of all types release once they become ischemic (starved for oxygen).

Once the kinins are released they cause a burning pain, and this burning pain is responsible not only for chest pain but also is, in fact, the basis of the painful sickle cell crisis, which is most common of the sickle cell crises. The myocardial ischemia that occurs in patients with sickle cell disease is just as detrimental as any other ischemia that affects the heart. It leads to muscle scarring and if one or more of the coronary arteries were to become occluded then acute myocardial infarction can occur.

Nevertheless, more commonly, what happens is that the small vessels that carry blood to the heart muscle is occluded, causing myocardial ischemic disease to occur.

Along with the ischemia of the myocardial muscle that occurs in women with sickle cell disease, the red blood cells of these people constantly hemolyze. The homolysis causes lots of iron to be deposited in the bloodstream, resulting in a serious condition called hemochromatosis. This secondary hemochromatosis results in elevated serum ferritin.

This storage iron gets deposited in many organs in the body, in particular the heart muscles, the liver, the pancreas, the joints, the testicles, etc. The iron, once it accumulates in the heart muscles, causes the heart to become enlarged (a condition called cardiomyopathy). When the iron breaks down, it releases free radicals, which damage myocardial tissues, as well as many other tissues.

The enlargement of the heart in turn makes blood pumping very difficult, resulting in congestive heart failure. Cardiac arrhythmias of different types can also occur in this situation. The pumping of the heart becomes so sluggish at times that blood within its chambers becomes stagnated, which can cause a clot to form, and this clot can be carried to different organs as emboli. An organ that is particularly vulnerable to this situation is the brain. If a clot gets loose and becomes lodged in the brain, then an acute stroke can occur. To prevent such a problem from arising, these patients with cardiomyopathy are frequently treated with Heparin or Coumadin (blood thinners) to thin the blood to prevent the development of emboli.

As just mentioned, these individuals frequently develop different rhythm irregularities of the heart and one of the most common rhythm disturbances seen in this situation is a condition known as atrial fibrillation. The reason why this particular rhythm abnormality is so serious is that in the acute setting it can make the affected woman quite sick. Atrial fibrillation can cause the heart to decompensate but it can also cause a stroke to develop. Digitalis is used to control the rate of the heart and Coumadin is used to prevent a clot from forming.

Hemochromatosis (too much iron in the body) in people with sickle cell disease is quite serious because of what it can do to the liver, pancreas, heart, and the joints, etc.
The two most effective treatments are phlebotomy (removing one unit of blood—500 cc—from the body at a time) and Desferal (a chelating agent). Desferal, when used in the proper fashion, chelates the iron, removing it from the body and passing the iron out in the urine, thereby decreasing the level of iron in the body. Also available to remove excess iron from the body is a new drug called Exjade (deferasirox).
It is used by mouth at 20-30 mg/kg/day on an empty stomach.

In addition to the problems just outlined, people who suffer from sickle cell disease (SS), sickle thalassemia, or sickle cell C disease, commonly have a spectrum of clinical manifestations of disease that causes them to be frequently quite sick.

What is the mechanism through which sickle cell disease causes stroke to occur?

Stroke occurs in sickle cell disease patients because the misshaped and sticky red cells clog the small vessels within the brain preventing oxygen from getting to vital parts of the brain. This lack of oxygen results in ischemia, which in turn causes ischemic stroke to occur, and depending on the extent and location of the stroke paralysis may result.

Other major problems that arise as a result of stroke induced by sickle cell disease, even in a child, are inability to control bowel and urinary functions, and aphasia may occur (the inability to speak), sometimes permanently. The stroke frequently causes difficulty in swallowing, which is quite common, and this can sometimes result in recurrent aspiration pneumonia, which may lead to lung abscesses, bronchiectasis, and, sometimes, pulmonary death is the result.

Other frequent complications are seizures. These seizures can be quite troublesome even when anti-seizure medications are used. Pulmonary problems are also quite common in sickle cell patients such as pneumonia, pulmonary embolism, congestive heart failure, causing marked difficulty in breathing with severe hypoxia (lack of oxygen).

Along with these new concepts and mechanisms in sickle cell disease are the proposed newer treatments of sickle cell disease. Hydroxyurea works in sickle cell disease by raising hemoglobin F. In addition, it decreases the level of white blood cells and platelets and helps to improve the symptoms of sickle cell disease.

So, sickle cell patients on hydroxyurea, even if their hemoglobin F level does not go up, benefit because of the lowering of white cells and platelets (Ref: American Society of Hematology Education Program Book, 1998).

Other proposed treatment modalities include inhalation of nitric oxide gas to dilate blood vessels, allowing for better tissue perfusion. Another proposed new modality of treatment for sickle cell disease is low-dose aspirin, which works as an anti-inflammatory medication against the effects of the adhesion proteins. Aspirin also works to prevent platelet aggregation, resulting in better blood flow through blood vessels and decreasing the incidence of sickle cell painful crises (Ref:. American Society of Hematology Education Program Book, 1998).

Another common problem that frequently occurs in blacks who suffer from sickle cell disease is gall bladder disease. If gall bladder disease is allowed to go undiagnosed it can cause severe problems for the patient. It usually presents with acute abdominal pain, nausea, and vomiting. This constellation of symptoms is usually due to acute cholecystitis. Because blacks with sickle disease and other chronic hemolytic diseases hemolyze constantly, they dump large amounts of bilirubin pigments into their bloodstream. These bilirubin pigments in turn form bilirubin-containing gall bladder stones.

Over time, these gall bladder stones cause the gall bladder to become inflamed and sometimes infected, resulting in a spectrum of acute and chronic gallbladder diseases. The diagnosis and treatment of gallbladder disease is described elsewhere in this book.

Other frequent problems that people with sickle cell disease have to cope with are things such as:

1. Sickle cell retinopathy (bleeding into the eyes) is seen more frequently in SC disease than in SS disease.
2. Leg ulcers
3. Aseptic necrosis of different bones, such as the shoulder joints, the elbow joints, the hip joints, and the knee joints.
4. Microscopic or gross hematuria due to papillary necrosis is quite common. It is seen more often from the left kidney than the right kidney. The reason why papillary necrosis is seen more frequently from the left kidney is that the anatomical position of the two kidneys is different. The left kidney is located higher than the right kidney.

The position of the left kidney places it in a situation where it is less able to receive appropriate amount of oxygen as compared to the right kidney. In normal people that doesn't matter but in people who have sickle cell disease, that becomes a major problem and in the left kidney where that situation occurs, papillary necrosis occurs frequently, resulting in gross hematuria.

People with sickle cell disease have the propensity of getting infected with capsular bacterial organisms such as pneumococci and Haemophilus influenzae.

It has been said that patients with sickle cell disease get infected in the bone frequently with salmonella bacteria, resulting in osteomyelitis.

The spleens of people with sickle cell anemia (SS) variety get destroyed by the time these people become teenagers, due to the recurrent insults of the sickling phenomena to the splenic circulation. The hyposplenic state that results causes these women to become immunoincompetent, thus causing them to get infected much more easily.

It is therefore recommended that these individuals get vaccinated with pneumococcal vaccine about every three years or so. It is also recommended that these people get treated with penicillin 250 mg daily as a prophylaxis against pneumococcal organisms.

These organisms are exquisitely sensitive to penicillin. If the patient is allergic to penicillin, Erythromycin 250 mg daily or twice a day can be used as a substitute. People with sickle thalassemia or sickle C disease tend to have large spleens.

People with sickle cell disease are prone to develop sickle hepatopathy (sickle cell liver disease), with large engorgement of the liver, which frequently causes right upper abdominal pain.

Another common problem that individuals with sickle cell disease suffer from is disease of the kidneys. At first the manifestation of the kidney disease appears as different degrees of renal insufficiency in the blood chemistry tests that evaluate kidney function. As the sickle cell disease progresses, chronic renal failure develop, forcing these individuals to be placed frequently on chronic hemodialysis.

Before the kidneys fail completely, hypertension frequently develops, complicating the picture even more because the hypertension can cause strokes or congestive heart failure. As outlined earlier in this chapter, people with sickle cell disease have the propensity to develop strokes and cardiomyopathy. When the blood pressure becomes elevated, it is superimposed on an already sick heart and sick brain, risking decompensation of these and other organs that are frequently affected by elevated blood pressure.

There are no definite treatments available to cure sickle cell disease presently. However, there are several medications and methods available to treat the disease. Hydroxyurea is being used to treat patients with sickle disease to improve the symptoms of the disease.

Hydroxyurea works to improve the symptoms of sickle cell disease in some patients by raising the level of hemoglobin F. Hemoglobin F is an excellent carrier of oxygen and by increasing hemoglobin it enables oxygen to be carried to tissues much more easily, thereby preventing ischemia from occurring.

The result is less pain and improvement in the overall symptoms of the affected patients.

Sodium butyrate has been shown in a recent setting to be able to increase hemoglobin F level as well. Recombinant human erythropoietin (Epogen or Procrit) is being used in combination with hydroxyurea to increase hemoglobin F and red blood cells levels.

Another common complication of sickle anemia is chronic sickle cell lung disease.

In spite of all the many millions of dollars that have been spent looking for a cure for sickle cell disease, no cure has been found as of this date. Bone marrow transplantation is being tried as a curative measure for sickle cell disease but it is in its infancy and the results so far have been few, although some reports appear to be quite encouraging. In for the future, it is hoped that stem cell—based gene therapy and RNA interference holds promise in helping people with sickle cell disease.

Genetic counseling remains the most worthwhile approach for those who are affected with sickle cell disease resulting in pulmonary fibrosis and restrictive lung disease and pulmonary hypertension. The best test to diagnose pulmonary hypertension is echocardiogram. Pulmonary hypertension exists when a mPAP >25 mmHg is present on the echocardiogram. Right heart catheterization is often done to cofirm the diagnosis of pulmonary hypertension.

Treatments of pulmonary hypertension include

Oxygen
Calcium channel blocker
Anticoagulation Source: American Society of Hematology Education Program Book
December 10-13, 2011

There exist a serious misconception in the literature regarding hemoglobin CC and hemoglobin AC. No where in the text books of hematology and text books on hemoglobin is it mentioned that hemoglobin CC and hemoblobin AC cause anemia.

The truth it both these conditions cause a microcytic anemia with erythrocytosis.
I have large number of black patients in my practive with hemoglobin AC with microcytic anemia with erythrocytosis. To resolve this falsehood once and for all, here are the CBC, serum ferritin and quantitative hemoglobin electrophoresis of a 63 year black female patient in my practice with classic hemoglobin AC.
WBC 8.000
HGB 11.0 grams
RBC 3.990.000
HCT 31.4%
MCV 76.7
Sreum Ferritin 78
Quantitative hemoglobin electrophoresis hemoglobin A 55.4% hemoglobin C 44.6%.

Chapter 35
THALASSEMIA

Alpha thalassemia

Alpha thalassemia affects several hundred million people in the world.

The areas of the world most affected by alpha thalassemia are Africa, North Africa, Mediterranean, Asia, South East Asia, India, Middle East and North America, and The Americas.

In alpha thalassemia, the silent carrier is missing one alpha globin chain, and the alpha thalassemia trait missing two alpha globin chains taken together is among the most common genetic disorder in the world. About 32% of black Americans carry the alpha thalassemia genetic abnormality. Of that figure, 30% are missing one alpha globin chain and 2% are missing two alpha globin chains.

Blacks don't have any symptoms from this abnormality. Those who are missing two alpha globin chains from opposite sides of the alpha globin chain may have a mild microcytic anemia and are said to have alpha thalassemia trait or alpha thalassemia minor. People with immediate African ancestral genes always miss the two alpha globin chains from opposite sides of the alpha globin chain. On the other hand, Asian people and others, when they are missing two alpha globin chains, always miss the chains from the same side of the alpha globin chain, creating an unbalanced alpha globin chain situation.

This is what happens in hemoglobin constant spring which causes anemia and symptoms in individuals who are afflicted with it. Individuals who are missing three alpha globin haplotypes have hemoglobin H and severely anemic. Hine's bodies are seen in the red blood cells of these individuals on blood smears. When four alpha globin chains are missing, that is Hemoglobin Bart's (hydrops fetalis) and the fetuses that these women carry die in utero, resulting usually in spontaneous abortion.

How to diagnose alpha thalassemia

The best way to diagnose alpha thalassemia is to do a CBC and a quantitative hemoglobin electrophoresis. In alpha thalassemia, the CBC shows microcytosis, low MCV, erythrocytosis, and high RDW. The erythrocytosis (elevated red blood cell count) differentiates thalassemia from iron deficiency. For every 10% of the hematocrit there is 1 million of red blood cells and where there is a discordance of about 400,000 or greater, there exists a thalassemia syndrome in the patient.

If all the aforementioned conditions exist and hemoglobin A2 and hemoglobin F are normal on the quantitative hemoglobin electrophoresis, then the patient has alpha thalassemia of one degree or another.

The treatments for alpha thalassemia are folic acid, blood transfusion, and Procrit/ Epogen when necessary.

Beta thalassemia/Cooley's anemia

Beta thalassemia affects about 3% or 201 million of the world population and its distribution are worldwide. The people who are most affected by Beta thalassemia are some Greeks, Italians, Turkish, Iranians, Syrians, Arabics, Pakistanis, Indians, Asians, Northen China, Southeast Asians; Kurdish Jews; and, in North America, Blacks and Hispanics. Beta thalassemia has also been reported in some Northern European people as well.

The cause of beta thalassemia is the deficiency in the beta globin chains of the hemoglobin molecule. Normal hemoglonin has 2 globin beta chains and 4 alpha globin chains.

In beta thalassemia the quantity of the beta chain is deficient and the degree of this deficiency determines the degree and severity of the disease.

Beta thalassemia has three clinical categories: beta thalassemia minor, beta thalassemia intermedia and beta thalassemia major.

Beta thalassemia minor causes no clinical manifestation or disease. Beta thalassemia intermedia cause a hypochromic microcytic anemia with moderate degree of iron overload, but growth is normal and life span is also not affected.

Beta thalassemia major causes a severe anemia, serious symptoms, and high iron overload, endocrine abnormalities with growth retardation, large spleen, large liver, large heart, and congestive heart failure along with cardiac arrhythmias etc. Without early, effective, and aggressive treatment, many individuals with thalassemia major die before reaching adulthood.

How to diagnose beta thalassemia

The CBC in beta thalassemia major shows low hemoglobin and hematocrit, low MCV, high red blood cell count, high RDW and the blood shows many target cells. The quantitative hemoglobin electrophoresis shows elevated hemoglobin A2 or F or both.

An example of what a CBC, serum ferritin and Hemoglobin electrophoresis of a person with beta thalassemia trait looks like. This person has the increased HGB A2 variant of beta thalassemia with normal HGB F level.

WBC	8.6	(4.0-10.5)	TH/MM3
RBC	6.37	(4.2-5.8)	MIL/MM3
HGB	13.4	(13.0-17.0)	G/DL
HCT	42.1	(38.0-50.0)	%
MCV	66.1	(80-96)	FL
MCH	21.0	(27-32)	UUG
MCHC	31.8	(33-35.5)	%
RDW	15.4	(11.0-14.5)	%
PLT	21.9	(130-400)	TH/MM3
MPV	9.0	(6.8-11.0)	FL
NEU	69.6	(43-75)	%
LYMPH	21.4	(15-45)	%
MONO	7.5	(3-12)	%
EOS	1.0	(0-5.5)	%
BASO	0.5	(0-2.0)	%
NEU#	6.0	(1.7-7.9)	TH/MM3
FERRITIN	673	(12-282)	NG/ML
hemoglobin A	93.4	(94.7-98.2)	%
hemoglobin a2	5.80	(1.8-3.3)	%
hemoglobin f	0.80	(0.0-2.0)	%

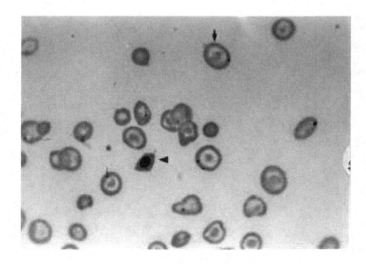

Figure 35.1-Thalassemia (arrow head) showing nucleated red cell, small arrow showing howel jolly body. Big arrow shows target cell.

How to treat beta thalassemia major

The most effective treatments for beta thalassemia major consist of:

1. Blood transfusion
2. Chelation therapy using Desferal, Deferiprone, or Exjade
3. Folic acid
4. Bone marrow transplantation
5. Prenatal diagnosis during the first 9-10 gestation can be done, using chorionic villus sampling for DNA fetal analysis. This procedure allows the parents of the unborn fetus to know whether the fetus is homozygous or heterozygous for beta thalassemia major.
6. Preimplantation genetic diagnosis (PGD) is also available for couples who acrry the the beta thalassemia genes and wish to use this modality to secure the birth of a child free of the beta thalassemia that can be used as a bone marrow donor for a sibling who is sick with beta thalassemia major.

The thalassemias as well as the major sickling diseases are in great measure responsible for the preservation of the new world from the old world because these diseases allowed some people who lived in the old world to survive the ravages of malaria, mainly because the malarial organism could not flourish inside these abnormal red blood cells.

Chapter 36
AUTOIMMUNE HEMOLYTIC ANEMIA

Autoimmune hemolytic anemia affects hundred of million people in the world.

Autoimmune hemolytic anemia develops when the body develops antibodies against its red blood cells. There are warm and cold auto antibodies. Fifty percent of warm antibodies are idiopathic and fifty percent are secondary.

In idiopathic autoimmune hemolytic anemia, immunoglobulin G (IgG) bins to red blood cells at 37 degree temperature (body temperature) and causes red blood cells hemolyse (burst).

The diseases that are associated with autoimmune hemolytic include:

Chronic Lyphocytic leukemia
Non-Hodgkin's lymphoma
Ovarian cancer
Systomic Lupus Erythematosis (SLE)
Multiple myeloma
AIDS
Hepatitis
Rheumatoid arthritis
Mixed collagen vascular diseases etc;

Drugs that are associated with autoimmune hemolytic anemia include:

Quinidine
Methyldopa
Hydralazine
Tylenol
Ibuprofen
Alfa interferon
Cephalothin
Insulin
Sulfa drugs like Bactrim
Hydrochlorothiazide
Rifampin
Streptomycin
Penicillin etc;

Secondary warm autoimmune hemolytic is associated with diseases like Lymphoproliferative disorders such as lymphoma and chronic lymphocytic leukemia
SLE
Rheumatoid arthritis
Mixed collagen vascular diseases
Ulcerative colitis
ITP/Evan's syndrome
Myasthenia gravis etc;

Cold autoimmune hemolytic anemia occurs because of autoantibodies of immunoglobulin M (IgM). The IgM antibodies bin to red blood cells causing the red blood cells to hemolyse (burst) when the body temperature dropps to 32˙C.

The diseases that are associated with cold autoimmune hemolytic anemia include:

Infectious mononucleosis
Mycoplasma pneumonia
Lymphoma
Paroxysmal cold hemoglobinuria
Syphilis
Mumps
Measles etc;

Symptoms of autoimmune hemolytic anemia include:

Fatigue
Weakness
Fever
Pale skin
Dizziness
Tiredness
Head ache
Low blood pressure
Enlarged liver
Enlarged spleen
Rapid heart rate
Flow heart murmur
Chest pain
Jaundice
Dark urine
Anemia
High reticulocyte count

Low platelets in Evan's syndrome etc;

Evaluations of autoimmune hemolytic anemia include:

History
Physical examination
Blood pressure
Pulse
Temperature
Respiratory rate
Oxygen saturation
CBC
Peripheral blood smear (shows rouleaux formation, spherocytes, macrocytes, polychromasia)
Direct coombs test
Serum complement level
IgG/C3 test
In warm autoimmune hemolytic anemia the IgG/C3 test is positive
In cold autoimmune hemolytic anemia C3 is positive
Lactic dehydrogenase
Indirect bilirubin
Haptoglobin
Urinalysis
Cold agglutinin titer (positive when >1:64)
Bone marrow aspiration and biopsy
Donath-Landsteiner test (to be done only when paroxysmal cold hemoglobinuria is suspected)
EKG
Chest ray
Abdominal CT scan with contrast both IV and by mouth

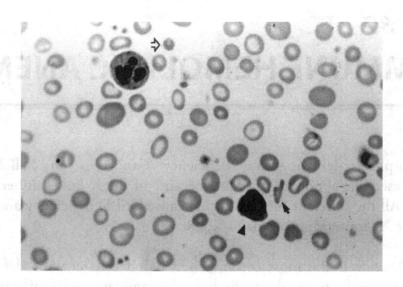

Figure 36.1-Hemolytic anemia (arrow head) showing nucleated red cell in a person. Arrow showing schistocyte (fragment of red blood cell). Open arrow showing spherocyte (very small red cell full with hemoglobin).

Treatments of autoimmune hemolytic anemia include:

Steroid
Folic acid
Intavenous Immunoglobulin
Blood transfusion (a person is having chest pain due to low blood count)
Slpenectomy (when all other treatments have failed)

Chapter 37
NONIMMUNE HEMOLYTIC ANEMIA

Glucose-6-phosphate dehydrogenase deficiency G6PD is an X-linked recessive hereditary disease. The abnormality occurs because of the X-linked inheritance pattern of the disease. All the different mutations that cause G6PD deficiency are found on the long arm of the X chromosome on band Xq28.

G6PD deficiency is the most common red blood cells enzyme deficiency in the world. About 400 million people in the have this problem and it affects people of all ethnicities.

This abnormality causes low level of G6PD, and men are affected more often than women are. Women get affected via the process of lyonization of the X chromosome.

G6PD deficiency is closely linked with favism. Favism is a condition that develops when people with G6PD deficiency eat fava beans.

Causes of hemolysis in G6PD deficiency include:

Anti malarial drugs like chloroquine, Pamaquine and, primaquine
Bactrim
Mafenide
Thiazolesulfone
Aspirin
Acetanilide
Nitrofurantoin
Isoniazid
Dapsone
Furazolidone etc;

The tests that are in use to diagnosis of G6PD deficiency include:

CBC
Complete chemistry metabolic profile
Reticolocyte count
Hatoglobin
Lactic dehydrogenase
Direct coomb's test
Peripheral blood smear to look for Heinz bodies

Beutler fluorescent spot test

Treatments of G6PD deficiency include

Blood transfusion
Folic acid

Similar to peole with sickle anemia, G6PD deficiency prevent people from dyeing from malaria because the spleens of people who are suffering from these two diseases filter out of the body red cels that are infected with the malarial orgnisms. It is said that this process plaid a major role in the preservation of the old world in the continent of Africa which, ultimately gave birth to the new world. The human race began in Africa, and all human beings can trace their ancestry to Africa.

Chapter 38

CIRRHOSIS OF THE LIVER AND HEMOLYTIC ANEMIA

Cirrhosis of the liver affects 20 million people worldwide
Source: WHO

The most common causes of cirrhosis of the liver include:

Alcoholism
Obesity
Hepatitis B
Hepatitis C
Hemochromatosis
Wilson disease
Primary sclorosing cholangitis
Biliary atresia
Parasitism
Exposure to toxins etc;

Everyone with cirrhosis of the liver if they live long enough will eventually an enlarged spleen. The enlarged spleen causes a condition called hypersplenism. Hypersplenism causes destruction of red blood cells, white blood cells, and platelets.

Evaluations of hypersplenism and hemolysis include:

History
Physical examination
CBC
Reticulocyte count
Complete chemical metabolic ptofile
Lactic dehydrogenase (LDH)
Indirect bilirubin
Urinalysis, including urobilinogen
Abominal ultrasound
CT scan of the abomen with contrast by mouth

Treatments of hemolytic anemia due to hypersplenism include
Folic acid 2 mg 4 times per day by mouth

Chapter 39
THROMBOTIC THROMBOCYTOPINIC PURPURA

The indidence of TTP is about 1 per 100,000 or 3.120.000 people in the U.S. (The U.S. population is 312 million) and about 4 per 100,000 or 12,480 people worldwide (The world population is 7 billion) and women are affected more than men.

TTP is a disease of the coagulation system that causes wide spread small clots to develop inside small blood vessels throughout the body. Most of the time, TTP develop because of the inhibition of the enzyme ADAMTS13, "a metalloprotease responsible for cleaving large multimers of VonWillerbrand factor into smaller units".

Several drugs have been associated with TTP and among them is Plavix.

The organs most frequently affected by TTP include:

Kidney
Brain
Heart
Blood

As blood passes trhough blood vessels, the small clots inside the vessels damage the red blood cells and platelets leading to fragmentation of red blood cells and low platelets. The red cells fragmentation causes the development of schistocytes.

The small clots inside the vessels that pass through the brain cause brain ischemia leading to seizures, stroke and hemorrhage. The small clots that pass through the kidneys cause kidney failure. The small clots that pass through the heart can cause ischemia, angina pectoris, and myocardial infartction. The damage that occurs to red cells as blood pass through blood vessels causes hemolytic anemia.

TTP occurs more often in women and it is seen more often in black women than women of other racial groups. Pregnancy and the postpartum states both increase the incidence of TTP.

Evaluations of TTP include:

History and physical examination

CBC
Periheral blood smear
Complete metabolic profile
LDH
Incomplete bilirubin
Direct coomb's
Haptoglobin
Reticulocytes count
PTT
PT
INR
Urinalysis
Chest Xray
Renal ultrasound
EKG
EEG
Brain CT scan
Brain MRI

Treatments of TTP include;

Steroid
Cytoxan
Vincristine
Tituximab
Aspirin
Plasmapherisis
Folic acid
Dialysis
Anti-seizure medications
Anti-Stroke medications
Anti-angina pectoris medications
Anti-myocardial infarction medications

Chapter 40
HEREDITARY SPHEROCYTOSIS

Hereditary spherocytosis is an autosomal dominant genetically transmitted hemolytic anemia. This disease is characrerized by sphere shaped red blood cells instead of the usual disk shaped (bi-concaved) red blood cells.

Hereditary spherocytosis is seen most commonly in people Northen European descent and Japanese. The incidence of hereditary spherocytosis in the U.S. is 1 in 5000 or 62,400 people (The U.S. population is 312 million) and 300 per million people in the world or 2, 100,000 (The world population is 7 billion) people in the world.

The red cells membrane proteins abnormalities responsible for hereditary spherocytosis are

Spectrin deficiency
Ankyrin defects
Band 3 deficiency
Protein 4.2 deficiency

Alpha-spectrin deficiency mutations are seen in the recessive forms of hereditary spherocytosis and beta-spectrin forms of hereditary spherocytosis are seen in autosomal dominant forms of hereditary spherocytosis.

Ankyrin defects in hereditary spherocytosis are seen in people with translocation of chromosome 8 or deletion of the short arm of chromosome 8. The ankyrin gene is located in the short arm of chromosome 8. About 75-80% of people with autosomal hereditary spherocytosis have a combination spectrin and ankyrin deficiency.

Band 3 deficiency is seen in about 10-20% in people who have mild to moderate autosomal dominant hereditary spherocytosis.

Protein 4.2 deficiency causes hereditary hemolytic. Spherocytes, elliptocytes or sphero-ovalocytes are seen on the peripheral smear. Protein 4.2 deficiency is very common in Japanese.

Signs and symptoms of hereditary spherocytosis include:

Weakness

Fatigue

Shortness of breath

Paleness

Head ache

Jaundice on the skin

Jaundice in the eyes

Anemia

Spleenomegaly (large spleen)

Cholelithiasis (gallstones)

Acute Cholecystitis

Abdominal pain

Nausea

Vomiting

Hypersplenism

Aplastic anemia

Low white blood cells

Low platelets

Low red blood cells

Evaluations of hereditary spherocytosis include:

History and physical examinations

Temperature

Pulse

Blood pressure

Respiratory rate

Examination of the skin

Examination of the eyes

Examination of the abdomen

Examination of the heart

Examination of the lungs etc;

CBC

Peripheral blood smear examination

Complete chemistry metabolic profile

Lactic dehydrogenese LDH

Total bilirubin

Indirect bilirubin

Reticulocytes count

Direct coomb's test

Serum Folic acid level

Serum B12 level

Osmotic fragility test

Bone marrow aspiration
Bone marrow biopsy
B19 human parvovirus blood test (this virus can cause pure red blood cells aplasia)
Chromosone analysis
Abdominal ultrasound
Abdominal CT scan
Chest xray
EKG

Complications of hereditary spherocytosis include:

Abdominal pain due to enlarged spleen
Abdominal pain due gall bladder disease
Aplastic anemia etc;

Medical treatments of hereditary spherocytosis include:

Blood transfusion
Folic acid 4mg 4 times per day by mouth
Pain medications as needed

Surgical treatments for hereditary spherocytosis include:

Spenectomy (surgical removal of the spleen)
Cholecystectomy (surgical removal of the gall bladder)

Chapter 41
MEGALOBLASTIC ANEMIAS

B12 deficiency:

B12 deficiency is a very common disease B12 is necessary in the myelination of nerve cells in the brain, and is also necessary in the maintenance of the myelination of these nerve cells for normal brain functions.

In addition, B12 is needed to mediation of nerve cells in the cervical, thoracic dorsal, lateral columns of the spinal cord, cranial and peripheral nerves. When B12 level is low in the body, degeneration of myelin sheets occurs. B12 deficiency also causes demyelination of the white matter of the brain. Myelin is lipid like substance that forms a sheet around the axons of nerve. All cells that grow in the body require B12 to grow, including red blood cells, white blood cells and platelets.

The different things that cause B12 deficiency are:

1. Nutritional deficiency (diet deficient of B12)
2. Parasitic infestation (Diphyllobothrium latum, a Fish tape worm)
3. Blind loop syndrome
4. Atrophic gastritis (being elderly)
5. Gastrectomy
6. Malabsorption
7. Pernicious anemia
8. Inhalation of nitrous oxide
9. Xerostomia
10. Inflammatory bowel disease
11. Divirticulosis (diffuse)
12. Sprue
13. Tropical sprue
14. B12 deficiency itself can cause malabsoprtion because low B12 causes the cells in the GI tract to become macrocytic resulting in malabsorption of B12.
15. Gastric bypass etc;

How do these different things cause B12 deficiency?

The total store in the body is about 5000 micrograms. The body loses about 1-4 micrograms of B12 per day and the daily requirement for B12 is in the range of 2 micrograms per day. B12 is found in liver, milk, eggs, cheese, and meats.

Nutritional B12 deficiency is usually found in strict vegetarians and in people who don't have access to the food products just mentioned.

Diphyllobothrium latum is the fish tapeworm most commonly associated with B12 deficiency. This worm causes malabsorption of B12 to occur.
The tapeworm takes up the B12; thereby preventing its absorption from the ileum, and the result is B12 deficiency.

Small bowel blind loops/bacterial overgrowth, small bowel diverticulosis, and other pouches and fistulae cause B12 deficiency because the bacteria eat the B12, making it unavailable for absorption. In this condition, the level of folate is quite high.

Atrophic gastritis causes B12 deficiency because as an individual age the stomach is less able to produce acid and an acidic milieu is necessary in order for intrinsic factor to properly work to allow B12 to be absorbed. Along the same line, the elderly are prone to develop B12 deficiency because of a deficiency that occurs in the mouth due to a lack of certain salivary enzymes that are necessary to begin the process of B12 digestion.

Millions of elderly individuals, who have macrocytic anemia, have B12 deficiency that can cause severe medical problems, including dementia. B12 deficiency state does not always mean B12 deficiency anemia. It takes years before B12 deficiency state becomes B12 deficiency anemia. Anemia is the last stage of the multiple stages of B12 deficiency disease. A person can be very sick from B12 deficiency and not yet develop macrocytic anemia. A good example of that is dementia.

Gastrectomy can cause B12 deficiency 5-10 years post gastrectomy because the bulk of the intrinsic factor-producing surface was removed during the gastrectomy, leaving very little or no intrinsic factor behind, so B12 cannot be absorbed, resulting in B12 deficiency. It would take that long to deplete the B12 store of about 5000 micrograms. Therefore patients who have undergone hemigastrectomy ought to receive B12 injection monthly for life about 5 years after the procedure.

Malabsorption of B12 occurs in chronic pancreatitis because of exocrine enzyme insufficiency. It also occurs in Zollinger-Ellison syndrome because of low pH in the ileum; it occurs as well in regional enteritis involving the terminal ileum in Crohn's disease. Chronic hemodialysis can also cause malabsorption of B12. Therefore, individuals who are affected by these conditions ought to receive B12 injection on a regular basis.

Pernicious anemia is an autoimmune condition involving an interaction between the stomach and intrinsic factor. This antigen-antibody reaction prevents intrinsic factor from attaching itself to B12 to allow it to be absorbed from the terminal ileum into the bloodstream, where it is taken to the bone marrow and incorporated in the early red cells for the production of red blood cells.

Pernicious anemia can be seen in association with hyperthyroidism, hypothyroidism, vitiligo, diabetes mellitus, Addison's disease, and sometimes cancer of the colon.

The previous standard way of making the diagnosis of pernicious anemia which, was by doing the Schilling test, is no longer practical because the radioactive B12 that is used to be employed to carry out this test is no longer routinely available in this country.

Using the patient's symptoms, the low serum B12, the high MCV, the megaloblastic features on the bone marrow smear and the positive intrinsic factor antibody, will suffice to establish the diagnosis of pernicious anemia.

If the diagnosis of pernicious anemia is established, then ANA, T4, TSH, fasting blood sugar, serum electrolytes, and colonoscopic evaluation of the patient in question ought to be done, for the reasons previously described.

Nitrous oxide interferes in the biochemical pathway of B12 in a way that leads to B12 deficiency and megaloblastic anemia. People who chronically inhaled nitrous oxide are likely to develop this form of anemia and all its medical complications if left untreated.

How to diagnose B12 deficiency

The first thing to do is to take good history and do a good physical examination.

The next thing to do is to order CBC, serum B12, serum homocysteine, and if the serum B12 is borderline or normal and the diagnosis is still suspected, then serum methylmalonic acid ought to be done.

The serum methylmalonic acid is much more accurate in making the diagnosis of B12 deficiency than the serum B12. Methylmalonic acid is elevated in true B12 deficiency. In B12 deficiency both the methylmalonic acid and the homocysteine are elevated but in folate deficiency, only the homocysteine is elevated.

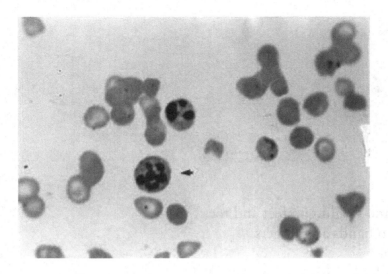

Figure 41.1-Folic acid deficiency and alcoholismin a person (big arrow showing segmented polynucleated white cell with 7 lobes, typical of macrocytic anemia). Small arrow showing macrocytes (large immature red blood cells).

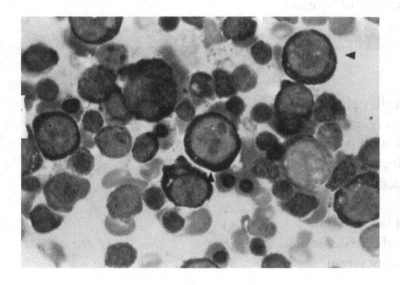

Figure 41.2-Bone marrow aspiration smear in a person (arrow heads) showing megaloblastic red cells (very large immature red cell and pernicious anemia due to B-12 deficiency).

Complications B12 deficiency include:
The brain:

Memory loss
Dementia
Depression
Mania (psychosis)
Paranoia

Irrititabilty
Delusison
Lability
Insomnia etc;

Spinal cord:

Myelopathy
Parasthesia
Numbness and tingling in feet and toes
Numbness in hands and fingers
Ataxia of gait
Weakness of legs
Incontinence
Hypotension when standing
Sexual impotence (ED)
Glossitis (redness of tongue)
Loss of taste
Optic atrophy
Infertility
Low WBC
LOW Red cells count
Low platelets count
Hypersegmented polys
Low reticulocytes count
High indirect bilitubin
High LDH
Decreased Haptoglobin
Elevated methylmalonic acid
Elevated homocystein
High MCV
Megaloblastic anemia
High megaloblasts in the bone marrow etc;

How to treat B12 deficiency in blacks who are B12 deficient

The first thing to do to treat is the underlying problem or problems responsible for the B12 deficiency:

1. In the case of nutritional deficiency, B12 can be given IM at first then added to the diet.

2. In the case of fish tapeworm infestation, treat with anti-tapeworm medication and replace B12 by injection at first, then by mouth until the macrocytic anemia is corrected and the store of B12 is replenished.

3. In the case of blind loops, treat the problem surgically if possible, give B12 by injection, give tetracycline by mouth (if the women are not pregnant), document by tests, physical examination and history that the malabsorption has resolved and add B12 by mouth till the store has been replenished.

As for atrophic gastritis, give injection of B12 monthly for life.

For post-gastrectomy, give injection of B12 monthly for life.

For malabsorption, treat the same as for blind loops.

For pernicious anemia, give 1 mg of B12 IM daily for 7 days, and then give 1 mg of B12 IM three times per week for three weeks and then give 1 mg of B12 monthly thereafter, for life.

It is prudent when treating truly B12-deficient patients with B12 injection to do the following in the beginning of the treatment.

1. Take the patient's baseline weight.
2. Weigh the patient weekly.
3. Listen to the patient's lungs carefully for evidence of heart failure (rales).
4. Listen to patient's heart for evidence of heart failure (S3 gallop).
5. Check the patient's serum potassium weekly for the first 4 weeks.

Patients with true B12 deficiency who receive B12 injection are likely to respond quickly by increasing their blood volume markedly, as though they have just been given 2-3 units of blood, which can throw them into acute congestive heart failure and death.

Acute weight gain would be an indication of water retention and congestive heart failure.

In order to make new red blood cells, potassium is needed to be incorporated into RNA; this process can cause an acute depletion of body potassium, resulting in chest muscle weakness with inability to breathe, as well as acute cardiac arrhythmia and death. Therefore, treating a person for true B12 deficiency is serious business and to be carried out by physicians experienced in dealing with this disease.

As for nitrous oxide, those who are exposed to it ought to find ways to decrease their exposure and those who use it, as an addicting drug ought to seek help to resolve their addiction and stop using it. B12 injection at first, followed by B12 by mouth, is the treatment of this form of B12 deficiency.

If anindividual who is B12 deficient remains untreated, he or she can develop severe megaloblastic anemia, combined system disease with severe neurological problems, dementia and psychosis. The neurological problems associated with B12 deficiency are not reversible after going untreated for 5 years.

Chapter 42
FOLIC ACID DEFICIENCY

The other common cause of macrocytic/megaloblastic anemia is folic acid deficiency. Folic acid deficiency occurs in

1. Nutritional deficiency
2. Alcoholism
3. Hemolytic anemia
4. Drug-associated folic acid deficiency
5. Tropical sprue, etc.
6. Non-tropical sprue
7. Cirrhosis of the liver
8. Gastric bypass
9. Chronic pancreatitis
10. Malabsoption
11. Nutritional deficiency etc
12. Chemotherapy treatments.

How folic acid deficiency occurs

Nutritional deficiency causes folic acid deficiency because of poor intake of folic acid. The total body folic acid store is about 5000 micrograms and in 2-4 months the body can become depleted of folic acid. The daily requirement for folic acid in an adult is about 400 micrograms. In fact the body is incapable in a normal individual to absorb more than 400 mcg of folic acid per day. The foods that are richest in folic acid are vegetables. Poor nutrition causes folate deficiency if a person stays on a folate-free diet for about 2-4 months.

Alcoholism causes folic acid deficiency via three main mechanisms:

1. Alcoholics as a rule eat a diet that is poor in folate.
2. Alcohol as a substance, when consumed in excess, poisons the folate biochemical pathway.
3. When the alcoholic develops cirrhosis of the liver, portal hypertension develops, which in turn causes hypersplenism with secondary hemolysis, making folic acid deficiency worst.

Medications such as Dilantin, Phenobarbital, Mysoline, and Methotrexate, to name a few, are known to cause folic acid deficiency. Both tropical and non tropical sprue is known to cause folic acid deficiency because of the malabsorption that they cause.

How to diagnose folic acid deficiency

To diagnose folic acid deficiency, do a serum folate, CBC and a reticulocyte count. In folic acid deficiency, the serum folate is low, the hematocrit is low, the MCV is high and the reticulocyte count is low. Sometime the folate level may be in the range even though the patient is folate deficient. That may happen because the folate level reflects the last folate-containing meal that the patient ate before the blood was drawn.

The most accurate test to do to measure folate level is red blood cells folate level, but this test is not routinely available and is therefore not practical. The bone marrow aspirate in folate deficiency shows megaloblastic changes in the red blood cells and a left shift in the early white blood cells.

How to treat folate deficiency

The best treatment for folate deficiency is folic acid by mouth or IV/IM.

If the patient is very anemic, then blood transfusion can be given. To treat tropical sprue and non-tropical sprue folic acid 1 mg per day, tetracycline 250 mg 4 times per day ought to be given. Chronic hemolytic anemia is treated with high doses of folic acid, up to 25 mg per day in order to keep up with constant destruction of red blood cells that is taking place.

Chapter 43

ANEMIA OF CHRONIC DISEASES/ INFLAMMATORY DISEASES

Anemia of chronic disease is mediated by cytokines IL1 and TNF⊠ (Interleukin 1 and Tumor Necrosis Factor alpha), these substances cause an inflammatory reaction to occur, which then result in the production of nitric oxide, which in turn suppresses the ability of erythroid blood progenitors (early red blood cells) from being able to make red cells. In this setting iron moves from the blood into to the tissues where it is stored and not made available for red blood cell production.

Apparently, this is the body's way of protecting itself from invading microorganisms, such as bacteria, viruses, and fungi, by depriving them of iron for their growth. In addition, the body seeks to protect itself from cancer by depriving the cancer cells of iron, which is necessary for their growth.

The second apparent advantage of anemia of chronic disease is to deprive cancer cells and microorganisms of sufficient oxygen needed for their growth and their proliferation by not making enough red cells to carry oxygen to them.

The third proposed advantage of anemia chronic disease is that the lack of circulating iron strengthens the cell-mediated immune system. The third advantage mentioned seems to make sense, since having cancer in the human body, by itself, creates an immune deficiency-type state (Source: American Society of Hematology Education Program Book, pages 42-45, 2000).

Evaluations of anemia of chronic diseases/inflammatory diseases include:

History
Physical examination
CBC with differential
Reticulocytes count
Serum ferritin
Soluble serum transferrin receptor level
Complete metabolic chemistry profile
Urinalysis
T4/TSH
Serum B12
Serum folate

PSA
Hemglobin electrophoresis
Chest Xray
Abdominal ultrasound
Abdominal CT scan
Chest CT Scan when indicated
PPD TB skin test
QuantiFeron TB Gold blood test
HIV/AIDS test
Hepatitis B screen blood test
Hepatitis C screen blood test
VDRL
ANA
ENA
Rheumatoid factor
ESR etc;

Treatments of anemia of chronic diseases /anemia of inflammatory diseases:

Treat the chronic diseases with medications or surgical means etc. as appropriate for each disease.

Use Procrit or Epogen to mobilize the iron from the reticuloendothelial cells into the pro-erythroblasts in the bone marrow to produce red blood cells to improve the hematrocrit level while remove the iron from the tissues to prevent the damage that iron causes when it degrades and releases free radical in the body's tissues.

The different chronic diseases that are treated with Procrit/Epogen and Aranesp are:

1. Hemochromatosis/Iron overloads both primary and secondary, when the
2. patient is anemic
3. Rheumatoid arthritis
4. End stage renal failure
5. Sickle cell anemia
6. Beta thalassemia
7. Alpha thalassemia
8. AIDS
9. Chronic hepatitis B with iron over overload and anemia
10. Chronic hepatitis C with iron overload and anemia
11. Chronic auto immune hemolytic anemia
12. Other chronic hemolytic anemia
13. Chemotherapy/radiotherapy associated anemia
14. Chronic osteomyelitis with anemia

15. Myelodisplastic syndrome
16. Sideroblastic anemia
17. All other diseases that cause anemia and iron overloads
18. Cirrhosis of the liver with iron overload
19. Mixed connective tissue diseases with anemia and iron overload

Chapter 44

HEMOCHROMATOSIS/IRON OVERLOAD

A very serious complication of chronic hemolytic diseases is iron overload, known as hemochromatosis, which was discussed earlier in the section on sickle cell disease.

Primary hemochromatosis is very common herediatary disease in the U.S. and around the world. It affects 1 million white Americans which is about 1 in 300 white

Americans. Several million Black, Latino and Asian Americans are also affected by hemochromatosis. The total number of hemochromatosis in these other racial groups is not known because most physicians are not testing nonwhites for hemochromatosis.

This is wrong because there are 3 more genes plus hepcidin deficiency that cause hemochromatosis other than the C282Y gene. The non hematology literature seems only Interested in talking about the C282Y gene seen in whites, if as tough whites are the only people in existence in America. Of course they did not say that, they just get their facts wrong.

Some articles the literature say "1 million Americans or 1 in 300 have hemochromatosis" and hemochromatosis is the most common hereditary disease in America". This is blatantly false.

The truth is that, while primary hemochromatosis is most common in white Americans, it is not the most common hereditary disease in the U.S.

For instance, there are about 52 million Latinos in America and 8.5% of them have sickle trait (representing 4.4 million) and tehere are about 44 million Blacks in America and 8.5% of the them have sickle trait (representing 3.7 million). In addition, 32% of Blacks in America have Alpha thalassemia either as silent carrier or as alpha thalassemia minor (representing 14 million). These diseases are all hereditary and can be transmitted from parents to their children.

Now you can clearly see how blatantly false the assertion that "hemochromatosis is the most common hereditary disease in the U.S." is. Worldwide hemochromatosis affects 1 in 400 people or 28 million people.

A serum ferritin of 500 or greater at some point during a person life time represents hemochromatosis. Hemochromatosis/iron overload must be treated with a low iron diet or phlebotomy to bring the iron level to below 200 if the

person is not anemic. If the person is anemic, Procrit or Epogen 10,000 units SC must given either every week or every 2 weeks to bring the serum ferritin down.

Genetic testing is positive for the C282Y gene (HFE) in less than 50% in Caucasians with hemochromatosis/iron overload. Genetic testing for the C282Y gene is hardly ever positive for hemochromatosis/ iron overload in known Caucasians.

There is only one reported case in the literature of the C282Y gene (HFE) having found in a black person and this author made such a discovery and published it. (see below)

The basis for the other cases primary hemochromatosis/iron overload has recently been published The Journal The hematologist ASH NEWS AND REPORTS August/September 2005 volume 2 issue 4. According to this article, it is a deficiency of hepcidin, which causes the level of ferroportin to remain unchecked resulting in both over absorption of iron from the small bowel and over production of iron from dying red blood cells under the influence of ferroportin.

Other genetic reasons to explain hemochromatosis/iron over load are:

1. Type 2 Hemochromatosis 2nd to G320V mutations
2. Type 3 Hemochromatosis 2nd to TFR2 receptor mutations
3. Type 4 hemochromatosis 2nd to 977 GYC mutations

The hemochromatosis seen in the individual who suffers from hemoglobinopathies is the secondary type as compared to the idiopathic type or primary hemochromatosis. About 10% of the U.S. population carries the gene for primary hemochromatosis, and in certain sub groups, as much as 1:200 or 1:2000 have hemochromatosis.

Primary hemochromatosis-affected people over-absorb iron because of a genetic defect that forces them to absorb too much iron. In secondary hemochromatosis, which is the result of hemoglobinopathies, the iron gets dumped into the bloodstream because of shortened red cell survivals, resulting in hemolysis. In the full-blown thalassemia, these children classically have bronze skins due to iron deposits under the skin.

The iron gets deposited in different tissues and organs in the body of these children who are suffering from thalassemia and sickle cell disease or any other chronic hemolytic anemia. The organs that are most affected by iron deposits are the heart, the liver, the endocrine organs such as the adrenal glands, the pituitary, the gonads and the pancreas. Iron deposits also affect the joints. Iron deposits cause damage to tissues and organs because as iron particles lie in the tissues they break down, releasing free radicals.

These free radicals are extremely toxic to human tissues, damaging the tissues, resulting in diseases such as cardiomyopathy with resulting heart failure. As the free radicals are released they damage the liver, resulting in cirrhosis, which results in scarring of the liver, which can result in hepatocellular carcinoma of the liver. One of the most sensitive ways to diagnose iron deposits in the liver is by doing an MRI of the liver, which, if positive with iron deposits, shows a starry sky-type picture.

Damage caused by iron deposits in the gonads can result in sexual dysfunction and sexual underdevelopment. Damage of iron deposits into the pancreas often result in diabetes mellitus Type II, because the beta cells within the pancreas get damaged and destroyed. These beta cells that are responsible for the production of insulin, and without insulin, sugar cannot be broken down to be used as fuel for proper body functions.

Osteoarthritis is a common disease in people who are affected by hemochromatosis, and women are particularly afflicted by this because women, as a result of their lower economic status, are forced to do heavier work to earn a living, which places their bone structure at most stress and also their musculoskeletal structures at most stress, causing osteoarthritis. When iron deposits are superimposed on this condition, osteoarthritis is made worse.

The free radicals that are released from the breakdown products of iron deposits in the joint spaces cause an inflammatory reaction to occur, which results ultimately in destruction of the joints, causing severe arthritis in these joints and chronic pain. Many blacks do not know that they have hemochromatosis and that is really a major issue.

The worst-case scenario is that oftentimes they are carrying abnormal hemoglobin which predisposes them constantly to smoldering hemolysis with secondary iron being dumped in their body. At the same time, they may be carrying the gene for hemochromatosis, which is also causing them to over-absorb iron, having, therefore, two problems affecting them simultaneously, resulting in more frequent problems associated with iron overload.

Primary hemochromatosis is believed by some to be a disease that is found usually in Caucasians of Scandinavian and European descent. This in fact turns out not to be so. While the disease is more common in whites, it does occur with significant frequency in blacks and other races. The gene that is responsible for primary hemochromatosis is located in the short arm of chromosome 6 and is on the HLA locus.

Many people with no abnormal hemoglobin frequently have high serum ferritin consistent with hemochromatosis/iron overload state with clinical features of primary hemochromatosis. **The author was the first in the world to discover the C282Y**

gene in a black woman, in the year 2000, documenting that this gene, which is responsible for primary hemochromatosis, is also found in Blacks in very rare instances. The so-called African Iron Overload Syndrome probably does not exist at all and never existed but rather those who described it were in fact describing hepcidin deficiency with ferrportin eccess.

There are in fact many whites who have primary hemochromatosis /iron over load and are treated for it and yet the C282Y (HFE) gene is absent in them and they are said to have primary hemochromatosis/iron over load. However, when Blacks have clear and unquestionable primary hemochromatosis/iron over load, many physicians would say that they have "African Iron Overload Syndrome".

This is nothing more than an attempt to say that Blacks cannot possibly have the same disease that Whites have. Which is total racial nonsense because the human race began in Africa and all human beings are the same from a DNA standpoint, except for a few minor differences, and since skin color happens to be one of these minor differences, some choose to make a big deal of it for their own psychosocial and economic advantages.

"Prevalence of Iron Overload in African-Americans—A Primary Care Experience—Revised" Prestige Medical News, February 2003, Vol. 5 No. 3 pp 1-22

By Valiere Alcena, M.D., FACP.

Le Negre Publishing

37 Davis Avenue

White Plains, NY 10605

The C282Y (HFE) test to diagnose primary hemochromatosis of different degrees is available in several commercial clinical laboratories. The best way to determine if someone has hemochromatosis is to do a serum ferritin. A serum ferritin costs about $56.00 to do and it is immensely important. The serum ferritin gives an evaluation of the total body iron. A serum ferritin of 500 or greater establishes a possible diagnosis of hemochromatosis.

Another organ that is frequently affected by hemochromatosis is the skin, which, in fact, is the largest organ in the human body. In primary hemochromatosis the skin has a bronze color to it. The easiest and best treatment for hemochromatosis is phlebotomy, which is removing blood from the body if the person is not anemic.

During that procedure 500 ml of blood is removed. Each time 500 ml of blood is removed, 250 mg of iron is removed with it. Each 1 cc of blood contains 0.5 mg of iron. It is important that the person whose blood is being removed is examined by a physician, to be certain that she is not anemic or has no active cardiac disease that can contraindicate the removal of that much blood from him or her.

The only other treatment available to remove iron from the body is a chelating agent called Desferal, which works to remove iron from the body by chelating the iron from the body and excreting it through the kidneys, into the urine. Desferal is given subcutaneously as a continuous infusion over 12 hours together with 100 to 200 mg of Vitamin C. The Vitamin C helps to mobilize iron in the tissues, making it easier for the chelating agent to remove it from the body into the urine and out.

This is a unique property that Vitamin C has. Because Vitamin C is able to mobilize iron from the body, it is dangerous for someone to take Vitamin C unless it is prescribed by a physician.

If an individual has hemochromatosis and does know it, and is taking Vitamin C, the Vitamin C would help to enhance the absorption of iron from the stomach. The vitamin C will help to mobilize a lot of iron into vital organs such as the heart, liver, pancreas the joints etc., resulting, in a multitude of diseases, such as diabetes mellitus, cirrhosis of the liver, cancer of the liver and cardiomyopathy, etc.

Vitamin C is plentiful in fruits, juices, bananas, and vegetables and, when consumed as food products, is both nutritious and helpful to keep the body in good Vitamin C balance.

People who have secondary hemochromatosis due to hemolytic diseases, such as sickle cell disease, thalassemia, or other diseases such as, rheumatoid arthritis, chronic renal failure with high body iron store. And blacks who have secondary hemochromatosis and are anemic at the same time, can be given injection of Procrit, 10,000 units SQ twice per week or Epogen, 10,000 units SQ, twice per week, to use the iron in their bodies to make red cells, thereby decreasing the iron level while at the same time treating their anemias.

Deferosirox (Exjade) is vailable to treat secondary hemochromatosis-iron overload.

The daily dose of Exjade is 17.3 mg /kg/day by mouth. This medication is very effective
In iron overload due to multiple blood transfusions.

Deferipone (Ferripox) is another medication in used to treat iron overload in thalassemia. The usual dose is 75-100 mg /Kg/day 3 times per day by mouth.

Chapter 45
AIDS

In 2012, 30.6 million adults and 3.4 million children were living with HIV/AIDS and 1.7 million people died of HIV/AIDS. Sources: WHO, UNAIDS and UNICEF. Sub-Saharan Africa is home for 12% of the world pulation but is responsible for 68% of all HIV/AIDS cases in the world.

Of the 34 million people living with HIV/AIDS in 2012, 22.9 millions of them were living in Sub-Saharan Africa, and 59% of them were women. In 2010, 2.7 million people including 390,000 became infected with HIV/AIDS.

The number of people living with HIV/AIDS in different regions of the world in 2011 was:

Sub-Sahara Africa 22.5 millions
East, South, and South Asia 4.1 millions
Eastern Europe and Central Asia 1.4 millions
East Asia 770,000
Middle East and North Africa 460,000
Central and South America 1.4 millions
Oceania 57,000
North America 1.5 millions
Carbbean 240,000
Western and central Europe 820,000 Source: WHO

As of the end of 2010, 1,142,714 people have been diagnosed with HIV/AIDS in the U.S. since the epidemic began and more than 500,000 people have died ftom AIDS. Close to 20% of people infected with HIV in the U.S. does not know that they are infected.

WHAT IS AIDS? AIDS STANDS for Acquired Immune Deficiency Syndrome (as opposed to Inborn Immune Deficiency Syndrome). AIDS is referred to as Acquired Immune Deficiency Syndrome because the virus, the HIV Type I or Type 2, a retrovirus, enters the human body and attacks and kills the T helper lymphocyte (T4 or CD4), causing a decrease in their numbers, resulting in immunodeficiency of the body and in turn causing vulnerability to a multitude of diseases.

Some of these diseases are caused by the HIV viruses themselves and some of the diseases are caused by different opportunistic organisms that enter into the body at different times in the course of the HIV/AIDS syndrome. The T4 helper lymphocytes are in the body to help the body to be healthy, while the T8 suppressor lymphocytes are in the body to cause it to be sick when their numbers increase.

Therefore, in HIV/AIDS, the number of T helper lymphocytes is lower than the number of the T suppressor lymphocytes, thereby inverting the T helper-to-T suppressor ratio. How does the AIDS virus cause immunosuppression? Answer:

The AIDS virus enters the bloodstream of the person being infected and quickly enters into the T cell CD4 lymphocytes. Once inside these lymphocytes, the virus multiplies by making copies of itself. Sometimes the virus can copy itself in numbers as large as a billion copies or several billion copies per day, until the body gradually becomes more and more immunosuppressed, stage by stage, leading ultimately to full-blown AIDS and all its associated problems and complications which, without treatment, or if the treatment fails, causes death of the affected person.

AIDS a historical perspective

The first reported cases of AIDS appeared in an article published in June 1981 in The New England Journal of Medicine, in which a group of homosexual men was found to be sick with Pneumocystis carinii pneumonia.

Further evaluation of these problems revealed that they were immunosuppressed and that the immunosuppressive state that they were suffering from had predisposed them to the development of Pneumocystis carinii pneumonia (PCP).

From that point on the AIDS epidemic was underway. Subsequently it was published that a young man who was retarded and who lived in the streets of St. Louis, Missouri, who was a vagrant in the street of that city and who had frequent contacts with homosexual men, became very sick with an unknown disease associated with fever, weight loss, and pulmonary infection. He went on to die in the early 1960s from complications of the disease.

After his death, an autopsy was performed on him and the pathologist wisely froze tissues and plasma that were taken from his body. In the 1980s after the AIDS epidemic was already underway, this pathologist evaluated these specimens that he had frozen and tested them for the AIDS virus and found that these specimens were teeming with the AIDS virus, which documented that this young man in fact had died of AIDS.

Therefore, in retrospect, the AIDS virus had been around in the United States, since the early 1960s, as documented by this case. Many of us, including this author who, while in training in the inner city of New York City, saw many drug addicts presented to the hospital with febrile illness associated with large lymph nodes, etc., and had no idea what they had. When these lymph nodes were biopsied and the pathologists would report them to us as lymphocytic hyperplasia.

We used to think that the different materials that were used to cut the cocaine or heroin that these drug addicts were using were responsible for the so-called lymphocytic hyperplasia. Little did we know that most probably these people had AIDS that killed them? We simply did not know of the existence of the disease at that time. Therefore, one does not have to go to Africa or to Haiti and other Third World countries to look for a scapegoat for the origin of the AIDS virus.

The AIDS virus was in the inner cities of the world, long before 1981 when the first cases of AIDS were published. According to the literature, the virus that muted into the HIV1 virus may have originated in certain specie of monkey indigenous in Africa.

Be that as it may, blame passing aside, scapegoating aside, name calling and finger pointing aside, AIDS is now worldwide and it knows no racial boundaries; it spares no social classes, spares no sexes and it affects people of all ethnic backgrounds and religious beliefs. AIDS is the largest epidemic that mankind has ever known.

Every few seconds a new person in the world is being infected with the AIDS virus and those infections are mainly being transmitted through sexual intercourse. As of the end of December 2001 there were 40 million cases of HIV/AIDS in the world and 28.1 million people in Sub-Saharan Africa live with the HIV virus (Source: UNAIDS/WHO, Dec. 2001). Source: UNAIDS

Why is AIDS so much more prevalent among blacks in the U.S., as compared to whites.

HIV/AIDS in African American men:

"There are 1.1 million people living with HIV/AIDS in the U.S. and more than 500,000of them are Blacks" "Black represents about 13.6% of the U.S. populations and about 2% of them are HIV positive and African American males had 8 times the rate of AIDS as whites in 2007". Source: The office of Minority Health U.S. Department of Health and Human Services.

The reason more blacks are infected with the AIDS virus than whites is because more blacks are using intravenous drugs than whites are. Once these blacks become infected with the AIDS virus, they quickly pass it on to their sexual partners.

Many black women get infected with the AIDS virus although they are not using IV drugs, but their drug-using sexual partners pass the virus on to them during unprotected sexual intercourse.

AIDS is causing a great deal of suffering in all communities, in all ethnic groups, all social standing, all economic status and in all genders. Since the HIV/AIDS began, 230,000 African Americans have died of AIDS representing 40% of the total deaths AIDS from in the U.S.

Sixty seven percent 67% of the HIV/AIDS cases in women in the U.S. is found among black women as compared to 19% in white women. 1 in 16 African American men are expected to be diagnosed with HIV and 1 in 30 African American women are expected to be diagnosed with HIV. About 50% of HIV/AIDS in the U.S. are found in blacks. Blacks represent 13.6% of the U.S. populations.

Over all the incidence of HIV/AIDS in the U.S. is on the rise. In the recent 12 month periods, it is reported that 63,000 individuals became infected with the HIV/AIDS virus. The rate of new HIV/AIDS infection has gone down across the world and the death rate From HIV/AIDS has also gone down in 2007.

There are several reasons why both the rate of new HIV/AIDS infection and the deaths from HIV/AIDS have gone down.

First and most important is the fact the program of male circumcision that has been implemented in several African countries is working to prevent to prevent the transmission of HIV/AIDS infections in Africa where both rate infection and deaths are
most numerous. Second, the wide spread distribution of condoms in several African countries is working.

Third, sex education programs which have been implemented with an emphasis on abstinence seem to be making a difference.

Fourth, the programs which have been implemented to treat some HIV/AIDS individuals with HAART medications are making a difference to keep some of these infected people alive.

The author is credited, as being the first person in the world to have proposed the idea that male circumcision would decrease the transmission of the HIV/AIDS by Eliminating balanitis, phimosis, paraphphimosis, and other mini-ulcerations of

the foreskin of the penis. The conditions represent an entry points for the HIV/ AIDS virus to enter the blood stream of men while engaging in intra-vaginal or intra-anal sexual intercourse.

1. "AIDS in Third World Countries"
NEW YORK STATE JOURNAL OF MEDICINE, Vol. 86 August 1986
By: VALIERE ALCENA, M.D., F.A.C.P.
"That male circumcision might reduce risk of HIV acquisition was first proposed in 1986" Alcena V. AIDS in third world countries. NY state J Med 1986; 86 446. MEDLINE
2. The Lancet, Volume 369, Number 9562, February 2007

This idea is being acclaimed as one of the most important contributions made since the HIV/AIDS epidemic began in 1981. It has already prevented the transmission of millions of HIV/AIDS infections and undoubtedly million of lives in Africa. According to the World Health Organization, seventy percent of men in the world are not circumcised. If a program of circumcision were carried out world wide, 3 million of HIV/AIDS infections could be prevented and millions lives could be saved says the WHO.

The different ways in which a person can get infected with the AIDS virus include:

1. Sexual intercourse; men who have sex with men
2. Men who have sexual intercourse with both men and women
3. Men or women who are injected with IV drugs
4. Women who have sexual intercourse with men who use IV drugs
5. Women who have sexual intercourse with bisexual men
6. Individuals who receive blood or blood products contaminated with the HIV virus
7. Women who use IV drugs
8. Some babies born to mothers who are infected with the HIV virus
9. Some health workers who get stuck with needles contaminated with the HIV virus
10. Being bitten by an AIDS-infected person
11. Using the same toothbrush as that used by an AIDS-infected person
12. Engaging in passionate kissing with an AIDS-infected person
13. Engaging in oral sex with an AIDS-infected person

What are some of the high-risk behaviors that can lead to the transmission of the AIDS virus from one person to another?

1. Anal intercourse, men with men, or men with women.
2. Intravenous drug use
3. Prostitution, males or females
4. Promiscuity, males or females
5. Having unprotected sexual intercourse with strangers

In order for a person to become infected with the AIDS virus, the virus must enter the bloodstream of the person at risk.

How does a woman become infected with the AIDS virus while having intra-vaginal intercourse with an infected man?

The natural vaginal milieu of a woman has a high pH that allows for growth and multiplication of the HIV virus. Further, during sexual intercourse, there is also microtrauma of the capillaries that occurs as part of the natural events, making it possible for the HIV virus to enter into a woman's bloodstream. The HIV virus is brought into the woman's vaginal environment in the semen that is deposited within it during unprotected sexual intercourse.

If a woman were to have open sores, such as genital herpes, syphilitic sores, and other venereal chancres, etc., and have sexual intercourse with an HIV-infected man, her chances of being infected increases several-fold, because the HIV virus can easily enter through these sores into the bloodstream of the woman. There is a very high correlation between STD and HIV infection.

What happens when the HIV virus first enters into a person's bloodstream?

When the HIV virus enters the blood, the virus goes into the T helper lymphocytes, also known as CD4. Inside the CD4 lymphocytes that are in the circulation, the HIV virus multiplies into millions at first then into billions of HIV virus copies per day. Within two to four weeks of the entry of the HIV virus into the bloodstream, the newly infected person often develops a flu-like syndrome with fever, general aches, chills, runny nose, and even a cough, simulating acute rhinovirus or influenza infection. These symptoms quickly disappear and the person feels fine.

The HIV viruses continue to multiply in the bloodstream and within the nodes of the person's body where they have entered. This represents the HIV stage 1 infection. During ten days to two weeks the P24 antigen level becomes elevated. However, the HIV RNA PCR becomes elevated within about a week of someone becoming infected with the HIV virus, making it the earliest test and the most sensitive test that becomes positive, indicating the presence of HIV infection.

The ELISA test becomes positive after the window period, which is from 6 to 12 weeks after infection. During the window period the ELISA for the HIV, the P24 antigen, and the HIV RNA PCR all will be positive, if the person is infected with the AIDS virus.

As the HIV viruses continue to multiply, the number of T4 lymphocytes decreases while the number of the T8 or T suppressor lymphocytes increases. This situation is what triggers the immunosuppressive states that occur in AIDS. As the infection progresses, the disease moves into different stages.

First the HIV infection moves from the HIV-infected stage to ARC (AIDS-related complex) stage and then to the AIDS stage. The HIV stage may be completely silent, except for some patients who may develop thrombocytopenia (low platelet count) with or without enlarged nodes. The second stage is ARC. In this stage the person will start to lose weight with diffuse lymph node enlargement, thrush in the mouth, diarrhea, fever, headache, oral hair leukoplakia, shingles, thrombocytopenia, molluscum contagiosum, recurrent herpes simplex, aphthous ulcer, condyloma, etc.

Some individuals take many years to progress from these stages to full-blown AIDS, 8 to 10 years, and still other individuals go quickly from these early stages to full-blown AIDS in 4 to 6 years. How fast the infected person becomes infected. The mode of infection and the stage of HIV infection that the person who is doing the infecting may play a role develops AIDS.

There is a discussion in the literature regarding chemokine receptors CCR5 and CX4 that seem to play a role in when certain individuals who are infected with the HIV virus progresses to full-blown AIDS. For that matter, certain individuals who have some of these chemokine receptors may be resistant to the HIV infection. This is a new concept yet to be fully elucidated, but it would appear that there are different effects of the CCR2 and the CCR5 variants on HIV disease.

This new concept will be further evaluated and elucidated in the future.

One of the important factors is the overall makeup of the infected individual, in terms of his or her immune strength, his or her ability to pay for medical care, to pay for anti-retroviral medication, his or her ability to afford good nutrition, etc. All these factors interplay on how well the AIDS-affected person does.

In order to say that a person has AIDS, clinically established criteria have to be met, as defined by the CDC. For example, a person with HIV infection whose CD4 count drops below 200 can be said to meet one of the criteria to have AIDS.

The list of AIDS-defining illnesses includes the following:

Diseases diagnosed definitively without confirmation of HIV infection in patients without other causes of immunodeficiency

Candidiasis of the esophagus, trachea, bronchi, or lungs
Cryptococcuses, extra pulmonary
Cryptosporidiosis > 1 month's duration
Cytomegalovirus infection of any organ except the liver, spleen,
or lymph nodes in patients > 1 month old
Herpes simplex infection, mucocutaneous (> 1 month's duration) or
of the bronchi, lungs, or esophagus in patients of 1 month's
duration Kaposi's sarcoma in patients < 60 years old
Primary CNS lymphoma in patients < 60 years old
Lymphoid interstitial pneumonitis (LIP) and/or
pulmonarylymphoid hyperplasia (PLH) in patients < 13 years old
Mycobacterium avium complex of Mycobacterium kansasii disseminated
Pneumocystis carinii pneumonia
Progressive multifocal leukoencephalopathy
Toxoplasmosis of the brain in patients > 1 month old

Diseases diagnosed definitively with confirmation of HIV infection

Multiple or recurrent pyogenic bacterial infections in patients
< 13 years old
Coccidioidomycosis, disseminated
Histoplasmosis, disseminated
Isosporiasis > 1 month duration
Kaposi's sarcoma, any age
Primary CNS lymphoma, any age
Non-Hodgkin's lymphoma (small, noncleaved lymphoma;
Burkitt or non-Burkitt type; or immunoblastic sarcoma)
Mycobacterial disease other than Mycobacterium tuberculosis, disseminated
M. Tuberculosis, extra pulmonary Salmonella septicemia.

Diseases diagnosed presumptively with confirmation of HIV infection

Candidiasis of the esophagus

CMV retinitis

Kaposi's sarcoma

LIP/PLH in patients < 13 years old

Disseminated mycobacterial disease (not cultured)

P. Carinii pneumonia Toxoplasmosis of the brain in patients > 1 month old HIV encephalopathy HIV wasting syndrome

CDC definition of AIDS

To diagnose AIDS in a patient, the first blood test that is often done is the screening test called ELISA. If the ELISA test is positive, then the Western Blot Test is done to confirm whether the ELISA test is truly positive. The Western Blot Test is an actual electrophoresis of the protein contained within the body of the virus itself. The problem with the ELISA test is that it does not become positive until about 8 to 12 weeks and it can be falsely positive.

Another problem is that during this so-called window period, the HIV test could be falsely negative. To deal with this problem, the P24 antigen test can be done because it becomes positive within a minimum of 10 days after the virus enters into the human body. In addition, the HIV DNA PCR test can be done to determine whether the HIV test is truly positive or not.

Among the tests that are available to diagnose AIDS are the following:

1. ELISA Test
2. Western Blot Test
3. HIV1 DNA PCR test
4. HIV1 RNA PCR test
5. P24

AIDS is a multi-systems disease in that it affects all systems in the body in one form or another or to one degree or another, leading eventually to certain death of the infected individual. The first system that is affected with the AIDS virus is the immune system, resulting in immunosuppression.

The immune system has three parts to it:

1. Cell-mediated
2. Humoral-mediated
3. The complement system

As outlined in the book ***AIDS,*** The Expanding Epidemic: What the Public Needs to Know A Multicultural Overview, by V. Alcena, MD, 1994

Cell-mediated immunity. This system is dominated mainly by T-lymphocytes. Macrophages also play a role in this system. There are different types of T lymphocytes such as CD4 or T helper lymphocytes, CD8 or T-suppressor lymphocytes. Delayed-type hypersensitivity plays a major role in the immune system CD4 or T helper lymphocytes and macrophages are necessary for the antigen specific part of this system.

Delayed—type's hypersensitivity is crucial in vaccination. CD4 or T helper lymphocyte is necessary to help the body maintain a normally functioning immune system. A decrease in the total T helper lymphocytes leads to immune deficiency state maybe congenital or acquired. When the level of CD4 goes down, the level of CD8 or T suppressor goes up, leading to further suppression of the immune system. The humoral-mediated immune system is dominated by B-lymphocytes.

These B-lymphocytes give rise to plasma cells, which then produce antibodies. These antibodies are known as immunoglobulins IgG, IgM, IgA, IgD and IgE. These antibodies have many functions, but paramount amongst them is to protect the human body from infections. When the level of antibody-producing B-lymphocytes goes down, as occurs in AIDS, then all sorts of infections can occur in the human body.

The third immune system that plays a major role in the fight against infection in the human body is the complement system. The complement system is divided into the classical pathway and the alternate pathway.

These complement systems have many components and these components work in concert with other immunoglobulins to lyse microorganisms, such as bacteria, viruses, fungi, parasites and protozoa to kill them, thereby preventing them from killing the human organism.

When there is a decrease in the level of complement in the human body, this can lead to a state of immunodeficiency that, if not corrected, can lead to different infections such as bacterial, viral, fungal, and parasitic infections, leading to many problems for the human organism and ultimately its death, if appropriate treatments are not provided.

Several more sophisticated systems that are known to play different roles in the immune system, but the three outlined above are the major ones that are responsible to fight infections and maintain good health.

Normal Immune Competence Profile in a person

Normal Values

% T cells (60.1-88.1%)
% B cells (3-20.8%)
% Helper cells (34 -67%)
% Suppress T cells (10-41.9%)
Lymphocytes (0.66-4.60 THO/UL)
T cells (644-2201 CELLS/UL)
B cells (82-392 CELLS/UL)
Helper cells (493-1191 CELLS/UL)
Suppressor cell (182-785 CELLS/UL)
H/S ratio 1 or greater

Abnormal Immune Competence Profile in a in person infected with HIV

T—and B-Cell Surface Markers:
T-Helper/T-Suppressor

Lymphocyte Ratio, Blood		Patient's	Normal
% T Cells		75%	60.1-88.1
% Helper Cells	L	16%	34-67
% Suppressor T Cell	H	60%	10-41.9
% B Cells		6%	3-20.8
Lymphocytes		3.0 thou/UL	0.66-4.60
T Cells	H	2250 cells/UL	644-2201
Helper Cells	L	480 cells/UL	493-1191
Suppressor Cells	H	1800 cells/UL	182-785
B Cells		180 cells/UL	82-392
H/S Ratio	L	0.27	1 or greater

The second most frequently affected system in HIV infection is the hematopoietic system (the blood). The routine blood system includes the white blood cells, the red blood cells, the platelets, and the coagulation system. The two earliest affected cells are the white blood cells and the platelets. Frequently, the first indication that someone is HIV infected is a low platelet count, known as thrombocytopenia. In this situation, the HIV virus directly infects the megakaryocytes, the cells that produce the platelets, which result in thrombocytopenia. Thrombocytopenia can also occur in AIDS because of idiopathic thrombocytopenia (ITP) or thrombotic thrombocytopenic purpura (TTP).

The mechanisms of idiopathic thrombocytopenic purpura, or thrombotic thrombocytopenic purpura as seen in HIV/AIDS, are most likely autoimmune in nature, in particular, the ITP.

Leukopenia, low white cell count, is due to a combination of HIV infection plus the different medications that people with HIV infection are treated.

The red blood cells are low (anemia) due to different reasons. One reason is that the HIV virus enters into the earliest red cells (erythroblasts), infect them, thereby preventing them from maturing, resulting in anemia.

Another reason is that the HIV infection is frequently associated with parvo virus B#19. The parvo virus enters into the early red blood cells, resulting in pure red cells aplasia, resulting in anemia. Still another cause of anemia in HIV-infected individuals (AIDS) is low levels of erythropoietin. Erythropoietin is a protein made by the kidneys whose job is to stimulate the production of red blood cells. AIDS patients with an erythropoietin less than 500 usually respond to erythropoietin injections to correct the anemia, usually in association with AZT.

Another reason HIV-infected individuals become anemic is chronic gastrointestinal blood loss, fungal gastritis, esophagitis, viral and other infections of the GI tract, resulting in chronic anemia. Patients with AIDS frequently have folate deficiency, and at times B12 deficiency, resulting in anemia. A condition called red cells aplasia can occur due to the HIV/AIDS infection.

The poor nutritional state of these patients can cause a low protein anemia. Further, the chronic infection state of these patients causes a cytokines-associated anemia of chronic diseases. The pulmonary system is commonly affected by different infections in patients with AIDS. Pneumocystis caranii pneumonia (PCP) is prominent among these infections of the lungs.

Other pulmonary infections seen in AIDS patients are pneumococcal infections, H. Influenza infections, pseudomonas infections, etc. Fungal infections of the lung are also quite common in AIDS patients.

Still other pulmonary infections seen frequently in AIDS patients are mycobacterium tuberculosis (MTB), mycobacterium avium intracellulare (MAI). Both MTB and MAI can be diffuse, affecting multiple organs in the body. About 80% to 90% of patients with full-blown AIDS who die are found at autopsy to have MAI.

People with AIDS are frequently infected with viruses of different types. Among these viruses that infect AIDS patients most frequently are herpes simplex, Herpes Zoster, Epstein-Barr virus, and cytomegalovirus (CMV). All of these viruses can infect different organs, resulting in severe morbidity and mortality.

A multitude of fungi can cause infections in AIDS patients. The most common ones are Candida histoplasma and cryptococcus. The brain, quite frequently, becomes infected with different microorganisms (see tables below).

AIDS patients frequently become infected with protozoal organisms, such as, Pneumocystis carinii and toxoplasma, etc. (Source: AIDS, The Expanding Epidemic: A Multicultural Overview, 1994, by Valiere Alcena, MD, FACP).
Valiere Alcena, M.D., F.A.C.P.

The different infections seen in AIDS patients and how they are treated.

Infecting Agent	Manifestations	Treatment	Prophylaxis	Drug Toxicities	Comment
Pneumocystis carinii			TMP/SMX 1 DS tablet daily or 3x/wk, or	Rash, fever, neutropenia	Begin once CD4+T cell count<200/uL or CD4%<15
	Mild to moderate pneumonia (Pao2≥ 70 mmHg and (A-a)dO2≤ 35 mmHg}	TMP/SMX 15-20 mg/kg/d PO		Bronchospasm	
		TMP 20 mg/kg/d PO qd+	Aerosolized pentamidine 300 mg/month,	Methemoglobinemia, neutropenia	Contraindicated in patients with G6PD deficiency
		Dapsone 100 mg PO qd Clindamycin 600 mg PO q6h+	or Dapsone 50 mg/d PO+	Rash, fever, neutropenia	Treat for 21 d if possible; no less than 14 d
	Severe pneumonia [Pao2 < 70 mmHG or (A-a)dO2> 35 mmHG]	Primaquine 15 mg PO qd IV Pentamidine 3-4 mg/kg/d	Pyrimethamine 50 mg/wk PO + Folinic acid 25 mg/wk PO	Methemoglobinemia C. *Difficile* colitis	Contraindicated in patients with G6D deficiency
		Atovaquone, 750 mg, PO, tid for 21 d		Rash, Neutropenia, nephritis, pancreatitis, hypoglycemia, diabetes	Contraindicated in patients with G6D deficiency
		Aerosolized pentamidine 300 mg/d		Bronchospasm	Provides no systemic effects. Not recommended but an option for multidrug-allergic
	Disseminated disease	TMP/SMX 15-20 mg/kg/d IV initially (total course 14-21 d)		Rash, fever, leukopenia, thrombocytopenia, hepatitis, nephritis, pancreatitis, hypoglycemia, diabetes, C. *Difficile* colitis	patient with mild pneumonia Prednisone, 40 mg bid for 2 d, then 40 mg/d for 5 d, then 20 mg/d to the end of therapy (21 d total) added to specific antimicrobial ASAP and no later than 36 h after diagnosis
		Pentamidine 3-4 mg/kg/d IV for 14-21 d Clindamycin 900 mg IV q 8h then 450 mg PO q6h+		Rash, neutropenia	
		Primaquine 30 mg PO qd for total of 14-21 d		Rash, neutropenia	Contraindicated in patients with G6D deficiency
		Trimetrexate 45 mg/m2 IV (over 60-90 min) qd x 21 d + Leucovorin 20 mg/m2 IV q6h x 24 d		Thrombocytopenia	For patients intolerant of other regimens. Less effective than standard therapy. Bone marrow-suppressive effects blunted by use of leucovorin
		Eflornithine (DFMO) 100 mg/kg IV q6h for 14 d followed by 75 mg/kg PO q6h for 4-6 wk Any of the systemic therapies outlined above			Call 1-800-TRIALSA for information

Organism	Manifestation	Treatment	Prophylaxis	Side effects	Comments
Toxoplasma tondii			TMP/SMX 1 DS tablet qd	Rash, fever, neutropenia	Alternative is dapsone, 50 mg PO qd.+ pyrimethamine, 50 mg, PO weekly + folinic acid, 25 mg, PO weekly
	Encephalitis, brain abscess, chorioretinitis, myocarditis	Sulfadiazine 1-2 g PO q6h + Pyrimethamine 25—100 mg qd + Folinic acid 10-20 mg PO qd Clindamycin initially 200-400 mg IV q6h		Crystalluria, rash	
				Rash, fever, neutropenia, C.*difficile* colitis	Treatment is generally for life. Leucovorin to minimize bone marrow suppression
Toxoplasma gondii— *(continued)*		Pyrimethamine 25-100 mg qd + Folinic acid 100-20 mg qd followed by Clindamycin 300-900 mg PO q8h+ Pyrimethamine 25-100 mg qd Atovaquone 250 mg PO tid+ Pyrimethamine 25-100 mg qe + Folinic acid 10-20 mg qd Macrolides (clarithromycin or azithromycin) + Pyrimethamine		Rash, fever, neutropenia Rash, fever, neutropenia	Leucovorin to minimize bone marrow suppression Leucovorin to minimize bone marrow suppression Early results disappointing
Ttospora Belli	Diarrhea	TMP/SMX 1 DS tablet PO qid for 10 d then bid for 3 weeks		Rash, fever, neutropenia	TMP/SMX 1 DS tablet PO 3x/week for maintenance NTZ;
Cryptosporidia Microsporidia	Diarrhea	No known specific therapy; supportive measures include parenteral nutrition			NTZ; bovine colostrum in trials
Mycobacterium avium complex			Clarithromycin 500 mg PO bid or Azithromycin 1200 mg weekly or Rifabutin 300 mg PO qd		Begin prophylaxis once CD4+T cell count <100/ uL or <50/uL. Treatment is generally for life. Macrolides + rifabutin may be more effective; however, mor toxic and costly
	Disseminated disease that may involve lung, bone marrow liver	Ethambutol 15 mg/kg qd+ Rifabutin 600 mg/qd + Clarithromycin 100 mg PO bid		Hepatitis, neuropathy (peripheral/optic)	

Mycobacterium tuberculosis	Asymptomatic, PPD test positive	Isoniazid 15 mg/kg up to 900 mg PO twice a week or 300 mg daily for 1 y+ Pyridoxine 50 mg/d		Hepatitis	
	Active disease	Isoniazid, 300 mg PO qd x 1y +		Hepatitis	Treat with 3 drugs for 2 mo. If isolate is sensitive to Isoniazid and rifampin, then switch to 2 drugs. Treat a minimum of 9 mo and at least 6 mo after third negative culture. Quinolones may also be considered as a fifth drug
	Active disease in a setting where there is a possibility of multidrug resistance	Rifampin 600 mg PO qd x 1y + Pyrazinamide 30 mg/kg/d in 2 doses		Hepatitis	
				Hepatitis	
				Neuropathy (peripheral/optic) Nephrotoxicity, hearing loss	
		Add ethambutol 15-25 mg/kg/d and Streptomycin or Amikacin			
Candida Albicans	Thrush, vaginitis	Clotrimazole troches, Nystatin prn Fluconazole 200 mg PO qd for 7-14 d Amphotericin B 0.25 mg/kg/d IV for 7-10 d	Fluconazole 200 mg PO qd (optional)	Hepatotoxicity Hepatotoxicity Nephrotoxicity, fever/chills	Primary prophylaxis generally not indicated. Treatment is generally prn
Cryptococcus neoformans	Meningitis, brain abscess, pneumonia, disseminated disease	Amphotericin B 0.3 mg/kg/d IV + Flucytosine 150 mg/kg/d PO for 6 wk followed by Fluconazole 100-200 mg PO qd indefinitely	Fluconazole 200 mg PO qd (Optional)	Hepatotoxicity Nephrotoxicity, fever/chills, bone marrow suppression Hepatotoxicity	Begin prophylaxis if CD4+ T cell count <50/uL (optional; depending on risk). Approximately 50% will need to have flucytosine held during therapy due to neutropenia. An alternative is amphotericin B alone at a dose of 0.8 mg/kg/d
Histoplasma capsulatum	Disseminated disease, pneumonia	Amphotericin B 0.6-1 mg/kg/d to a total 1 g then Itraconazole 200 mg qd indefinitely		Nephrotoxicity, fever/chills	
Bartonella henselae (quintana)	Nodular skin lesions, peliosis hepatitis, trench fever	Erythromycin 500 g PO or IV qd for 2 months			
Penicillium marneffei	Disseminated disease, umbilicated skin lesions	Amphotericin G, 0.6-1 mg/kg/d to a total of 1 g then Itraconazole 200 mg qd indefinitely		Neurotoxicity, fever, chills, hepatitis	

Cytomegalovirus	Retinitis, esophagitis, colitis, and pneumonia	Ganciclovir 5 mg/kg q 12h for 14 d followed by 5 mg/kg qd IV indefinitely Foscarnet 90 mg/kg q 12h for 14 d followed by 90-120 mg/kg qd IV indefinitely	Ganciclovir 1.0 g PO tid with food (optional)	Neutropenia Intestinal nephritis, seizure, hypocalcemia	Expensive, marginal efficacy. Neutropenia may be ameliorated by colony-stimulating factors Retinitis may also be treated with ocular implant Oral ganciclovir, 1 g PO tid with food may be used for maintenance Should be preceded by saline infusion to minimize nephrotoxicity
Herpes simplex virus	Recurrent perioral, perirectal, or genital ulcers Esophagitis; acute retinal necrosis	Acyclovir 200-400 mg PO 5id as needed Acyclovir 5 mg/kg IV q8h for 10-14 c			Foscarnet 60 mg/kg q8h x 14 d for patients with acyclovir-resistant herpes simplex or zoster
Varicella-Zoster virus	Cutaneous (local or disseminated); retinal necrosis	Acyclovir 800 mg PO 5id or 10 mg/kg IV q8h for 10-14 d or longer			Famciclovir 500 mg PO q8h x 7 d is an alternative
Treponema pallidum	Early syphilis Late or neurosyphilis	Benzathine penicillin G 2.4 million units IM weekly for 3 wk Aqueous penicillin G 12-24 million units IV daily for 10-14 d + probenecid 500 mg PO qid Ceftriaxone 1-2 g IM or IV aq 10-14 d			Approximately 20% relapse, need retreatment. Immunologic abnormalities may cause inaccurate serology

Source: *AIDS, the Expanding Epidemic: A Multi-Cultural Overview,* 1994 by Valiere Alcena, MD, FACP

Different diseases of the brain in AIDS Patients

Opportunistic infections
    Toxoplasmosis

Cryptococcosis
Progressive multifocal leukoencephalopathy
Cytomegalovirus
Syphilis
Mycobacterium tuberculosis
HTLV-1 infection
Neoplasms
    Primary CNS lymphoma
    Kaposi's sarcoma
Result of HIV-1 infection
    Aseptic meningitis
    AIDS dementia complex (HIV encephalopathy)
    Myelopathy
    Vacuolar myelopathy
    Pure sensory ataxia
    Paresthesia/dysesthesia
    Peripheral neuropathy
    Acute demyelinating polyneuropathy
    Mononeuritis multiplex
    Distal symmetric polyneuropathy
    Myopathy

Disease	Clinical Features	Characteristic CSF Findings	Characteristic Radiologic Findings
HIV encephalopathy (AIDS dementia complex)	Personality changes, dementia, unsteady gait, seizures	Nonspecific increases in cells and protein	Cortical atrophy, ventricular dilation, bright spots on T2-wieghted MRI
Toxoplasmosis	Fever, headache, focal neurologic deficits, seizures, + antibodies in 95%	Nonspecific	Single or multiple ring-enhancing lesions in multiple locations
Cryptococcal meningitis	Fever, nausea, vomiting,	Elevated protein, low glucose,	Nonspecific

	confusion, headache	positive cryptococcal antigen or culture	
Progressive multifocal leukoencephalopathy	Multiple focal deficits without changes in level of consciousness	Nonspecific	Multiple white matter lesions on T2-weighted MRI images
Neurosyphilis	Meningitis, neuroretinitis, deafness, focal neurologic deficits	Positive VDRL, elevated protein, increase in cells	Nonspecific
Lymphoma	Seizure, focal neurologic deficits, headache	Nonspecific in primary CNS lymphoma; malignant cells in systemic lymphoma	Single or few ring-enhancing lesions
Tuberculosis meningitis	Fever, headache, confusion, meningitis, cough	Elevated protein, low glucose, pleocytosis, positive smear/culture for acid-fast bacilli (AFB)	Mass lesions in approximately 50%, abnormal chest x-ray

Source: AIDS, The Expanding Epidemic: What the Public Needs to Know—A Multi-Cultural Overview, 1994 by Valiere Alcena, MD, FACP

Clinical management of HIV stage infection

The decision as to when to start treatment in a person who becomes HIV positive is quite controversial. Most clinicians, however, start patients who are HIV positive on AZT and, to prevent resistance, frequently add 3TC (Epivir) to that regimen. This thinking, however, has changed in recent years. Up to now, in most cases, treatment is being withheld till the CD4 count reaches the range of 300, at which point, HAART (Highly Active Antiretroviral Treatment) or Combivir medication is started. In addition, Bactrim DS, 1 tablet per day, is started as prophylaxis against PCP (Source: Joel E. Gallant, et al., HIV Forefront, Vol. 2, No. 1, April 2000). If the CD4 is 200, even if the patient is asymptomatic, HAART must be started (Source: Report of the Panel on Clinical Priorities, Department of Health and Human Services, Feb. 2001).

Now in 2013, WHO recommends starting anti-retroviral medications (HAART) at CD4 of 500 cells/mcl.

A recent report came out that shows that treating HIV stage disease early decreases transmission of HIV to a person's sexual partner. Source: CDC

A new report just came out that shows that starting "ART treatment for the HIV stage when the CDC cell counts reaches 350 cells/mcl and 499 cellls/mcl was associated with slower disease progression compared with a deferral stragedy." Source: ARCHIVE of Internal Medicine 2011; 171:1560-1569

Seizure is a common problem seen in patients with AIDS, due to either fungal infection of the brain, lymphoma of the brain, or possibly PML. After appropriate evaluation with brain CT scan or brain MRI, followed by lumbar puncture with evaluation of the cerebrospinal fluid, chemically and bacteriologically, the doctor looks for microorganisms and, in the case of lymphoma, looks for cancer cells. Once these things are done then appropriate treatments are given for the specific problems discovered or empirically for whatever the treating physician feels clinically appropriate for the particular circumstances.

Toward the end of full-blown AIDS, the wastage stage usually sets in. Few people, if any, ever recover from this stage of AIDS, in spite of expensive nutrition and androgenic steroid treatments. Megace in high doses works well to increase AIDS patients' appetite.

However, using Megace in treatment of full-blown AIDS patients is risky because many of these patients have nephrotic syndrome through which they lose Protein C and Protein S and anti Thrombin III in their urine, resulting in a hypercongealable state, which, by its very nature, can lead to clot formation and thrombosis. Even in those patients who have no evidence of renal disease, a loss of Protein S in the urine is known to occur, resulting potentially in the same syndrome as just described.

It is a known fact that Megace and other estrogenic-like hormones can cause a hypercoagulable state through the loss of anti-thrombin III. Therefore, it is prudent to use Megace in AIDS patients or any patient very carefully and when necessary to avoid the development of deep vein thrombosis (DVT) and its possible associated complications, which can result in morbidity and mortality.

While there is no cure and no vaccine available for people infected with HIV Type I or Type II and full-blown AIDS, there are many medications available. The first category of medications made to treat AIDS patients was the reverse transcriptase inhibitors.

Examples of reverse transcriptase inhibitors are Zidovudine (AZT), didanosine (ddI), zalcitabine (ddC) and stavudine (D4T).

AZT, ddI and ddC can be used both as combination therapy and as mono therapy in early HIV disease. D4T is best used in people with advanced AIDS who are not able to tolerate the other medications.

These reverse transcriptase inhibitors work to prevent the multiplication of the HIV virus by blocking the production of the enzyme reverse transcriptase, thereby preventing the synthesis of RNA and DNA and in so doing preventing viral multiplications. Lamivudine (Epivir, 3TC) is used in combination with AZT to treat HIV infections.

The importance of this combination is that HIV virus becomes resistant to AZT reasonably quickly in many individuals who are treated with the AZT alone. When 3CT is added to the AZT, the DDI, or the DDC it enhances the sensitivity of the reverse transcriptase that is used along with it to kill the HIV virus. 3TC by itself has very little effect against the HIV virus.

A new drug for the treatment of HIV was just approved by the FDA. It is a combination of AZT and 3TC and it is named Combivir. It has the advantage of being used two times per day. The newest invention in the treatment of AIDS that has shown the most promise in the last few years is triple therapy, HAART. The key component of the triple therapy is the addition of a protease inhibitor. The protease inhibitors in use are Saquinavir, Ritonavir, Indinavir, and Nelfinavir. The so-called AIDS cocktail is usually made of a reverse transcriptase inhibitor, such as AZT, with 3TC and a protease inhibitor such as Indinavir.

Once it becomes clear that the patient has gone into the full-blown AIDS stage, and then the whole way of clinically managing the patient is dictated by the particular AIDS-defining signs, symptoms, and disease that affect the patient. If the patient has PCP, she is to be treated for PCP using PCP-effective medications. If the patient has MAI, she is to be treated for MAI using MAI-effective medications.

If the patient has gastroenteritis, diarrhea, she is to be evaluated and treated for the diarrhea based on the clinical and laboratory findings. If the patient has blurry vision and CMV retinitis is suspected, then an evaluation must be carried out by an ophthalmologist, to document whether this is so or not. Ganciclovir is used IV to treat CMV retinitis.

If the patient has herpes simplex infection, appropriate culture ought to be taken and sent to the lab, and treatment with Zovirax IV or PO is to be started, depending on the severity of the herpes infection and which organ system is affected. If the patient has community-acquired pneumonia, treatment with IV antibiotics must be given. If the patient is severely anemic, transfusion of red blood cells must be given.

Epogen or Procrit is very effective in treating anemia in AIDS patients if the serum erythropoietin level is low. If the patient has fungal infections of either the GI tract or the brain, antifungal treatment must be given using either Ketoconazole or Amphotericin B IV.

The most recently recommended combinations of antiretroviral medications for patients with known HIV infection is as follows:

1. Indinavir + Stavudine + Lamivudine
2. Efavirenz + Stavudine + Didanosine
3. Nelfinavir + Zidovudine + Didanosine
4. Ritonavir + Indinavir + Zidovudine
5. Ritonavir + Saquinavir + Zidovudine
6. Ritonavir +Lopinavir + Zidovudine
7. Viracept (Nelfinavir Mesylate)

Different Suggested Dosages of Anti-Viral Medications
Nucleoside Reverse Transcriptase Inhibitors

Zidovudine (AZT)—200 mg 3 times a day
Combivir (300 Mg. ZDV and 150 mg. Epivir)—1 tablet twice a day
Didanosine (ddI)—250 mg. twice a day
Zalcitabine (ddC)—0.75 mg. three times a day
Epivir—150 mg. twice a day
Abacavir (ABC)—300 mg. twice a day (or Trizivir—ZDV 300 mg, Epivir 150 mg., Abacavir 300 Mg.)
Stavudine (Zerit)—40 mg. twice a day
Non-nucleoside Reverse Transcriptase Inhibitors
Nevirapine (Viramune)—200 mg. by mouth daily for 14 days, then 200 mg. by mouth twice a day, thereafter
Delavirdine (Rescriptor)—400 mg. 3 times a day
Efavirenz (Sustiva)—600 mg. by mouth at bed time
Protease Inhibitors
Indinavir (Crixivan)—800 mg. every 8 hours

Ritonavir (Norvir)—600 mg. every 12 hours

Nelfinavir (Viracept)—750 mg. 3 times per day or 1250 Mg. twice a day

Saquinavir (Invirase)—400 mg. twice a day

Fortovase—1200 mg. 3 times a day

Amprenavir (Agenerase)—1400 mg. twice a day

Lopinavir + Ritonavir (Kaletra) Lopinavir 400mg/day and. Ritonavir 100mg twice a day Atazanavir 400mg/day with AZT 100mg and Epivir 150mg twice per day.

Efavirenz 600mg/day with AZT 100mg and Epivir 150mg twice per day.

Atripla which is a combination efavirenz, emtricitabine and tenofovir is the world top selling AIDS medication. The FDA has just approved Tivicay to be used in combination with other AIDS medications.

(Source: Panel & Clinical Practices for Treatment of HIV Infection, Dept. of Health & Human Services, 2001 and HIV News Line, Volume 8, Issue 2 October 2003, Feb. 2001)

Different antiretroviral medications have different side effects and must be used under different types of clinical circumstances using physician's advice. There are many more combinations of treatment of antiretroviral medications available but the ones just listed are the most commonly used. Valiere Alcena, M.D., F.A.C.P.

As outlined by the CDC. HIV-infected pregnant women give birth to about 60% of infants who are born infected with HIV virus. However, when these pregnant women are treated during pregnancy with AZT, most of these women give birth to HIV-negative infants. AZT is the only one of the reverse transcriptase inhibitors that is safe to use during pregnancy. The protocol for treating women who are pregnant and infected with the AIDS virus is as follows:

Start treatment with Zidovudine at 14-34 weeks of pregnancy and the treatment must be continued throughout the pregnancy. The Zidovudine can be given 100 mg.5 times per day or 200 mg. 3 times per day or 300 mg. 2 times per day. During labor the Zidovudine must be given at 2 mg. per kg intravenously over 1 hour followed by a continuing infusion of 1 Ml per kg until the baby is delivered. After delivery, Zidovudine, also known as AZT, is given to the newborn in syrup form at 2 Ml per kg every six hours for the first 6 weeks of life. The medication must be started 8-12 hours after birth.

Health professionals who get stuck with needles contaminated with blood from AIDS patients are treated with triple therapy of AZT, 3TC and Indinovir. Once the injury occurs, the wound must be cleansed and antiseptic applied immediately. These individuals usually get their blood taken for baseline HIV and hepatitis B, C and VDRL. In 4-6 weeks they must get tested again using the ELISA/Western Blot blood tests or, better still, using the HIV RNA PCR test. The incident must be reported to the appropriate authorities where the person works and then the person must be seen by the employee health physician to be examined and treated.

Two blood tests are used to evaluate the status of HIV patients. They are the CD4 and the HIV viral load. Ideally, one looks for CD4 of 500 or greater and a viral load of less than 500 copies. A sign of HIV disease progression is a CD4 count of less than 200 and a plasma HIV RNA level of greater than 20,000 copies. HIV-infected patients with a viral load of 100,000 copies have a tenfold greater risk of progressing into full-blown AIDS than patients with 10,000 copies of viral load per ml. Although a CD4 count of less than 200 is usually seen in patients with full-blown AIDS, the viral load test is much more sensitive in evaluating the status of HIV infections.

If the viral load is 20,000, even if the CD4 is in the normal range, it is recommended that HAART treatment be started. The addition of a protease inhibitor to the regimen of AZT or any of the other reverse transcriptase inhibitors and 3TC frequently can lead to an undetectable level of HIV in the blood of the infected person. This does not mean that HIV infection has gone. It just means that the level is low but the infected individual still has the infection and can still transmit it to an uninfected person, thereby giving him or her AIDS.

The turnover of the HIV virus in an infected person is tremendous. On any one day about 10 billion viral particles can be produced and cleared from the HIV-infected person. About 2 billion CD4 lymphocytes are produced and destroyed from the HIV-infected person daily.

Cancer is one of the multitudes of complications that can afflict the HIV-infected person. Among the cancers that AIDS-infected people would have to contend with is Kaposi's sarcoma, said to be caused by herpes virus #8.

Women who are infected with HIV are prone to the development of invasive cervical cancer. This syndrome of cervical cancer, as seen in HIV-infected women, is associated with the human papilloma virus (HPV). HPV is associated with an invasive form of cervical cancer in women infected with the AIDS virus.

Another common form of cancer seen in AIDS patients is large cell lymphoma.

Blacks and other minorities are at higher risk to become infected with HIV than other racial groups in the United States and around the world because more blacks and other are using IV drugs, thereby exposing themselves to a higher risk of contracting the HIV infection through sharing dirty needles.

Further, since most black and other minority women have sexual intercourse with black men and other minority men, and since black men and other minority men have the highest incidence of HIV infection, many black and other minority women get infected with HIV by having sexual intercourse with their HIV-infected black and other minority men sexual partners.

The take-home lesson for all people is not to involve themselves in high-risk behaviors, such as, using IV drugs, having sexual intercourse with multiple sexual partners without the protection of a condom, and having sex with men or women whom they have just met, without a condom, etc. These changes in behavior will decrease the incidence of HIV infection in all individuals.

AIDS in third world Countries:

The notion that the AIDS virus had its genesis from Africa is a controversial topic. In my opinion, the data are not at all convincing as to where the virus originated.

It is my opinion that because the majority of men from Central Africa and Haiti are not circumcised, they constantly develop balanitis as a result of the heat and other problems, leading to breakage of the skin. This leads to chronic infections such as phimosis and paraphimosis. In this setting, there is frequent mini-ulceration of the foreskin of the penis. This represents an easy portal of entry for the virus during coitus with, let us say, an infected prostitute. Another possibility arises because the women in that part of the world do not shave the pubis. Thus there is the possibility of mini-lacerations occurring during coitus as the foreskin comes into contact with pubic hair. This is another possible portal of entry for the virus. This, to me, seems a more plausible explanation for female-to-male transmission in Central Africa and Haiti.

By
Valiere Alcena M.D.F.A.C.P.
N.Y. State J Med 1986: 86. 446

Valiere Alcena,MD.,M.A.C.P.

Male circumcision and HIV/AIDS

Dear Editor:

I have been reading with interest the recent spate of articles on findings that link circumcision of men in certain African countries with the incidence of the HIV/AIDS virus. One reporter in *The New York Times Magazine* has even described male circumcision as possibly the best method of eliminating the AIDS virus – superior even to an AIDS vaccine, which may still be several years in development.

You may be interested in knowing that in August 1986, in a letter to the editor of *The New York State Journal of Medicine,* Vol. 86, page 446, I first discussed the significance of male circumcision in lowering the incidence of the HIV/AIDS virus in Africa, Haiti and other developing countries. In my published letter, I wrote in part:

"It is my opinion that because the majority of men from Central Africa and Haiti are not circumcised, they constantly develop balanitis as a result of the heat and other problems, lead-ing to breakage of the skin. This leads to chronic infections such as phimosis and paraphimosis. In this setting, there is frequent mini-ulceration of the foreskin of the penis. This represents an easy portal of entry for the virus during coitus with, let us say, an infected prostitute. Another possibility arises because the women in that part of the world do not shave the pubis. Thus, there is the possibility of mini-lacerations occurring during coitus as the foreskin comes in contact with the pubic hair. This is another possible portal of entry of the virus. This, to me, seems a more plausible explanation for female-to-male transmission in Central Africa and Haiti."

Later, I repeated my theory in my two books that were published in 1992, "The Status of Health of Blacks in the United States of America: A Perspective for Improvement" and "The African American Health Book." I again described the significance of male circumcision in possibly eliminating the HIV/AIDS virus altogether in a sub-sequent book that was published in 1994 entitled "AIDS: The Expanding Epidemic: What the Public Needs to Know: A Multi-Cultural Overview."

I would be happy to discuss with the researchers for these most recent articles this most exciting subject in the future if needed.

Valiere Alcena, MD, FACP

WHITE PLAINS, NY

I am grateful to Dr. Alcena for his letter. He purports therein to be the first to suggest that male circumcision might somehow play a role in reducing the risk of heterosexual transmission of HIV, then known as HTLV-III. A brief search on PubMed suggests that he may indeed be correct; other authors made such suggestions several years later, in 1988 and thereafter. Thus, the spate of publications in recent years offering proof of that hypothesis represents solid support of his earlier thinking.

Source:
Infectious Disease News
Vol; 20, number 3
March, 2007

That Male circumcision might reduce risk of HIV acquisition was first proposed in 1986. 3
Reference 3
Alcena, V AIDS in third world countries. NJ State J of Med 1986; 86: 446

Male circumcision for HIV prevention in young men
In Kisumu, Kenya: a randomized controlled trial
The Lancet 2007, 369:643-656
24 February 2007

WHO, UNAIDS recommend male circumcision world-wide to decrease the incidence HIV/AIDS transmition by 60% and save 3 million lives.
WHO, UNAIDS estimate that worldwide only 30% men are circumcised

According to the WHO, 70% of men in the world are not circumcised. The vast majority of black men in the developing world and largely in the developed world are not circumcised. Male circumcision to reduce the spread of HIV/AIDs first suggested By Dr Valiere Alcena on August of 1986 has made the biggest difference so far in controlling the AIDS epidemic and preventing deaths from AIDS.

When an uncircumcised man has sexual intercourse with HIV an infected individual, be it a female or a male sexual partner, the foreskin of the penis is frequently the entry point for the HIV virus to enter the blood stream.

Circumcision of male babies and men in the world and in particular in the developing world will continue to decrease the incidence of HIV/AIDS and deaths from this terribly deadly diease.

According to a study carried out by the Institute for Global Health and Infectious Diseases which was began in April of 2005, funded by the National Institute of Allergy and Infectious Diseases, and reported in May 12, 2011. 1, 763 people (890 men, 873 women) were entered in the study. HIV infected sexual partners from Botswana, Brazil, India, Kenya, Malawi, South Africa, Thailand, the United States, and Zambabwe participated in the study. The CD4+ T-cell levels were between 350 and 550 cells per cubic millimeter (mm2)

> Eleven HIV drugs were used in various combinations to treat these people
> Involved in the study including
> "atazanir 300 mg once daily
> didanosine 400 mg once daily
> efavirenz 600 mg once daily
> emtricitabine/tenofir disoproxil furmarate 200 mg emtricitabine/300 mg tenofovir mg twice daily (BID)
> nevirapine 200 mg taken once daily for 14 days followed by 200 mg taken twice daily
> ritonavir 100 mg once daily, used only to boost atazanavir
> stavudine (weight dependent dosage)
> senofovir disoproxil fumarate 300mg once daily
> zodovudine/lamivudine (150 mg lamivudine/300 mg zidovudine taken orally twice daily)"

The risk of sexually transmitted HIV was reduced by 96% in the people in the study because of the anti-retrovirus drugs."

The AIDS epidemic which was officially first reported in The U.S in June of 1981
is 30 years old this year and yet no cure has been found. 60 million people have been infected with HIV since the epidemic was first recognized. 25 million people have died of AIDS world wide including 650,000 people in the U.S. 33 million people are in the world are living with HIV/AIDS. While sopme progress has been made by using

anti-trevirus (ART) drugs, this epidemic is still unfolding in the U.S. and worldwide. Source:

Annals of Internal Medicine 7 June, Volume 154 Number 11

ART are very expensive and must be taken for life. On top of the list of prevetive measures to take to protect one selves from getting infected with HIV 1&2 is male circumcision. It might as well be called the "AIDS vaccine" or better still the "Dr Valiere Alcena AIDS vaccine" Male circumcision is Dr Valiere Alcena's AIDS vaccine.

Dr Valiere Alcena first proposed using male circumsicion to prevent HIV/AIDS In August of 1986 as described in this chapter above. Male circumcision has decreased the total HIV/AIDS infection in the world from 39 million in 2006 to 33 million and has brought the yearly deaths from AIDS down to close to 1 million per year. No other factors have made such a big difference and no other physicians beside Dr. Valiere Alcena in the world have made such a major contribution in the prevention and deaths from HIV/AIDS.

Chapter 46
OSTEOPOROSIS

Osteoporosis causes softening of bones that causes pain, arthritis, and fractures. The bones become soft due to decrease in bone mass. When looking under the microscope at a bone in a person suffering from osteoporosis, what is seen is a decrease in what is called cortical thickness of the bones. Osteopenia is the beginning of the softening process that leads ultimately to osteoporosis.

Osteoporosis / osteopenia affect about 44 million Americans and 55 percent of the U.S. population 50 years or older have osteopenia. Worldwide 200 million people have osteoporosis.

The percentage of whites and Asians affected by osteoporosis is greater than the percentage of blacks who are affected by this disease. Women are affected more from osteopenia/ osteoporosis than do men. Blacks have higher bone density than whites do and as such, blacks have stronger bones.

However, blacks suffer significantly from osteopenia/osteoporosis because 90% of blacks and other people with dark have vitamin D insufficiency and about 70% have vitamin D deficiency risking them to the development of osteoporosis/ osteoporosis. 90% of Hispanics have low vitamin D, 75% of Whites and 75% of Asians have low vitamin D.

The fact blacks and other people with dark skin make it harder for them to produce vitamin when they are exposed to the sun's rays. The sun's rays activate Ergosterol under the skin to produce vitamin D. Other sources of vitamin D include egg yolk, milk, cheese, butter, salmon, and cod liver oil.

In addition, 75% of blacks have lactose lactose intolerance and this further adds to them propensity to developing osteopenia/osteoporosis.

The fragile bone fractures associated with osteoporosis amount to about 1.5 million per year in the USA. Between the ages of 40 and 50 years, cortical bone loss is somewhere in the range of 0.2% to 0.5% per year. Loss of bone mass per year ranges anywhere from about 40% to 50% in some individuals.

Women tend to lose bone mass much earlier than men do, and this loss of bone mass seems to progress more rapidly after menopause. The difference in the incidence of osteoporosis in black versus whites and other racial groups seems to be due to the fact that blacks have higher bone minerals than other racial groups, hence the lesser incidence of osteoporosis seen in blacks.

Risks of osteoporosis include:

1. Smoking
2. Alcohol abuse
3. Low dietary calcium
4. Vitamin D
5. Lack of exercise
6. Malabsorption
7. Malnutrition
8. Postmenopausal
9. Heparin use chronicaly
9. Primary hyperparathyroidism
10. Secondary hyperparathyroidism
11. Chronic use of steroid
12. Kidney failure
13. Cushing syndrome
14. Thyrotoxicosis
15. Calcium deficiency
16. Systemic mastocytosis
17. Rheumatoid arthritis
18. Scurvy
19. Rickets
20. Homozygous osteogenesis imperfecta
21. Heterogygous osteogenesis imperfecta
22. Hemochromatosis
23. Marfan's syndrome
24. Gigantism

There is a form of osteoporosis called idiopathic, which occurs in children and adolescents of both sexes. The two most common forms of osteoporosis are Type I osteoporosis, which occurs in postmenopausal women between the ages of 51 and 75. It causes loss of trabecular bones, and fractures of vertebral body and distal forearm are quite common. Type II osteoporosis is seen in people over the age of 70 and these people suffer frequently from fractures of the femoral neck, proximal humeral, proximal tibia and pelvis. Collapse of vertebral bodies frequently occurs, resulting in kyphosis, scoliosis and other deformities as these people get older, and fractures of the hips are quite common, as well.

Five to ten years after menopause women can lose up to 4% of bone density per year. This can cause them to lose up to 35% of their bone density.

Cancers that may be associated with osteoporosis, bone pain, and vertebrae fractures. Among these cancers are the following:

1. Multiple myeloma
2. Leukemia
3. Lymphoma
4. Metastatic cancer to bones

Multiple myeloma is the most common cancer that is associated with osteopenia/osteoporosis. To diagnose multiple myeloma using x-rays, skeletal survey is the most accurate. Bone scan is the most sensitive test to diagnose metastatic cancer to the bones. Plain x-ray study is the best test to diagnose multiple myeloma, because multiple myeloma causes an osteolytic process.

Bone scan is the best test for metastatic cancer to the bones because metastatic cancer to bone is an osteoblastic process. MRI of bones will show cancer in bones, in both osteolytic and osteoblastic processes. However, MRI is an expensive test and is not routinely done to diagnose cancer to the bones, but is done when either the bone scan or the plain x-rays are not definitive. Still a better test to diagnose bone cancer is PET scan.

Another common disease that causes osteoporosis is primary hyperparathyroidism. The reason why primary hyperparathyroidism is associated with osteoporosis is because of bone resorption.

The bleaching of calcium from the bone causes the bone to become soft and painful, and because the bones are soft, they break easily, resulting in even more pain.

Still, another more common cause of osteoporosis is steroid treatment Steroid treatment has many major and minor side effects, and prominent among these side effects is osteoporosis. Among the reasons why steroid treatment causes osteoporosis is the fact that it reduces calcium absorption from gastrointestinal tract and increases calcium loss in the urine. As calcium is lost in the urine, the bones become calcium deficient, which ultimately causes soft bones (osteoporosis).

Estrogen is a hormone that is required for strong bones and because of that fact, the postmenopausal state, and either natural or surgical, is associated with osteoporosis. It appears that people who are not black, have smaller frame, and have higher incidence of osteoporosis than larger frame people.

Non-black people weighing in the 127-pound range are roughly two times more likely to have fractures of the hip, pelvis, and ribs, as compared to non-black whose weight is in the 161-pound range. Blacks with small frame are not at higher risk for fractures of the arm, elbow, wrist, ankle, and foot.

Bone density measurement is the best test to diagnose osteoporosis. This is a painless test, which is quite accurate in diagnosing bone loss of different degrees. In addition to the bone density study, regular bone x-ray is capable of showing osteopenia/osteoporosis and different degrees of fractures that occur because of osteoporosis.

The following are two examples of osteoporosis as seen on x-rays and MRI done on individuals suffering from osteoporosis:

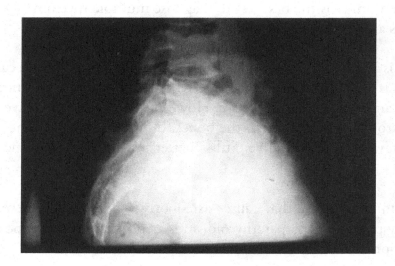

Figure 46.1-Plain x-ray of the lumbar spine of a person with osteoporosis; multiple wedge compression on osteoporosis with mark osteopenia at L1, L2, L3 and L4.

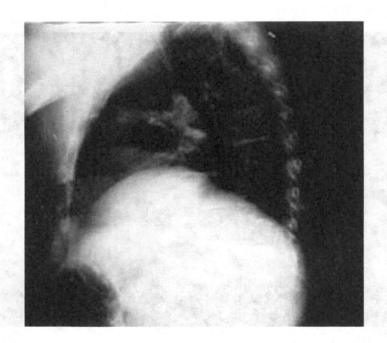

Figure 46.2-Plain x-ray of the thoracic spine of a person with osteoporosis; multiple wedge compression on osteoporosis with mark osteopenia at T9, T10, T11, and T12.

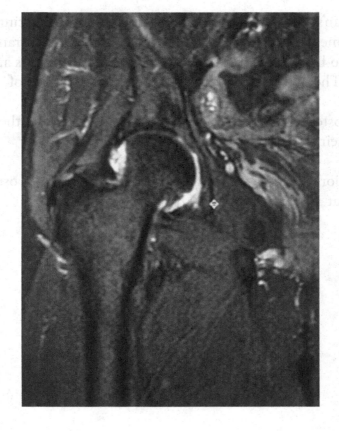

46.3 Osteoporosis and inflammation of the hip bone of a person with adult Ricket's/ Oeteomalacia

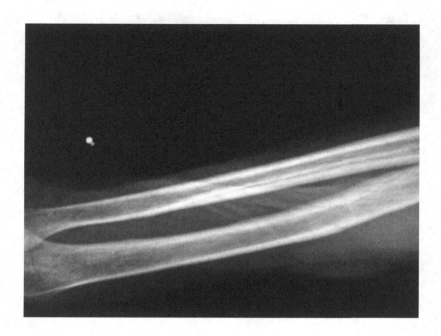

46.4 Osteoporosis and inflammation of the forearm of a person with adult Ricket's/ Osteomalacia

An adult woman's body contains roughly 700 grams of calcium phosphate; 120 grams of that is elemental calcium. An adult needs to take in 0.8 grams of calcium daily in a diet, in order to be in calcium balance. During pregnancy, this amount increases to 1.3 grams per day. The body of an adult male contains 800 grams of calcium.

Prevention of osteoporosis is extremely important to avoid the complications of osteoporosis and their associated morbidities and mortality.

Diet plays a major role both the cause and in the prevention of osteoporosis.
Other Foods that are rich in vitamin D and calcium include:
Cheese
Yogurt
Beans
Eggs
Kale
Cauliflower
Chard
Molasses
Rhubarb
Beets
Almonds
Cabbage,
Bran

Carrots
Celery
Dates
Chocolate
Figs
Lettuce
Lemons
Oranges
Oysters
Pineapples
Raspberries
Shell fish
Spinach
Walnuts
Watercress
Parsnip etc;

While several of the aforementioned do have good calcium source, it must be kept in mind that because some of them are very rich in cholesterol, they must be consumed in moderation. Some of these cholesterol-rich foods are milk, cheese, egg yolk, oysters, shellfish, etc. It is a good idea to consume skim milk, as well as cheese made with skim milk, to decrease the amount of cholesterol intake.

The human skin contains a substance called ergosterol, and sunlight, as well as ultraviolet radiation fron the sun, activates this substance, which leads to the production of Vitamin D, hence, the importance of sunlight exposure.

Many people are not exposed to sun light on a regular basis because they work in offices. In addition, elderly people are confined to their places of residence and have no sun exposure. In addition, people who cannot tolerate dairy products because of lactose intolerance, depriving them of an importance of source of vitamin D and calcium.

Another important reason why blacks and others with dark skins have such high rate of vitamin D insufficiency/deficiency is because their skins have high concentration of melanin making it very difficult for the sun ray to penetrate their skins to stimulate vitamin D production.

As mentioned above ninety pervcent of blacks, ninty percent of Hispanics, South Asians, Arabs, other people with dark skins, and senty-five percent of whites have vitamin D insufficiency in the U.S. Accordng to a published report by the CDC on March 30ᵗʰ 2011, "one third of Americans are not getting enough vitamin D".

Vitamin D deficiency can cause osteoporosis, rickets, caries, secondary hyperparathyroidism, low magnesium, low phosphorous, renal tubular acidosis, congestive heart failure, uncontrol essential hypertension (low vitamin D causes over activation of the rinin-angiotensin-aldosterone system which can lead to elevated blood pressure), increase infection by suppression of the immune system, and a multitude of possible other skeletal malformations. Increase exercise plays a major role in the prevention of osteoporosis.

The normal vitamin D-25 OH level in the blood is between 30-100 NG/ML.

Vitamin D is insufficient when the level of D-25 OH in the blood is between 10-29 NG/ML and vitamin D-25 OH is deficient when the level in the blood is between 1-9 NG/ML.

When the vitamin D OH is deficient in the blood, it is necessary to check the levels of magnesium, phosphorous and parathyroid hormone in the blood to rule out Adult Rickets /Osteomalacia. In Rickets/Osteomalacia, the serum magnesium and phosphorous will be low and the parathyroid hormone level will be elavetated. It is always necessary to do a bone debsity test in people 50 years and older.

The effects of low level of vitamin to the kidney are significant. Low vitamin can cause the kidney to excrete magnesium and phosphorous in the urine and elevated parathyroid hormone in the blood, which in turn can lead to renal tubular acidosis.

Renal tubular acidosis is a serious kidney disease.

This combination of medical problems affecting the kidney prevent the kidney from properly metabolize vitamin D 25 OH which takes place in the kidney.

The form of vitamin D in the liver is vitamin D 125 OH. Vitamin D 125 OH must go the kidney to be activated to vitamin D 25 OH to be used in the body for normal functions.

Therefore, a disease kidney cannot do this, hence the reason kidney failure causes low vitamin D, and low vitamin can cause kidney insufficiency/failure. Both conditions lead to osteoporosis.

Treatments of osteoporosis

Medications that are available in the USA to treat osteoporosis include:

1. Fosamax
2. Actonel
3. Evista

4. Miacalcin
5. Calcium supplements, and
6. Vitamin D in age-appropriate dosages.
7. Zoledronic injection once per year

The National Academy of Sciences, in 2002, recommended the daily intake of Vitamin D to be:

0-50 years 200 IU/day (International Unit)
51-70 years 400-600 IU /day
71 years and older 600-800 IU /day

and the National Academy of Sciences in 2002 also recommended the following daily intake of calcium:

0-6months	200 mg/day
7-12 months	270 mg/day
1-3years	500 mg/day
4-8 years	800 mg/day
9-18 years	1,300 mg/day
19-50 years	1000 mg/day
51 years and older	1,200 mg/day until menopause
51 years and older	1,500mg/day after menopause

In people whose vitamin D level is abnormally low, it is necessary to treat them with 50,000 units of vitamin D 2 tablets per week for either for 4 weeks, 8 weeks or 12 weeks denpending on how low the vitamin D level is. Once vitamin D level is corrected to normal, the person can be placed maintenance dose of vitamin D of either 1000 units per day or 2000 units per day for life.

Understanding the different causes of osteoporosis and knowing the different subgroups of individuals in society who have a predisposition to deloping it, will help to prevent it by providing the right diet and treatments for these people.

Chapter 47
OSTEOARTHRITIS ARTHRITIS

WHAT IS ARTHRITIS?

Arthritis is an autoimmune/inflammatory condition that affects mainly joints resulting in swelling, pain, restriction of movement and, ultimately, deformity of the joints and bones, as a result. In addition, chronic bony destruction and edematous destruction also occur. However, certain types of arthritis, at times, can be multi-system, affecting a multitude of organs such as the heart, the lungs, the kidneys and the blood system, etc.

The most common forms of arthritides are:

1. Osteoarthritis
2. Rheumatoid arthritis
3. Gouty arthritis
4. Ankylosing spondylitis
5. Psoriatic arthritis
6. Reiter's dyndrome with arthritis
7. Systemic lupus erythematosus associated with arthritis
8. Polymyalgia rheumatica
9. Infectious arthritis
10. Lyme disease associated with arthritis
11. Sickle cell disease-associated arthritis, etc.

Different types of arthritis affect 50 million Americans, but osteoarthritis is the most common form of all the arthritides. Twenty seven million Americans suffer from osteoarthritis and six hundred millions people in the world have osteoarthritis. The process that ultimately leads to osteoarthritis begins in the cartilage.

The cartilage apparently releases a certain enzyme, which causes its destruction and in time causes breakdown of the joints to occur. Cartilage is a gelatinous substance whose function is to provide cushion in between joints. Once the cartilage dries out, overtime; the areas in between the joints rub against each other, resulting in bone destruction and deformities.

Worldwide, about 60% of the population ages 60-70 have osteoarthritis of one joint or another. Certain ethnic groups seem to be affected with arthritis of some part of their body structure to a lesser degree than others do. For example, Africans and southern

Chinese's have less arthritis in their hip joints. The knees seem to be the joint most frequently affected by osteoarthritis in all ethnic groups. Hundreds of million of people in the world are affected by osteoarthritis.

A study published in 2008 showed that 33.8 percent of blacks have osteoarthritis compared to 26.6 percent whites. 57.9 percent black women have osteoarthtritis as compared to 32.9 percent white women. The aging process plays a major role in the development of osteoarthritis. In most cases, people over age 40 will develop osteoarthritis by virtue of getting older.

Obesity plays a major role in causing osteoarthritis of the knees in older individuals leading to morbidity and mortality. Black and Hispanic women are more affected by this. Source: Annals of Internal Medicine, February 15, 2011, Volume 154, Number 4

The joints, most frequently affected by osteoarthritis are

Knees
Hips
Hands
Fingers
Spine
Feet
Ankles
Shoulders
Neck
Wrists
Jaws
Ribs
Toes

Osteoarthritis is classified as primary or secondary.

Table 1: Classification of Osteoarthritis
"

I. Primary-Idiopathic
   A. Localized
1. Hip, superolateral, superomedial, medial, inferoposterior
2. Knee, medial, lateral patellofemoral
3. Spinal apophyseal
4. Hand, interphalangeal, base of thumb
5. Foot, first metatarsophalangeal joint, midfoot, hindfoot
6. Other, shoulders, elbows, wrists, ankles

B. Generalized
1. Hands, Heberden's nodes
2. Hands and knees; spinal apophyseal generalized osteoarthritis

II. Secondary
A. Dysplastic
1. Chondrodysplasia
2. Epiphyseal dysplasias
3. Congenital joint displacement
4. Developmental disorders, Perthes' disease, epiphysiolysis

B. Post-traumatic
1. Acute
2. Repetitive
3. Postoperative

C. Structural failure
1. Osteonecrosis
2. Osteochondritis

D. Post-inflammatory
1. Infection
2. Inflammatory arthropathies

E. Endocrine and metabolic
1. Acromegaly
2. Ochronosis
3. Hemochromatosis
4. Crystal deposition disorders

F. Connective tissue
1. Hypermobility syndromes
2. Mucopolysaccharidoses

G. Etiology obscure
1. Kashin-Beck disease"

Primary osteoarthritis occurs as part of the aging process; secondary arthritis occurs because of some form of abnormality that occurs in the joint causing it to be misaligned, resulting in the abnormalities that ultimately result in the formation of arthritic changes. Sometimes these changes are the result of injuries to the joints or the result of a person's occupation, which exposes the joints to repeated stress, resulting in the development of arthritis.

If a joint becomes infected and the infection is not treated quickly, then that joint can develop post-inflammatory changes, which could develop arthritic changes ultimately.

Both primary and secondary hemochromatosis are conditions that cause iron to be deposited in joints and breaks down within the joints into free radicals that can cause breakdown of the tissues and the bones in the joints. The result is the development of arthritis. Blacks and Hispanics have a high percentage of secondary hemochromatosis, because of such diseases as sickle cell anemia and thalassemia that cause a large amount of iron to be deposited in their bloodstream from hemolyzed red blood cells. Many Italians, Greeks, Arabics, Indians, Whites and Asians men, and women also suffer from primary and secondary hemochromatosis with resulting high incidence of osteoarthritis.

People who suffer from sickle cell disease can develop aseptic necrosis of joints such as the hips, shoulders, elbows, etc. This occurs because the sickling phenomenon impedes the ready flow of blood with oxygen to these joints, resulting in ischemic changes in the bony parts of these joints, which can lead to the development of aseptic necrosis and different stages of arthritis. People who use steroid chronically frequently develop aseptic necrosis of the hip and other joints.

There are many other people of different ethnic background who, because they suffer from thalassemia, either beta or alpha, have secondary hemochromatosis, which can cause them to develop osteoarthritis due to the deposition of iron in their joints.

Obesity is a major predisposing factor in the development of osteoarthritis. The knees are most prone to the development of arthritis because of the stress placed on them by the excess weight. About 76% of black Americans are overweight/obese and 2/3 of Americans adults are obese/overweight. Worldwide there are 502 million obese adults. As a result, osteoarthritis is quite common in these groups

The chances of a person developing osteoarthritis of the knees can be determined by the body mass index of that person. The greater the body mass index of a peson, the greater his or her chances of developing osteoarthritic changes in her knees, hip, ankles, and feet.

TABLE 2:
Determining Body Mass Index (BMI) from Height and Weight Body Mass Index*
(kg/m2)

Body Mass Index* (kg/m2)													
19 20 21			22	23	24	25	26	27	28	29	30	35
Height (in) Body weight (lb)													
58	91 96 100		105	110	115	119	124	129	134	138	143	167
59	94 99 104		109	114	119	124	128	133	138	143	148	173
60	97 102 107		112	118	123	128	133	138	143	148	153	179
61	100 106 111		116	122	127	132	137	143	148	153	158	185
62	104 109 115		120	126	131	136	142	147	153	158	164	191
63	107 113 118		124	130	135	141	146	152	158	163	169	197
64	110 116 122		128	134	140	145	151	157	163	169	174	204
65	114 120 126		132	138	144	150	156	162	168	171	180	210
66	118 124 130		136	142	148	155	161	167	173	179	186	215
67	121 127 134		140	146	153	159	166	172	178	185	191	223
68	125 131 138		144	151	158	164	171	177	184	190	197	230
69	128 135 142		149	155	162	169	176	182	189	196	203	236
70	132 138 146		153	160	167	174	181	188	195	202	207	243
71	136 143 150		157	165	172	179	186	193	200	208	215	250
72	140 147 154		162	169	177	184	191	199	206	213	221	258
73	144 151 159		166	174	182	189	197	204	212	219	227	265
74	148 155 163		171	179	186	194	202	210	218	225	233	272
75	152 160 168		176	184	192	200	208	216	224	232	240	279
76	156 164 172		180	189	197	205	213	221	230	238	246	287

Body mass index, or BMI, is the measurement of choice to determine obesity. BMI is a formula that takes into account both a person's height and weight. BMI is a person's weight in kilograms divided by height in meters squared (BMI=kg/m2). The table printed above has already done the conversions. To use the table, find the appropriate height in the left-hand column. Move across the row to the given weight. The number at the top of the column is the BMI for that height and weight.

In general, a person age 35 or older is obese if he or she has a BMI of >27. For people age 34 or younger, a BMI of >25 indicates obesity. Obesity is an indication for further clinical evaluation.

The BMI measurement poses some of the same problems as weight-for-height tables. BMI does not provide information on a person's age or body fat or take into consideration the person's body fat distribution.

As published by the American Diabetes Association

To evaluate pain in a particular joint or joints, a history and physical examination must be carried out. Once that is done, then, certain blood tests ought to be done. Included among these blood tests are

CBC
Complete blood chemistry profile
Serum uric acid
Urinalysis
Erythrocyte sedimentation rate (ESR)
Rheumatoid factor
Anti-nuclear antibody (ANA)

In addition, radiological evaluation of the joint or joints in question must be done.

These tests include
Plain x-ray
Ultrasound
CT scan
MRI

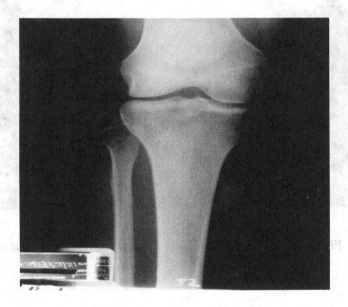

Figure 47.1-X-ray of a normal knee

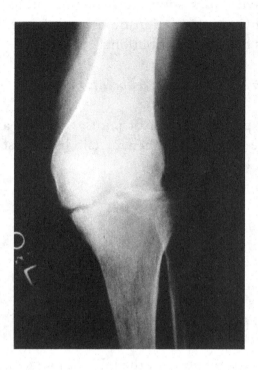

Figure 47.2-X-ray of a knee affected with osteoarthritis

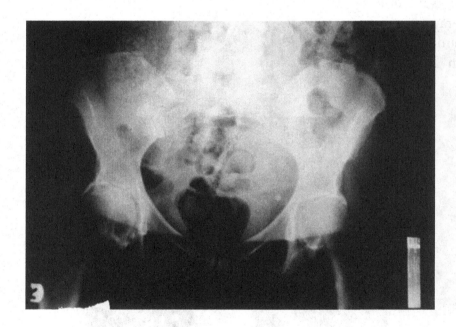

Figure 47.3: X-ray of hip joint affected with osteoarthritis

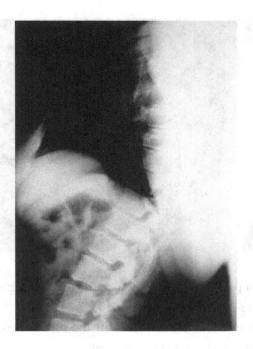

Figure 47.4: X-ray of lumbar spine affected with osteoarthritis

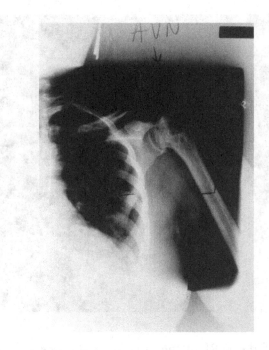

Figure 47.5: X-ray of shoulder joint showing aseptic necrosis in a patient with sickle cell anemia

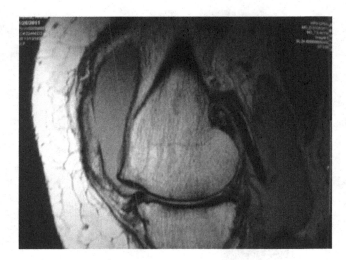

47.6 MRI of right of a patient with severe osteoarthritis showing a large joint
Effusion, a large Baker's cyst measuring 4.5 x 2.0 x 7.2 cm
High grade tear of the anterior cruciate ligament, and partial tears of the
posterior cruciate ligament and collateral ligament.

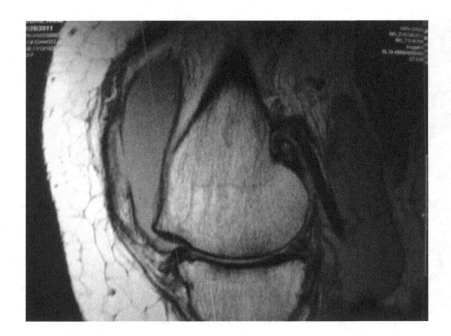

47.7 Another view of the MRI of the same knee showing a complex tear of the
posterior horn of the meniscus and many degenerative arthritic changes.

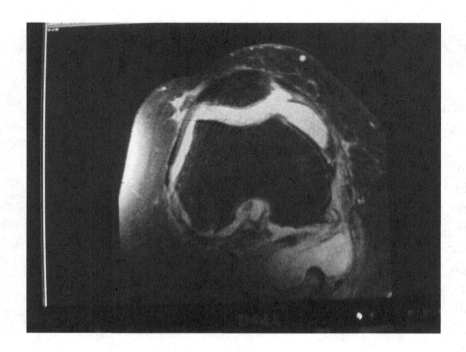

47.8 MRI of hip in a patient with adult Rickets showing osteoporosis and inflammation and ratrhitic changes

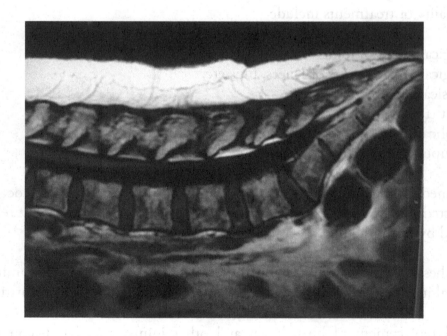

47.9 MRI of lumbar spine in a patient with adult Rickets Osteomalacia showing degenerative changes.

Osteoarthritis is a painful condition, and it can be very disabling disease.

The medications in use in the U.S. to treat osteoarthritis are

Motrin

Advil

Aleve

Naprosyn

Anaprox

Daypro

Relefan

Indocin

Celebrex (COX2)

Aspirin

Athrotec

Voltaren

Flector

Toradol

Mobic

Tylenol

Steroid

Ultram etc;

Other modality of treatments include

1. Surgical repair of joints
2. Surgical replacements of Knees, hips etc;
3. Physical therapy
4. Heat treatments
5. Application of different cream/ointments to affected bony parts
6. Accupuncture

These medications work by interfering with the inflammation that occurs locally in the affected joints, thereby easing the pain. Physical therapy works by relieving the stiffness and by strengthening the affected joint or joints.

When these treatments are no longer effective and the pain and discomfort persist, then surgical intervention is often considered as an option to treat the arthritic joint.

Surgical replacement of hips, knees and other joints, etc., has become common practice these days, provided the affected individual is not too obese to allow for the operation to have a chance of success, or provided there are no other contraindications, such as associated major medical problems, etc.

Osteoarthritis is both more common and more severe in minorities than whites are. Many minorities work as factory workers, housekeepers, construction workers, sanitation workers, farmers etc; and these types of work require a lot of physical activity, which places a lot of stress on the joints of the fingers, shoulders, elbows, knees, lumbar spine, cervical spine and the hip joints. Low back pain is one of the most common causes of work related disability in the world causing hundred of billions of dollars in lost income worldwide.

Osteoarthritis, as a disease, is also common in athletes, no matter what form of athletic activities they are engaged in. Preventive measures such as eating a proper diet to maintain an ideal weight and wearing proper sports equipment during athletic activities would help to decrease the incidence of osteoarthritis.

Paget's disease of the bone is another type of arthritis that is frequently seen in some people with osteoarthritis.

Chapter 48
RHEUMATOID ARTHRITIS

Rheumatoid is an autoimmune/inflammatory disease that affects close to 2.1 million Americans. Rheumatoid arthritis is 2-3 more common in women than in men. People who smoke seem to have a higher incidence of rheumatoid arthritis. Blacks with RA develop serious complications. RA affects people of all ethnic back grounds.

Worldwide 140 million people are afflicted with Rheumatoid Arthritis and 1.3 million people in the U.S. have rheumatoid arthritis.

When left untreated, or when treatment fails, causes chronic deformity of the bones with destruction of the affected joints. In point of fact, even when appropriate and effective treatments are provided to a person suffering with rheumatoid arthritis, joint deformities ultimately develop in the majority of patients with rheumatoid arthritis.

The joints frequently affected by rheumatoid arthritis are

Feet
Ankles
Hands
Fingers
Elbows
Wrists
Shoulders
Hips
Neck
Lumbar spine
Thoracic spine

The cause of rheumatoid arthritis is unknown. Although many theories have been proposed, none has so far been proven.

Rheumatoid arthritis is a multi-system disease, but the joints, bones, muscles, skin, and blood system are affected most frequently.
Other organs that can be affected by RA include
Heart
Lung
Brain

Blood system
Kidney
Skin
Neurological system,

In the beginning, the symptoms of rheumatoid arthritis can be insidious and difficult to discern. At times, a person may present with vague symptoms such as

General malaise
Fatigue
Weakness weight loss
Aches and pains
Head ache
Fever

Morning stiffness in different joints that improves as she starts to move around, doing daily chores.

As the disease progresses, then the signs of synovitis with swelling of the joints with pain and warmth become evident.

The disease affects women between the ages of 20 and 50 years, although some women are afflicted earlier and some are afflicted at a later age. Women are affected three times more often than men with R A. R A also affect children, resulting in juvenile arthritis,

TABLE 1: Classification of Rheumatoid Arthritis
Revised, as Published by the American College of Rheumatology

1. Guidelines for classification
    Four of seven criteria are required to classify a patient as having rheumatoid arthritis
    Patients with two or more clinical diagnoses are not excluded

2. Criteria
    a. Morning stiffness: Stiffness in and around the joints lasting 1 hr before maximal improvement.
    b. Arthritis of three of more joint areas: At least three joint areas, observed by a physician
       Simultaneously, have soft tissue swelling or joint effusions, not just bony overgrowth.
       The 14 possible joint areas involved are right or left proximal interphalangeal,

metacarpophalangeal, wrist, elbow, knee, and ankle and metatarsophalangeal joints.

c. **Arthritis of hand joints: Arthritis of wrist, metacarpophalangeal joint, or proximal interphalangeal joint.**
d. Symmetric arthritis: Simultaneous involvement of the same joint areas on both sides of the body.
e. Rheumatoid nodules: Subcutaneous nodules over bony prominences, extensor surfaces, or juxtaarticular regions observed by a physician.
f. Serum rheumatoid factor: Demonstration of abnormal amounts of serum rheumatoid factor by any method for which the result has been positive in less than 5% of normal control subjects.
g. Radiographic changes: Typical changes of RA on postero-anterior hand and wrist radiographs, which must include erosions or unequivocal bony decalcification localized in or most marked adjacent to the involved joints.

*Criteria a-d must be present for at least 6 weeks. A physician must observe criteria b-e.

Taking a thorough and detailed history is crucial in a person in whom the physician suspects rheumatoid arthritis. Equally important is a thorough physical examination. Eliciting the fact that other immediate members of the family have rheumatoid arthritis or symptoms suggesting rheumatoid arthritis is quite important, because there is clear evidence that rheumatoid arthritis can run in the family.

No one test is diagnostic of rheumatoid arthritis, but a series of blood tests together with x-ray examination of certain joints, such as the hands and the fingers, may add up to confirming the diagnosis of rheumatoid arthritis. X-rays of the proximal interphalangeal, metacarpal phalangeal, metatarsal phalangeal, have distinct characteristics that are seen mainly in rheumatoid. Chronic changes of the hands and wrists resulting in swan neck deformity is classic for rheumatoid arthritis but these are late bony changes.

X-ray of the wrist and hand joints showing arthritic changes in a patient with rheumatoid arthritis

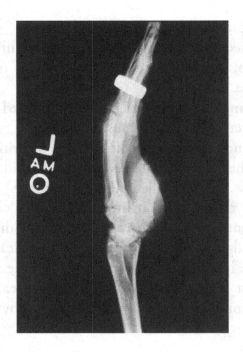

Figure 48:1

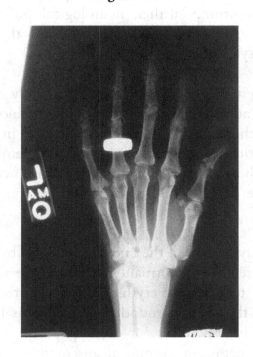

Figure 48:2
Deformed finger's joints in person with rheumatoid arthritis

Other systemic involvements of rheumatoid arthritis include:

1. Vasculitis involving medium-sized vessels.
2. The lungs may become involved because of pleural effusion, resulting in shortness of breath, and diffuse interstitial fibrosis may develop, resulting in chronic lung disease.
3. The eyes may become involved with a condition called keratoconjunctivitis sicca (also known as Sjoren's Syndrome) causing dry eyes.
4. In about 10% of individuals with rheumatoid arthritis, the spleen is enlarged. Frequently, when the spleen is enlarged in rheumatoid arthritis, the white blood cell count is also low. (This is called Felty's Syndrome.)
5. Some adults with rheumatoid arthritis develop a clinical picture similar to children with rheumatoid arthritis called Still's disease, with fever spike, polyarthralgia, myalgia, a maculopapular rash, pericarditis, pneumonitis, sore throat, large spleen, lymphadenopathy and pain in the abdomen.
6. The heart can, at times, be involved and pericarditis can occur. Aortic regurgitation and conduction abnormalities of the rhythm of the heart can also occur.

People with rheumatoid arthritis may develop peripheral neuropathy because of vasculitis of the vasa nervorum. Further, neurological problems may result when, because of tenosynovitis of the wrists, compression of the median nerve occurs, resulting in carpal tunnel syndrome.

The hematopoietic system (blood system) is markedly affected by rheumatoid arthritis. Anemia is the most serious and most common blood abnormality seen in rheumatoid arthritis. A characteristic of the anemia seen in rheumatoid arthritis is normochromic, normocytic (meaning the sizes and the hemoglobin contents of the red cells are normal but there are not enough red cells produced, resulting in anemia). The serum iron is low, the TIBC (total iron binding capacity) is normal but the serum ferritin is high.

Although there is plenty of iron in the body, as reflected by the high serum ferritin, anemia exists because there is an abnormality involving the release mechanism of the iron from the transferrin to the early erythroblasts (early red blood cell precursors). The iron accumulates in the reticulo-endothelial cells. This failure to release iron to the erythroblasts is what is responsible for the hypoproliferative anemia that is seen in rheumatoid arthritis (anemia of chronic disease/anemia of chronic inflammatory diseases).

In effect, the rheumatoid person suffers from iron deficiency anemia because she has an inability to use the iron in the body (iron-deficient dyserythropoiesis).

Recent evidence in the literature suggests that some cytokines play a major role in this process of anemia of chronic disease (now also referred to as anemia of inflammatory diseases).

Leukopenia (low white blood cell) is frequently seen in rheumatoid arthritis and in particular when there is splenomegaly (known as Felty's Syndrome as mentioned earlier).

Other blood tests that are frequently abnormal in rheumatoid arthritis are:

1. Elevated ESR (erythrocyte sedimentation rate)
2. Elevated rheumatoid factor (latex fixation)
3. ANA (antinuclear antibodies) is elevated in up to 60% of patients with rheumatoid arthritis.
4. Anti-cyclic citrullinated peptide (anti-CCP)

An ESR of 100 mg/hr or greater, together with a high latex fixation and rheumatoid nodules as seen in some joints represents not only severe rheumatoid arthritis but also a very poor prognosis.

The symptoms of rheumatoid arthritis and the overall clinical course of rheumatoid arthritis is worse in blacks than in whites because most blacks are engaged in heavier physical work than their white counterparts. Poverty and heavier physical work and poor working conditions in the factories, housekeeping and domestic work are more closely associated with black women.

Therefore, people whose life circumstances place them in these poor working conditions, while at the same time being afflicted with rheumatoid arthritis, have a harder task to cope with it. Trying to work to earn a living using stiff, painful, and swollen joints of the hands, elbows, shoulders, knees, feet and lower back is a very difficult task, to say the least.

There are several modalities available to treat rheumatoid arthritis although there is no cure for this disease. Rheumatoid arthritis is primarily treated with medications such as:

Aspirin
Indocin
Motrin
Naprosyn
Clinoril
Feldane
Daypro
Relafen

Anaprox
Celebrex
Methotrxate
Arava
Minocin
Steroid
Imuran
Cytoxan
Orencia
Kineret etc;

Physical therapy as a modality plays a major role in the treatment of rheumatoid arthritis to prevent weakness, contractures, atrophy, and other assorted problems affecting the joints of people suffering with rheumatoid arthritis.

At times, surgical intervention must be carried out to help alleviate some of the deformities that rheumatoid arthritis causes in the joints of its victims. Anti-inflammatory medications, such as aspirin, Indocin, Excedrin, and all the NSAIDS, can cause gastrointestinal bleeding in up to 10% of individuals taking them with major medical complications. A higher number, up to 30%, of individuals taking these medications chronically develop a multitude of stomach symptoms, such as heartburn, etc.

People with kidney disease, such as renal insufficiency, ought to be very careful with NSAIDS because not only can these medications themselves cause kidney disease, de novo, they can make kidney disease worse. When taking these medications, these individuals ought to be supervised closely by a physician, in order that their blood counts, their liver function tests, and their kidney functions test can be closely monitored.

The most effective and the only medication approved by the FDA to prevent bleeding from the stomach (gastric ulcer) caused by aspirin and NSAIDS is misoprostol (Cytotec). Cytotec is used as 100 mcg three times per day with food. Cytotec is a prostaglandin analog. Its mode of action is to:

1. Increase the pH of the gastric juice;
2. Increase mucous production by the stomach; and
3. Increase blood flow to the lining of the stomach, thereby preventing erosions and ulcerations of the stomach wall.

Because Cytotec is a prostaglandin analog, it can induce abortion. Therefore, women of childbearing age ought not to take this medication when pregnant, as per the FDA and the makers of Cytotec.

Methotrexate has major side effects to the liver and bone marrow, so physicians must observe individuals taking Methotrexate closely with blood count and liver function tests, etc. Methotrexate also ought not to be taken by women who are pregnant because it can cause abortion and deformities in the fetus.

The Author was the very first person in the world to have shown that Methotrexate prevented the production of antibobies when injected in mice while working as medical a technologist as a supervisor of an immuno-heamotoplgy laboratory in a Hospital in Brooklyn New York in 1966-68. This research was published by the Physician in whose laboratory I was working without any credit given to me. I gave him all my research data as I was leaving to go to medical school.

I am therefore entitled to the legitimate credit every time Methotrexate is used to treat any rheumatological diseases any where in the world. All the new biologic medications in use on the market presently to treat RA were most likely based on that original reseach idea.

Chapter 49
SYSTEMIC LUPUS ERYTHEMATOSUS

Systemic lupus erythematosus (SLE) is an autoimmune/chronic inflammatory disease of unknown cause that most commonly affects women of childbearing age, though a small percentage of adolescent girls and other women and men can also be affected.

According to the National Institute of Health, 9 out 10 individuals affected with lupus are women. This disease is more common in black women than white women are. SLE is diagnosed 3 times more frequently in black women than in white women, but SLE affects both men and women of different ethnic groups.

The incidence of SLE varies from 15 per 100,000 populations to 50 per 100,000 populations. According to the Lupus Foundation of America, 1.5 million people in the USA are affected with lupus. Worldwide 5 million people have SLE.

The prevalence of SLE is 40 cases per 100,000 in Whites and 200 cases per 100,000 in Blacks. Ninety percent of patients with lupus are female. The number of SLE in the US is about 1.5 million. Source: Washington Post.Com 3/9/11

Risk factors for SLE include
Race
Age
Sex
Sunlight
Epstein Barr infection
Smoking tobacco
The following medications can cause lupus like syndrome
Apresoline
Isoniozide
Procainamide
Quinidine

Methyldopa
Compozine

SLE affects many organs in the human body including
Skin
Joints
Kidneys
Blood
Heart
Lungs
Brain
Blood vessels
Hair
Mouth

The symptoms of SLE include
Skin rash over sun exposure of the skin
Butterfly rash over the face, nose, or cheeks
Alopecia—hair loss
Morning stiffness
Joints pain
Swelling of joints
Fever
Weight loss
Fatigue
Loss of appetite
Sores in the mouth
Easy brusing
Chest pain
Shortness of breath
Raynaud's phenomenon-fingers and toes turning blue on exposure to cold
dry eyes etc;

Morning stiffness with swelling and pain in the joints is a frequent presentation of SLE. As the term implies, SLE affects many organs, and disease in any one of these organs may be the first manifestation of SLE. In addition, patients with SLE may present with fatigue, malaise, fever, anorexia, weight loss and nausea, etc. The musculoskeletal system may be affected by myalgias, arthralgias, and polyarthritis with bony erosions, deformities of the hands, myositis, myopathy, and ischemic necrosis of bones.

The skin may be affected with a melar rash over the cheeks. A discoid rash may be seen on the skin. Photosensitivity may be seen. Ulcers of the mouth may be seen. Any number and types of other rashes may be seen such as a maculopapular rash, urticarial rash, bullous rash, alopecia, and vasculitis, etc.

The hematopoietic system (blood system) may be affected with anemia, both chronic and hemolytic. Leukopenia (low white blood cell count), thrombocytopenia with circulating anticoagulant, large spleen; large liver, lymphadenopathy (large lymph nodes) may be seen.

SLE frequently affects the neurological system. Among the neurological symptoms manifested in patients with SLE are memory loss, acute psychosis, seizures, peripheral neuropathy vasculitis, and stroke, etc.

The lungs are frequently affected in patients with SLE. Patients can develop pleurisy, pleural effusion, pneumonitis, interstitial fibrosis, pulmonary hypertension, and ARDS (adult respiratory distress syndrome).

Evaluation of people suspected of having SLE include
History and physical examination
Blood tests in use to diagnose SLE are
Antinuclear antibody-ANA
dsDNA
Anti-Extractable Antibody
Anti-Ribonucleic Acid-RNP
Anti-Smith Antibody
Erythrocyte sedimentation rate-ESR
Rheumatoid factor
Anti-phospholipin Antibody
Lupus Anticoagulant
D-Dimer
CBC
Complete metabolic profile-SMA20
Urinalysis

In people with SLE, the anti-dsDNA is positive, the anti—Smith antibody is positive, the ESR is high, the HCT is low, the WBC may be low and the total lymphocyte count is low and the urinalysis may show microscopic hematuria and protenuria etc;

Other tests that must be done are
Chest X-ray
CT of chest
CT of different joints
MRI of different joints

MRI of the brain
Renal ultrasound
Echocardiogram
EKG Skin biopsy as indicated etc;

The heart can also be affected by SLE

Among the problems that affect the heart in SLE are the following:

1. Pericarditis
2. Myocarditis
3. Endocarditis
4. Arrhythmias, and
5. Heart blocks (electrical disturbances of the heart)

The kidneys are frequently affected in patients with SLE with

1. Nephritis
2. Hematuria
3. Neprotic syndrome
4. Renal failure

Proteinuria greater than 500 mg/24 hours, along with nephrotic syndrome, which can ultimately result in renal failure, frequently occurs in patients with SLE.

Anti-cardiolipin/anti-phospholipid syndromes are frequently seen in SLE with associated thrombosis of different organs, such as the brain, the lungs, the vascular system, and the placenta in women, resulting in frequent spontaneous abortions. Any woman who has had frequent spontaneous abortions ought to be evaluated for the anti-cardiolipin/anti-phospholipid syndromes. Because of protein loss, as part of the nephrotic syndrome, anti-thrombosis III, protein C and protein S levels are low resulting in an hypercoagulable state (thick blood), causing formation of clots (DVT) or pulmonary embolism-clot in the lung.

The brain is frequently becomes affected in people with SLE resulting in
Head ache
Diziness
Vascullitis
Transient ischemic attacks—TIA
Cerebrovascular accident (stroke)
Seizure
Depression
Psychosis
Dementia

Many gastrointestinal symptoms are manifested in patients who have SLE. Among these symptoms are nausea, vomiting, diarrhea, gastrointestinal bleeding, abnormal liver function tests, etc. Both venous and arterial thrombosis frequently occur in patients with SLE and the Prednisone that is used as the main treatment of SLE can also cause a state of hypercoagulation, which itself is a frequent cause of thrombosis. The eyes in patients with SLE can develop retinal vasculitis, conjunctivitis, and the SICCA syndrome with dry eyes.

People with SLE frequently develop blood diseases such as
Autoimmune hemolytic anemia
Anemia of inflammatory diseases
Leukopenia-low white blood cells
Thrombocytopenia-low platelet count

SLE frequently is associated with different types of infections because SLE causes immunosupression by itself, plus the fact steroid is usually used to treat Lupus and steroid causes immunosuppression as well, and among these infections are

Viral infections-herpes, cold, sinusitis, shingles, viral gastroenteritis, viral pneumonia, viral meningitis etc;
Fungal infections-yeast infection, meningitis etc;
Bacterial infections—bacterial pneumonia accounts for 1/3 of deaths from lupus, urinary tract infection, pyelonephritis, sepsis, infectious gastroenteritis etc;

SLE is frequently associated with different types of cancers and among these cancers are Lung cancer and Non-Hodgkin lymphoma.

SLE is also associated with significant bone problems resulting in arthritis and aseptic necrosis of the
Hips
Shoulders
Elbows
Knees
Wrists
Ankles
Lumbar spine
Cervical spine

Women with lupus erythematosus have a very high propensity of suffering spontaneous abortion when pregnant. This occurs because women with SLE frequently develop antiphospholipin antibody. Antiphospholipin antibody causes a state of hypercoabulity resulting in clotting of the vessels carrying blood to the placenta resulting in spontaneous abortion.

In addition, this same process causes pre-ecclamsiam/ecclampsia to develop.
Further, women with SLE who become pregnant have the propensity of experiencing
severe flare up when pregnant.

There is another form of lupus called discoid lupus. Discoid lupus affects the skin of the face, neck, arms, and scalp. It causes chronic scarring with severe disfigurement.
Very few of these patients with discoid lupus go on to develop SLE. On the other hand, 20% of patients with SLE develop discoid lupus lesions and 5% of patients with discoid lupus go on to develop SLE.

Another form of lupus that can be seen is drug-induced lupus. The drugs that are generally associated with the development of a lupus-like state include Procanamide, hydralazine, Isoniazid, chlorpromazine, methyldopa, and Quinidine, among others. The symptoms of drug-induced lupus include fevers, skin rash, arthralgias, polyarthritis, pericarditis, etc. These symptoms usually disappear after a few days or up to 1 week to 10 days once the offending drug is stopped.

Evaluation of lupus includes a history and physical examination, laboratory tests and sometimes x-ray examinations.

Laboratory tests that are the most helpful in diagnosing lupus are ANA, ENA, anti-double-stranded DNA, anti-Ro antibody, anti-La and anti-Sm., serum complement levels, erythrocyte sedimentation rate, CBC, platelet count, urinalysis and blood chemistries. Usually the ANA test is positive in lupus. Then the next tests to order are the anti-double-stranded DNA and the ENA. The ENA has two parts to it. One part is the RNP (ribonuclear protein) and the other part is the SM (Smith antibody). If the SM part is positive then SLE is most probably present.

If the RNP is positive then mixed connective tissue disease is present. Examples of mixed connective tissue disease (MCTD) include overlap syndrome of SLE, rheumatoid arthritis, polymyositis, in association with scleroderma and high titers of RNP and clinical features of SLE.

The anti-double-stranded DNA and the anti-SM are specific for SLE. Tests such as the serum complement levels and the ESR are used to monitor the activity of the disease.

A positive ANA is found in association with many conditions and is therefore not specific for lupus. A significant percentage of the U.S. population has positive ANA and these individuals are not sick with anything.

SLE is more common in women than men by about a 9:1 ratio. Black women seem to have a particular predilection to get sicker with lupus than other women. Pregnancy can cause an acute flare-up of SLE and, as such, it is not advisable for women to get pregnant when suffering with lupus.

Two new susceptible gene have been identified as being possibly responsible for SLE BLK-C8orf13 on chromosome 8 and ITGAM-ITGAX on chromosome 16 (NEJ of Med
358;9 Feb 28,2008)

Treatments of SLE
Medications
Aspirin
Motrin
Naproxen
Advil
Aleve
Hydroxychloroquine
Steroid
Rituxan
Cytoxan
Imuran
Benlysta (just approved by the FDA on 3/9/11 to treat SLE by injection)
"Benlysta reduces the disease's level of activity by inhibiting a bodily protein called the B-lymphcyte stimulator, which at elevated levels can contribute to the creation of antibodies. Autoantibodies are cells that attack otherwise healty tissue, such as the skin, kidneys, heart, and joints."

Other treatments include:
Skin rashes are treated with topical steroid cream or ointment
CNS lupus and other aggressive forms of SLE are treated with IV steroid.

Prednisone is the main drug used to treat lupus and its multitude of complications. Cyclophosphamide (Cytoxan) and Azathioprine are also quite effective in treating SLE. Lupus has no cure but can be treated and managed for a very long time. Many patients with SLE can go on to develop renal failure, requiring chronic dialysis.
People with SLE usually die of Stroke, Heart attack or Infection.

The death rate from SLE in blacks is quite high, and among black women in the age range 45 to 64, the death rate increased to 70% between 1979 and 1998.

In 1950, the median survival people with SLE were 4 years. Presently the median survival is about 15 years from diagnosis because better medications and better overall management.

Chapter 50
MIXED CONNECTIVE TISSUE DISEASES/OVERLAP SYNDROME

Another series of rheumatological diseases that are very common are mixed collagen vascular diseases MCTD also called overlap syndrome. About 5 million people in the U.S. have MCTD and 1 in 100,000 people in the world have MCVD. Frequently these diseases are seen in conjunction with SLE, scleroderma, polymyositis, dermatomyosis, rheumatoid arthritis, polymyositis, sjogren' syndrome and psoriatic arthritis.

MCTD is an autoimmune disease of unknown cause. MCTD affects people of all ethnicity but, is more common in women than men and is more common in Blacks, Chinese, and Japanese than Caucasians. MCTD affects 1 in 100,000 or 70,000 people in the world.

The symptoms of MCTD include

Malaise
Fatigue
Fever
Joints pain
Pain in muscles
Swelling of hands, fingers, wrists ankles, feet, and elbows
Raynaud's disease

MCTD can affect several organs including lungs, heart, joints, bones, skin, eyes, mouth, esaphogus, stomach, small bowel, large bowel, blood system etc;

Evaluation of MCTD include

History
Physical examination
CBC
Complete metabolic profile (SMA20)
Urinalysis
ESR
Rheumatoid factor
ANA
Anti-dsDNA

ENA
Anti-RNP
Anti—Ro/SSA antibody
La/SSB antibody
Anti-Jo 1 antibodies
Anti-Smith antibodies
Anti-Scl 70 antibodies

Other tests to do in evaluating a person for MCTD include:

Chest x-ray
CT of the chest
MRI of the chest
Esaphogram
Endoscopy
Esaphogram motility study
Colonoscopy
Abdominal CT etc;

Treatments of MCTD include

Motrin
Advil
Aleve
Naproxen
Anaprox
Celebrex
Steroid etc;

Because MCTD is often an overlap syndrome with other diseases
Such as SLE, RA, Scleroderma, Dermatomyositis, Polymyositis, Sojgreen syndrome, treatments are usually prescribed based on associated diseases and symptoms.

Scleroderma is an autoimmune disease of unknown cause anover growth of collagen to develop. Three hundred thousand people in the U.S. have scleroderma. More women than men have scleroderma. According to the literature, "the risk systemic sclerosis is 4-9 times higher in women than in men" Two third of people with scleroderma have the limited form of the disease and one third have the systemic form. Systemic sclerosis is 10 times higher in blacks and other minorities than as compared to whites.

Scleroderma/systemic sclerosis affects the skin, muscles, blood vesels, lungs, esophapus, stomach, small bowel, large bowel, heart, hands, fingers, kidneys, genitourinary, endocrine system, neurological system etc.

Some of these different symptoms can lead to a condition called CREST syndrome.
CREST syndrome stands for
Calcinosis
Raynaud's phenomenon
Esophageal dysfunction
Sclerodactyly
Telangiectasias

However, CREST usually occurs in the systemic part of scleroderma.
Scleroderma usally develops in people who are between ages of 30-50.

Symptoms of scleroderma include:

Hardness of skin
Hair loss
Tickening of skin
Stiffness of fingers, hands, arms
Sores and ulcers of fingrs and toes
Bleuness, redness, blanching of fingers, toes to heat, and cold
Weight loss
Fatigue
Weakness
Shortness of breath
Joints pain
Chest pain
Numbness of hands and feet
Swelling of joints, hands, arms, wrists and feet
Cough
Wheezing
Difficulty swallowing
Bloating
Heartburn (GERD)
Diarrhea
Costipation
Diziness
Malabsorption
Hypertension
Congestive heart failure
Pulmonary hypertension
Pulmonary fibrosis
Kidney failure
Cardiac arrhythmias (heart block etc;)

Erectile dysfunction

Hypothyroidism

Anemia of Chronic diseases

Menstrual irregularity

Vaginal drydness

Fibrosis of the urinary bladder ect;

Evaluations of scleroderma/systemic sclerosis include:

History and physical examination

CBC

Complete metabolic profile

ESR

Urinalysis

Antinuclear antibody

Rheumatoid factor

Anticentromere antibody

Anti-SCL-70 antibody

Radiological examinations to in evaluating scleroderma/systemic sclerosis include:

Chest x-ray

Chest CT

EKG

Echocardiogram

Pulmonary function test

Skin biopsy

Treatments of sclereoderma/systemic sclerosis include

Steroid

Imurin

Cytoxan

Methotrexate

NSAID

In addition, people with scleroderma/systemic sclerosis are treated for different medical complications that individual patients may suffer from.

Sometimes, individuals with scleroderma/systemic sclerosis have no external signs of the disease. Therefore, it is important to always be vigilant to look for internal symptoms like heart, lungs, kidneys, esophagus, small bowel, large bowel etc;.

Several years ago, I received a long distant phone call on a late Friday afternoon from lady. A patient of mine referred her to me. Her complaint was many years of diarrhea, with 20-30 bowel movements per day and marked weight loss. Her weight was down to 65 ponds. She was had been admitted to hostipals in her home town, Washinton DC and Atlanta Georgia and no one could tell her what was wrong with her.

I admitted her to a Hospital in White Plains N.Y. on a Monday and bgan to evaluate her. I odered CBC, SMA20 chemistry profile, urinalysis, ESR, ANA, ENA, RNP, anti-dsDNA, anti-Centromere antibody, EGK, Chest X-ray, stools culture, stools ova and parasites, stools for clostridium difficile and skin biopsy. In addition, I started her on IV fluid with glucose/normal saline with added potassium chloride.

Two days later, the results came back with positive ANA, positive RNP and positive anti—centromere antibody, establishing the diagnosis of systemic sclerosis of the small bowel causing malabsorption and diarrhea.

Subsequently, the skin biopsy which was sent to a special laboratory confirmed scleroderma/systemic sclerosis as the diagnosis.

I treated her with IV solu-Medrol and 2 days later, her bowel movements becreased to 6 bowel movements per day. She responded well to treatments and discharged home on tapering dose of prednisone and 50mg of cytoxan. To this day, she remains on daily cytoxan, off prednisone. Her normal weight has returned and she has returned to work having been on disability for several years.

Another common autoimmune/MCTD is Sjogren's syndrome. Sojgren's syndrome frequently overlaps with other diseases such as SLE, RA, and Scleroderma.

Sojgren's syndrome affects four million American. Nine out of ten people affected are women.

Half of Sojgren's syndrome occurs alone and is called primary Sojegren's and half occurs in combination with other connective tissue diseases and is called secondary Sojgren's.

The cause of Sojgren's syndrome is unknown. It affects all racial groups equally. Most people affected are in the age range of 30 to 60 years.

Symptoms of Sojgren's syndrome include:

Dry eyes
Dry mouth
Sores in the mouth

Diseases of the gum
Oral cavities
Joints pain
Arthritis
Raynaud's phenomenon
Heartburn (GERD)
Throiditis
Vascullitis
In addition, Sojgren's symptoms affected the lungs, the kidneys, the pancreas, the liver, the nervous system the GI tract etc;

Evaluations of Sojgren's include:

History and physical examination
Examination by an ophthalmologist
Examination by a dentist
ANA
Anti—Ro/SSA antibody
Anti-Ro/SS-B antibody
Anti-jo 1 antibody
Anti-RNP antibody
Anti-Smith antibody
Anti-dsDNA antibody
Rheumatoid factor
ESR
CBC
Complete meatabolic profile
LDH
CPK
Aldolase
Urinalysis
T4
TSH
Anti-thyroid antibody
Serum B12
EKG
Chest X-ray etc;

Treatments of Sjogren's Include:

Eye drops
Steroid
Cytoxan

Azothioprine
Plaquenil

Dermatoyositis is an inflammatory disease, which cuases muscle weakness. The cause of drematomyositis is not known. It affects more women than me. It occurs in all age groups but it is seen more frequently in ages 40 to 60.

Symptoms and complications of dermatomyositis include:

Muscles weakness
Aspiration pneumonia
Difficulty swallowing
Gastrointestinal problems
GERD
Bleeding from the stomach
Shortness of breath
Skin rashes
Calcium deposits on the skin
Raynaud's phenomenon
Recurrent infections
Myocarditis
Cardiac arrhythmias
Congestive heart failure
Lung fibrosis
Lung cancer (increase incidence)
Breast cancer (increase incidence)
Cervical cancer (increase incidence)
Pancreatic cancer (increase incidence)
Colon cancer (increase incidence)

Overlap /syndrome MCTD that can be seen in dermatomyositis include:

SLE
RA
Scleroderma
Sjogren syndrome etc;

Blood tests in use to help in the dianosis of dermatomyosistis include:

CPK
Aldolase
ANA
ENA

Rheumatoid factor
Anti-dsDNA
Antitransfer RNA synthetases
ESR
Skin biopsy

Radiology tests in use to help in the diagnosis of dermatomyositis include:

MRI of muscles
Electromyography (EMG)

Treatments of dermatomyosis include:

Steroid
Imuran
Cytoxan
Methotrexate
Azothioprine
Plaquenil
IV immunoglobulin
Prograf
Enbrel
Remicade
NSAID
Physical therapy
Speech therapy
Surgical removal of calcium deposits from skin.

Chapter 51
GOUT

Gout is a very common disease that affects eight millions of people in the U.S. and many more millions people in the world are affected by gout.

Three are other forms of arthritis are interconnected in that their symptoms are similar, and must be differentiated one from the other all the time.

They are as follows:
1. Acute gouty arthritis
2. Acute pseudo-gout
3. Septic arthritis

High serum uric acid affects 43.3 million American adults, representing 21 per cent of the U.S population. Diseases such as obesity and hypertension are associated with increased incidence of gout.

Acute gouty arthritis is one of the most painful conditions known in the field of medicine and to mankind. It usually occurs in a single joint such as the big toe, the ankle, the knee, the foot, or the wrist, etc.

The affected joint is usually markedly swollen, painful, and tender. Gouty arthritis occurs because of either too much production of uric acid or a decreased excretion of uric acid. Thirty two million people in the U.S. have levated uric acid. Source: International Medical news December 2010. In addition, 8 million Americans suffer from Gout and many of them are women.

Primary overproduction of uric acid occurs because of deficiency of hypoxanthine-guanine-phosphoribosyltransferase.

This enzyme deficiency causes an increased level of 5-phosphoribosyl-1-pyrophosphate (PRPP), which accelerates purine biosynthesis and results in an increased production of uric acid.

The reduced excretion of uric acid leads to uric acid accumulation. Reduced filtration, enhanced resorption, and decreased excretion are three other processes that lead to accumulation of uric acid in the blood.

Several other conditions can cause elevated uric acid.
Diuretic treatment
Lymphoma
Leukemia

Rapid cells turn over can cause acute and massive release of purines into the bloodstream as a result of chemotherapy-induced cells breakdown, resulting in marked increase of serum uric acid.

This is a crucial point to remember when treating patients who present with this form of cancer requiring acute chemotherapeutic treatment, so that IV fluid must be provided together with Allopurinol to prevent acute renal failure because of purine accumulation in the blood from clogging up the kidney tubules, causing them to fail.

Gout, which is the disease responsible for gouty arthritis, is an interesting disease but it is not under discussion here, but one of the many problems that it can cause, namely arthritis, is under discussion.

Gout causes the production of monosodium crystals, which accumulate in joints. These crystals cause an acute inflammation leading to swelling, warmth, and severe pain of the affected joints. When this attack occurs in the big toe, it is called podagra.

Acute gouty arthritis is one of the most painful conditions known to humanity. Another gouty condition that causes acute and chronic pain in joints is pseudo-gout. Pseudo-gout occurs most frequently in older women.

The inflammatory reaction that occurs in pseudo-gout is due to calcium pyrophosphate dihydrate crystals. These crystals are seen under the microscope as weakly positive birefringent using polarized light. Similarly, the monosodium urate crystals are seen in synovial fluid taken from the joint and examined under the microscope.

The blood test that is elevated in gout is uric acid. The uric acid can be tested in the blood as part of the blood chemistry profile. The normal uric acid in the blood is 2.8 to 6.0 mg/dl. The higher the level of uric acid in the blood the more likely that it will accumulate in joints, causing inflammation to occur. The repeated inflammatory reactions that occur in the joints can result in chronic destruction of these joints to different degrees.

It is important to realize that in an acute gouty arthritic attack the uric acid level may be normal to low. The reason is that the uric acid is moving from the blood to the joints, thereby reducing its level in the blood. When someone presents with an acute, swollen, hot, and painful joint, there are really three major considerations:

1. Gout
2. Pseudo-gout
3. Septic arthritis or
4. Trauma

Septic arthritis can occur because of bacteria in the blood settling into a joint, causing inflammation to occur. Many clinical conditions can be associated with septic arthritis:

1. Gonorrheal infection is probably the most common in sexually active individuals;
2. Pneumonia with bacteremia;
3. Sub-acute bacterial endocarditis (SBE) as seen frequently in IV drug-abusing individuals or any non-IV drug addict with SBE;
4. Penetrating trauma in a joint, etc.

To differentiate gouty arthritis in the joint from septic arthritis, one must tap synovial fluid off the joint and send it to the laboratory for evaluation. In the laboratory, the fluid will be evaluated for:

1. Turbidity or cloudiness
2. The total number of white blood cells
3. The level of protein
4. The bacterial content of the fluid by gram stain
5. Bacterial growth on bacterial cultures
6. The presence or absence of crystals in the fluid, etc.

Further evaluations include history and physical examinations and x-ray studies of the affected joint.

To treat gouty arthritis the physician has to determine the extent and severity of the symptoms. The most effective treatment to treat acute gouty arthritis includes:

Colchicine
Colcrys
Indocin
Motrin
Naprosyn
Anaprox
Steroid

Allopurinol during an acute attack of gout might lead to an idiosyncratic reaction, worsening the condition.

Once the acute attack has been brought under control, Allopurinol 300 mg per day is given to lower the level of uric acid in the blood and colchicine 0.6 mg two times per day is given along with it.

NSAIDS or Indocin may be given clinically to prevent acute attacks from occurring. For reasons that are not quite clear, acute gouty arthritic attacks seem to occur in spite of the fact that the patient is on a good dose of prophylactic medications.

Both gout and pseudo-gout can lead to markedly deformed joints with chronic arthritic pain. It is said that a diet that contains sweetbread, shellfish, too much red meat and red wine can all contribute to bring about acute attacks of gout. Therefore, dietary management with a decreased intake of this type of foods is a reasonable approach in the management of patients with gout and frequent gouty arthritic attacks.

As for septic arthritis, this diagnosis must be made without failure, or the affected joint will be destroyed. The treatment of choice for septic arthritis is antibiotics given intravenously. Once the suspicion is strong that septic arthritis may exist, the joint must be tapped and fluid sent to the lab for studies and IV antibiotics must be given to the affected individual immediately. The type of antibiotics given depends on the clinical profile of the patient involved. Physicians are trained to know precisely what to do, and how to do it in these circumstances.

Chapter 52
FIBROMYALGIA

Although there are no cures for these different arthritic conditions, there are many treatments that are available to relieve their symptoms. Blacks and other minorities for a multitude of reasons as just outlined, have a higher propensity of developing certain types of arthritis as compared to whites. Therefore, it is important that individuals remain vigilant as to the presence of these different arthritic conditions and seek medical attention as quickly as possible to help alleviate their arthritic symptoms.

Fibromyalgia is chronic diffuse painful disease that affects 5 million people in the U.S.

It is more common in women than men with a ratio of 9-1 women vs men. Blacks have more diffuse pain than do whites From Fibromyalgia and black women and other minority have more severe pain from FM do white women. Fibromyalgia affects people of all ethnicities and 1 in 20 people or 350 million people in the world are affected by fibromyalgia.

The cause of Fibromyalgia is not known. The symptoms of FM include
Diffuse chronic pain in muscles
Diffuse joints pain
Fatigue
Head ache
Imsomnia
Depression etc;

The diagnosis is made clinically by physicians by ruling out other conditions such as
Ossteoarthritis
Rheumatoid arthritis
Lupus
Gout
MCVD etc;
Evaluations of FM include
History
Physical examination
CBC
Chemistry profile
T4 and TSH
ESR

Rheumatoid factor
ANA
CRP
Urinalysis
B12
Serum Ferritin
Vitamin D level
Lyme disease blood tests
Chest Xray
EMG
Xray of affected joints
MRI of affected joints

Medications available to treat FM include
NSAIDs
Lyrica
Analgesics
Ati-depression medications
Sleeping medications
Sometime psychiatric evaluation and treatments as needed maybe necessary.

Chapter 53
PSORIATRIC ARTHRITIS

The cause of psoriatic arthritis is not known and psoriatic arthritis is a chronic inflammatory disease of the skin that affects both skin and joints. There is a genetic component to psoriatic arthritis.

In addition, psoriatic arthritis can be systemic and affects the eyes, lungs, heart, and kidney. Psoriasis affectcs about 2 % of whites in the U.S. It affects about 8% of people with psoriasis and is less common in blacks as compared to whites.

It usually found in people between the ages of 40-50 years. Most of the time, psoriasis precedes psoriatic arthritis by 15-20 years. However, sometime arthritis precedes psoriasis by as much as 20 years. 7.5 million People in the U.S. have psoriasis and 30% of people with psoriasis develop psoriatic arthritis.

About 5 million people in the U.S. have psoriatic arthritis and 125 million people in the world have psoriasis and about 30% of them have psoriatic arthritis. People of all racial back grounds have psoriatic arthritis.

Symptoms psoriatic arthritis include

Swollen and pain in knees
Swollen and pain in ankles
Swollen and pain wrists
Swollen, stiffeness and pain hands
Pain and stiffness in shoulders
Pain and stiffness in neck
Pain and stiffeness in lower back
Pain and stiffness in upper back
Pain and stiffness in buttocks
Pain and stiffness in the elbows
Shortness of breath
Chest pain
Blurry vision etc;

The diagnosis of psoriatic arthritis is made clinically.
Evaluations of psoriatic include
History

Physical examination
CBC
Chemistry profile
ANA
ESR
RF
CRP
T4 and TSH
B12 level
Vitamin D level
Serum Ferritin
HIV blood test (some patients with AIDS do develop a sporiatic rash)
RPR
Serum uric acid
Blood test for HAL-B27 gene (50% of people with psoriatic arthritis are positiove for this gene)
Skin biopsy
Chest xray
EKG
Echocardiogram
Eye examination by an Ophthamologist (some people with psoriatic arthritis develop iristi and become blind)

Medications available to treat psoriatic arthritis include
NSAIDs
Steroid
Methotrexate
Plaquenil
Celebrex
Endrel
Exercise etc;

Chapter 54
SARCOIDOSIS

Sarcoidosis is a disease of unknown cause, which is very common among blacks and other minorities. In the United States, the ratio of blacks to whites who have sarcoidosis is about 17:1. In other words, more blacks are affected by sarcoidosis than whites are. Blacks and other minorities are affected at an earlier age and the disease is more sever in blacks as compared to whites. In addition, the death rate is higher in blacks and other minorities as compared to other racial groups. Sarcoidosis occurs in the age's range 20 to 40. Worldwide the incidence of sarcoidosis is 20 per 100,000. or about 1.4 million people. The incidence of sarcoidosis is very high in Scandinavian people.

The disease is a multi-system disease, although the lungs are the most frequently affected organ. The disease is characterized pathologically by forming what is called non-caseating granulomas with derangement of the normal tissue architecture of the nodes.

The organs that are frequently affected in sarcoidosis are:

Lungs
Skin
Eyes
Heart
Kidney
Liver
Spleen
Bone marrow
The exocrine system
The hematopoeitic system (blood system)
The gastrointestinal tract etc
Upper respiratory tract
Neurological system
Musculoskeletal system

The symptoms of sarcoidosis include:

Fever
Malaise
Anorexia

Weight loss
Dry cough
Shortness of breath
Redness in the eyes
Blurry vision
Bell palsy
Skin rash
Muscles pain
Joints pain
Chest pain
Dry mouth
Anemia
Low white blood cells
Low platelets
Enlarged liver
Enlarged liver
Cardiac arrhythmias
Enlarged lymph nodes etc;

In acute sarcoidosis, the affected person may have fever, malaise, and anorexia with weight loss. The vast majority of individuals who develop sarcoidosis are younger than 40 years old. Patients with pulmonary sarcoid often have shortness of breath, cough, and sometimes chest pain. The chest x-ray in sarcoidosis often shows bilateral hilar adenopathy in association with pain in the joints.

Biopsy of the hilar node done via bronchoscopy examination shows non-caseating granulomas. About 50% of individuals with pulmonary sarcoid develop permanent pulmonary disease and about 15% go on to develop pulmonary fibrosis. Other organs that are frequently affected by sarcoidosis are as follows:

Lymph node enlargement is quite common in sarcoidosis. Enlargement of nodes inside the chest is seen in about 75% to 90% of individuals affected with sarcoidosis. Enlargement of cervical, inguinal and axillary nodes are quite common in sarcoidosis. Biopsy of any of these peripheral nodes is likely to show the classic lesions seen in sarcoidosis, namely non-caseating granuloma.

The classic lesions seen over the skin of individuals with Sarcoidosis is something called erythema nodosum. Other skin lesions that can be seen include a maculopapular rash, subcutaneous nodes and lupus pernio (indurated blue/purple swollen lesion on the nose, cheeks, lips, ears, fingers, etc.).

Erythema nodosum is frequently accompanied by symptoms such as polyarthralgia. Eye problems occur in about 25% of people who have sarcoidosis. Usually the iris and the uveal tract are involved, etc. Anterior uveitis occurs in approximately 75% of patients with sarcoidosis and posterior uveitis occurs in about 25% of affected patients.

Blurry vision, photophobia, and tearing occur frequently in patients with sarcoidosis. The conjunctival involvement is quite common as well as the lacrimal gland. If the lacrimal gland is involved, then frequently dry and sore eyes can develop. If sarcoidosis of the eyes is left untreated or treated too late, total blindness can result.

The upper airway can be involved in up to 20% of patients suffering with sarcoidosis. Hoarseness, nasal stuffiness, dyspnea, stridor, and wheezing can occur.

The heart can be involved in up to 5% of patients with sarcoidosis. The conduction system of the heart can be involved, leading to complete heart block. Cardiac arrhythmias are common and the left ventricle is frequently involved. Pericarditis and congestive heart failure can occur.

The nervous system is affected in about 5% of patients with Sarcoidosis. Any part of the nervous system can become involved with sarcoidosis. The seventh nerve is frequently affected by sarcoidosis, causing unilateral facial paralysis. Other nervous system involvement may include optic nerve dysfunction, papilledema, hearing difficulty, pituitary and hypothalamic dysfunction, etc.

The endocrine system can be involved in sarcoidosis, causing diabetes insipidus. The adrenal glands can also be involved, resulting in an Addison-like syndrome.

The reproductive system can also be involved with sarcoidosis, but women can get pregnant while suffering with the disease. The disease seems to improve during pregnancy, only to flare up after delivery.

The disease can involve the bone marrow in up to 40% of patients. Anemia, neutropenia and thrombocytopenia can occur as a result of bone marrow involvement. The spleen can become enlarged in sarcoidosis.

The liver is involved up to 90% of the time in sarcoidosis. The liver may be enlarged 30% of the time. The kidneys can be involved in a small percentage of patients with sarcoidosis.

More commonly, patients with sarcoidosis can have high serum calcium, and high calcium in the urine can cause calcium kidney stones.

The musculoskeletal system is frequently involved in sarcoidosis, with bone, joint and muscle pain. Bones of the hands and feet are most commonly involved. Nevertheless, any bone can be involved.

Sometimes the first presentation of sarcoidosis is painful and swollen joints and bone pains. Arthritis and arthralgias frequently occur in large joints. Deformities may occur in joints and bones in sarcoidosis. Muscle weakness and symptoms of polymyositis may occur, confusing sarcoidosis with collagen vascular diseases or mixed collagen vascular diseases.

How to diagnose sarcoidosis:

First and foremost, it is important to take a good history from the patient.

Second, x-ray tests such as chest x-ray showing bilateral hilar adenopathy may be seen. If the presenting symptoms refer to the eye, then an eye examination is important; uveitis is a frequent finding in patients with sarcoidosis with eye symptoms.

Laboratory tests in use to diagnose sarcoidosis include:

CBC
Complete metabolic chemistry profile
ESR
Angiotensin-I-converting enzyme which is elevated in about 2/3 of patients with sarcoidosis. Serum calcium, 24-hour urinary calcium is also elevated in patients with sarcoidosis.
Urinalysis
Non-caseating granuloma on lymph node or other tissues on biopsy

Therefore, if the complex of symptoms fits the profile, the angiotensin-converting enzyme is elevated, and the tissue biopsy shows non-caseating granuloma, then the patient has sarcoidosis.

Other tests in use to diagnose sarcoidosis include:
Chest xray
CT of chest
MRI of chest
Pulmonary function test
EKG
Echocardiogram
Renal ultra sound
Examination by eye doctors
Examination by pulmonary specialists

It is important to keep in mind that in clinical medicine things do not always fit into a neat package which means that clinical judgment must be brought into play to arrive at a diagnosis even though all the pieces of the puzzle may not fit.

Medications in use to treat sarcoidosis include:

Steroid
Methotrexate
Imuran
Cytoxan
Remicade
Azothiaprine

In up to 50% of cases, the disease resolves spontaneously. However, clinically, it may not be wise to take a chance and not treat, because the disease can go on to cause permanent damage to vital organs such as the eyes, the heart, the lungs, etc., which in some instances may be fatal (see the chapter on lung diseases for further discussion about sarcoidosis).

Chapter 55
EYE DISEASES

The incidence of eye diseases and blindness are more common in blacks and other minorities than in their white counterparts. Many of the diseases that predispose the development of diseases in the eye are much more common blacks and other minorities.

For example, diseases such as hypertension, diabetes mellitus, and glaucoma are much more common in blacks than in whites and other racial groups.

"285 million people are visually impaired worldwide, 39 million are blind and 246 million have low vision. About 90% of the world visually impaired live in developing countries. "Source: WHO

The incidence of glaucoma is five times higher in blacks and other minorities than in whites. 60.5 million People in the world are diagnosed with glaucoma yearly.

Diabetes is among the most common causes of blindness. Tewnty six million Americans have diabetes. According to the American College of Ophthalmology, about 5 million Americans have glaucoma. Both hypertension and diabetes mellitus predispose a person to the development of glaucoma. Of the 5 million or so Americans who have glaucoma, a very large percentage of them are blacks. For reasons that are not yet clear, blacks have a higher propensity to develop glaucoma than whites do.

Glaucoma runs in families. About 80,000 individuals go blind in the U.S. because of glaucoma yearly. What makes glaucoma so dangerous is the fact that it causes no pain. So, a person whose intraocular pressure is high, which is the first step to the development of glaucoma, will not know that the pressure inside the eye is high unless she goes to the ophthalmologist to have her eye pressure tested.

As is the case for many other diseases, blacks and other minorities often present for medical evaluations when the disease they are suffering from have already gone too far. Sometimes, these conditions are too far gone to be helped, even with the best medications or the best of medical procedures.

There are four different types of glaucoma:

1. Primary open angle glaucoma
2. Secondary glaucoma

3. Angle closure glaucoma
4. Congenital glaucoma

One-fourth of all cases of glaucoma presents at birth and are due to congenital reasons. According to the Center for Health Statistics, in Bethesda, Maryland, 1.2 out of every 100 individuals have some form of eye disease. Though this is a high percentage, the incidence is much higher among the blacks and other minorities than in whites.

The reasons are:

> The higher incidence of hypertension, leading to hypertensive retinopathy with hemorrhage inside the eyes, which, if left untreated, will cause permanent blindness,

> The higher incidence of diabetes in blacks and other minorities and in particular obese Blacks, Hispanics, American Indians, and Alaskan Natives who have the propensity to develop diabetes mellitus because of obesity, which then leads to diabetic retinopathy with different degrees of bleeding inside the eyes that can lead to blindness if left untreated

> The high incidence of trauma to the eye which occurs much more frequently in blacks and other minorities as compared to whites because blacks and other minorities are more likely to get exposed to riskier jobs that predispose them to a higher likelihood of being injured in their eyes on the job.

Besides glaucoma, diabetes mellitus, and hypertension, other diseases that affect the eyes include cataracts, syphilis, sarcoidosis, sickle cell disease, AIDS, temporal arteritis, vitamin deficiency, and malignant tumor, etc.

In adults there are three different types of glaucoma:

1. Primary open angle glaucoma
2. Angle closure glaucoma
3. Low tension glaucoma

There are about 5 million reported cases of glaucoma in the United States. Glaucoma is the third leading cause of eye problems leading to blindness in blacksand other minorities in the United States and around the world. It is the number one cause of blindness in the world.

The incidence of blindness because of Glaucoma is 7 to 8 times higher in blacks and other minorities than in whites. Blacks and other minorities between the ages of 44 and 65, and in particular, those who are hypertensive and have a family history of glaucoma have a 15 to 17 times greater possibility of developing glaucoma than whites. According to published reports, 30% of glaucoma patients have family history of glaucoma.

Open-angle glaucoma

The cause of open angle glaucoma is an inherited defect in the function of the endothelial cells of the cellular meshwork inside the eyes. The result is increased production of aqueous humor fluid inside the eyes on the one hand, and on the other hand, failure of drainage of the aqueous humor fluid, resulting in increased pressure inside the eyes.

The normal intraocular pressure is 13 to 20 mm/Hg. While an intraocular pressure of 13-20 mm/Hg is normal for whites, it is not necessarily normal for blacks and other minorities. This fact must be kept in mind because blacks and other minorities have a higher incidence of glaucoma; it is also true that glaucoma is much more aggressive in its progression in blacks and other minorities than it is in whites. Therefore, an intraocular pressure above 14 in a minority person must be watched closely and evaluated more frequently.

When the pressure inside the eyes is elevated, it damages the optic nerve. The optic nerve is the nerve that allows the eyes to see. Once the optic nerve is damaged, vision becomes impaired. Though the intraocular pressure is elevated, it causes no pain, and therefore, a person suffering from elevated intraocular pressure has no way to know about it until he or she is examined by an ophthalmologist.

The test done to evaluate the pressure inside the eye is called tonometry. The test used to evaluate the optic nerve is called a visual field. Elevated intraocular pressure does not mean glaucoma. If the intraocular pressure is allowed to remain high for an extended period of time months to years the optic nerve will become damaged. Once the optic nerve is damaged, then glaucoma ensues.

Open-angle glaucoma is responsible for more than 90% of all cases of blindness. The first sign that a person has glaucoma is when the person loses his or her peripheral vision. About 5% of first-degree relatives of people with open angle glaucoma 50 years or older develop open angle glaucoma, as compared to 1% of people in the general population.

Three things happen clinically in open angle glaucoma:

1. Intraocular pressure of 24 mm/Hg or greater
2. Cupping of the optic disc
3. Visual field loss

Typically, the first modality of treatment in someone with open angle glaucoma is eye drop medication to either reduce the production of aqueous humor fluid and/or increase the drainage, thereby lowering the intraocular pressure.

Some frequently used eye drops include:

1. Pilocarpine
2. Timoptic
3. Ocupress
4. Trusopt
5. Carbachol
6. Phystignine salicylate
7. Desmocranium bromide (Humorsol)
8. Acetazolamide (Diamox)
9. Isofurophate (Floropryl)
10. Btaxololhydrochloride (Betoptic)
11. Optipranolol
12. Propine
13. Latanoprox solution (Xalatan)
14. Betagan,
15. Cosopt
16. Alphagan P
17. Travatan etc;

If maximum eye drop treatment fails to bring the intraocular pressure down and visual field abnormality starts to develop, then laser treatment is carried out to facilitate drainage of aqueous humor fluid from the eye, thereby reducing the intraocular pressure.

As stated before, the peripheral vision is the first vision to go when increased intraocular pressure damages the optic nerve.

Angle-closure glaucoma

It is reported that angle closure glaucoma occurs mostly in individuals who are farsighted and are above age 55. About 5% of first-degree relatives of people with angle closure glaucoma are affected with the same condition in their later years.

There are three different stages of angle closure glaucoma:

1. Sub-acute angle closure glaucoma
2. Acute angle closure glaucoma
3. Chronic angle closure glaucoma

As just outlined, angle closure glaucoma occurs principally because of blockage to the proper drainage of the aqueous humor fluid that is produced inside the eyes.

In sub-acute angle closure glaucoma, the drainage is occurring in an insidious way so that the patient's eyes find ways to compensate, keeping the intraocular pressure intermittently normal.

In acute angle closure glaucoma, the intraocular pressure rises suddenly, resulting in a painful red eye, with reduced ability to see in that eye. When the examining physician places his or her finger on the affected eyeball, it is rock-hard and quite painful. On tonometric examination, the intraocular pressure may be as high as 50 mm/Hg. The affected patient feels very sick, with pain and nausea, and may even vomit.

Next to trauma to the eye, acute angle closure glaucoma is the severest emergency seen in the field of ophthalmology.

The first step in the treatment of acute angle glaucoma is to try to bring the intraocular pressure down as quickly as possible. To do that, a doctor is likely to treat the eye with Pilocarpine eye drops 2% to 4% for five minutes. Later 0.5% Timolol solution is placed in the affected eye. If this does not work then 500 mg of Diamox IV is given to bring the pressure down.

If the intraocular pressure fails to come down in spite of these treatments, then IV Mannitol can be given to reduce the intraocular pressure, while the eye doctor is getting the patient ready for surgery to open the eye to allow the aqueous humor fluid to drain, bringing the intraocular pressure down to save the eye. Frequently after surgery, eye drops are used to maintain a normal pressure in the eye.

As angle closure glaucoma affects both eyes, in treating acute angle closure glaucoma, the non-affected eye must also receive immediate treatment with 0.5%-1% Pilocarpine, followed by Timolol or other beta-blocker like eye drops.

The Pilocarpine is used every four hours and the beta blocker twice a day until prophylactic laser surgery can be done to that eye to prevent a similar event from occurring as that which has occurred in the acutely affected eye.

Other forms of glaucoma include:

1. Low-tension glaucoma
2. Congenital glaucoma
3. Secondary glaucoma, which can result from using iridocyclites, steroid treatment, either directly into the eye or when taken by mouth for long periods of time.

Low-tension glaucoma is seen most often in elderly individuals who suffer from severe circulatory diseases impeding blood flow. Glaucoma occurs more frequently in blacks and other minorities than in whites. The ratio is about 5-6:1 black versus white.

Glaucoma also occurs in blacks and other minorities at a younger age than in whites and it is more aggressive in blacks and other minorities and leads to blindness more rapidly than in whites. The most important thing to do is to get the eyes examined in order that if the pressure inside the eye is found to be elevated then appropriate treatments and other measures can be instituted to prevent progression to blindness.

Cataract

Another common disease of the eye is cataract. The most common form of cataract is age-related cataract or senile cataract. Cataract is an opacification of the lens of the eyes. 24.4 million Americans have cataracts and 50 million people worldwide are diagnosed with cataracts yearly.

The second form of cataract is a congenital cataract, which is usually the result of maternal rubella or cytomegalovirus infection during the first trimester of pregnancy.

Other causes of cataract include diabetes mellitus, systemic use of steroids, myotonic dystrophy, uveitis, cigarette smoking, heavy alcohol consumption, etc.

Trauma to the eye is also a common cause of cataract. Traumatic cataract is more common in blacks and other minorities than in whites because the economic circumstances of blacks and other minorities is worse, as compared to that of whites, exposing blacks and other minorities to more work-related trauma to the eyes.

The first sign of cataract is blurry vision, which progresses over months to years, with no pain, or redness to the eye and obvious clouding of the lens of the eyes when examined with the ophthalmoscope.

There are three types of cataract:

1. Posterior subcapsular cataract
2. Cortical cataract
3. Mixed cataract

Treatment of cataract

Once the diagnosis of cataract is established, the first mode of treatment is glasses to improve vision. This is the conservative management. When this treatment fails, then surgical removal of the cataract is recommended to the patient. There are two types of surgical cataract removal procedures:

1. Extracapsular cataract removal with implantation of an intraocular lens.
2. Intracapsular cataract removal

The second type of surgical procedure is much less popular because of the advent of microsurgery, which facilitates the first procedure. Cataract removal surgery is carried out in the operating room with the patient being able to go home in a few hours after the operation has been completed with a patch on the operated eye, to be followed by the surgeon in his or her office. The patient is fully awake during the time of the surgery. Only the eye being operated on is anesthetized.

Hypertensive retinopathy:

Hypertension has many complications associated with it and if left untreated will cause serious damage to occur in many organs. Prominent among these organs are the eyes. The increase in pressure within the vessels of the eye causes different degrees of damage to occur within the lumen of these vessels. The damaged vessels then trap platelets and other materials from the blood on the inner surface of these vessels, starting a nidus, which leads to plaque formation.

Leakage of fatty material occurs out of these damaged vessels, making the situation more complicated. This process perpetuates itself over time, causing different vascular abnormalities to occur inside the eyes, resulting in hypertensive retinopathy.

Hypertensive retinopathy is graded as 1, 2, 3, and 4, depending on the severity of the vascular abnormalities.

Grade 1 shows arteriolar narrowing.
Grade 2 shows arterio-venous nicking, some exudates, and hemorrhages.
Grade 3 shows retinal edema, hemorrhage, and cottonwool spots. Grade 4 shows a combination of Grade 3 plus papilledema.

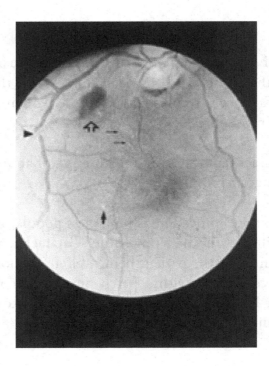

Figure 55.1: Showing different types of abnormalities in the eye of a hypertensive patient (hypertensive retinopathy). Small arrow showing silver wiring. Big arrow showing hand yellow exudates. Open arrow head shoing blot hemorrhage. Arrow head shoing A-V nicking.

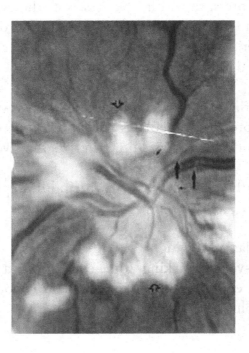

Figure 55.2: Showing different types of abnormalities in the eye of a hypertensive patient (hypertensive retinopathy). Small arrows showing early papilledema. One big

arrow pointing to vein engorgement (larger vessel). The other big arrow pointing to arterial attenuation (smaller vessel); open arrow showing cotton wool exudates.

If proper treatment is not provided for these abnormalities, the patient often develops blindness. Hypertension is a very common disease, according to the latest estimates, occurring in about 73 million individuals in the United States. About 42% of these individuals go untreated for hypertension. Hypertension is the number-one disease among blacks in the United States.

The percentage of hypertension is higher among blacks and other minorities than whites are because there are many more obese blacks. In fact, 76% of black Americans are overweight/obese, and obesity has a major impact in both the causation of hypertension and in making it worse.

It is common knowledge that many blacks and other minorities with hypertension are being treated inappropriately because many of them are receiving the wrong medications, namely they are not being treated with water pills. Thiazide water pill (diuretic) is the most appropriate and the most effective medication to treat blacks with hypertension the world over.

According to a recent report that appears in the literature, it costs about 7-10 cents per day to treat patients with diuretic, as compared to an ACE inhibitor and calcium channel blocker that costs about $1000 per year each. This amount of momey represents about 8% of the Social Security income of many people who are on Social Security.

This report confirms the inappropriateness of the treatment that some people are receiving for their hypertension. The result is that they are getting treatments for their blood pressures that cause their blood pressure to go without proper control, resulting in end organs damage. The eyes are one of the end organs. The medication prescribed is often too expensive to buy, so the condition goes untreated, resulting in progression of their hypertension.

Therefore, the percentage of people with untreated hypertension is much higher in blacks and other minorities than it is in whites, as most blacks and other minorities often are forced to do without adequate health care. It is, therefore, not difficult to see why there is such a high incidence of glaucoma and other hypertension-associated lesions in the eyes of many blacks, leading to their very high incidence of blindness.

Diabetes mellitus and its effects on the eyes

Type II diabetes mellitus is very common among blacks and other minorities and this is in part due to the fact that the incidence of of overweight/obese among blacks and other minorities is very high, and obesity is highly associated with diabetes. According to the American Diabetic Association, there are roughly 24 million individuals diagnosed with diabetes mellitus in the United States.

Worldwide there 1.9 billion people who are overweight and 2.1 billion people who are obese.

All diabetics are at risk of developing diseases of the eyes, such as cataracts, glaucoma and diabetic retinopathy with hemorrhage inside the eyes. One out of every 14 African-Americans is likely to develop diabetes. This rate is 30% to 40% higher in blacks and other minorities than that seen in whites. Therefore, blacks and other minorities are 30% to 40% more likely to have diabetes eye diseses compared to whites.

Diabetic retinopathy

Diabetic retinopathy is a very serious disease, which causes blindness in a significant number of blacks and other minorities who are diabetics. The same is true for any individuals who suffer from diabetes mellitus. Some of the lesions that can be seen in patients who are suffering from diabetes mellitus are as follows:

1. Micro-aneurysm
2. Arteriolar narrowing
3. Retinal edema
4. Hard exudates
5. Venous abnormalities
6. Soft exudates
7. Vitreus hemorrhages
8. Retinal hemorrhages
9. Retinal detachment, etc.

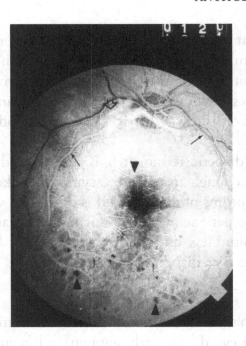

Figure 55.3-Showing different degrees of abnormalities in the eye of a patient with diabetes mellitus (diabetic retinopathy). Fluorescein angiogram shortly after injection of dye in patient's eye. Dye in arteries (white) and just starting to enter veins (large arrow). White area off NH is neovascular tuff (open arrow). White spots are hemorrhages (arrow heads). Tiny white spots are micro-aneurysms (small arrow).

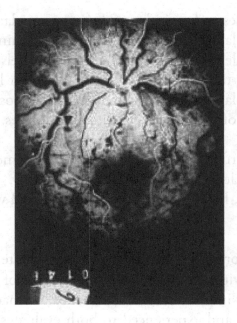

Figure 55.4-Showing different degrees of abnormalities in the eye of a patient with diabetes mellitus (diabetic retinopathy). Large arrows showing dilated veins. Arrow heads showing hemorrhages inside the eye.

517

It should be noted that eye symptoms and abnormalities may be the first signs that a person is suffering from diabetes mellitus. Very often, the patient presents to the ophthalmologist complaining of blurry vision, and the examining ophthalmologist, if he or she suspects diabetes mellitus as a cause of the blurriness of the eyes, can then order the blood sugar to confirm whether it is elevated blood sugar that is causing the blurry vision.

As just stated, if the diabetic retinopathy is not very advanced, the fact that the blood sugar is elevated is enough to cause eye symptoms like blurry vision. Once the patient presents with symptoms of diabetes and is diagnosed with diabetes, the treating physician should refer the patient to an eye doctor for an appropriate eye evaluation to prevent unnecessary blindness due to diabetes mellitus. Because the incidence of diabetes mellitus is on the rise, diabetes-associated blindness is also on the rise among all people.

It is very important that individuals with diabetes mellitus understand that if they present themselves to the eye doctor early enough and keep their blood sugar under tight control, and remains under constant care of a qualified ophthalmologist; they can prevent eventual blindness secondary to the effects of diabetes mellitus to the eyes.

Diabetes and ischemic diseases of the eyes

Diabetes mellitus causes ischemia because it causes plaque depositions to occur, the same way it causes plaque depositions to occur within vessels of the legs. The same process also causes deposition of plaque in the vessels of the eyes. When these very delicate vessels within the eyes have plaque within their lumens, and lipid material leaks out of these vessels, platelet deposition and plaque deposition take place, resulting, gradually, in the occlusion of these vessels to different degrees.

The occlusion causes rupture of these vessels and hemorrhage to occur, leading to different types and degrees of diabetic retinopathy. That is the underlying pathophysiology as to why, how these conditions occur, and why they lead to blindness if left untreated.

The eye is the only organ in the human body where an examining physician can actually see a vessel with the naked eye and the use of an instrument called the ophthalmoscope. It is very important that all referrals are made to an ophthalmologist, who is a physician trained and experienced to both evaluates and treats diseases of the eyes.

Hemoglobinopathies and eye disease

Sickle cell disease is the number-one abnormal hemoglobin disease that causes eye disease in those affected. Many three different types of sickle cell diseases that can cause retinopathy:

1. Sickle cell disease retinopathy (SS)
2. Sickle cell-C retinopathy (SC)
3. Sickle thalassemia retinopathy

The most severe retinopathy among these three conditions is seen in sickle cell-C disease. There are two types of retinopathies seen in sickle disease: the proliferative type and the non-proliferative type. The proliferative type is more common in SC disease and sickle thalassemia than in SS disease.

The problems occur because of sludging of red blood cells inside the small vessels of the eyes. The red cells in sickle cell disease are mal-shaped and sticky, making it difficult for them to pass through these vessels. The result is occlusion of these vessels, resulting in a multitude of vascular abnormalities within the eyes.

The types of vascular abnormalities range from arteriovenous anastomosis and neovascularization that result in leakage of blood through these newly formed vessels and cause different degrees of hemorrhages.

Retinal tear and detachment commonly occur as well. Flurocescin angiography is used to demonstrate these abnormalities. Photo-coagulation can be used as a treatment modality and laser is used to treat these conditions in the eyes of sicklers with retinopathy

Sarcoidosis and its effects on the eyes

Sarcoidosis is quite common in blacks and the eyes are frequently affected in this condition. In fact, eye symptoms are often the presenting symptoms of sarcoidosis. Redness and swelling of the eyes with blurry vision are often seen. The eye doctor usually looks for anterior uveitis, which is often present when sarcoidosis involves the eyes.

Slit-lamp examination is usually carried out to evaluate the eyes when sarcoidosis is suspected. If sarcoidosis is not recognized and treated early with Prednisone, the end result often means total blindness in the affected eye. Glaucoma is also seen in chronic untreated sarcoidosis of the eye. The angiotensin-1-converting enzyme blood test is often elevated in individuals affected with sarcoidosis, and the serum calcium may be elevated as well.

AIDS and eye disease

AIDS, as a viral illness, frequently affects the eyes. The most common infection that is seen in the eyes of AIDS patients is cytomegalovirus (CMV). CMV causes an infection of the eyes called retinitis. Blacks are affected more than whites with AIDS-associated CMV retinitis are because the percentage of blacks with AIDS is much higher than that of whites.

CMV retinitis in AIDS is quite difficult to treat and eradicate. The most effective medication is Ganciclovir. This medication has serious side effects and must be given IV in the hospital setting.

Temporal arteritis and eye disease:

Temporal arteritis (giant cell arteritis) is a condition seen in middle-aged to elderly individuals The diagnosis of temporal arteritis cannot be missed, and, in fact, must not be missed, for if it is missed, the end result is permanent blindness in the affected eye.

Usually, the patient comes to see the physician with headache, general malaise, and visual abnormality, and may report having a low-grade fever. Following a physical examination, a diagnosis can quickly be established by doing an erythrocyte sedimentation rate (ESR). If the ESR is very high (normal ESR is from 10- 30 ml/hr) then the diagnosis of temporal arteritis is very likely.

The next step is to admit the patient to the hospital for treatment with high-dose IV steroids. The ophthalmologist always must always be involed in the care of the patient, to carry out a thorough eye examination of the patient.

The next step is to call a surgeon in to do a temporal artery biopsy. It is not necessary to wait for the biopsy before starting steroid treatment. If the physician waits for the results of the biopsy, it may be too late to save the eyes. A negative temporal artery biopsy does not rule out the diagnosis of temporal arteritis (giant cell arteritis) because this disease is often a segmental disease and a normal segment of artery could easily have been biopsied, leaving behind the abnormal segment.

Vitamin deficiency and eye disease

As alcoholism is quite common among all people, and certain vitamin deficiencies are likely to occur. One of the frequent vitamin deficiencies that occur in this setting is Vitamin B6 (thiamine). Thiamine deficiency can cause ocular motor palsy. It can also lead to Wernicke's disease, which is associated with nystagmus, ptosis, retinal hemorrhage, diplopia, and internal strabismus.

Treatment consists of injection of thiamine to replete the store, followed by B-complex vitamins by mouth, which contains all the B vitamins, and abstinence from alcohol is the key. Thiamine by mouth can also be given following the acute repletion of the stores.

Malignant tumor and eye symptoms

Malignant tumors, such as primary melanoma, tumor of the lid of the eye (associated with xeroderma pigmentosum), can affect the eye. The eye can also be affected by sarcoma.

Malignant melanoma is a particularly troublesome disease that can lead to the demise of the patient if not diagnosed quickly and treatment started right away.

Metastatic cancer may first show signs of its presence in the eye. This is believed to be due to an autoimmune phenomenon (the body reacting to the cancer as a foreign agent), thereby producing an antibody against it, causing an inflammatory reaction to occur in the eye, resulting in eye symptoms.

Sexually transmited diseases and eye diseases include:

AIDS (see CMV retinitis above)
Syphilis
Herpes simplex infection

Syphilis and eye problems

In the latter stage of syphilis, a variety of different eye problems can occur. One problem may be small, irregular pupils that sometimes react to accommodation, but does not react to light. Another problem might be the Argyle-Robertson pupils (the result of atrophy of the iris), which is seen in neurosyphilis. Neurosyphilis is common in people
suffering from AIDS.

Other problems that can occur in neurosyphilis include iritis and photophobia. Adhesion of the iris to the lens of the eye can also occur, which can cause a fixed pupil. These problems can all be picked up through a good eye examination by an internist who can then refer the affected person to an ophthalmologist for further evaluation and treatments.

According to The Center for Disease Control and Prevention (CDC) guidelines, treatment for neurosyphilis must include blood VDRL and FTA-ABS. A lumbar puncture ought to be done to obtain cerebrospinal fluid (CSF). The CSF fluid must be sent for VDRL and FTA-ABS. If it is positive, then treatment for neurosyphilis must be started by giving 10 to 20 million units of aqueous penicillin daily IV for ten days.

In addition, a three-week course of 2.4 million units of Bicillin for 7.2 million units must be given. If the patient has HIV infection (AIDS) and a positive VDRL, FTA-ABS in the blood, even if the CSF is negative or if the patient refuses a lumbar puncture, the same protocol as just outlined ought to be employed to treat the patient.

This ought to be done because neurosyphilis is quite prevalent in individuals with AIDS. If a person is allergic to penicillin, then Erythromycin 2 grams by mouth daily for 30 days or Tetracycline 2 grams daily for 30 days should be prescribed to treat the syphilis. Keep in mind that if a person is pregnant she ought not to be treated with Tetracycline.

In summary, eye diseases are very common in blacks, for the reasons outlined in this chapter. Diseases such as diabetes mellitus, hypertension, trauma in the workplace to the eyes, sickle cell disease, sarcoidosis, AIDS, Syphilis, all of which participate in the rising incidence of glaucoma that is five times higher in blacks than whites. (see the section on sarcoidosis in the previous chapter above)

The overall economic and educational situations of the majority of blacks will have to be improved drastically if it is expected that a real impact can be made to decrease the accelerated rate of blindness from which some blacks are suffering.

Chapter 56
HYPERTENSION

Hypertension is one of the most common diseases in the world and a disease that is associated with other diseases such as obesity, diabetes mellitus, and high lipid in the blood. When left untreated or poorly treated, it causes conditions like stroke, coronary artery disease, heart attack, congestive heart failure, kidney failure, blindness, and dementia.

Seventy-six million people in the U.S. have hypertension and, 67 million adults in the U.S. or 31% (1 in 3) have prehypertension. 1.5 billion People in the world have high blood pressure. By 2025, it is said that half a billion more people will develop high blood pressure.

Presently, one in four people in the world has high blood pressure. In the U.S., the ratio is one in three adults have hypertension. Hypertension is more common in blacks and other minorities as comapered to whites and other racial groups in the world, and the disease begins at an earlier age in these subgroups and is much more aggressive. 4 out of every 10 black Americans have hypertension. Worldwide, 7.5 million people die of high blood pressure every year. "Every year, hypertension contributes to one out of every seven deaths in the United States and nearly half of all cardiovascular disease related deaths, including stroke." If all hypertensive patients were treated sufficiently to reach the goal specified in current clinical guidelines, 46,000 deaths might be averted each year in the U.S."

"Thirty percent of patients with hypertension in the U.S. are not being treated pharmacololically, and only 46% of individuals with hypertension have their blood pressure under control." The direct and indirect cost of hypertension is $93.5 billion per year. Sources: CDC, MMWR. 2011; 60:103-108, National Health and Nutrition Examination Survey (NHANES).

More blacks and other minorities have hypertension than do whites. The incidence of the disease is 41% among black Americans and 27% among white Americans.

Forty-eight percent of black males and 41.4 percent of black women in the U.S. have high blood pressure. The incidence of high blood pressure in blacks in the U.S. is higher than in any other ethnic group in the world. Blacks represent 13.6 % or forty-two million one hundred and sixty thousand (42,160,000) of the U.S. population and 15.6 million blacks in the U.S. have high blood pressure.

High blood pressure develops at an earlier age in blacks and other minorities and the complications it causes are more severe and aggressive compared to whites. Fifty percent of blacks with hypertension die of stroke and eighty percent die of heart disease.

Among the U.S. population with high blood pressure, 78.7 percent are aware that they have the disease, 69% are being treated for the disease, 45.4 % have the blood pressure under control, and 54.6% do not have the blood pressure under control. Roughly 63% of whites, 58% of Hispanics, and only 40% of blacks have normal blood pressure readings when taking medications for high blood pressure. Source: U.S. Department of Health and Human Services.

Since 2005, the death rates for high blood pressure rose from 25.2% in 1995 to 56.4% in 2005. In 2005, the death rates per 100,000 from high blood pressure were 15.6 for white males, 52.1 for black males, 15.1 for white females, and 40.3 for black females.

Source: American Heart Association—Heart Disease and stroke Statistics Update 2009.

What is hypertension?

The kidney is the organ responsible for the development of hypertension. Hypertension occurs when the systolic part of the blood pressure is higher than normal and the diastolic part of the blood pressure is higher than normal.

What is the systolic blood pressure?

The systolic blood pressure is the upper number in the blood pressure reading machine.

What is the diastolic blood pressure?

The diostolic blood pressure is the lower number in the blood pressure reading machine

What is a normal systolic blood pressure?

A normal systolic blood pressure ranges from 100 to an upper limit of 130

What is normal diastolic blood pressure?

A normal diastolic blood pressure ranges from 60 to an upper limit of 80

CLASSIFICATION OF BLOOD PRESSURE IN ADULTS AGE 18 YEARS AND OLDER

New blood pressure Classifications			
Classification	*Systolic*		*Diastolic*
Normal	<120	and	<80
Pre-hypertension	120-139	or	80-89
Stage 1	140-159	or	90-99
Stage 2	160+	100+	

Source JAMA Volume 289, No 19 May 21, 2003 the JNC-7 Report

What instruments are needed to take the blood pressure?

The instruments that are needed to take the blood pressure are:

1. A blood pressure cuff, which is attached to a manometer on which is listed different numbers from 20 mm/Hg to 300 mm/Hg.
2. A stethoscope, which is placed on a pulsating artery, most often at the bend and on the inside part of the arm.

What are some of the pitfalls in taking the blood pressure?

If the cuff is too small the blood pressure can be falsely high, as much as 10 to 20 mm/Hg systolic or diastolic. If the cuff is too large, the reverse can happen, namely the blood pressure can be too low by as much as 10 to 20 mm, /Hg. The person taking the measurement should make sure the blood pressure cuff is neither too large nor too small. That person should also make sure that the blood pressure cuff is functioning properly before using it. In particular, the blood pressure cuff should not be leaking, because if it is leaking air, then it is sure to give a false reading.

Both errors can have a serious negative impact in the care of a person being treated for hypertension, in that either she can receive too much or too little medication, which in either case can be harmful.

A small cuff should be used for a person with a small arm, a medium-size cuff for a person with a medium-sized arm and a large cuff for a person with a large arm. There are also very large cuffs made to suit the needs of very obese individuals, and as just stated above, using an undersized cuff to take the blood pressure of a person with a very large arm can cause a false reading in the blood pressure of that person.

An example of such an error in a blood pressure reading is a person with a large arm with a blood pressure reading of 140/90 measured with an undersized cuff, when in fact the blood pressure is 130/80 when a large blood pressure cuff is used. This type of error must be avoided because the woman's psyche can be quite seriously affected when she has been told that her blood pressure is high when in fact the pressure is perfectly normal when it is taken with the proper cuff. When the person in this situation applies for life insurance, this particular error can adversely affect her ability to be insured. If insurance is obtained, higher premiums are likely to be charged because of the falsely taken blood pressure.

One should make sure that the stethoscope being used to take the blood pressure is in good working order, because if it is not, this can also cause improper blood pressure readings. One should be certain that there are no holes in the diaphragm of the stethoscope—the bottom part—and be certain to check the rubber tubing for holes and cracks. If these problems are found in the stethoscope or the blood pressure machine, it should not be used because air will escape while the doctor is trying to listen to the blood pressure, resulting in false blood pressure readings.

Automatic blood pressure machines are suitable if one knows how to use them. The blood pressure should always be taken in three positions:

1. When the person is lying down.
2. When the person is sitting down.
3. When the person is standing up for at least 3 to 5 minutes.

Why is it important to take blood pressure in this manner?

It is important to take the blood pressure in this manner because most active individuals are either sitting up or standing up most of the time during the day and lie down only to sleep at night or to take a nap during the day. Several antihypertensive medications work best when the person is standing up. It is, therefore, important to know what these individuals' blood pressure readings are when they are standing up, sitting down or lying down. If an individual is bleeding or dehydrated, his or her blood pressure will drop when he or she is sitting up or standing up compared to when he or she is lying down.

The pulse rate of the person who is sitting up or standing up who has lost a lot of blood or fluid is likely to go up. This is the cause of orthostatic hypotension. That is, the pulse goes up and the blood pressure goes down. The pulse rate going up is a much more sensitive sign of orthostatic hypotension than the blood pressure dropping by itself. Of course, this maneuver depends on the age of the person because the older the individual, the weaker will be the tone within the wall of their vessels.

When one stands up, this can itself cause one's blood pressure to drop. Such individuals tend to have what is called a wide pulse pressure and all this has to be taken into consideration when one is talking about volume loss that is either blood or fluid from the body.

It takes a minimum of 1200 to 1800 cc of either fluid or blood loss for orthostatic hypotension to occur.

Again, it depends on the age and the size of the woman, because an older individual who has lost between 800 and 1000 cc of either blood or fluid may have her blood pressure drop significantly. This is because a person's intravascular volume becomes contracted as the person ages.

Therefore, a diagnosis of orthostatic hypotension has to be made taking into account the person's size and age. A younger individual is more likely to tolerate the loss of 1800 cc of either blood or fluid with only slight evidence of orthostasis, compared to an older individual who might in fact develop cardiovascular collapse due solely to 1800 cc of either blood or fluid loss.

Other conditions that can cause an acute drop in blood pressure include:

1. Too much anti-hypertension medications;
2. Acute heart attack;
3. Certain abnormal rhythms of the heart—either too fast or too slow a heart rate;
4. Severe infection in the blood, such as sepsis;
5. Oversensitivity of the carotid bodies, which are located in both sides of the neck, can frequently cause orthostatic hypotension to occur.

Vasovagal reaction can also cause a person's blood pressure to drop. In fact, it can also cause the person to collapse based on certain emotional factors, foe example when someone receives bad news such as the loss of a loved one or some other major crisis. Such events can cause a person to collapse because of vasovagal reaction. In addition, a vasovagal reaction in an older person with underlying cardiac disease can actually cause her blood pressure to drop when having a bowel movement, due to the straining that activates the vasovagal reaction mechanism.

In addition, acute and severe vomiting with retching can also cause an older individual to collapse because of the activation of the vasovagal reaction mechanism of the human body.

The system just described is closely associated with the control of posture in the human body, referring specifically to the carotid body is located in the neck—sensitivity. Many other factors or conditions exist that can cause a person's blood pressure to drop which can result in collapse.

It is mandatory and necessary to take blood pressure in the elderly in both arms, and when feasible, lying down, sitting down and standing up as described above. The reason for this is that as a person gets older, he or she loses muscle elasticity within the blood vessels, resulting in what is called wide pulse pressure (the term for a large difference between the systolic and diastolic blood pressure). A drop in blood pressure can occur in the standing position as a natural physical phenomenon in elderly individuals.

This phenomenon is partly responsible for the higher systolic blood pressure seen frequently in the elderly. Although it is important to treat hypertension in the elderly, it is prudent to make all efforts not to be too aggressive with antihypertensive medications in the elderly so as not to cause too great a drop in the systolic blood pressure. The elderly need the systolic blood pressure to remain in the range of 130 to 140 for proper perfusion to take place in the brain.

As the blood vessels of the veins get stiffened and narrowed due to plaques that occur due to aging, a higher systolic pressure head is needed to push blood to the brain circulation to deliver the necessary oxygen for proper brain functions.

Dropping the systolic blood pressure too low in the elderly can lead to a stroke and this is something that must be avoided. On the other hand, if the systolic blood pressure is allowed to remain too high in the 170 to 180 range, for example for too long a period, the result can be a stroke, a heart attack, or congestive heart failure, and even death can result.

The root causes of essential hypertension in people are many and chief among them are the following:

1. Genetic predisposition
2. Salt sensitivity
3. Salt-rich diet
4. Obesity
5. Stress

6. Genetic component of the salt sensitivity being transferred from the forebears of women in Africa to those who are now living in the New World and also those who are still living in Africa.

Among these factors, salt sensitivity and retension is the most important as the genesis of hypertension. Salt sensitivity and retension is a genetic phenomenon. The gene responsible for causing salt retension and sensitivity originated in Africa. Salt retention in the body of blacks living under the severest conditions that existed in Africa millions of years ago, and to some degree still existing today, was and is necessary for survival.

Working in the hot sun in the fields of Africa was associated with massive salt loss due to sweating through the skin that existed then and that exists today for those who still have to toil the land under the hot sun in Africa and tropical coutries of the world. This massive salt loss leads to water loss resulting in dehydration.

To prevent death, which would have been the result of this severe water loss, the body developed a gene located in the kidneys to retain salt in the body, thereby retaining water and preserving life.

Incidentally, on October 1, 2009, scientists at the University of California—Berkeley published information about the discovery of Ardi 4 feet tall that lived 4.4 million years ago in Ethiopia. Once more, this discovery confirms that the human race began in Africa and that all human beings are to one degree or another Africans, no matter the skin color or other physical characteristics.

This lifesaving gene located in the kidneys, was a necessity in the Old World in Africa but, is a detriment to health in the New World and results in the disease of essential hypertension. The salt-sensitive gene is extremely strong and highly penetrating. The diet contributes significantly to the development of many of the most common diseases. The interplay of hypertension, diabetes mellitus, obesity and high cholesterol, referred to as metabolic hypertension, or Syndrome X, is quite common in people wordlwide. All four components of hypertension are genetically transmitted.

When babies start out in life with this abnormal genetic package, by the time they grow up and are forced to live through all the psychosocial and other stresses of living in this fast paced world they are certain to suffer from the adverse effects of metabolic hypertension.

The history of salt sensitivity and secondary fluid retention resulting in elevation of blood pressure did not start millions of years ago as a disease but rather as a God-given measure to maintain life and prevent deaths, as described above.

Living conditions in ancient Africa millions of years ago, and to a significant extent in present-day Africa, are quite harsh with people working in extremely high temperatures. Under these conditions, the human body loses a lot of salt through the skin and in so doing loses water along with salt through the skin as sweat.

Wherever salt goes in the human body, water goes with it. When a person loses salt and too much water with it, the body can become dehydrated quickly. Once the intravascular system is depleted of fluid the body risks being collapsed.

It takes between 1800 cc to 2500 cc of fluid lost ordinarily to cause the blood pressure to fall in a 70 kg man or a normal-sized woman.

Once the kidneys sense that the blood pressure is falling, their normal tendency is to prevent salt from going out of the body in the urine, thereby attempting to maintain the blood pressure in the normal range. Through this mechanism, salt remains in the body and keeps water with it to maintain blood pressure and to prevent the body from collapsing. The kidneys are able to do this because there are special genes that are located in the kidneys that enable them to hold on to salt.

This gene, called G protein-coupled receptor kinase 4, (GRK4⊠,) was discovered in 2002 at the University of Virginia and Georgetown University after eighteen years of research using specimens taken from kidneys of some Caucasian American, Ghanaian, and Japanese individuals. The same quantity of GRK4 was found in all three racial groups. This study documents that GRK4 is responsible for the salt retention that occurs in essential hypertension and therefore is the basis of this disease. Source: Proceedings of National Academy of Sciences (2002; 99:3872-3877).

As far as the kidney is concerned, people are still living in the same conditions that the forbearers of the human race lived in Africa six millions years ago and need to hold onto salt constantly to preserve the human body from dehydration.

Essential hypertension has the same genesis in people of all racial stripes, without regard to skin color. All human beings are salt sensitive to one degree or another.

Blacks, Hispanics and Asians are more salt sensitive than other racial groups. Blacks and Hispanics are salt sensitive because they are born with low renin.
Asians are salt sensitive because they eat a salt rich diet that suppresses their rennin level.

These three racial groups when there are hypertensives have what is called high volume high blood pressure.

The kidney is the center of the cause of essential hypertension and the center where some of the most important medications are used to treat high blood pressure work. Two examples of these medications are thiazide diuretic and angiotensin receptor blocker.

Hypertension causes significant problems for people because it affects such important organs as the heart, brain, kidneys, and eyes—the four organs commonly referred to as the end organs. The damage done to people's heart by hypertension causes arteriosclerotic plaques to be deposited within their coronary arteries resulting frequently in heart attacks and death, congestive heart failure and hypertensive heart disease.

Hypertension can also cause the heart to become enlarged because the heart has to pump against a high load, the high load being the high blood pressure. Over time, the muscles around the heart become hypertrophied, resulting in enlarged ventricles. Once hypertrophy sets in, because the heart muscle only has a finite length to which it can be stretched, it can no longer stretch, and the heart then begins to pump ineffectively. The ineffectivity of the heart muscle reflects in what is referred to as cardiomyopathy with secondary congestive heart failure. Many people develop congestive heart failure due only to high blood pressure.

At this point, the heart is unable to push the blood away from the ventricles (heart chambers), the blood/ water backs up into the lungs and accumulates as fluid, and then congestive heart failure causing shortness of breath, tiredness and other symptoms of conestive heart failure.

If not treated quickly it can result in what is referred to as pulmonary edema (acute congestive heart failure), the result of which, when it is not treated quickly and acutely, is immediate death.

In the less dramatic way, the enlarged heart sets in and the person suffering from it begins to develop lassitude, inability to walk down the block without stopping several times, inability to sleep at night on one pillow and constant coughing at night.

This condition is referred to as nocturnal coughing. All these are signs that the heart is failing. If the person gets to a physician quickly, the condition can be discovered and treatment can be started with appropriate medication to prevent the aforementioned acute condition from occurring.

Another organ that suffers immensely from the effect of hypertension is the kidney. Hypertension damages the kidney resulting in kidney failure.

The way this happens is that the pressure rises within the vessels that run through the substance of the kidneys. All the different tissues of the kidney need blood vessels of different sizes to carry blood and oxygen to them.

As the pressure rises within the kidneys, there are structures within the kidneys referred to as glomeruli, which are small capillary blood vessels, which need to be fed blood and oxygen. As the blood pressure rises, these very delicate capillary blood vessels begin to rupture. They are rupturing without the person realizing that this is occurring.

After a while, these vessels rupture and die out and the tissues to which they are responsible to bring blood and oxygen will no longer be there and, as a result, these areas of the kidneys die. Eventually, the person loses so many glomureli that the kidneys cannot function properly affecting the renal tubules, (the filtering system inside the kidneys) resulting in renal insufficiency/kidney failure.

Once all the glomureli die, the kidneys can fail suddenly. Once the kidneys fail, waste materials accumulate within the body, resulting in swelling of the legs with smelly breath and salty skin, and a condition referred to as chronic renal failure with uremia develops. At this point either peritoneal dialysis or hemodialysis on a chronic basis must be used to clean the blood free of toxic materials to maintain life.

If a person is fortunate enough that he or she can get a kidney transplant, and the transplant succeeds, then he or she can go back to normal kidney function and a normal life. High blood pressure that goes untreated can damage the kidney to the point of kidney failure. Typically, the kidneys fail slowly, losing function gradually.

Another organ that is very sensitive to the effects of hypertension is the eye. When the blood pressure rises in the body, the pressure also rises within the vessels in the eyes. The vessels inside the eyes are quite fragile and as a result they can get damaged easily. The damage that occurs to the vessels inside the eyes of untreated or poorly treated hypertension causes different degrees of leakage to occur. If left untreated, blindness is usually the result. Hypertension is also associated with an increased incidence of glaucoma, a common disease of the eye seen hundred of millions people throughout the world.

The brain is yet another organ that suffers the effects of hypertension to verying degrees. Over time, the effects of elevated blood pressure cause plaques to develop within small vessels and large vessels of the brain. The damage that occurs within the small vessels in the brain results in multiple small vessel infarctions. This condition inevitably leads to the condition referred to as multi-infarct syndrome. Multi-infarct syndrome is the most common cause of senility in people in the world (organic brain syndrome).

Hypertension affects 1.5 billion people in the world. The incidence of hypertension is highest among among people of immediate African ancestry as compared to Whites. 4 out of 10 black Americans are hypertensive.

Blacks and other minorities across the world are more prone to the development of early senility due to untreated hypertension or poorly treated hypertension. Elevated blood pressure can cause three different types of major strokes to occur (cerebrovascular accident). The first type is called ischemic stroke; the second type is called hemorrhagic stroke; and the third type is known as embolic stroke.

Ischemic stroke occurs because of the chronic narrowing of the affected vessel with plaques and/or the rupture of plaques within the affected vessels, resulting in bleeding, with clot formation acutely closing off the vessel, cutting off blood flow, resulting in a stroke.

Elevated blood pressure can cause hemorrhagic stroke to occur due to chronic damage that takes place affecting the vessels, resulting in acute rupture of those vessels, causing hemorrhage to occur inside the brain. Hypertension-associated embolic stroke can occur because of hypertensive heart disease with enlargement of the heart. This can cause atrial fibrillation to develop, and if the atrial fibrillation is not treated with anticoagulants such as Heparin, Coumadin, Prodaxa, or Xaralto to prevent clot formation, then the clot can get dislodged from the atrium to the brain, causing an embolic stroke.

Frequently, hypertension is intertwined with obesity, diabetes mellitus, and elevated lipids in the same individuals. These conditions interplay in a significant percentage of people. About 81% of black American women are obese/ overweight and 69% of black American men are overweight/ obese. Overall, 73% of black men and women are overweight/obese in the U.S. Two third of the adults in the U.S. are obese/overweight and one third of children in the U.S. are obesew/overweight, and 3.3 billion people in the world are obese/overweight.

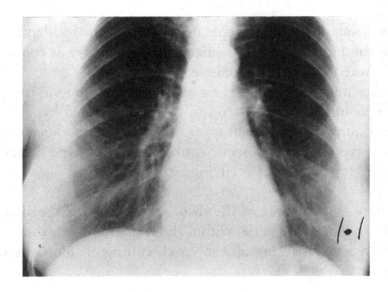

Figure 58.1—normal chest x-ray in a patient

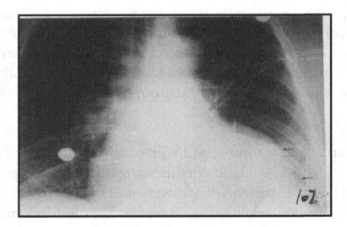

Figure 58.2—An abnormal chest x-ray in a patient with hypertensive cardiovascular disease, showing heart failure as a result of chronic hypertension with secondary coronary artery disease, leading to an enlarged heart and heart failure, with arrow showing enlarged border of the right heart and arrows showing enlarged border of the left heart with pleural effusion (fluid in lower left lung).

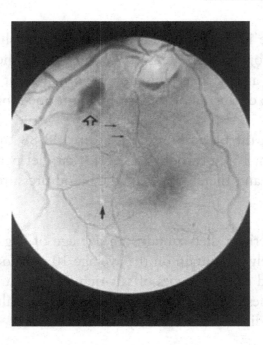

Figure 58.3—Showing different degrees of abnormalities in the eye of a hypertensive patient (hypertensive retinopathy). Small arrow showing silver wiring; big arrow showing hard yellow exudates; open arrowhead showing hemorrhage; arrowhead showing A-V nicking.

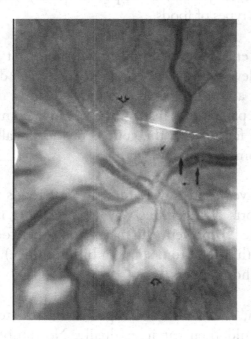

Figure 58.4-Showing different types of abnormalities in the eye of a hypertensive patient (hypertensive retinopathy). Small arrows showing early papilledema, one big arrow pointing to engorgement of (larger vessel). The other big arrow pointing to arterial attenuation (smaller vessel): open arrowheads showing cotton wool exudates.

If the blood pressure in a person is 138/88, and he or she is overweight, and he or she has a family history of hypertension (that is, either her mother or father has hypertension), then the approach to this upper normal limit of blood pressure is to repeat the blood pressure during an office visit in about one month.

If in the second visit, the blood pressure is again 138/88, and then the treatment is 4 g sodium, 90 g protein, 160 g carbohydrate, 31 g fat diet per day along with exercise to try to lose the weight and thereby prevent the blood pressure from creeping up even higher.

The usual daily American diet contains an average of 7 g of sodium. The diet of African Americans is likely to contain on the average 10 g of sodium. This is so because of the so-called soul food or other types of salt-rich foods that many blacks like to eat. The salt adds taste to these foods. Whites also eat a lot of salt because they consume many fast foods and the diet of Asians is very rich in salt.

These foods typically are rich in salt, and if one is accustomed to eating food that is salty, no matter what type of food one eats one tends to add more salt in order to satisfy one's taste for salt. The vast majority of African Americans live under substandard economic conditions in which they consume fast foods, because that is the type of foods most can afford. Fast foods, in general, are of poorer quality. To enhance taste, a lot of fat and salt are added to these types of foods.

Fast foods, therefore, end up containing much more salt than would normally be the case. The greater the level of poverty, the more likely is a diet of poor quality. Since the diet is of poor quality, a lot of spices and salt are added in order to enhance the taste and make the foods more palatable. This is not a negative comment. This is a comment based on known facts. In fact, this is the genesis of the so-called "soul-food", which is really a legacy left over from slavery days.

During the time of slavery, slaves were forced to eat foods that were of poor quality and so they devised all sorts of ingenious ways of preparing meats and other foods to make them more palatable. To prevent the meats and other foods from getting spoiled, they cured these foods with juices from sours (a bitter orange), lime juice, plenty of salt and other spices, crushed hot peppers, etc.

Slaves would then put the meat on a rope in the sun to dry to prevent it from getting spoiled. They would then eat it gradually. No doubt these foods tasted very good, but unfortunately they were very bad for their bodies particularly because of the salt content. These foods are still bad for the human body today especially when eaten on a regular basis. So, when the statement is made that the poorer the individual, the poorer the quality of food is likely to be, that is a statement of fact, because the foods that are of higher quality cost much more money which is unaffordable for poor people.

One can only eat what one can afford, balanced with the numerous other financial demands with financially limited resources.

The DASH Diet ("Dietary Approaches to Stop Hypertension") recommends eating nuts, legumes, seeds, fruits and vegetables four to five times per week, along with a low fat dairy intake. The results show lowering of both systolic and diastolic blood pressures (Source: Internal Medicine News, June 1, 2003). The present recommended daily salt intake is 1.5 grams or a maximum of 2.3 grams per of sodium. Therefore, adherence to a good diet is very important as both prevention and management of hypertension.

Treatment of high blood pressure should be started early. Once the blood pressure reaches 140/90 in a salt-sensitive person, treatment with medication ought to be started, particularly if the person is obese. The best and most effective medication for hypertension is a water pill (diuretic). It does not matter what the racial make-up of the person is, so long as his or her kidneys are functioning. Water pills work to control high blood pressure by preventing salt from being reabsorbed by the kidneys back into the blood stream, taking water with it, which results in raising the blood pressure. Some of the common diuretics that are available in the United States are:

Hydrocholorothiazide
Clorthalidone
Dyazide
Moduretic
Aldactone
Lozol
Maxzide
Lasix
Bumex, etc;

All these medications are effective in removing salt and water from the body. The cost of Hydrocholorothiazide at 25 mg per day is low (30 generic tablets cost $10.00). However, if one were to buy a more expensive medication, the blood pressure would be treated much less effectively (using it as mono-therapy meaning by itself) and yet the person would spend four times more money for that medication. A good example is Procardia XL 30 mg, 30 tablets Brand costs $75.00. Another example is Zestril 10 mg 30 tablets Brand cost $52.00. Because it is an angiotensin-1-converting enzyme (ACE) inhibitor (meaning that it needs the presence of an elevated level of renin to be effective in bringing down the blood pressure), it does not work in blacks to treat hypertension.

The reason Zestril and other ACE donot work to treat blood pressure is because blacks Asians, Hispanics and other minorities is because these people genetically have low renin in their blood. Zestril and other ACE inhibitors such as Accupril, Capoten, Vasotec, Monopril, Altace, Mavik, etc. are great medications to treat hypertension when used in some whites. These medications are also extremely effective in the treatment of congestive heart failure and certain cardiac arrhythmias.

Overall, the basic reason for essential hypertension is salt retention and the water retention that goes with it and this phenomenon applies to all individuals who suffer from essential hypertension which, accounts for about 98% of people with hypertension without regards to ethnicity. The gene responsible for essential hypertension has been discovered and it is located in the kidneys and it is the same in all individuals without regard to race.

Therefore, all individuals who suffer from hypertension and have functioning kidneys need water pills to treat their hypertension.

Water pills work to control high blood pressure by preventing salt from being reabsorbed by the kidneys back into the blood stream. A water pill /diuretic forces salt out in the urine taking water with it. This decreases the amount of water in the intravascular compartment resulting in lowering of the blood pressure.

The first medication that must be used in the treatment of high blood pressure in a person with functioning kidneys is a thiazide diuretic.

There is a substance made by the human kidney called renin. Renin, once made by the kidneys, enters into a biochemical reaction leading ultimately to another substance called aldosterone, which causes salt retention leading to water retention, which in turn causes expansion of water within the intravascular compartment, leading to elevation of blood pressure.

This system is called the renin angiotensin aldosterone system.

However, blacks, Hispanics, Asians, and other people of color have low renin in their bloods as a genetic fact. So prescribing medications that work to attack the renin angiotensin system to decrease blood pressure in these individuals is useless and makes no clinical sense. Furthermore, these medications have a lot of side effects and are very expensive.

Examples of these medications are beta-blockers, such as Inderal, Lopressor, Tenormin, Toprol XL to name a few, and ACE inhibitors such as Capoten, Zistril, Vasotec, etc. Beta-blockers are excellent medications for treating angina, migraine headaches, cardiac arrhythmias, congestive heart failure, etc., in people of all ethnic make-ups and work very well in these circumstances.

The only situation in which a beta-blocker might have some effect in a salt-sensitive person in controlling hypertension is when the person is under stress and is secreting a lot of adrenalin. The beta-blocker might transiently shut off the sympathetic system in this setting to decrease the blood pressure.

However, when a salt-sensitive low-renin-secreting person's kidneys fail and the person develops chronic renal failure, the renin level goes up by necessity, and then a beta-blocker becomes a necessity in the treatment of hypertension because the renin level is always elevated in chronic renal failure.

Another circumstance in which the beta-blocker might work to decrease blood pressure although the individul may be classified as salt-sensitive is in reno-vascular hypertension.

When plaques or fibrous substances within the vessels obstruct the circulation of the kidneys, then the renin level at that point is elevated. In this circumstance, beta-blockers would work via the renin angiotensin system and the beta-receptors within the kidneys to decrease the blood pressure.

Beta-Blockers also work to decrease high pressure in pheochromocytoma.

Pheochromocytoma is a benign tumor of the adrenal gland that secretes catecholamines resulting in elevated blood pressure.

Still another important use for a beta-blocker occurs when a person's blood pressure is critically high—for example, in the 200/120 range. In this situation, Labetalol IV can be used to acutely bring the blood pressure down.

The reason that Labetalol works to acutely decrease blood pressure when given intra-venously is that via the rennin-angiotensin system, angiotensin-2 is released causing stimulation of the adrenal medulla resulting in the release of catecholamines which raises the blood pressure. Labetalol blocks the release of catecholamines and decreases the blood pressure.

However, this is a minor effect of the rennin-angiotensin system on the overall causation of high blood pressure. This is the reason that beta blockers given by mouth do not work to decrease blood pressure. There are specific circumstances when beta blockers are used to treat specific medical conditions that cause blood pressure to go up. Source: "Beta-blockers for hypertension going out of style", Cleveland Clinic Journal of Medicine, Volume 76, Number 9, September 2009.

The ASCORT-BPLA (Anglo-Scandinavian Cardiac Outcomes Trial—Blood Pressure Lowering Arm) shows that beta-blockers, as monotherapy, do not work to treat high pressure.

Some of the beta-blockers in use in the U.S. are:

Inderal
Tenormin
Corgard
Timolol
Labetalol
Visken
Tenormin
Toprol XL
Coreg
Bystolic

As has been just stated, ACE inhibitors are very good medications in the treatment of the blood pressure in Caucasians and in the treatment of cardiomyopathy with associated congestive heart failure, myocardial infarction in diabetics with associated high blood pressure, diabetics with microalbuminuria and in all individuals, regardless of their ethnic background, who suffer from these conditions.

ACE inhibitors can be used with caution in blacks with chronic renal failure to treat high blood pressure because in this setting, the renin level is high. The reason for the caution is because ACE inhibitors can cause an increase in the BUN and serum potassium, and the elevated serum potassium is a major problem unless the patient is on chronic dialysis, in which case the potassium can be removed during dialysis.

It is best to treat Blacks, Hispanics, Asians and other racial minorities with high blood pressure with an angiotensin—2-receptor blocker (ARB) because ARB blocks the entire rennin angiotensin Aldosterone system to prevent the production of Aldosterone which, when elevated, causes salt and water retension resulting in elevation of blood pressure. ARB works effectively in all ethnic groups. Everything that an ACE can do, ARB does it better for high blood pressure, microalbuminuria in diabetics, post myocardial infarction, congestive heart failure, etc.

The following are some of the ARBs in use in the U.S.:

Cozzar
Avapro
Diovan
Aceon
Atacand
Benicar
Micardis

As already mentioned, the second most common form of hypertension is reno—vascular hypertension which represents about 2% of all types of hypertensions. As individuals age, plaques may develop within the blood vessels carrying blood to the kidneys, resulting in elevation of renin, causing a state referred to as hyperenemia and high blood pressure.

Frequently, in renovascular hypertension, a sound referred to as a "bruit" can be heard over the flanks of the patient's abdomen using the stethoscope, either on the right side or the left side of the abdomen. However, in a certain percentage of patients with renovascular hypertension, a bruit is not heard. In this situation, either the so-called Capoten test or renal angiography has to be done to determine whether renovascular obstruction exists or not.

The other family of medications in use in the U.S. to treat high blood pressure is calcium channel blockers. These medications work by relaxing the smooth muscles in the human body. Relaxing the muscles causes the blood pressure to drop. Constriction of blood vessels causes blood pressure to rise. In order for any muscle to contract, calcium is needed for the contraction to occur and the absence of calcium inside the blood vessels results in relaxation of muscle.

The following are some of the calcium channel medications in use in the U.S.

Verapamil
Cardizem CD
Vorvasc
Procardia
Adalat
Caduet

These medications are expensive but they are very effective to treat hypertension not only in all ethnic groups.

Still another family of anti-hypertension medications in use in the U.S. is Alpha-blockers such as:
Hytrin
Cardura
Clonidine
Aldomet
Hydralazine

Aliskiren is a newly approved family of medications. Angiotensin—2 is a vasoconstrictor which causes the release of catecholamines from the adrenal medulla and prejunctional nerve endings and causes the secretion of aldosterone to occur resulting in reabsorption of salt raising the blood pressure. This reaction occurs under the influence of rennin which is made by the kidney. Aliskiren works to decrease blood pressure by blocking renin directly.

None of the anti-hypertensive medications listed above works as monotherapy to treat high blood pressure. For any of these medications to work to treat high blood pressure, a water pill (Thiazide diuretic) must be added to the regimen. As explained above, the reason it is necessary to use a diuretic in the treatment of high blood pressure is that the basis of essential hypertension is salt retention and water retention resulting in high volume hypertension with expansion of the intra-vascular compartment with elevation of the blood pressure.

Modiuretic, Dyazide, Maxzide, etc., contain triamterene, which prevents potassium loss in the urine. In addition, potassium chloride can be prescribed by mouth along with the water pills, if on testing the blood, the potassium is found to be low. It is the standard practice to prescribe potassium supplement for any elderly patient on water pills to prevent low serum potassium. Elderly individuals frequently have a diet that contains less than 80 mg of potassium per day.

In addition, elderly individuals have a higher propensity of losing potassium in their urine when taking water pills. For these, and all the other aforementioned reasons, when an elderly person is on water pills and particularly if that elderly person is on Digitalis, close attention must be paid to the serum potassium.

Potassium replacement ought to be provided to prevent potassium loss which alone can cause severe cardiac dysrhythmias.

The argument that water pills cause blood sugar to rise is, in fact, a false argument because replacing potassium restores insulin receptor sensitivity, which then keeps the blood sugar at a normal level. The benefit of having well-controlled blood pressure far outweighs the questionable slight increase in cholesterol that might be seen in some rare instances in individuals taking water pills.

All that needs to be done is to advise the individual to stay on a low-fat diet and monitor the serum cholesterol as often as possible.

The incidence of high blood pressure is on the decrease in whites but is on the increase in blacks and is continuing to increase steadily in this group.

There is a rare tumor of the adrenal gland called pheochromocytoma that secretes substances called catecholamines. Catecholamine causes a characteristic elevation in blood pressure. Because 95% of the time when a person has high blood pressure, it is due to the so-called essential hypertension, it is more cost effective to do a few simple tests following a complete physical examination and start treatment for the blood pressure. It is inappropriate to do extensive and expensive tests before trying treatment with antihypertensive medications in a woman with hypertension.

The basic tests that are necessary in the initial evaluation of hypertension in blacks include:

1. Complete blood count
2. Blood chemistries, such as blood sugar, blood urea nitrogen, serum electrolytes, serum creatinine, lipid profiles such as cholesterol, triglycerides, high-density lipoprotein, low-density lipoprotein
3. Urinalysis
4. EKG
5. Chest x-ray.

The tests for pheochromocytoma are expensive and very tedious to do. It requires serum catecholamines; 24 hours urine catecholamines, and a specific diet that must be adhered to for several days before these tests can be done. It is simpler to do an abdominal CT scan to evaluate the adrenal glands looking for abnormality, rather than doing these very extensive blood tests looking for pheochromocytoma, which is quite rare. Most of the time, people with pheochromocytoma have sustained elevated blood pressure rather than the blood pressure that goes up and down as is being taught in medical schools and residency training.

To determine the extent of damage that the hypertensive state has done to the different end organs of hypertensive women, a series of basic tests ought to be done. The end organs are the brain, heart, eyes, and kidneys.

These basic tests are not only inexpensive but also clinically rationale. The Complete Blood Count (CBC) can tell whether a person is anemic or not, and in renal failure associated with long-time hypertension, the red blood cell count is low because the kidneys are damaged and not able to make erythropoietin. Erythropoietin is a hormone made by the kidneys to stimulate the production of red cells by the bone marrow—the organ within which red blood cells are made in an adult.

The urinalysis is abnormal in kidney disease associated with hypertension. When high blood pressure damages the kidneys, the urine specific gravity is low. The urine is likely to have protein in it and the urine sediment, when examined with the microscope, is likely to have substances called casts, indicating intrinsic kidney damage.

In the blood chemistry tests, the BUN, the creatinine, the serum potassium and the bicarbonate may all be abnormal in high blood pressure-associated kidney disease. If the blood sugar is elevated, this means the patient, in addition to having hypertension, may have diabetes mellitus. The serum lipids such as cholesterol, triglycerides, LDL, are elevated and if the woman is hypertensive, the blood sugar is elevated, and if the woman happens to be obese, this is also very important; this is called syndrome X or metabolic hypertension.

Metabolic hypertension or syndrome X is a very serious condition in which there is interplay between obesity, hypertension, hyperlipidemia, and diabetes in the same individual. This very deadly combination needs to be handled extremely expertly and carefully. The chest x-ray is important to determine whether the heart is enlarged or not, or whether the lungs have fluid in them, a condition known as congestive heart failure. If the heart is enlarged, it gives the physician a very good idea as to how long the person has been hypertensive. The electrocardiogram (EKG) is very important, in that it allows the physician to have an idea as to the different types of damage that the high blood pressure may have caused to the heart muscle over a long period.

These basic tests having been done, then the physician has sufficient information at hand to organize a sensible, rational, safe, and cost-effective treatment plan for the hypertensive patient. Examining the eyes using the ophthalmoscope allows the physician to see the fundi of hypertensive women, which shows small blood vessels in the eyes, and if found to be damaged, reveals that these women have been hypertensive for a long time and most probably without effective treatment.

In order for people to keep their blood pressures normal, in addition to appropriate medications such as diuretics, they must follow a diet that is low in salt, fat, and simple carbohydrates and high in fiber, protein, vitamins, iron, and minerals. They also must control their weight and exercise regularly.

Another common hypertension-associated problem that is frequently seen in women is toxemia of pregnancy, pre-eclampsia, and eclampsia. When a woman is pregnant, the kidney function changes.

The rate of glomerular filtration inside the kidneys and the so-called renal plasma flow are both increased by anywhere from 30% to 50%. If the blood urea nitrogen (BUN) and the serum creatinine levels start to increase from the normal range in a pregnant woman, an investigation must be started by doing a renal sonogram and a 24-hour urine creatinine clearance and protein.

Similarly, if the diastolic high blood pressure goes up to 80 mm/Hg in the second trimester and above 85 mm/Hg in the third trimester, corrective measures are necessary at this point to prevent the patient from going into toxemia.

Toxemia of pregnancy usually starts in the third trimester of pregnancy. Different components of this syndrome include hypertension, protein in the urine, elevated serum uric acid, edema (that is, swollen ankles), salt retention, consumptive coagulopathy (abnormal coagulation tests of the blood which can lead to bleeding) and hyperreflexia (on examination of the reflexes they are brisk and increased).

This constellation of problems is called pre-eclampsia. If seizure develops, then the patient is said to have eclampsia. Pre-eclampsia exists when the blood pressure remains 140/85 or greater for several hours. If the woman had high blood pressure before becoming pregnant, pre-eclampsia can become accelerated quickly into eclampsia.

Treatment of the toxemia syndrome includes bed rest in an area that is quiet, and administration of magnesium sulfate to treat the neurological abnormalities.

Medications that will decrease the blood pressure by dilating the blood vessels such as methyldopa and hydralazine must be given. Diuretics are contraindicated in toxemia of pregnancy and ought not to be used.

People must endeavor to exercise regularly, stop smoking, and abstain from abusing alcohol, if they are to decrease their incidence of high blood pressure. These measures can lead to decreasing some of the adverse consequences of high blood pressure such as stroke, heart attack, and kidney failure.

All these factors contribute to decrease the median survival age in black women of 77 years compared to the white women's median survival age of 81 years as well as black men's median survival age of 70 years compared to that of white men's median survival age of 76 years.

There is a need for a change of lifestyle of individuals to help decrease the incidence of hypertension. This change in lifestyle is not always realistic because of the poor economic circumstances of most poor people in the U.S. and in the world.

The stress brought on by a multitude of problems associated with poverty plays a major role in the elevation of blood pressure. If the stress that is common in poor people is not significantly diminished, it makes it that much more difficult to control the elevation of their blood pressures.

Hypertension is among the leading causes of morbidities and mortalities in people in the U.S. and in the world. However, education and an understanding of this most serious disease can delay its onset by many years, and therefore, can decrease its incidence in in all racial groups. It is important to understand that essential hypertension has the same genesis in all racial groups and therefore must be treated the same in all these groups.

Doing otherwise guarantees the development of major difficulty in controlling blood pressure in all ethnic groups. Treating high blood pressure in all individuals with a proper regimen of medications is essential to decrease hypertension associated deaths.

Hypertension is an easily treatable disease if the right medication or medications are provided to hypertensives. Treatment with the right medications would mean that this highly treatable disease would be dealt with much more effectively; the result is the prevention or at least the significant decrease of the devastation it causes on the health of people in the U.S. and in the world.

Chapter 57
STROKE

Stroke is one of the leading diseases that kills and disables people in the United States and around the world. Each year, 795,000 people suffer a new or recurrent stroke in the United States; 600,000 of these strokes are first strokes and 185,000 are recurrent strokes. Worldwide, 12.7 million people suffer a stroke yearly because of high blood pressure. Source: WHO.

Every 53 seconds someone suffers a stroke in the U.S. and every 3.3 minutes someone dies of a stroke. Alltogether, 7 million Americans have had a stroke. Each year, 60,000 more women than men have a stroke. Every year, 143,579 people die from stroke in the U.S. Worldwide, 15 million people have a stroke each year, 5 million people die from a stroke, and 5 million people are permanently disabled from a stroke.

The rates of stroke are higher in blacks and other minorities than in whites, and stroke develops in blacks and other minorities at a younger age than it does in whites. Eighty-seven percent (87%) of strokes are of the ischemic type, 10% are of the intracerebral hemorrhage type, and 3 % are of the subarachnoid hemorrhage type.

Blacks and other minorities have twice the incidence of a first stroke compared to whites. The rates of stroke in ages 45-84 are 6.6 per 1,000 in black males and 3.6 in white males.

For black females in the same age range, it is 4.9 per 1,000 and 2.2 in white females. Source: National Heart, Lung, and Blood Institute, 2006, Bethesda, M.D.

According to report presented on 2/7/13 at the American Stroke association's conference in Honolulu, people who eat deep fried foods and who drink a lot sugary drinks have a high incidence of stroke. In addition, people who eat traditional southern diet have a 41% increase of stroke and African Americans who eat this diet have a 63% higher risk of stroke.

"The so-called Stroke Belt" of the U.S. consists of Alabama, Akansas, Georgia, Indiana, Kentucky, Lousiana, Mississipi, North Carolina, South Carolina, Tennessee and Verginia, according the National Heart, and Lung, and Blood Institute," 10 of which are Soutern states.

Stroke is responsible one of every 16 deaths in the U.S. Stroke is the third leading cause of deaths in the U.S. after heart disease and cancer.

Every year, 140,000 people die of a stroke in the U.S. and 5 million people die of stroke in the world. About 7.6% of the individuals who suffer ischemic strokes and 37.5% of those who suffer a hemorrhagic stroke die within 30 days.

In 2004, the overall death rate from stroke was 50.0 percent: 74.9 percent for black males, 48.1 percent for white males, 65.5 percent for black females, and 47.2 percent for white females. Source: NCHS, CDC.

There are 4,600,000 survivors of strokes in the U.S. Blacks and other minorities have the highest prevalence of large vessels/small vessel strokes than whites. The incidence of intracranial strokes is 19% in black women and 6% in white women. The incidence of lacuna strokes is 10% in black women and 2.7% in white women. Black males have 19% prevalence of small vessel stroke compared to 6% for white males and black males have 10% of lacuna strokes compared to 2.7% for white males.

Small vessel strokes (TIA) and large vessel strokes are associated with a high incidence of dementia. Therefore, the incidence of stroke related dementia is highest for blacks than any other racial group.

Because blacks and other minorities have a higher incidence of high blood pressure than any other racial groups and poorer treatments or no treatments at all for this disease, they suffer more strokes and other serious complications of high blood pressure.

Risk factors for stroke include:

1. Being men or women
2. Hypertension
3. Diabetes mellitus
4. Hyperlidemia/High cholesterol
5. Obesity
6. Metabolic syndrome
7. Hypercoagulable state
8. Primary polycythemia
9. Esential thrombocythemia
10. Kidney failure
11. Sickle cell disease
12. Atrial fibrillation
13. Cancer
14. Cigarette /Tobacco smoking
15. Trousseau disease

16. Elevated Lipoprotein-a
17. Elevated homocysteine
18. Vitamin B12 deficiemcy
19. Folic Acid deficiency
20. Low protein C level in the blood
21. Low protein S level in the blood
22. Nephrotic symdrome
23. Secondary polycythemia
24. Decreased anti-thrombin lll level in the blood
25. Obstructive sleep apnea
26. Taking birth control pill
27. Taking Estrogenic hormone
28. Elevated anti—phospholipin anti body
29. Elevated circulating lupus anticoagulant
30. AIDS
31. Factor V liden mutation
32. Prothrombin G20210A mutation
33. Hyperviscosity in patient with multiple myeloma
34. Hematocrit level 40% or greater in patients with chronic renal failure can cause stroke to occur
35. Hematocrit level 40% or greater in patients with sickle cell anemia can cause stroke to occur
36. Racial discrimination
37. Poverty
38. Stress
39. Pregnancy
40. Alcoholism
41. Elevated factor VIII level
42. Elevated fibrinogen level etc;

What is a stroke?

A stroke occurs when an obstruction of blood flow occurs within the blood vessel, preventing blood flow to an area of the brain which then becomes damaged.

This damage results in what is called a stroke. Another terminology frequently used to describe a stroke is a "cerebrovascular accident".

This obstruction of blood flow can be either caused by plaques within a vessel or by a clot from the heart brought through the vessel by the bloodstream to the brain. Another type of stroke occurs when a vessel inside the brain ruptures and leaks blood inside the brain. The rupture of a vessel in the brain is either due to a vessel filled with atherosclerotic plaques or the elevation of blood pressure within the vessel, which causes the membrane of this vessel to rupture and leak blood into the brain, leading to a stroke.

This type of stroke is called a "hemorrhagic stroke". Brain aneurysms, which are a meshwork of vessel malformations due to genetic defects, can rupture and leak blood into the brain when the blood pressure is too high. Aneurysms of the brain can rupture and cause a hemorrhagic stroke within the brain whether the blood pressure of the individual is elevated or not.

Another frequent cause of bleeding into the brain is hemangiomas, or arteriovenous malformations. These are a group of small arteries and veins in a mesh, which form an abnormal network of vessels, which can bleed easily in the brain, leading to hemorrhagic stroke.

There is a form of stroke called a transient ischemic attack (TIA). In TIA, there is a transient occlusion of a small vessel by a clot or a clump of platelets, which are trapped within the vessel, preventing free flow of the blood to pass to deliver oxygen to that part of the brain. This temporary lack of oxygen to the brain causes a clinical condition, which can temporarily lead to loss of consciousness, seizures, weakness, lassitude, and a feeling of being sick, which sometimes can last for several hours or several days.

Frequently these people have what is called "presyncope" or a full-blown "syncopal episode" because of the TIA. This condition usually occurs in the setting of what is referred to as multi-infarct syndrome which is the result of many years of either poorly treated or untreated hypertension. In multi-infarct syndrome, different parts of the brain deep within it are affected with this condition.

The most common types of stroke or cerebrovascular accident include:

1. Arteriosclerotic or ischemic stroke 61% of all strokes.
2. Lacunae stroke 20%
3. Embolic stroke, which represents 24% of all strokes.
4. Hemorrhagic stroke associated with high blood pressure 10% of all strokes.
5. Ruptured aneurysms.
6. Bleeding arteriovenous malformations.
7. Transient ischemic attacks.
8. Subarachnoid hemorrhage 7% of all strokes.
9. Occlusion of carotid arteries by plaque, causing stroke to occur because of lack of blood flow to the brain.

Arteriosclerotic-type strokes and hypertension-associated strokes are the two most common types seen. Stroke is one of the leading diseases that cause deaths among people of all ethnic back grounds. The combination of salt sensitivity, salt retention and water retention and the elevated high blood pressure are responsible for such a high incidence of strokes.

As far as the risk of having a stroke is concerned, even people who are rich and have the best of everything face the same fate if they fail to take good care of themselves. That is to say, obesity, diabetes mellitus, hypertension, stress, and domestic turmoil also affect individuals of good financial means, high education, and esteeemed professions as well.

The human brain is in total control of all activities associated with being a human being. The ability of the brain to think is what differentiates the human animal from all other animals.

The following outlines, in part, some of the facilities that the human brain controls:

1. The ability to think
2. The ability to gather information and process such information logically, rationally to formulate judgments rightly or wrongly.
3. The ability to breathe
4. The ability to see
5. The ability to hear
6. The ability to smell
7. The ability to feel
8. The ability to taste
9. The heartbeat and other crucial functions of the heart
10. Lung functions
11. Hunger
12. Lack of desire for food
13. Thirst
14. Lack of desire to drink
15. Sleep
16. Insomnia
17. Happiness
18. Unhappiness
19. Moods
20. Good moods
21. Bad moods
22. Elation
23. Motivation
24. Lack of motivation
25. Hardworking habits
26. Laziness
27. Neatness

28. Sloppiness
29. Anger
30. Aggressive behavior
31. Antisocial behavior
32. Pleasant and friendly behavior
33. Lying as a habitual behavior
34. Honesty
35. Dishonesty
36. Criminal behavior and other antisocial behaviors
37. Sexual orientations/preferences
38. Sexual desires
39. Erectile functions for both men and women
40. Ejaculatory functions and satisfactions for both men and women
41. Bowel functions
42. Urinary functions
43. Chewing
44. Swallowing
45. Sneezing
46. Coughing
47. Yawning
48. Lying down
49. Sitting
50. Bending
51. Standing
52. Walking
53. Running
54. All other motor body functions
55. Writing
56. Reading
57. Speaking, etc.

Different parts of the human brain are in control of these different functions, so when the brain is damaged by a stroke, or accidents of one type or another, infections or other abnormalities that interfere with its normal functions, one, or several of these vital functions become impaired in one way or another.

Hypertension causes a stroke to occur through three basic mechanisms:

1. Increased blood pressure in the vessels within the brain which causes the inside part of these vessels to become damaged, and over time, the damaged areas of these vessels trap platelets and other material as they pass through the blood. A nidus of these different materials develops within these vessels and the result is plaque formation.

The formation of plaques within these vessels leads to narrowing of these vessels, impeding blood flow. Superimposed on the plaque frequently is a clot which can acutely close off a vessel, resulting in a cerebrovascular accident stroke. A plaque within a vessel can cause a stroke through different mechanisms:

The plaque can cause the vessel to become narrowed, impeding blood flow and oxygen delivery to a particular part of the brain. (b) The plaque that sits inside that vessel can break off, causing either an embolus or a clot to start forming, resulting in a stroke as has just been outlined.

2) Another mechanism through which hypertension causes stroke is acute intracerebral bleeding secondary to very elevated blood pressure causing rupture of a blood vessel, resulting in bleeding within the brain. Bleeding inside the brain can result in a coma because of edema (swelling) within the brain, and if the coma lasts too long, then the result can be death of the affected person. Another type of stroke syndrome that can occur, is people who have been hypertensive for a long time, and in particular if the blood pressure has not been treated or not treated properly as mentioned before, is multiple small vessel infarctions (microvascular disease) of the brain.

The following are radiological examples of strokes.

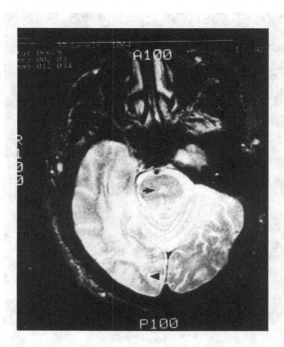

Figure 57:1-MRI of the brain in a person patient with hypertension: small infarct in the pond (arrow) and right occipital white matter (arrowhead).

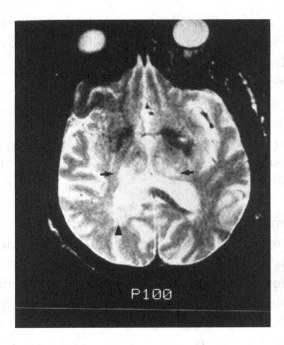

Figure 57:2-MRI of the brain in a person with hypertension: infarction of thalamus (arrows) and right parietal white matter (arrowhead).

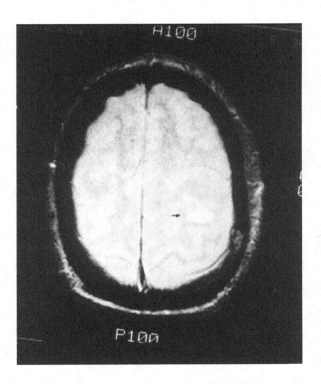

Figure 59:3-MRI of the brain in a person with hypertension: left parietal small infarction (arrow).

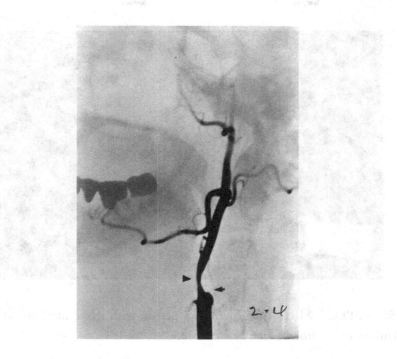

Figure 57:4-Arteriosclerotic disease of carotid artery in a peson with hypertension causing transient ischemic attacks (pre-stroke syndrome). Carotid angiogram: occlusion of internal carotid artery at its origin (arrow); narrowing of proximal internal carotid artery (arrowhead).

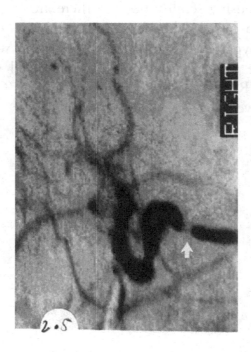

Figure 57:5-Cerebral angiogram 95% occlusion of internal carotid artery in a person with hypertension (arrow).

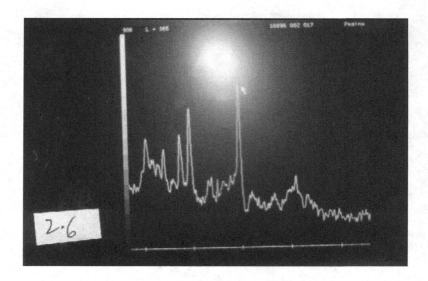

Figure 5:6—SPECT MRI of the brain of a person with Alzheimer's disease showing hypoperfusion of the frontal lobe of the brain.

These small vessels are located deep inside the brain and supply blood to very vital structures within the brain. This condition is associated with early memory loss resulting in organic brain syndrome. Multiple small vessel infarctions are second only to Alzheimer's disease as a cause of senility. In fact, it is probably more common than Alzheimer's in terms of causing senility because there are so many more hypertensive patients than people who have Alzheimer's. It is common to see 40-year-old black women who have been hypertensive since their 30s or 20s who are having difficulty remembering very simple things because of multiple small vessel infarctions of the brain, as seen on brain MRI (magnetic resonance imaging). (CT of the brain does not show this syndrome very well.)

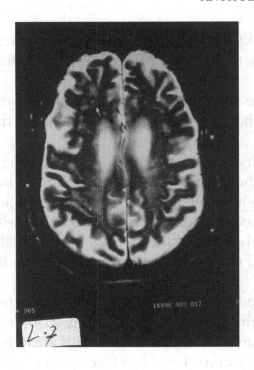

Figure 57:7-MRI of the brain of a person with Alzheimer's disease and longstanding hypertension showing multiple small vessel infarctions of the brain.

In evaluating memory loss in a 40—to 60-year-old hypertensive person, the following tests need to be done:

1. A complete history and physical examination by a competent internist, primary care physician or neurologist
2. CBC with differential
3. SMA20
4. Urinalysis
5. Thyroid tests such as T4, TSH, and T3
6. B12/ Folate levels
7. Complete lipid profile
8. Lipoprotein-a
9. Homocysteine level
10. VDRL
11. HIV test
12. Chest x-ray
13. EKG
14. Brain CT scan
15. MRI of the brain
16. Carotid Ultrasound

If the tests mentioned above are normal and the neurological examination is normal, then a SPECT scan of the brain must be done to look for hypoperfusion in the frontal lobe of the brain. (Hypoperfusion in the frontal lobe of the brain is seen in

Alzheimer's disease on SPECT MRI of the brain.). Enlargement of the temporal horns of the lateral ventricles when present on MRI of the brain is diagnostic of AD.

Each one of these tests is done for a particular reason. The history gives the physician a profile as to what sorts of exposures or conditions the patient may have had.

The physical examination allows the physician the opportunity to find abnormalities that may shed light on the poor memory. The complete blood count tells the physician if the white blood cell count is either too low or too high. Both too low and too high white blood cell counts may be associated with conditions that might explain the memory loss. It is important to realize that there is a difference in the level of white blood cell (WBC) counts in Caucasians compared to Blacks and Hispanics.

The normal white blood cell count in whites is 4,500 to 10,000. In Blacks and Hispanics, the normal white blood cell count is from 3,500 to 10,000. In Blacks from the Caribbean, and Ashkenazi Jews, the normal WBC may be as low as 2.500. If the WBC is found to be 3,500 or even lower in a Black person, and the differential count is normal, then there may not be a need to do anything further other than ANA, ESR and rheumatoid factor to rule out collagen vascular disease or connective tissue diseases.

However, low WBC/leukopenia is a very important finding and may have serious medical implications. It is up to each individual physician to decide what to do when the WBC is in a particular clinical setting.

The red blood cell count tells the physician whether the poor memory is due to low red cell count (anemia) or too high red blood cell count (polycythemia). When the red blood cell count is too low, oxygen cannot be delivered easily to the body's vital organs, including the brain. Poor oxygen delivery to the brain is one of the causes of poor memory (organic brain syndrome).

When the red blood cell count is too high such as in polycythemia, the high viscosity of the blood results in stagnation of blood flow within blood vessels making it difficult for oxygen to get to the brain for proper functioning.

The thicker the blood, the more difficult it is for oxygen to get to the memory center in the brain for good memory to occur. The platelet count, which is part of the CBC, is also very important.

If the platelets drop to less than 10,000 (normal platelet count is 130,000 to 400,000), spontaneous bleeding can occur anywhere in the body, including the brain. Bleeding in the brain can result in serious brain malfunctions including stroke and poor memory. If the platelet count is too high—750,000 to 1,000,000 or greater—both stroke and bleeding can occur within the brain, resulting in poor brain functioning including poor memory. **(This occurs only if the high platelet count is associated with a myeloproliferative disorder.)**

Abnormalities in the differential blood count may indicate many different abnormalities, including leukemia or lymphoma, both of which frequently affect the brain, resulting in poor brain functioning. The blood chemistry and its component parts are very important in determining whether a person's poor memory is due to abnormality or abnormalities of the body's chemistry.

Abnormalities in the electrolytes can cause poor brain function. The electrolytes are sodium, potassium, chloride, and bicarbonate. Severe acidosis (too low bicarbonate) or severe alkalosis (too high bicarbonate) can lead to abnormalities that can cause brain abnormalities and brain malfunction. Too high blood sodium (a condition called hypernatremia), the normal sodium being 135 to 140, can cause brain malfunction, including confusion, to occur. Too low blood sodium 110-120 can cause low blood pressure, confusion, poor memory, and, at times, seizures to occur.

One of the frequent abnormalities in the blood chemistries that can cause brain malfunction is too low blood sugar, known as hypoglycemia. The normal blood sugar is between 60 and 112. When the blood sugar falls to less than 60 or lower, this situation can lead to confusion, poor memory, or seizure. Starvation is a common cause of low blood sugar. Medications such as blood sugar-lowering pills and insulin are the most common medications that frequently cause too low blood sugar to occur.

When the blood sugar is too high 400 or greater it can lead to a condition called diabetic ketoacidosis, which can cause severe brain malfunction and, if not treated quickly and properly, can cause the person to go into a coma and die. What happens in diabetic ketoacidosis is that the person is unable to use sugar as fuel, due to lack of insulin; therefore, fat is being used as fuel, resulting in breakdown products of fat, which are ketone bodies. These ketone bodies are toxic to the body, leading to severe brain malfunctioning, including confusion and sometimes seizures.

There is another condition involving high blood sugar called non-ketotic hyperglycemia, which frequently can lead to coma if left untreated for very long. In this condition, there is no high level of ketones, but the blood sugar rises very high, and sometimes greater than 2,000, and frequently in people who never before had trouble with elevated blood sugar.

High blood sugar acts as diuretic and affected individuals pass a large quantity of urine daily and experience extreme thirst. After a while, the volume of urine that he or she passes is far in excess of the fluid he or she takes in, resulting in severe dehydration, including dehydration of the brain, causing coma to develop, and death if left untreated.

When the kidneys are malfunctioning, many abnormalities can be detected in the blood and in the urine, but some of the earliest and most important abnormalities that can be seen when the kidneys start to fail are:

1. High BUN
2. High creatinine
3. High potassium
4. High phosphate
5. Low bicarbonate
6. Anemia
7. Too much protein in the urine
8. Low 24-hour urine creatinine clearance
9. Low GFR
10. High microalbumin level in the urine

When the kidneys fail, waste products which are very toxic cannot be removed from the blood, resulting in malfunctioning of the brain including confusion and seizures.

Another important series of blood chemistry tests that are used by physicians to detect diseases in the human body are the liver function tests. In particular, liver function tests such as serum calcium, serum phosphate, serum LDH, serum SGOT, serum SGPT, GGTP, serum uric acid, serum bilirubin, and alkaline phosphatase and prothrombin time and uric acid.

Abnormalities seen in these different tests may indicate association with different diseases such as hepatitis, cancer involving the liver, etc. Complete liver failure causes mental confusion and, at times, seizures. If the urinalysis is abnormal, it may indicate infection in the bladder or kidneys. If sugar is found in the urine, it may indicate diabetes mellitus.

If a substance called acetone is found in the urine, this may indicate dehydration or the presence in the body of the condition called diabetic ketoacidosis as mentioned above, seen in people who are diabetic, when the diabetes is out of control.

If protein is found in the urine, it may indicate different degrees of kidney failure. When sediment of the urine is examined under the microscope, different crystals may be seen in association with kidney stones. Materials called casts of different types may be seen in these sediments representing association with different diseases of the kidneys. Prominent among these diseases include hematuria, (blood in the urine both gross and microscopic), urinary tract infection, kidney stone, sickle cell disease, cancer of the bladder, cancer of the kidney.

When the kidneys fail, urine output ceases and different degrees of mental confusion can be seen and if dialysis is not carried out to cleanse the blood of toxic substances, coma may ensue, which may result in death. Blood tests to evaluate the functions of the thyroid glands are very important. Both hypothyroidism (low function of the thyroid gland) and hyperthyroidism (high function of the thyroid gland) can cause mental aberration, resulting at times in memory loss, confusion, and many times, coma.

Evaluating serum magnesium, serum phosphorus, parathyroid hormone and vitamin D3 levels are extremely important to rule out secondary hyperparathyroidism and Rickett's disease/osteomalasia.

Low Vitamin B12 can cause a multitude of problems, such as numbness, pain and needle symptoms over the legs and the fingers. Memory loss and neurological damage can occur because of low B12. If the B12 level remains low for five years or more, permanent brain and neurological damage are certain to occur.

The conditions that can cause low Vitamin 12 include:

Diet deficient in vitamin B12
Atrophic gastritis
Malabsorption
Tropical sprue
Non-tropical sprue
Crhon's disease
Ulcerative colitis
Blind loop syndrome
Fish tape worm infestation
Gastrectomy
Pernicious anermia
Xerostomia
Inhalation of Nitrous oxide
Chronic pancriatitis with secondary malabsorption.

More recently, a condition has been discovered the low B12 syndrome occuring in the elderly population. It is, therefore, very important to do a B12 level when evaluating a person for memory loss. It is also important if one has evidence physically that a person is suffering from B12 deficiency and the B12 level comes back normal, to do a urine or blood test for methylmalonic acid. It is a very sensitive test because if someone has B12 deficiency the methylmalonic acid will be elevated.

A test for syphilis, using the RPR or VDRL, is very important because syphilis, when involving the brain, can cause severe brain damage resulting in memory loss, etc. The VDRL test is used to detect syphilis in the human body; if it is positive, it is very important to do the confirmatory blood test, FTA-ABS (Fluorescent Treponoma Antibody-Absorption Test). In true syphilitic infection, this test stays positive for life. When neurosyphilis is suspected, then a CT scan ought to be done, and if the CT scan appears normal, then a lumbar puncture ought to be conducted to examine the cerebrospinal fluid for the presence of syphilis.

In the evaluation of poor memory (organic brain syndrome) the HIV Type I or Type II test is very important and ought to be done. Frequently, in AIDS, loss of memory is a presenting symptom. This is due either to HIV infection of the brain tissue itself or infections of the brain such as toxoplasmosis, cryptococcus of the brain or herpes infection of the brain, etc.

In evaluating poor memory or organic brain syndrome, the chest x-ray is very important because the chest x-ray may show evidence of cancer in the lungs, which if allowed to spread to the brain, can result in memory loss, confusion and, at times, coma.

There are many infectious processes that can be seen in the lungs on chest x-rays which may affect the function of the brain, resulting in poor memory, confusion and sometimes coma.

Doing an electrocardiogram in evaluating a patient with poor brain function is important because the EKG may show evidence of recent myocardial infarction during which the patient may have become hypotensive and that situation may have affected brain function transiently. The EKG may show cardiac arrhythmias or other rhythm abnormalities that may interfere with proper pumping of the heart, preventing adequate oxygen delivery to the brain, causing transient ischemic attack, and its associated brain malfunctions.

When a person presents to the emergency room or to the doctor's office with symptoms of brain malfunction manifesting as acute confusion or acute memory loss, this could at times be due to a syncopal episode. A syncopal episode can be caused by a number of different things, among them malfunctioning of the heart, which can oftentimes be seen on an EKG or 24-hour holter.

When a person presents with symptoms that are consistent with stroke, several things need to be done. A thorough history ought to be taken from the patient if she is able to speak, and if she cannot speak, the history should be taken from a family member. The next thing to do is to carry out a complete physical examination. It is crucial that the patient's airway be quickly evaluated to be certain she is breathing properly and that she has control over her saliva to prevent aspiration.

It is also crucial that all precautions are taken to watch out for seizures that can occur because of the damage to the brain. Oxygen ought to be administered, IV access ought to be established, and a foley catheter ought to be inserted. Blood must be drawn for blood tests such as CBC, SMA20, PT, PTT, ANA, ESR, B12, serum folate, lipid profile, serum liprotin a level, serum homocystein level, serum immunoglobulins levels and serum protein electrophoresis.

Other tests that need to be done are a chest x-ray, EKG, urinalysis and a brain CT. In acute stroke, the CT scan of the brain is used right away to see whether there is blood within the substance of the brain or whether the brain is swollen, the ventricles of the brain are pushed to one side or another, or whether there is a brain tumor.

Any one of these findings can cause symptoms consistent with a stroke. Sometimes evidence of old strokes can be seen on the same brain CT scan. When contrast material is injected into the patient's blood stream, through an arm vein, more can be seen within the brain, such as metastatic brain tumor or fungal infection such as toxoplasmosis, as seen in patients with AIDS.

Frequently, nothing is seen on a non-contrast brain CT in someone who has an acute stroke. That is not to say that the person does not have a stroke. It simply means it takes one to two weeks to see evidence of a non-bleeding stroke on a brain CT, but doing it eliminates the presence of both acute bleeding and brain tumor.

Elimination of these findings in the brain when someone presents with an acute stroke is not only important in diagnosing the cause of the acute stroke, but it also allows the treating physician the possibility to proceed with a test such as a lumbar puncture to rule out subacute bleeding.

It also allows the treating physician to use medications such as TPA (tissue plasminogen activator), heparin and aspirin, if he or she thinks that this is an evolving stroke. Heparin or TPA can help to prevent an acute stroke in this setting. The CT scan of the brain does all these things, in addition to being a diagnostic instrument. MRI of the brain can be used to evaluate the brain immediately after a stroke and it will show either the stroke or whatever else may be causing the patient's symptoms of a stroke.

Once the initial evaluations of the patient are completed, blood must be drawn for CBC, PT, PTT SMA20 (blood chemistry profile), lipid profile and urinalysis.

Depending on the severity of the stroke, a Foley catheter may be inserted into the bladder to insure that the patient can pass her urine and monitor her urine output.

If the blood pressure is very high, heparin ought not to be used to avoid bleeding into the brain. In this case, the blood pressure must be brought down very carefully to avoid worsening the stroke or to prevent the precipitation of a new stroke by dropping the blood pressure too fast.

If bleeding in the brain has been ruled out, then the patient ought to be given 325 mg of aspirin to chew and swallow. If she is not able to do these things, she then can be given the aspirin in suppository form rectally.

The decision that must be made is whether the patient should be given heparin intravenously or whether she should be given tPA IV in an attempt to dissolve the clot that is causing the stroke.

These are very difficult decisions and can only be made by the treating physicians who are at the bedside.

Then, one might ask why not do an MRI right way on everybody who has a stroke, bypassing the need for a brain CT? For one thing, the brain MRI is very expensive; it costs about $1,500 with contrast and $950.00 without contrast.

Brain CT with no contrast costs about $520. Another reason is that not every community hospital has MRI available and not everybody is suitable for an MRI study. Some people are claustrophobic; they just do not want to go into the MRI machine, and some people are too obese to fit into an MRI machine. The maximum weight that can fit in the MRI machine is about 300 lbs. Sometime in the future they might be able to make a machine that can fit these individuals.

Some facilities now have open MRI available which makes it easier for individuals who are claustrophobic to be able to undergo the MRI test. In addition, there are certain individuals who have metals implanted in them due to a previous accident or other surgical procedure, making them unsuitable for the MRI machine.

The list of metals found in the body that can prevent an MRI from being done is quite long, but the most important ones include:

1. Aneurysm and haemostatic clips
2. Biopsy needles
3. Carotid artery vascular clamps
4. Dental implant devices and materials
5. Halo vests
6. Heart valve prosthesis
7. Intravascular coils, filters, and stents
8. Ocular implants
9. Orthopedic implants, materials, and devices
10. Otologic implants

11. Pellets and bullets
12. Penile implants
13. Vascular access ports, etc., as published in the literature

Some of these devices may, in fact, be dislodged or moved by the magnetic field of the MRI machine, with possible disastrous consequences. All of the above tests and procedures may be necessary, at any one time, in any patient who presents with a stroke.

Blacks and other minorities are at higher risk of having strokes compared to whites because of their higher incidence of hypertension, obesity, and diabetes mellitus. Blacks and other minorities are five times more likely to have a stroke and dying from that stroke compared to whites.

Some of the predisposing factors for developing a stroke:

1. Blacks and other minorities are many times more likely to be hypertensives than whites are and hypertensive blacks and other minorities are less likely to seek medical care for their hypertension. When treatment is given, it is less likely to be appropriate and, therefore, less effective.

2. The incidence of obesity is quite high among blacks. Approximately 81% of black women in the United States are obese/overweight and 68% of black men are obese/overweight, two third of the adults in the U.S. are obese/overweight and obesity plays a major role in the elevation of blood pressure.

3. The high salt content diet of many people eat plays a major role in the elevation of the blood pressure and its devastating propensity in causing stroke.

4. Another factor that plays a role in an increased incidence of stroke in is stress. Most blacks and other minorities are under stress because of racial discrimination, their poorer educational status, poorer economic status, poorer social status, and their overall poorer living conditions, which cause a constant state of stress, resulting in elevation of adrelanin, such as epinephrine and norepinephrine. These can cause a rise in blood pressure with subsequent development of stroke.

Until these conditions are vastly improved in blacks and minorities, the incidence of stroke in blacks and other minorities in the world and in the United States, can be expected to continue unabated.

People can decrease their incidence of dying from stroke simply by decreasing the amount of salt, fat, and simple carbohydrates in their foods and by exercising regularly.

Stress is something over which blacks and other minorities in the world have no control over. Presently, blacks other minorities and poor people in the world eat the types of foods they can afford to eat. In the U.S. 50 million people go hungry every day, and 17 million children in the U.S. go hungry daily. Worldwide, 1 billion people go hungry every day. Twenty five thousands people die every day in the world because of hunger and fifteen million children die every year in the world because of hunger and in total, thirty five million people die every year in the world because of hunger.

It is a known fact that the poorer the individual, the less likely it is that he or she is able to afford the proper nutritional types of foods that are necessary to maintain good health. Sometimes it is not so much the quantity or quality of the food itself, but a combination of poor quality, high quantity, and poor preparation. The way one prepares one's food goes a long way in keeping one healthy.

Many blacks and other minorities in the world donot have access to foods of good quality. However, there are many simple things that can be done to prepare the foods in a healthier way. They should be careful to avoid some of the negative consequences of eating foods that are too salty, greasy, or too studded with simple carbohydrates. They ought to try to eat a lot of vegetables and fruits and whole grains if at all possible. Obviously this not aleways possible and to satisfy hunger, people eat what they have access to.

Treatments of strokes include aspirin, heparin, tPA, control of hypertension and physical therapy with rehabilitation therapy. These are used in different stages of the stroke syndrome.

One of the important things to do for the stroke patient is to provide him or her with prophylactic anticoagulant treatment with either Coumadin or heparin to prevent DVT (deep vein thrombophlebitis).

Patients who suffer hemorrhagic strokes ought not to be given anticoagulation to prevent DVT or pulmonary embolism because this type of treatment would cause more bleeding into the brain. In these cases, a sequential compression device ought to be used in their legs to prevent DVT and a Greenfield filter ought to be placed in their inferior vena cava to prevent the migration of clot into the lung, which can cause pulmonary embolism.

Every year in the USA, 2.5 million people have DVT (clot in the leg) and 600,000 people develop pulmonary embolism (Source: Internal Medicine World Report, Vol. 18 No. 6, and June 2003). The direct and indirect cost of stroke in 2010 was $73.5 billion.

In summary, it is clear that diet and weight management, exercise, and appropriate anti-hypertensive are important factors in the prevention of high blood pressure and stroke and in the prolongation of the life of people.

Chapter 58
DEPRESSION

Mental illness is one of the most common illnesses in the world. One in every four individuals or 25% of people in the world suffers from some types of mental illnesses.

The world population in 2013 is 7,103,804 people and 25% or 1,775,951,000 of them suffer from mental illnesses. 350, 000,000 in the world suffer from depression, in the world 25, 000, 000 suffer from schizophrenia, 2.4 % people in the world suffer from bipolar disorder, 5.7 000,000 American adults suffer from bipolar disorder, 24, 000,000 suffer from schizophrenia, 20,000,000 Americans suffer from depression and worldwide 140, 000,000 million suffer from alcoholism. Source: WHO

According to the Surgeon General, there are 44 million Americans with mental illness one in 4 Americans suffers with a diagnosable mental illness. Every year 19 million Americans suffer from some form of mental illnesses.

Mental illness affects all racial groups, both sexes and all social strata. However, Black Americans, Hispanic Americans other American minorities and other minorities in the world are affected by depression more than whites are. Mental is the number one cause of suicide. Every day 3000 people in the world commit suicide because of depression and 90% of suicide is due to mental illness.

Depression is more common than cancer, heart disease and HIV/AIDS combined.

There are different types of depression:

1. Transient situational depression
2. Permanent or chronic situational depression
3. Depression associated with taking medications for a medical condition
4. Depression associated with alcohol abuse or drug abuse
5. Minor classical depression
6. Major classical depression
7. Depression associated with anxiety reaction and panic attacks
8. Manic depression, etc.

(The concept of permanent or chronic situational depression is the author's own developed concept.)
Incidence of depression

Depression is 3 to 4 times more common in black men and other minority men than black women and other minority women. In the U.S. more than 17 million individuals (about 1 in 10 adults) suffer from a depressive episode at least once per year and more than 80% of the time these episodes go untreated.

According to some study, blacks and other minorities suffer more from mental illnesses than whites are.

Blacks, Hispanics and other minorities experience more depression, anxiety and panic attacks than whites do. Being poor is a depressive state of being and, therefore, 100% of poor people suffer from one form of depression or another, at one time or another worldwide. The difference is in the cultural expression of these symptoms and the cultural conditioning and reluctance to express the symptoms of these illnesses for fear of being ostracized by their communities. Being poor, it is a miserable state, however, is not a shame and many people have worked themselves out of poverty.

In any African ancestral society, mental illness is taboo because it is seen as a sign of weakness. A failure to be able to endure whatever it is that the majority of society can dish out and not only surviving it, enduring it and to be able to live long enough to tell one's children and grandchildren about it, is an essential part of the indigenous black culture.

Blacks and Hispanics and other minorities see mental illness as a label that can be used to discriminate against them by the medical community, the job market, the legal community and, by the law enforcement community to prevent them from getting ahead. Because these people do not want any mention of mental illness on their records if they can help it, they hide their symptoms of depression and suffer in silence.

When an interviewer tries to elicit mental illness from them, they would not tell him or her about it. They frequently do not tell a physician/therapist about their mental illness either, unless they absolutely have to.

Table 1

Some of the symptoms of major depression:

Five (or more) of the following symptoms have been present during the same 2-week period and represent a change from previous functioning: at least one of the symptoms is either depressed mood or loss of interest in pleasure, excluding symptoms that are due to medical illnesses.

(1) Depressed mood most of the day, nearly every day as indicated by either subjective report (e.g., feels sad or empty) or observation made by others (e.g., appears tearful). **Note:** In children and adolescents, can be irritable mood.

(2) Markedly diminished interest or pleasure in all, or almost all activities most of the day, nearly every day (as indicated by either subjective account or observation made by others.)

(3) Significant weight loss when not dieting or weight gain (e.g., a change of more than 5% of body weight in a month), or decrease or increase in appetite nearly every day. **Note:** In children, consider failure to make expected weight gains.

(4) Insomnia or hypersomnia every day

(5) Psychomotor agitation or retardation nearly every day (observable by others, not merely subjective feelings of restlessness or being slowed down)

(6) Fatigue or loss of energy every day

(7) Feelings of worthlessness or excessive or inappropriate guilt (which may be delusional) nearly every day (not merely self-reproach or guilt about being sick)

(8) Diminished ability to think or concentrate, or indecisiveness, nearly every day (either by subjective account or as observed by others).

(9) Recurrent thoughts of death (not just fear of dying), recurrent suicidal ideation without a specific plan, or a suicide attempt or a specific plan for committing suicide.

B. These symptoms do not meet criteria for a mixed episode.

C. The symptoms cause clinically significant distress or impairment in social, occupational, or other important areas of functioning.

D. The symptoms are not due to the direct physiological effects of a substance (e.g., a drug of abuse, a medication) or a general medical condition (e.g., hypothyroidism).

E. The symptoms are not better accounted for by bereavement, i.e., after the loss of a loved one, the symptoms persist for longer than 2 months or are characterized by marked functional impairment, morbid occupation with worthlessness, suicidal ideation, psychotic symptoms, or psychomotor retardation.

As modified from DSM IV

Depression as seen in blacks is a very complex disease with many associated components. Classical minor depression is defined as 3 or 4 depressive symptoms for 2 weeks or longer. Major depression is defined as 5 or more depressive symptoms for 2 weeks or longer.

TABLE 2

Some symptoms of minor depression:

A. A distinct period of abnormally and persistently elevated, expansive, or irritable mood, lasting at least 1 week (or any duration if hospitalization is necessary).

B. During the period of mood disturbance, three (or more) of the following symptoms have persisted (four if the mood is only irritable) and have been present to a significant degree.

(1) Inflated self-esteem or grandiosity

(2) Decreased need for sleep (e.g., feels rested after only 3 hours of sleep)

(3) More talkative than usual or pressure to keep talking

(4) Flight of ideas or subjective experience that thoughts are racing

(5) Distractibility (i.e., attention too easily drawn to unimportant or irrelevant external stimuli)

(6) Increase in goal-directed activity (either socially, at work or school, or sexually) or psychomotor agitation

(7) Excessive involvement in pleasurable activities that have a high potential for painful consequences (e.g., engaged in unrestrained buying sprees, sexual indiscretions, or foolish business investments)

C. These symptoms do not meet criteria for a mixed episode.

D. The mood disturbance is sufficiently severe to cause marked impairment in occupational functioning or in usual social activities or relationships with others, or to necessitate hospitalization to prevent harm to self or others, or there are psychotic features.

E. The symptoms are not due to the direct physiological effects of a substance (e.g., a drug of abuse, a medication, or other treatment) or a general medical condition (e.g., hyperthyroidism).

Blacks, Hispanics and other minorities worldwide can suffer from the classic forms of depression such as:

1. Minor depression.
2. Major depression.
3. Manic depression.

1. A mixed form of depression associated with anxiety and panic attacks.
2. Transient and permanent situational depression.
3. Depression associated with alcohol abuse and drug abuse.

Criteria used to make the diagnosis of major depression:

Blacks, as well as Hispanic, are extremely reluctant to go to the psychiatrist because of the fear of being labeled "crazy" in the case Hispanics "loco". Both these groups culturally deal with mental illness the way in which mental illness is dealt with in the African culture.

In the African culture, when a person of African ancestry is troubled with a mood disorder, he or she goes to an elder or group of family members within that family for advice in order to deal with the problem. Sometimes this group is organized as a committee, as is done frequently in the third world. Never in this setting is the word mental illness used. In fact, in the third world it is unlikely that a man would marry into a family that has an immediate member with a history of being mentally ill.

Because of racism, different degrees and different types of racial insensitivity and the suspicion and distrust that it causes, Blacks and Hispanics in the U.S. and in the world are almost exclusively reluctant to seek help for mental illness, and in particular depression, because most of the psychiatrists-therapists are Caucasians.

The reasons Blacks, Hispanics and other minorities give for refusing to see Caucasian or non-minority psychiatrists-therapists are as follows:

"Why should I go to the white and non-Hispanic, non-black psychiatrist-therapist to open up my innermost secrets to them, when they are partly responsible for my problems to begin with?"

Q. *"You mean the psychiatrist-therapist is the source of your problem?"*
A. "No, not him or her in particular, but he or she belongs to the group of people that is the underlying cause of my depression in the first place."
Q. "How so, could you elaborate?"
A. "Well, you know, racial insensitivity and bigotry are so pervasive and widespread you don't know who to trust and who not to trust."
Q. "Is it that you have a problem trusting anyone?"
A. *"No, I just have difficulty opening up my inner soul to the people who I know don't like me in the first place." And have a predetermined negavite notion about me.*

It is a known fact that when Blacks, Hispanics and other minorities are evaluated for mental illness by white psychiatrists-therapists, oftentimes the diagnosis made is wrong. The literature outlines cases of Blacks, Hispanics and other minorities that were diagnosed as schizophrenics, when in fact they were not.

Because of subjectivity that is often involved in the diagnosis of mental illnesses, very frequently psychiatrist-therapists and others involved in dealing with Blacks, Hispanics and other minorities who have mental illness tend to give them a worse diagnosis rather than a better diagnosis, and clearly racism, racial insensitivity, bigotry, racial insensitivity and intellectually condescendency play a major role in that particular situation.

Transient situational depression occurs in all groups regardless of ethnic background. In what normally would have been transient situational depression because of a loss of a job, a boyfriend, a girl friend, a death in the family, or the death of a close friend, etc. can sometime ends up in a severe form of depression.

The depression would seem to last longer because underneath exists a mental fragility born out of constant exposure to racial injustices, making it easier to cross over the line to a more permanent situational depressive state.

Permanent and chronic situational depression in blacks in the U.S. is a condition born out of constant and relentless barrages of daily exposure to racial discrimination and injustices at all levels of American society. Many several sub-cultures in the world communities whose poor people have been conditioned or brainwashed into the belief that their poverty is the result of divine will.

These folks then are coerced through different means to pray to God for easing of their earthly suffering to get to heaven, to get their divine rewards. This concept does not seem to be as prevalent among blacks in the U.S. as elsewhere in the world.

It does not matter if a black person in America works as a sanitation worker or as physician or a judge in a court of law; he or she has to deal with racial discrimination and racial confrontations, be it in different forms and different circumstances.

Granted, the less educated and less financially able a person is, the more he or she feels the stings and often the bites of racism eating away at his or her flesh, heart and soul. Because racism has become an accepted part of the American culture, Blacks and Hispanics and other minorities feel a sense of constant persecution that is "real" and, therefore, they are more prone to become chronically situationally depressed.

Most Caucasians and most non-blacks individuals leaving in America constantly discriminate racially against blacks in America. They do it because they see white Americans doing it, so they do it too. In particular, black men are the most discriminated against human beings in the U.S. by all other racial groups.

Some blacks in America and around the world have developed coping mechanisms to both survive racism and its depressive nature. Some blacks have chosen to excel at whatever it is that they do; they go beyond that which is necessary as a mechanism of coping, not just to be accepted necessarily, but also to be respected.

Professional respect means a lot to any professional person, but more so to blacks and other minorities. Professional blacks and other minorities typically would say, "Though you don't like the color of my skin and many other things about me, but

I dare you to doubt my ability to beat you at your own game and do my work with excellence" and more often than not, much better than you.

Some blacks and other minorities have chosen to become activists and community organizers, to wake up other blacks and minorities, to fight for their rights. Still, others have chosen to give up and allow racism to engulf all aspects of their beings by becoming welfare recipients and part of the culture of the have-nots.

Many people are on welfare because of physical or mental disabilities, and this is both acceptable and understandable, but many minorities have become so chronically passive, and dependent, they do not care a damn anymore, so welfare has become a way of life for them.

Still many blacks and other minorities have allowed their anger and despair to cause them to fall into the trap of drug, alcohol and other substance abuse, which have totally taken over their lives to a degree that their very humanity represents nothing to them. Thefore, the lives of other individuals have not much value to them either. It is this state of being, that causes some of them to commit unspeakable crimes against their neighbors, and their communities (see the chapters on drug abuse and alcohol abuse).

Depression, associated with anxiety and panic attacks, is extremely common in minorities. However, this type of depression is much more common in minorities than in whites based on the fact most minorities have more reasons to be anxious, and even more reason to be panicky.

This is so because blacks and other minorities have to face racism, poor education, and lack of jobs, lower economic status, raising children without a father around to help, and many other unspeakable injustices to cope with. All the above problems create a constant state of negative anger, disappointment, uncertainty, and the result is anxiety, panic attacks, and depression.

> THE WAY TO SUCCEED AS A BLACK PERSON IN THE U.S. AND THE WORLD IS TO AVOID THE NEGATIVE ANGER SYNDROME RATHER, IS TO BE POSITIVELY ANGRY.
> NEGATIVE ANGER IS DESTRUCTIVE AND POSITIVE ANGER IS CONSTRUCTIVE.

What makes this whole situation even more serious is the fact that more often than not, these Blacks, Hispanics and other minorities go without being diagnosed and without being treated for their mental illnesses. A small sub-group of educated and professional Blacks, Hispanics and other minorities does seek help and are receiving psychological treatment.

How to evaluate a Black, Hispanic and a minority person who comes in for evaluation of depression to the primary care physician

In the black community, the primary care physician is likely to be the one who is most likely to see the vast majority of blacks with depression. This is so because these blacks are extremely resistant to the concept that they may have a need for psychological care. This reluctant to admit mental illness is a cultural fact and it must be understood, respected and dealt with, with the greatest of care and ethnic sensitivity.

TABLE 3

Some of the most common symptoms of depression:

Depression
Persistent sad, anxious, or "empty" mood
Loss of interest or pleasure in activities, including sex
Feelings of hopelessness, pessimism
Feelings of guilt, worthlessness, helplessness
Sleeping too much or too little, early-morning awakening
Appetite and/or weight loss or overeating and weight gain
Decreased energy, fatigue, feeling "slowed down"
Thoughts of death or suicide, or suicide attempts
Restlessness, irritability
Difficulty concentrating, remembering, or making decisions
Persistent physical symptoms that do not respond to treatment, such as headaches, digestive disorders, and chronic pain
Mania

Abnormally elevated mood
Irritability
Severe insomnia
Grandiose notions
Increased talking
Racing thoughts
Increased activity, including sexual activity
Markedly increased energy
Poor judgment that leads to risk-taking behavior
Inappropriate social behavior

A thorough diagnostic evaluation is needed if five or more of these symptoms persist for more than two weeks, or if they interfere with work or family life. An evaluation involves a complete physical checkup and information gathering on family health history.

(As published by the National Institute of Mental Health)

Some of the symptoms of panic attack:

1. Palpitations, pounding of heart, or accelerated heart rate
2. Sweating
3. Trembling or shaking
4. Sensation of shortness of breath or smothering
5. Feeling of choking
6. Chest pain or discomfort
7. Nausea or abdominal distress
8. Feeling dizzy, lightheaded, or faint
9. Derealization (feelings of unreality) or depersonalization (being detached from oneself)
10. Fear of losing control or going crazy
11. Fear of dying
12. Paresthesias (numbness or tingling sensation)
13. Chills or hot flashes
14. Abdominal pain
15. Diarrhea
16. White-out spells
17. Urinary frequency
18. Hyperventilation
19. Leg cramps
20. Insomnia

Partially modified from DSM IV

The first step in evaluation someone with depression includes a complete history and physical examination. The next step is a series of specific laboratory tests such as:

1. CBC
2. Chemistry profile (SMA 18)
3. Thyroid profile T4, TSH
4. Urinalysis
5. Serum ferritin
6. Serum B12
7. Chest x-ray
8. EKG
9. Mammogram, if the woman is 40 years or older; or younger if a mass is felt in the breast or if there is a family history of breast cancer

10. A CT scan of the brain or MRI of the brain, if there is headache, dizziness, and forgetfulness, or symptoms of neurological signs are found during the history and physical examination. In fact, it may be important to do a CT scan anyway, even though there may be no obvious neurological signs or symptoms.

Other specific blood tests may become necessary based on the physician's assessment of the case.

Approaching the patient in this way allows the physician to ascertain whether or not the patient's signs and symptoms of depression, anxiety or panic attacks have no organic basis (that is, nothing medical can explain her symptoms).

Diseases such as diabetes mellitus, hyperthyroidism, hypothyroidism, cancer, iron deficiency anemia, kidney failure, heart disease such as mitral valve prolapsed, atherosclerotic heart disease with angina pectoris, congestive heart failure with low cardiac output and poor brain perfusion, B12 deficiency, etc. (if a person remains B12 deficient for 3 to 5 years, he or she may develop permanent neuropsychiatric problems).

It is not unusual to find a patient in a psychiatric hospital who is permanently committed as a result of B12 deficiency that either was not diagnosed at all or was diagnosed too late, resulting in permanent neurological and mental disease.

Brain tumor may first present with symptoms of psychiatric disease. It is, therefore, always necessary for a person who manifests symptoms of depression to undergo a thorough medical evaluation by a primary care physician before any definite statement can be made regarding the proper psychiatric diagnosis of that woman.

Both hyperthyroidism and hypothyroidism can manifest symptoms of depression. As part of the evaluation of depression, serum B12, T4, TSH, and brain CT ought to be done.

It is important that prior to starting any psychotropic medications, a CBC, liver function tests and EKG be done, because many of the psychotropic medications have many side effects that can cause the white blood cell count, the platelets, the red blood cell count as well as the EKG and liver function test to be abnormal.

Some of these medications can affect the rhythm of the heart in different ways, so a baseline EKG must be done before starting these medications. In fact, periodically CBC, kidney function tests such as BUN, creatinine, electrolytes, liver function tests, T4, TSH must be done during the course of psychotropic medication therapy.

Treatments of depression

Depression is treated usually with medications, psychotherapy and, at times, with ECT.

Some of the medications used to treat depression are the following:

Serotonin-specific reuptake inhibitors such as:
1. Zoloft
2. Paxil
3. Prozac
4. Celexa
5. Lexapro
6. Paxil
7. Celexa
8. Luvox etc;

Serotonin non-selective reuptake inhibitors such as:
1. Effexor
2. Effexor XR
3. Cymbalta etc;

Other anti-depression medications:
1. Wellbutrin
2. Wellbutrin SR
3. Remeron
4. Ludiomil, which is basically a dopamine-active medication
5. Norpramin.
6. Serzone
7. Symbyax
8. Desyrel
9. Pristiq
10. Serzone etc;

Anti-Anxiety medications include
1. BuSpar
2. Klonopin
3. Xanax
4. Lithium
5. Ativan
6. Valium
7. Serax
8. Valium
9. Klonorpin

10. Centrax
11. Serax
12. Librium
13. Tranxene etc;

Tertiary amines such as:
1. Elavil
2. Tofranil
3. Anafranil
4. Sinequan
5. Tofranil
6. Pamelor
7. Ascendin
8. Anafranil
9. Surmontil
10. Vivactil etc;

MAOIs or monoamine oxidase inhibitors such as:
1. Parnate
2. Eldepryl
3. Nardil etc;

The usual dosages and side effects of these medications are:

1. **Zoloft**—The initial dose is 50 mg per day; this dose can be increased up to 200 mg per day. There are several tolerable side effects of Zoloft, and liver function tests and EKG must be closely monitored along with blood levels while the patient is on Zoloft.
2. **Paxil**—The usual starting dose of Paxil is 20 mg per day and this dose can be increased up to 50 mg per day for those people who fail to respond to the 20 mg dose. Paxil can cause several tolerable side effects, but liver function tests and EKG must be monitored along with Paxil blood level.
3. **Prozac**—The usual dose of Prozac is 20 mg per day. If a patient fails to respond to 20 mg per day, the dose can be increased up to 80 mg per day. Prozac has several side effects, and liver function tests and EKG ought to be monitored along with blood level of Prozac.
4. **Effexor**—The usual starting dose of Effexor is 25 mg three times per day. The dose may be increased up to 150 mg per day in divided doses, and in rare circumstances, the dose may be raised to as high as 275 mg per day in divided doses. Effexor has many tolerable side effects, but liver function tests and periodic EKG ought to be done along with blood level of the medication.

5. **Wellbutrin SR**—The usual dose of Wellbutrin SR is 150 mg two times per day; at times a dose of 200 mg two times per day can be given. Wellbutrin SR has several tolerable side effects, but is important to monitor liver function tests, EKG and blood level of Wellbutrin SR.

6. **Ludiomil**—The usual dose of Ludiomil is 75 mg per day. In the elderly, as little as 25 mg per day may be effective. Doses as high as 150 mg to 225 mg may be used in hospital patients. Ludiomil has several tolerable side effects, but periodic EKG, liver function tests should be done.

7. **Norpramin**—The usual dose of Norpramin is 100 mg to 200 mg per day. This dose may be increased to as high as 300 mg per day. This medication is not recommended for use in children. Norpramin is not to be used in conjunction with MAO inhibitors. In fact, it cannot be used up to two weeks after stopping MAO inhibitors. Norpramin has several tolerable side effects, but CBC, liver function tests, EKG; and blood thyroid function must be done before starting this medication. These same tests must be done periodically while a patient is on Norpramin.

8. **Pamelor**—The usual dose of Pamelor is 25 mg 3-4 times per day. At times, the dose may be raised up to 150 mg per day. Pamelor has several tolerable side effects. While on this medication, EKG, CBC, liver function tests ought to be done along with blood level of Pamelor.

9. **Lithium**—The usual maintenance dose of Lithium is 450 mg, two times per day but, doses as high as 1,350 mg per day may be given. Lithium has several tolerable side effects. Before starting a patient on Lithium, CBC, liver function tests, kidney function tests, blood thyroid function tests, and EKG must be done. While on Lithium, these same tests must be done and monitored closely. Blood level of Lithium must also be monitored. The kidneys are particularly sensitive to the effects of Lithium, and at the first signs of blood kidney function test abnormalities, the treatment must be stopped. Lithium can cause thyroid function tests to become abnormal. The WBC can sometimes go down as a result of Lithium.

10. **Desyrel**—The usual starting of Desyrel is 150 mg in divided doses, but a dose up to 600 mg per day in divided doses can be used. Desyrel has several tolerable side effects; therefore, an EKG ought to be done before starting this medication and periodically ought to be done while the person is on this drug.

11. **Asendin**—The usual dose of Asendin is 200-300 mg per day in divided doses. Asendin has several tolerable side effects. Blood chemistry tests, CBC and EKG should be done while the patient is on Asendin.

12. **Klonopin**—The initial dose of Klonopin is 1.5 mg per day in divided doses. Sometimes the dose can be raised to as high as 20 mg per day. This medication is quite effective in individuals with anxiety reaction associated with depression. It allows the patient to get a good night's sleep. CBC, liver function tests and EKG ought to be done before starting the medication and the same tests should be monitored while the patient is on the medication.

13. **BuSpar**—The usual dose of BuSpar to treat anxiety is 10 mg two times per day and the dose can be raised up to 30 mg per day in divided doses.

14. **Xanax**—The usual dose of Xanax to treat anxiety is 0.25 mg three times per day. A dose up to 4 mg per day can be used in divided doses, in certain cases. In treating panic disorder, the dose can be as high as 4 mg in divided doses. Xanax has several tolerable side effects, but laboratory tests are not required during the treatment of patient on Xanax.

15. **Elavil**—The usual dose of Elavil is 75 to 300 mg per day in divided doses. Elavil has several tolerable side effects. EKG, CBC, liver function tests, along with Elavil blood level should be done periodically while the patient is on Elavil.

16. **Tofranil**—The usual dose of Tofranil is 75 mg per day. The dose may be increased up to 150 mg per day. Tofranil has several tolerable side effects; EKG, CBC, liver function tests along with Tofranil blood level should be done periodically.

17. **Anafranil**—The usual starting dose of Anafranil is 25 mg per day and the dose may be increased up to 200 mg per day in divided doses. EKG, CBC, liver function tests, along with Anafranil blood levels, should be done periodically while a patient is on Anafranil.

18. **Doxepin**—The usual starting dose of Doxepin is 75 mg per day. The dose may be increased up to 300 mg per day. EKG, CBC, blood chemistry tests should be done periodically while the patient is on Doxepin.

19. **Parnate**—The usual starting dose of Parnate is 30 mg per day in divided doses. The dose may at times be increased to as high as 60 mg per day in divided doses. Frequent monitoring of blood pressure, EKG, CBC, blood chemistry tests ought to be done while the patient is on this medication. Parnate has a long list of medications that it cannot be used with. Further, there are several food products that must be avoided while on Parnate; among those are cheeses, foods high in tyramine, sour cream, Chianti wines, sherry, beer, liquors, caviar, anchovies, pickled herring, canned figs, raisins, bananas, avocados, chocolate, soybean, sauerkraut, yogurt, yeast extracts, etc.

ECT remains an effective modality of treatment for depression. ECT is used under a general anesthesia and muscle relaxants, decreasing convulsions and eliminating the possibility of fractures and other injuries to the patient. ECT is most appropriate for patients who cannot take medications or whose associated illnesses contradict them taking an antidepressant medication. In addition, in certain life-threatening situations, when all other antidepressant medications fail, then ECT is most appropriate and useful.

Psychotherapy

Psychotherapy is a non-medication effective modality of treatment for certain types of depression. Psychotherapy involves counseling. The mental health professionals who provide psychotherapy treatments are psychotherapists, psychiatrists, and certified social workers. Primary care physicians are well equipped to provide psychotherapy counseling, if they have the time to do it. The incidence of depression is 3 to 4 times more common in blacks than in their male counterparts.

Many people fear being stigmatized with mental illness and refrain from seeking psychiatric treatment for depression, until the depression is too far advanced and more difficult to treat.

These people avoid going to the psychiatrist for treatment of depression because of the stigma associated with mental illness. This situation is gravest among working poor and working Blacks, Hispanics and other minorities and poor people the world over. This is true for all minority people no matter their status.

Upper-class Blacks, Hispanics and other minorities are less concerned about going to the psychiatrist because they have money and enjoy a high social standing, they do not fear the stigma of mental illness, and the economic and social negativities associated with it.

In addition, most of these individuals seem to have high trust in the Caucasian therapists who dominate and control the field of psychiatry, psychology and social work.

It is common for Blacks, Hispanics and other minorities to seek counseling from their priests, pastors and their elders. The primary care physician of color is the first one to diagnose and treat depression in minorities, because these affected minorities feel more comfortable with him or her whom they have known for a long time and trust. Therefore, primary care physicians of color are providing the bulk of the treatment for depression in minorities because these minorities feel more comfortable with these doctors as just outlined.

Depression is a very common disease and much more so in minorities than in whites. Depression has many bases, many causes, and many manifestations. In minorities, depression can be gravest because of the penetrating and pernicious nature of racism, which fosters so much distrust of those in control of U.S. and the world societies, that it makes it difficult for minorities to seek help for their depressive illnesses.

Minorities have a higher propensity for the development of depression as compared to whites, as already stated, and the fact that they are under more stress and many of the have a lesser level of education, lesser economic status and a lower social standing, creates a situation that makes their depression more grave, more serious, more multifactorial and much more difficult to treat.

What can be done to lessen the propensity of minorities to develop depression?

It is crucial to educate these Blacks, Hispanics and other minorities about the seriousness of mental illnesses. The fact is that 80% or more of individuals who suffer from depression can be successfully treated and the best people to seek treatment from for depression are those who have the professional training and expertise to treat these treatable diseases.

It is also important to sensitize the professionals who are in the position to treat minorities, by considering their cultures, their daily economic and social strugles and other things that trouble them.

Different and more racially sensitive approaches must be undertaken in order to provide appropriate and better treatments for minorities with mental illnesses.

It is foolish and potentially harmful to attempt to impose the majority's views, hypocritical values, and traditional treatment modalities to minorities whose psychiatric problems are uniquein many instances.

The bases and factors that are contributing to their state of mind are themselves unique because of their unique societal circumstances. So if the professionals from the majority community do not take it upon themselves to familiarize themselves with the culture, and the circumstances of life and other different dynamics that inter—play leading to these depressive illnesses, they will fail most of the time in their attempt to treat them for these very serious, but treatable, mental diseases.

The training programs whose job it is to train these individuals must include several components of the cultural diversity as it relates to minorities and minority people's issues in general, into their training programs. Future mental health professionals need to acquire special skills and techniques that are necessary to deal with the psychological problems of mionorities and their unique features.

Those in charge of organizing training programs in the field of psychiatry, psychology, etc., ought to set up a required sub-specialty in cultural diversity of minority people and in their mental health training programs.

This will prepare their trainees for the real world of the twenty-first century, using a model that mirrors the reality of those individuals and all aspects of their lives.

The number of people of color in the mental health profession needs to be increased significantly to help in correcting the problems just outlined.

In so doing, many of the barriers of mistrust will be lowered to a significant degree, making it easier for Blacks, Hispanics and other people of color in the U.S. and around the world to be more receptive to the care that the mental health professionals are providing for them.

Chapter 59
ALCOHOLISM

Alcoholism is a very commomly abused sudstance in the United States and in the world. 18 million people in the U.S. and 140 million people in the world abuse Alcohol. One in twelve adults in the U.S. abuses alcohol. However, more people abuse alcohol than those who are registered. Worldwide 2 billion people drink alcohol. Source: WHO

Alcohol abuse affects all segments of society. At any one time, there are roughly 18 to 21 million individuals in the United States receiving one treatment or another for alcohol abuse and its multitude of associated medical and psychosocial problems.

The racial break down of the number people who drank alcohol on a regular basis in the year 2001, were white females 61%, black female 38.6%, American Indian and Alaska Native 38.6%, Asian 30.1%, Native Hawaiian and other Pacific Islanders 30.l% and 38.4% Hispanics drank alcohol.
(Source: CDC and National Center for Health Statistics, National Health Survey, family core and sample adult questionnaires, 2003).

"The ten countries with highest per capita consumption of alcohol are
1. Luxembourg
2. Ireland
3. France
4. Hungary
5. Denmark
6. Czech Republic
7. Spain
8. Portugal
9. Austria
10. Switzerland"

The annual cost of alcohol abuse and its associated medical complication is 223.5 billion dollars and alcoholism causes 79,000 deaths annually in the U.S.: N Engl j MED 368; 4 January 24, 2013. Worldwide 2.5 million people die from alcohol abuse yearly Source: WHO

Alcohol abuse is one of the most serious medical problems known to humankind. What makes alcohol use so easy and so widespread is that a person does not need a prescription to buy it. Alcohol is sold in liquor stores, bars, restaurants, airport shops, supermarkets, etc. Some people start drinking alcohol in their teens, as a recreational habit or because of peer pressure.

Frequently, teenagers see their parents abusing alcohol at home and getting drunk in front of them and they think it is OK for them to do the same thing (obviously it is not).

It is not too difficult to see how some teenagers can drink alcohol, are not reprimanded by their drinking parents, because the parents do it in front of them, so they think it is all right, and "cool" to do the same thing.

It is said, according to the literature, that some form of alcoholism is hereditary. Parents, it is said, transfer an alcoholism gene to their offspring, resulting in them becoming alcoholics as well. The evidence is quite compelling that this may indeed so.

On average, it would appear that whites start drinking at an earlier age than Blacks, Hispanics and other minorities do. Whites on the aggregate have a high incidence of alcohol abuse than do Blacks, Hispanics and other minorities do but, Blacks, Hispanics and other minorities suffer more from the physical effects of alcohol abuse than do whites.

For example, Blacks, Hispanics and other minorities seem to have a greater incidence of cirrhosis of liver due to alcohol abuse than do Whites. In fact, the death rate from cirrhosis of the liver is two times as high for Blacks, Hispanics and other minorities as compared to Whites.

Blacks, Hispanics and other minorities suffer from more health problems because of alcohol abuse, than do Whites. Diseases such as cancer, hypertension, malnutrition, birth defects, and obstructive pulmonary disease are much more prevalent in alcoholic Blacks, Hispanics and other minoroties as compared to alcoholic Whites.

The risk of fetal alcohol syndrome (FAS) is seven times higher for Black, Latinos and other minority babies than it is for white babies. In 2013, it was estimated that 17 million Americans have alcohol-related health problems and worldwide 75 million people have alcohol related health problems. In the U.S. every year 85, 000 people die from alcohol related health problems and worldwide 2.5 million people die every year from alcohol health related problems. Alcohol consumption costs 188 billion dollars annually in theU.S.

The estimated annual cost for alcohol health care in the U.S. was 223 billion dollars in 2013.

Alcohol abuse is a multi-system disease. The organs that are most frequently affected by alcohol are the following:

1. The brain
2. The heart
3. The lungs
4. The liver
5. The spleen
6. The pancreas
7. The breasts
8. Female genital organs
9. Male genital organs
10. Male erectal functions
11. Females fertility
12. Males fertility
13. The gastrointestinal system
14. The blood system
15. The endocrine system
16. The mouth, throat, and esophagus
17. The neurological system
18. The psychological system
19. The skin
20. Frequently, many of the organs and systems are affected in combination in the same person.

When a person drinks alcohol, the brain is the first organ to be affected. When a person drinks alcohol, first it is absorbed from the stomach into the bloodstream. Once in the bloodstream, the alcohol goes to the brain. The effect of alcohol on the brain depends on the level of alcohol in the blood of the person drinking alcohol and the length of time that person has been drinking alcohol.

The level of alcohol that causes drunkenness in one person is different in another individual. In other words, different individuals respond differently to the effect of alcohol. The weight of a woman or a man determines how quickly she becomes intoxicated. Blood alcohol concentration (BAC) is measured as milligrams of alcohol per deciliter of blood.

This same number can be converted in percent of alcohol concentration in the blood: 100 mg of alcohol per deciliter in the blood equals 100 mg percent or 0.1 percent of alcohol in the blood. For example, a person weighing 200 lbs., who drinks six drinks of hard liquor in one hour, will likely develop a blood alcohol level of 100 mg per deciliter. A person who weighs 150 lbs. will reach a blood alcohol concentration of 100 mg per deciliter by drinking four drinks of hard liquor in one hour.

Alcohol is both a stimulant and a neuro-suppressor (brain suppressor). The first thing that happens when alcohol reaches the brain is to calm the person who drinks it. It relaxes the person at first. Then as more alcohol is consumed, a feeling of elation or euphoria ensues. Associated with this level of drinking is a mild form of excitement, and the person may become talkative and giddy.

Mild social drinking of 2-3 glasses of wine, or 1-2 drinks of hard liquor, or 2-3 twelve-ounce bottles of beer per day should not be harmful to the human body. Further consumption of alcohol can create a state of drunkenness associated with excitation, rude behavior, and physical dis-coordination. Another way of saying the same thing is that a standard drink of alcohol is usually expressed as a can of twelve ounces of beer, 1½ ounces of liquor/whiskey, vodka, etc., or 5 ounces of wine.

Different individuals metabolize alcohol differently, and when taken with food in the stomach, alcohol absorption is slowed. If alcohol is consumed on an empty stomach, its full effects are felt quicker.

Impairment due to the effects of alcohol occurs in a person when the alcohol concentration reaches 50 mg per deciliter. Blacks and elderly individuals show impairment from drinking alcohol at lower concentration, probably 25-30 mg per deciliter.

The risks of causing an automobile crash starts to occur when the blood alcohol concentration reaches 40 mg per deciliter. This risk rises when the blood alcohol concentration reaches 100 mg per deciliter. When the blood alcohol concentration reaches between 50-70 mg per deciliter, most drivers are alcohol impaired and are unsuitable to drive.

At this blood alcohol concentration, a person loses coordination (he or she cannot walk straight). At an alcohol level concentration of 100 mg per deciliter, a person has a more pronounced inability to walk, and would be stumbling around, and if that person attempts to drive, that person would be driving while drunk.

When the blood alcohol concentration reaches 200 mg per deciliter, the person becomes confused, disoriented and may actually lose consciousness (alcohol blackout). When the blood alcohol concentration reaches 400 mg per deciliter, coma may ensue and death may occur.

Blood alcohol levels that are deem unsafe for driving a car is different in different states in the USA. Examples of different blood alcohol levels from different states in the in the U.S. that are considered safe or unsafe to drive a motor vehicle:

TABLE 1

Alaska	0.10/0.00	90 days	after 30 days	Yes
Arizona	0.10/0.00	90 days	after 30 days	No
Arkansas	0.10/0.02	120 days	Yes	Yes
California	0.08/0.01	4 months	after 30 days	Yes
Colorado	0.10/0.02	3 months	No	Yes
Connecticut	0.10/0.02	90 days	Yes	No
Delaware	0.10/0.02	3 months	No	Yes
District of Columbia	0.10/0.02	90 days	Yes	No
Florida	0.08/0.02	6 month	Yes	No
Georgia	0.10/0.02	1 year	Yes	Yes
Hawaii	0.08/0.02	3 months	after 30 days	Yes
Idaho	0.08/0.02	90 days	after 30 days	Yes
Illinois	0.06/0.00	3 months	after 30 days	Yes
Indiana	0.10/0.02	180 day	after 30 days	Yes
Iowa	0.10/0.02	180 days	Yes	Yes
Kansas	0.08/0.02	30 days	No	Yes
Kentucky	0.10/0.02	—	—	No
Louisiana	0.10/0.02	90 days	after 30 days	Yes
Maine	0.08/0.00	90 days	Yes	Yes
Maryland	0.10/0.02	45 days	Yes	Yes
Massachusetts	None/0.02	90 days	No	No
Michigan	0.10./0.02	—	—	Yes
Minnesota	0.10/0.00	90 days	after 15 days—	No
Mississippi	0.10/0.08	90 days	No	No
Missouri	0.10/0.02	30 days	No	Yes
Montana	0.10/0.02	—	—	Yes
Nebraska	0.10/0.02	90 days	after 30 days	Yes
Nevada	0.10/0.02	90 days	after 45 days	Yes
New Hampshire	0.08/0.02	6 months	No	No
New Jersey	0.10/0.10	—	—	No
New Mexico	0.08/0.02	90 days	after 30 days	No
New York	0.10/0.02	variable	Yes	Yes
North Carolina	0.08/0.00	10 days	No	Yes
North Dakota	0.10/0.02	91 days	after 30 days	Yes
Ohio	0.10/0.02	90 days	after 15 days	Yes
Oklahoma	0.10/0.00	180 days	Yes	Yes
Oregon	0.08/0.00	90 days	after 30 days	Yes
Pennsylvania	0.10/0.02	—	—	No
Rhode Island	0.10/0.02	—	—	Yes
South Carolina	None/—	—	—	No
South Dakota	0.10/—	—	—	No

Tennessee	0.10/0.02	—	—	Yes
Texas	0.10/0.00	60 days	Yes	Yes
Utah	0.08/0.00	90 days	No	Yes
Vermont	0.08/0.02	90 days	No	No
Virginia	0.08/0.02	7 days	No	Yes
Washington	0.10/0.02	—	—	Yes
West Virginia	0.10/0.02	6 months	Yes	Yes
Wisconsin	0.10/0.02	6 months	Yes	Yes
Wyoming	0./10/—	90 days	Yes	No

(Insurance Institute for Highway Safety)

What is alcoholism?

Alcoholism is a disease. It is a disease that affects the human mind and the human body. Alcoholism is a serious disease causing both psychological and medical complications of all sorts to the human body. The psychological dependence on alcohol is real and has devastating consequences on the affected individual and his or her family and society.

People who suffer from alcohol dependency have great difficulty stopping being dependent on alcohol. These people are addicted to alcohol and crave it when they stop drinking. There are different patterns of alcohol dependency.

Some people drink alcohol in excess every day and feel the need to drink every day. A significant percentage of these blacks are able to go to work and function reasonably well on the job. They usually start drinking at lunchtime.

They often consume 2-3 drinks with lunch, after work they will drink 3-4 more drinks, in a bar on their way home or at job-related functions, and when they get home they will again have 2-3 more drinks with dinner. This is about 10 drinks of hard liquor per day. On weekends, that number quadruples. These people are what are called functioning alcoholics. They work, they make money, and they support their families. These people are found at all levels of society from the very rich to the poor, and to the middle class. They are referred to as people who can handle their alcohol.

There is another group of people who are working alcoholics, who must drink as soon as they get up in the morning to get going and they drink hard liquor at different times throughout the working day. Very often, people know that these people are alcoholics but tolerate them or cover up for them because they are oftentimes polite, very nice, and jovial, and when sober, they are productive at their work. Frequently, these people miss work because of heavy alcohol drinking and very often come up with very creative excuses as to why they were absent from work.

There is still a larger group of blacks who drink alcohol in large quantities and on such a regular basis that they become sick so frequently that they are unable to maintain a job. These are the hardcore, non-functioning alcoholics, who are entirely preoccupied with alcohol drinking on a daily basis. People in this group are found also in all segments of society, in all professions and most religious groups.

Alcohol abuse and peer pressure

Peer pressure plays a significant role in alcohol abuse in teenagers, as there is peer pressure to get them involved in illicit drugs. There is also peer pressure to force other young teenagers to drink alcohol. Peer pressure also exists among adults to get together in a bar after work for a drink or two. The incidence of alcohol abuse is quite high among blacks of all ethnic backgrounds.

Alcohol abuse among people starts at an early age (from adolescence to teenage years). Poor people drink alcohol for the same reasons that other rich people drink alcohol, to socialize with their friends and to be less inhibited. This use of alcohol frequently increases to drinking alcohol alone at home on a daily basis.

Eventually, these individuals become dependent on the alcohol, and once that happens, they become preoccupied with alcohol drinking, resulting in alcoholism. Frequently, these individuals grow up in homes where there is either a father or mother who abuses alcohol. They have either a husband who drinks alcohol, or a boyfriend who drinks alcohol, and they drink in order to please their husbands or boyfriends.

They drink because they saw their mothers or fathers doing it and they thought it was all right for them to start doing it also.

Some of these people are heads of the household, single parents with children to bring up with no fathers around and all the stress associated with running a house alone.

In addition, all the problems associated with poverty, racism, low level of education, unemployement etc; leads to heavy alcohol use in some people.

The working-class people group also has many alcohol abusers among it. The people in this group have similar problems with alcohol abuse, and the reasons are the same stress, single parenthood, poverty, racism and all its associated perniciousness, and in more instances, domestic violence and all the awful things that are associated with it.

Middle-class people who abuse alcohol do so for similar reasons as just outlined. The main difference is that this group of blacks has financial means, which help them to be able to cover up their alcoholism. As for upper-class people, most of them are professionals, business men and women, athletes, entertainers and entertainers' wives, husbands and daughters/sons.

The wealthy and privileged people who abuse alcohol do so for similar reasons, except that they are not poor and undoubtedly suffer less discriminations (in fact, reasonably frequently they do a significant degree of the discriminating themselves that occurs in society). Yes, some minority folks do discriminate against other minority folks, especially light skin minorities people frequently discriminate against dark skin minorities in America and elsewhere in the world.

Because of their money, social and professional status, doors are frequently open for them, etc., that allow their alcoholism to appear more acceptable to their friends, colleagues and their associates. The effects of alcohol on their bodies, however, is the same as that of the poorest minority people, because alcohol cares not how much money a person has, or for that matter, how privileged he or she is or how well a person is able to eat.

The best caviare, the best cheeses, or the finest filets mignons in the world cannot protect the human body from the ultimate devastation of alcohol abuse. Alcoholism affects the human body to the same degree, regardless of a person's nutritional state, with a few minor transient circumstances.

For example, if a person is undernourished and went on an alcohol binge and does not eat, the fact that he or she has low storage of carbohydrates in his or her liver from poor eating over an extending period of time, this person may develop hypoglycemia (low blood sugar) quicker than the person who drinks heavy, but eats a better diet. That being said, the long-term toxic effects of alcohol are the same in everyone who drinks alcohol heavily.

Even though blacks and Hispanics and other minorities start drinking alcohol at a later age than their white counterparts do, the signs of alcoholism seem to appear earlier in them than in whites. Undoubtedly, poverty and racism play a major role in these differences.

Poor folks do not have as much money as rich folks to go to the doctor for check-ups. White folks have more money than blacks do. (The top 2 per cent of the

U.S. population most of whom whites, owns 98 per cent of the wealth in the U.S. totaling 45 trillion dollars) Whites get physical examinations more often than do Blacks, Latinos and other minorities do.

Diseases such as cancer of the mouth, throat, esophagus, liver, and pancreas, which are quite common in alcoholics, get picked up earlier in rich white alcoholics than they get picked up in poor black, Hispanic and other minority alcoholics.

Alcohol is one of the most frequently abused drugs because it is legal to buy alcohol without a prescription. Alcohol is readily available and any person over age 21 who whishes to dink it. Different states set up different age limits at which a young person can legally buy alcohol. On a yearly basis, alcohol abuse and its associated problems lead to more than 100,000 deaths in the United States.

Of this number, close to 40,000 is due to cirrhosis of the liver and other associated medical complications of alcohol on the human body. The rest are due to alcohol-associated accidents on the highway (DWI) and homicides, liver cancer, pancreatic cancer, cancer of mout, throat esophagus etc;

The amount of alcohol that a person must drink on a long-term basis to cause damage to the liver is 80 grams of alcohol per day over an extended period, anywhere from 7 years to 15 years. Eighty grams of alcohol can almost be found in a six-pack of 12 ounces of beer, because each 12-ounce can of beer has 13.1 grams of alcohol. If one multiplies this, it adds up to 78.6 grams of alcohol, and some blacks drink twice that much beer per day. As stated above, if a person drinks this amount of alcohol on a regular basis, that person will develop liver disease, as time goes on.

If a person drinks wine regularly (3.5 fluid ounces of wine), which is a glass of wine, it has 9.6 grams of alcohol. A bottle of wine usually has about 5-6 glasses of wine in it. People who drink 2-3 glasses of wine with dinner every night do not develop liver disease. It takes a minimum of 80 grams of alcohol per day on a regular basis over several years to develop fatty infiltration of the liver, which leads to metamorphosis of fat, leading to necrosis, resulting in alcoholic liver disease with subsequent development of cirrhosis.

The same thing applies to champagne. One glass of champagne has 11 grams of alcohol in it; some champagne has 13 grams of alcohol per glass, depending on how dry the champagne is. Therefore, it would take a tremendous amount of champagne consumption to add up to 80 grams of alcohol. About 11-plus glasses of champagne daily over many years can cause a person to develop alcoholic cirrhosis. Most people do not drink that much champagne.

However, if a person drinks martinis, this is a different situation. Each martini has 18.5 grams of alcohol. If he or she drinks five martinis per day, he or she is already drinking what is in fact in excess of the minimum amount of alcohol that is needed to cause liver disease. Five martinis equal to 92 grams of alcohol.

A Manhattan, for instance, has 19.9 grams of alcohol in it. Five Manhattans equal to 99.65 grams of alcohol. A gin Ricky has 21 grams of alcohol. Five gins Ricky equal 105 grams of alcohol. A High Ball has 24 grams of alcohol in it. Five High Balls equal 120 grams of alcohol. A mint julep has 29.2 grams of alcohol in it. Five mint juleps equal 146 grams of alcohol, etc. Therefore, it does not take very many of these alcoholic drinks on a daily basis for a woman to develop alcoholic liver disease. The organs most affected by alcohol abuse are the following:

1. The brain
2. The liver
3. The pancreas
4. The spleen
5. The GI system
6. The blood system
7. The bones
8. The reproductive organs
9. The coagulation system
10. The skin
11. The behavioral system etc;

As described here, alcohol is very toxic to the brain. Acute alcohol ingestion alters a person's behavior by creating a state of excitation, restlessness, and poor social behavior. The agitated state leads to poor physical coordination, which frequently progresses to a state of drunkenness, leading to stupor and, at times, to coma.

When intoxicated, the alcoholic is a danger to herself or himself, and a danger to others around him or her. The adult brain is affected by alcohol in many ways. For instance, a person who abuses alcohol risks losing his or her ability to function properly on her job. He or she is likely to develop serious psychological problems, which can cause disruption of his or her family life, which often results in break-ups of personal relationships such as marriages, etc.

Serious damage to the brain tissues leading to dementia is quite common in chronic alcoholics. Chronic alcohol abuse can lead to Korsakoff syndrome, because of long-term vitamin B deficiencies. It is also known to be associated with acute episodes of encephalopathy, such as Wernicke's encephalopathy due to thiamine deficiencies.

Chronic alcohol abuse is also associated with other neurological abnormalities, such as ataxia (inability to walk in a straight line), altered mood functions with suicidal ideations, and peripheral neuropathy. A chronic alcoholic is prone to develop seizures, either because of alcohol withdrawal, or because of recurrent traumas to the brain.

The chronic alcoholic is often deficient in folic acid, all the B vitamins, magnesium, protein, and phosphate.

Alcohol affects the liver, because it is a direct toxin to the liver tissues. In other words, because alcohol is directly toxic to liver tissues, therefore, the amount of alcohol consumed, the frequency of that consumption, and the length of time an individual abuses alcohol determines the extent of the liver damage.

In some individuals, the damage to the liver occurs quicker than in others, but one thing is certain, as long as a person abuses alcohol, his or her liver will be damaged by it. In some instances, the liver becomes acutely swollen, which can in turn lead to acute enlargement of the spleen due to acute elevation of the portal pressure and the consequence can be acute rupture of the spleen, endangering the life of the affected person, if it is not diagnosed properly and treated surgically quickly.

More chronically, however, alcohol causes tissues within the liver to become inflamed and the recurrent inflammatory reaction in time leads to scarring of the liver tissues, resulting in cirrhosis of the liver.

Once the liver becomes cirrhotic, a multitude of clinical problems can occur. The liver is needed to synthesize (produce) different proteins, which are needed for good body functions. The liver is needed to make most of the coagulation factors required to prevent bleeding from occurring. The liver is needed to store carbohydrates and to break down carbohydrates into usable sugars to use as fuel in the body.

The liver is needed to produce bile, which is needed to break down fats that humans eat, plus a multitude of other essential functions. The liver is the largest organ in the body next to the skin and the skeletal system and it contains the largest supply of reticuloendothelial cells that are needed to participate in the immune system, etc.

In addition, the liver is needed to help remove a multitude of breakdown products that the human body produces constantly. So when the liver is sick and is unable to produce needed materials for proper body functions, and is too sick to help remove waste materials from the body, the human person becomes very sick.

In other words, when the liver is too sick to function properly and fails, life cannot go on. Another way of putting it is when the liver fails, the person dies, and alcohol abuse can frequently cause the liver to fail.

The pancreas is another organ that is quite sensitive to the toxic effects of alcohol. Pancreatitis is a common complication of heavy and chronic alcohol abuse. It is not exactly clear as to the number of years a person has to abuse alcohol before her pancreas becomes sick some say, after seven years of alcohol abuse.

However, again, different individuals have different degrees of resistance and tolerance to the effects of alcohol. Alcohol damages the pancreatic tissues, causing at first acute inflammation to occur. The inflammation causes marked swelling of the pancreas, resulting in acute pancreatitis. After repeated attacks of acute pancreatitis, over several years, scarring of the pancreatic tissues occur which in turn results in chronic pancreatitis?

The third scenario is when the chronicity of the pancreatic disease causes destruction of the pancreatic tissue, leaving empty spaces within the pancreas, causing pancreatic pseudocysts to develop. Quite often, these pancreatic pseudocysts become infected, which in turn can lead to abscesses within the pancreas. Still other sequelae of chronic pancreatitis is pancreatic failure, meaning the pancreas is so damaged that it is no longer able to produce the different enzymes that it was able to produce before it became damaged.

These enzymes are necessary to aid in the digestive process of ingested fat that humans eat. Failure of the pancreas to produce these necessary enzymes causes the development of greasy diarrhea to occur. To further cause matters to get worse, if the woman with pancreatic failure now becomes diabetic, because the pancreas has failed, it is not able to produce insulin for sugar metabolism; not to mention the constant and intense left-sided abdominal pain this person has to endure.

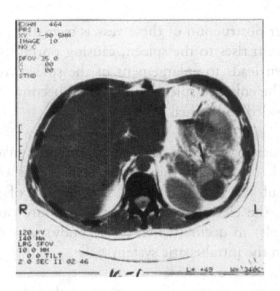

Figure 59:1—CT of acute pancreatitis. CT of the abdomen showing acute pancreatitis with a pseudocyst of the pancreas (arrow showing swollen pancreas with pseudocyst).

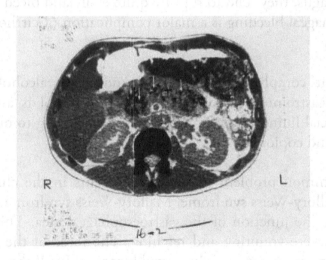

Figure 59:—CT of chronic pancreatitis.
CT of the abdomen showing chronic pancreatitis with calcifications. Arrows showing swollen pancreas in a patient who abuses alcohol.

The effects of alcoholism on the spleen

The spleen becomes sick with chronic use of heavy alcohol intake because of cirrhosis of the liver. When alcohol damages the liver, this damage occludes the blood vessels that run through the liver. These damaged vessels cause narrowing and obstruction of the circulation inside the liver to occur.

Because of intra-liver obstruction of these vessels over time, the pressure within the liver and the portal system rises to the spleen, causing portal hypertension to develop. Portal hypertension then leads to enlargement of the spleen, resulting in a condition called hypersplenism. The enlarged spleen can at times become quite bulky, resulting in severe and chronic left-sided abdominal pain.

The upper gastrointestinal system is quite frequently involved in this scenario and becomes quite sick because of the effects of cirrhosis of the liver and portal hypertension. Because of the destruction and obstruction of these intrahepatic and (intra-liver) circulation, the elevation of the portal pressure causes neovascularization (formation of new vessels) to occur (which is the body's way of trying to bypass the obstructed circulation in the intrahepatic system).

The new vessels, however, are superficial, meaning that they grow on the surface of the esophagus, resulting in esophageal varices.

Because these new vessels, called varices, are superficially located on the outer surface of the esophagus, they tend to rupture quite easily and bleed profusely.

Therefore, esophageal bleeding is a major complication of cirrhosis of the liver with portal hypertension.

Another frequent complication of chronic and heavy alcohol abuse is gastritis, resulting in upper gastrointestinal bleeding. Because alcohol is an irritating drug, it damages the superficial lining of the stomach, causing bleeding to occur, which at times can be quite severe and copious.

Still another common problem that at times occurs in the chronic alcoholic is a condition called Mallory-Weiss syndrome. Mallory-Weiss syndrome develops because of a tear that occurs at the junction of the gastroesophageal area. This occurs because of alcohol abuse and severe vomiting and retching. The force of the retching causes the tear to occur, resulting in upper gastrointestinal bleeding. In all these cases, the bleeding can be severe enough to cause the patient to go into shock with all its multitudes of complications.

Another frequently affected system is the hematopoietic system (blood system). The effects of alcohol on the blood system are many and varied. Acutely, alcohol can suppress the bone marrow, resulting in the lowering of white blood cells, red blood cells, and platelets.

Chronic alcoholism can cause anemia because of recurrent upper gastrointestinal bleeding on the one hand, and on the other hand, alcohol abuse always leads to folic acid deficiency, resulting in folic acid deficiency anemia. In other instances, chronic alcohol abuse can result in a condition called hypersplenism, as mentioned earlier, which causes hemolysis of red blood cells, causing anemia.

Hypersplenism can also cause leukopenia (low white blood cells) and thrombocytopenia (low platelet count). These abnormalities in the blood system are the result of splenic sequestration (because the spleen is enlarged, it soaks up these cells within it and destroys them). Chronic alcoholism with liver disease (cirrhosis) causes the white blood cells to not function well; as a result, affected blacks are not able to fight infection properly.

Chronic alcoholic abuse also affects the endocrine systems. For instance, the sick alcoholic liver is unable to break down estrogen effectively, which then allows the excess estrogen to remain in the blood, resulting in overstimulation of the uterus, causing breakthrough vaginal bleeding, worsening their iron deficiency state. Through this same mechanism, estrogen, resulting in swelling and pain in their breasts, over stimulates alcoholic's breast tissues.

Women, because of the overstimulation of estrogen, have a high propensity for developing both breast and uterine cancers.

The effect of excess circulating estrogen causes skin changes to develop in alcoholics (spider angiomata). The heart suffers a great deal from the effects of alcohol abuse.

The most frequent cardiac problem that occurs in alcohol intoxication is abnormal rhythm of the heart, such as "fast heartbeat" (tachycardia):

1. Atrial fibrillation
2. Super-ventricular tachycardia
3. Multifocal ventricular contractions (PVCs)
4. Atrial premature contradictions PACs.
5. Heart blocks, etc.

Chronic effects of alcohol on the heart cause damage to the heart muscles, resulting in enlargement of the heart (alcoholic cardiomyopathy). Alcoholic heart disease frequently results in congestive heart failure

Lung disease in alcoholics

Blacks who abuse alcohol frequently develop aspiration pneumonia. Pneumonia develops because when these people get drunk, they lose control of their gag reflux and the consequence of that is that they aspirate their vomitus into their lungs, causing aspiration pneumonia. The overall poor nutritional and health state of people who abuse alcohol predisposes them to community-acquired pneumonias. Smoking cigarettes or cigars is part of the alcohol abuse subculture.

The result of the tobacco abuse/ alcohol abuse that some blacks are involved with is that, here is a high incidence of lung cancer in alcoholic blacks who smoke. There is also a high incidence of head and neck cancer in this subgroup of blacks as well; there is a high incidence of cancer of the esophagus in this subgroup of blacks because of the adverse effects of alcohol and cigarette on esophageal tissue.

The take-home lesson is not to use tobacco in any form and not to abuse alcohol.

Alcohol is a drug and can be quite addicting when used in large quantities over a long period. Alcohol has the potential to be toxic to the entire human body. The literature clearly shows that alcohol in moderate quantities, such as one or two glasses of wine with dinner, is good in the prevention of coronary artery heart disease. Alcohol does so through different mechanisms:

1. It makes platelets less sticky, thereby, preventing them from aggregating and in so doing lowering the possibility of clot formation.
2. It increases the level of high-density lipoprotein, the good cholesterol. However, it is prudent that anyone with a propensity to alcohol abuse refrain from alcohol altogether.
3. Both white wine and red wine help to decrease the incidence of coronary artery heart disease when consumed in moderate quantity. It is believed that the phenols found in red grapes function as antioxidants and prevent the damage to coronary arteries.

Clinical management of alcohol-induced clinical problems:

Clinically, acute alcohol intoxication causes the intoxicated alcoholic to be agitated, unreasonable, sometimes violent, and frequently confused. This set of symptoms and behavior can cause intoxicated people to get into fights and other altercations that can cause problems for their spouses, their children and other members of society with whom they meet.

Alcoholics frequently are brought to the emergency room after fights during which they were traumatized, or brought to the emergency room due to upper gastrointestinal bleeding or due to fever and abdominal pain and other alcohol-associated problems. Once the intoxicated alcoholic arrives in the emergency room, he or she must be evaluated immediately.

Vital signs, such as blood pressure, pulse, temperature, and respiratory rate must be quickly taken and documented. It is very important to examine the abdomen, the head, the eyes and inside the ears, looking for evidence of blunt trauma.

Then, an intravenous access must be quickly established. Blood must be drawn and sent for CBC, SMA 20, serum magnesium, serum amylase, lipase, B12, folate, blood alcohol concentration, and urine, must be sent for drug screening. The urine also must be sent to the laboratory for urinalysis to make sure that there is no blood in it, which may indicate that the patient has had some trauma to the kidneys during a fight.

The examining physician must pay particular attention to the examination of the head area, looking for signs of trauma. It is important to examine inside the ears, looking for signs of blood coming out of the inner ears. The examination must be complete and must include a rectal examination, looking for signs of blood grossly, and if none is found, the stool must be tested for blood using the hemoccult test.

The neurological examination is extremely important, looking for signs of agitation, confusion, hallucinations, stupor, etc.

It is necessary to do a CT SCAN of the brain on alcoholics who present to emergency room for medical to rule out intracranial bleeding.

As soon as the physical examination is completed, the alcoholic must be started on the so-called alcoholic cocktail. The alcoholic cocktail is composed of:

1. IV glucose (50% in one ampule)
2. Thiamine 100 mg IV or IM
3. Folic acid 1 mg IV, IM, or PO if the patient can take PO
4. Magnesium sulfate 1-gram IV or IM
5. B complex vitamin IM, IV, or PO
6. Ativan IV or IM

It is crucial that thiamine is given before the glucose is infused. If the glucose is infused before the administration of thiamine, this will lead to an acute depletion of whatever trace of thiamine is left in the body.

This acute thiamine depletion will lead to a condition called Wernicke's encephalopathy. Acute Wernicke's encephalopathy causes acute agitation, confusion, hallucination and combativeness. The reason why acute Wernicke's occurs when 50% of glucose is infused in the alcoholic is because the alcoholic is frequently deficient in carbohydrates and all B-complex vitamins such as thiamine and folic acid.

Alcoholics do not eat enough foods that contain these vitamins. Thiamine is a necessary biochemical vitamin in the metabolism of glucose (the Krebs cycle, a biochemical pathway reaction that contains many substances that are necessary to metabolize sugars) to help make this reaction.

Therefore, the acute depletion of thiamine causes Wernicke's encephalopathy to occur. Sugar is needed in the acutely intoxicated alcoholic because she is likely to be starved and therefore has hypoglycemia (low blood sugar).

The acutely sick alcoholic needs folic acid because he or she is always folate deficient, and because he or she does not eat enough foods that contain folic acid. Further, alcohol as a drug poisons the folate biochemical pathway. As a result, all alcoholics by definition are folate deficient.

The acutely sick and intoxicated alcoholic needs magnesium, because all chronic and heavy alcoholic users are magnesium deficient, even though the laboratory may report the blood magnesium level as normal. Alcohol is a form of diuretic and as such, the alcoholic loses large quantities of magnesium in the urine.

Low magnesium can cause low serum calcium. Both low serum calcium and low magnesium in an individual can cause seizures, muscle cramps, and (in some cases) rhythm abnormalities of the heart. Hypoglycemia (low blood sugar) can cause seizures to occur. Another frequent substance that chronic alcoholics are frequently deficient in is phosphate.

Phosphate is a by-product of protein breakdown and since the alcoholics are too preoccupied with alcohol to eat properly, they are frequently deficient in protein and phosphate. Further, the alcoholic urinates frequently because of the diuretic effect of alcohol, and thereby loses large quantities of phosphate in the urine, causing hypophosphatemia (low serum phosphate).

Low serum phosphate can cause acute seizures and chronically can cause hemolytic anemia. This is so because phosphate is needed to provide for a normal level of 2-3 D-PG (2-3 diphosphoglycerate).

In some instances, low serum phosphate can cause severe rhythm disturbances of the heart.

Once the alcoholic passes through this first stage of her stay in the hospital, the next step is to evaluate her for acute or chronic disease in the usual manner. If it is decided that the alcoholic needs to be hospitalized, then all the medications in the alcoholic cocktail must be continued for several days except for the magnesium and the 50% dextrose.

The next step in providing acute care for the alcoholic is to watch for the possible development of delirium tremens (DTs). Both the blood alcohol concentration level and how the patient looks clinically are important in deciding when to start anti-DT treatment. Equally important is to try to ascertain when the patient last drank alcohol.

Most alcoholics will start showing signs of DTs 36-48 hours after they had their last drink of alcohol. It is important to keep in mind the fact that chronic alcoholics can have a blood alcohol concentration of 100-200 mg per deciliter in the blood and do not appear drunk. Because of this fact, the chronic alcoholic can go into DTs with an alcohol level concentration that is this high because their bodies are accustomed to having a higher concentration of alcohol in it.

Delirium tremens is a clinical syndrome that results from the craving for alcohol that occurs when an alcohol abuser has been kept away from alcohol for several days. The part of the brain that controls addiction misses the alcohol and the alcoholic goes into withdrawal, due to the loss of alcohol in her bloodstream to satisfy the brain's need for the alcohol.

DTs have several stages: Stage I, Stage II, Stage III, Stage IV and Stage V.

Stage I:	The first stage of DTs manifested with tremors (the shakes), restlessness, increased heart rate, insomnia, diarrhea, and irritability.
Stage II:	The second stage is all of the Stage I signs, plus sweaty palms and confusion.
Stage III:	All the symptoms of I and II plus sweating, rise in blood pressure, rise in pulse, palpitations and hallucinations.\
Stage IV:	All the preceding signs, plus seizures.
Stage V:	All of those in the preceding stages, plus coma.

To prevent DTs from developing, it is recommended that the patient be given Ativan 1-2 mg four times per day, prophylactically by mouth as soon as the patient gets to the emergency room and consciousness level has been evaluated to be clinically satisfactory. If the patient cannot take medication by mouth, Ativan can be given IM or IV.

Alternatively, the patient can be treated with Librium 10 mg PO, four times per day IM or PO. Librium is not absorbed well IM and is not a medication to be used if the patient has severe liver disease, because the liver metabolizes Librium.

The liver metabolizes Ativan differently and, therefore, it can be used even if the liver is severely sick.

Other things that are essential in the treatment of DTs are fluid and electrolyte replacement intravenously. It is very important to keep the sick alcoholic in an anabolic state, by making sure there is always sugar in the IV fluid being given to him or her. D5 ½ normal saline or D5 normal saline is preferred. If the patient is hypertensive, the IV can be D5 ¼ normal saline, along with specific medications to treat the hypertension. If seizure develops, then the patient must be treated first with IV Valium then with Dilantin. A brain CT scan without contrast, followed by an EEG at the appropriate time, must always be done.

Two medications in use to help alcoholics stop drinking are Antabuse (Disulfiram) and Naltrexone. Naltrexone is available to be used intramuscularly as well. Both of these medications have side effects and a person who is drinking alcohol must not take them. If a person drinks alcohol and takes Antabuse, he or she can become acutely ill and in fact can die as a result. Naltrexone works apparently on the brain to decrease the desire of the alcoholic to drink alcohol. Antabuse (Disulfiram) works by converting acetaldehyde, which is a breakdown product of alcohol to acetic acid in the liver that causes an increase in serum acetaldehyde anywhere from five to ten times the normal level.

Because of that, the woman can hyperventilate and can develop flushing of the skin, nausea, vomiting, headache, and respiratory distress along with anxiety, alpitations, and sometimes hypertension.

That is why it is important that people do not drink alcohol and take Disulfiram at the same time. The usual dose of Disulfiram is 250 mg. A 500 mg dose is also available, but frequently the 250 mg dose is sufficient to prevent someone from craving alcohol. The usual dose for Naltrexone (ReVia) is 50 mg daily for about 12 weeks as a prophylactic treatment against alcohol abuse.

Driving while intoxicated remains a major safety problem in the United States, and every year many thousands of people die because of accidents resulting from DWI. Drunken drivers remain a menace to society, and different states have different laws defining what DWI is.

The following is a complete list of the different listings of the blood alcohol concentrations that are considered legal for any person to drive a car, as published by the Insurance Institute for Highway Safety (see Table 1).

Women, drinking alcohol while pregnant is a serious problem and it leads to a condition called alcohol fetal syndrome. One in a hundred babies born to woman alcoholics suffers from the effects of alcohol. This is known as alcohol fetal syndrome (AFS).

Drinking alcohol during pregnancy is dangerous. Ten out of every one thousand babies born to women alcohol abusers suffer from alcohol-related neuro-developmental disorder (ARND) and fetal alcohol syndrome (FAS).

Alcohol affects two parts of the fetal brain more severely, the hippocampus and the cerebellum. A breakdown product of alcohol called acetaldehyde causes the bulk of the problem.

Acetaldehyde damages the DNA of the developing tissues in the fetal brain; therefore, alcohol and acetaldehyde are teratogenic to the unborn babies.

Women who abuse alcohol while pregnant are doing serious damage to their unborn babies. Many of these babies born to these women alcoholic are born with mental retardation, growth retardation, craniofacial abnormalities, and brain damage.

These babies also suffer ocular anomalies and hearing disorders such as hearing loss and recurrent serous otitis media. These children oftentimes develop speech impairment. These children frequently have learning disorders and have to be sent to a school for retarded children. These children, in effect, cannot grow up to become productive members of society.

It takes a lot of money to care for them and society is left to pay the bill to care for these fetal alcohol syndrome babies. Between 37,000 and 40,000 children in the U.S. are born each year with some form of alcohol-related problem and million of children in the world are born with alcohol related health problems due to Alcohol Fetal syndrome Nevertheless, even more devastating than the fetal alcohol syndrome just described is the fact that some mothers drink alcohol and take illicit drugs, causing their babies to die.

The United States is the richest country on the planet, and yet 19 of 1,000 babies born to blacks, compared to 9 babies per 1,000 babies born to whites, die. So many babies born to blacks die because of alcohol abuse, drug abuse, cigarette smoking, poverty, lack of prenatal care, and stress-related racial insensitivity, which is known to be associated with spontaneous abortion, all of which are more prevalent among blacks as compared to whites.

This is a catastrophe, because these pregnant black women either do not receive or do not seek prenatal care. Therefore, when they do present to the hospital emergency room to deliver their babies, they usually have many serious medical problems, such as diabetes, hypertension, anemia, preeclampsia, eclampsia, syphilis, gonorrhea, chlamydia, genital herpes, HPV, Step B, chronic hepatiotis B or C, HIV infection, etc.

Frequently, both the babies' and their mother's lives are at risk in these circumstances. Babies born to mothers affected with these conditions are likely to be born prematurely and are just as likely to develop several serious medical problems such as mental retardation, congenital heart problems, and a whole host of other permanent medical problems, guaranteeing lifelong suffering and dependence not only on their families, but also on society for financial support, etc.

Many individuals who abuse alcohol also abuse cocaine, heroin, and prescription drugs, such as Valium, Librium, Ativan, Xanax, etc. Drinking alcohol and taking these drugs is quite dangerous and can cause a person to die. Alcohol is a neurological, cardiac and pulmonary suppressant, so when a person has too much alcohol in his or her bloodstream, and adds illicit or prescription drugs on top of the alcohol, he or she increases the possibility of cardiac arrhythmia, respiratory failure, coma, and death. Drinking alcohol and then taking drugs is to be avoided, because it can be lethal.

Alcohol abuse is quite prevalent among blacks, and in the United States, 58% of whites drink alcohol and 36% blacks' abuse alcohol.

It is variably reported that there is 18 million registered alcoholics in the USA, plus anywhere from eight to ten million other individuals who abuse alcohol to different degrees.

Alcohol abuse contributes to about 100,000 deaths per year in the United States, making it the third leading cause of preventable death in the United States, after tobacco and obesity and its associated health risks. Based on statistics provided by the National Institute of Alcohol Abuse and Alcoholism (NIAAA), the cost of caring for alcohol and substance abuse problems in the United States is 166 billion dollars in 2010.

Presently in the USA, this great, powerful, and wealthy country with 10 million millionaires, every night about 17 million children go to bed hungry, and altogether 50 million Americans live in poverty and over all11 million children have no health insurance coverage, and overall about 52 million Americans have no health insurance.

While according to a recent report, the U.S. has 10 million millionaires, 50% of the U.S. population is reported to be poor and 45 trillion dollars of the U.S. wealth are in the hand of the top 2% of the U.S. population.

How can this happen in the U.S.? The answers are multifaceted and complex but lie mostly in the philosophy that the rich are to supposed get richer and the poor are suppose to get poorer.

How sad! And how awful! How a great and generous country like the United States of America can allows such a condition to exist? Poverty in the U.S. and around the world affects all racial groups, although minorities bare the heaviest burben.

Whites abuse alcohol many more times than Blacks, Latinos and other minorities in the U.S. and around the world do, and some of the reasons people drink alcohol are the same, while others are different. Most minorities abuse alcohol in part because of the stress associated with racial discrimination, broken homes, raising children without a man in the home, loneliness, stress in the workplace, unemployment, and pain associated with chronic diseases such as arthritis, depression, anxiety, panic attacks, other mental illnesses etc.

Many people abuse alcohol as the drug of choice to use while partying because this is socially acceptable. Since whites possess more money than minorities do, they spend more time partying and drinking more alcohol in the process. Many people also resort to alcohol abuse as a way of coping with their problems.

Alcohol, when used in small quantities, can be helpful in increasing the good cholesterol (HDL) one drink of hard liquor per day, or two glasses of wine with dinner, red or white wine, both of which can increase the HDL.

Furthermore, it is clear that alcohol decreases the stickiness of platelets (a cell in the blood necessary in forming clots); in so doing, there is less probability of clot forming in the coronary arteries, thereby decreasing the incidence of heart attacks.

When alcohol is used in excess, the advantage is nullified, because alcohol abuse can cause disease to develop in the heart muscles (cardiomyopathy). In addition, alcohol abuse can cause elevation in the blood pressure, which over time can cause hypertensive heart disease along with coronary artery heart disease.

Light to moderate alcohol consumption can be helpful, while heavy alcohol consumption is harmful to the human body.

Anyone at risk for alcohol abuse ought not to drink alcohol in any amount, because it might get them to start drinking alcohol heavily again.

The vast majority of blacks and other minorities in the world live in poverty of different degrees and also suffer from racial discrimination of different types, along with ethnic and religious bigotry, social depredation, domestic abuse of different types, male chauvinism, second-class citizenship, etc., and yet many of these individuals do not abuse alcohol.

Women ought to stop using alcohol, drugs, and cigarettes while pregnant so that their unborn babies can have a better chance of being born healthy.

By stopping alcohol abuse, an alcohol-abusing people will have a healthier livers, hearts, brains, nervous systems, endocrine systems, reproductive systems, gastrointestinal systems, pancreases, blood systems, psychological systems, emotional systems and overall a healthier, less painful and longer lives.

Chapter 60
DRUG ADDICTION

Drug addiction is a common addictive habit in the United States and around the world. According to published reports there are 22 million drug addicts in the United States and 200 million drug addicts worldwide in 2013. About 800,000 addicts are addicted to heroin in the U.S. and 15 million people in the world are addicted to heroin, opium or morpine resulting in annual market of 65 billion dollars and the total illicit drug industry costs 320 billion dollars per year worldwide.

According to some report, the U.S. spends about 1 trillion dollars annually on the war on drug to no avail.

"The vast majority of grug users are whites" Source: Huffington Post January 4, 2011

Many more millions of people in the world use and abuse illicit drugs of different types; they are also considered addicts.

Every year 200,000 people in the world die because of illicit drug use and in the U.S. every year 19,000 people die from illicit drug use.

The part of the brain stimulated by drugs that results in pleasurable feelings is the dopamine center, which is located at the base of the brain. Drugs such as heroin, cocaine, marijuana, opiates and amphetamines activate dopamine to release neurotransmitter substances, resulting in a pleasurable feeling called a "high," which drug addicts crave to experience.

The dopamine center also functions to allow for the experience of sexual pleasure, enjoyment of foods, music, art, and beautiful things, and other aesthetic things that are pleasing to the ears and the eyes. Once an individual becomes addicted to any drug such as heroin, cocaine, crack-cocaine, marijuana, etc., he or she craves these drugs when the level of the drug decreases in the bloodstream. The craving for the drug oftentimes is quite painful.

Drug craving can lead to severe withdrawal symptoms such as sweating, headache, runny nose, abdominal cramps, diarrhea, poor appetite, insomnia, nightmares, etc. So, addiction to a drug, in particular cocaine, heroin and crack-cocaine, can drive addicts to do anything to get money to buy the drugs in order to satisfy the drug craving on the one hand, which is the more powerful and intense feeling, and to avoid going into drug withdrawal feelings.

On the other hand, once a person becomes addicted to drugs, it is very difficult to give it up. The addicted person becomes dependent on the drug and spends a great deal of time preoccupying himself or herself with finding money to get the next fix. He or she will spend rent money, food money, mortgage money, or she will lie, steal, and commit crimes of different types and magnitude in order to get the money to pay for the drug. Frequently, she prostitutes herself to get money to pay for the drug and, at times, he or she will get involved sexually either with a man or with a woman for drugs or money.

Drug addiction is quite common among all racial groups in the U.S. and around the world. Drug addiction is common in all social and economic status. Wherever there is poverty and ghettos, there is a high incidence of illicit drug use.

However, illicit drug use has become prevalent in the suburbs of the United States, around the world and elsewhere, involving middle—and upper-class people. More than 15 millon people in the U.S. abuse prescription drugs and many more million worldwide abuse preceription drugs. Statistically, more whites' abuse prescription drugs than Blacks, Latinos and other minorities in the U.S. and around the world.100, 000 people in the U.S. die every year from prescription drugs.

In 2009, the U.S. population was 307,006,000 and 47.1% of the population abused drugs and 118,705,000 used illicit drugs.
The most frequently abused illicit drugs in the U.S. are:
Marijuana usage 104,446,000
Cocaine usage 36,599,000
Crack usage 8,359,000
Heroin usage 3,683,000
Methamphetamine usage 12,837,000
Psychotherapeutics usage 51,771,000
Ectasy usage 14,234,000
Hallucinogens usage 37,256,000
Pain killers usage 35,046,000
Alcohol usage 208,545,000
Heavy alcohol abuse 17,129,000 (In 2010 17.6 million people registered as alcoholic in the U.S.) Source: Substance Abuse and Mental Health Services Administration, (2009).

Illicit drug abuse is common in every community in the United States, around the world and in all communities. The people involved in abusing illicit drugs include the very poor who reside in the inner cities of the United States, and around the world in the working class, to the middle class and all the way up to the upper class.

Illicit drug abuse is common in all professions to one degree or another and all sexes are involved in the illicit drug subculture. Blacks use more heroin and crack-cocaine, and whites use more cocaine, marijuana, and amphetamines.

Cocaine has, however, made an entry into black, Hispanic, Asian, Native American, Pacific Islander and Latino ghettos in recent years, because the price of cocaine has gone down to a point where some poor people can now afford to buy it.

Outside forces from the communities fuel the illicit drug subculture where these drugs are produced. People who do not live in these communities are bringing the drugs into these communities. The big question is who are these people? What are their motives? Is it just for the money, or is it something else?

Some have said that infiltration of illicit drugs into the minority communities is a well-planned conspiracy to destroy generations of young people of color. Whether or not proof exists to substantiate these allegations is not quite clear. One thing is certain is that the illicit drug subculture is highly associated with criminal behavior of different types and different degrees. The result is that communities where illicit drugs are prevalent also are beset with high crime rates.

Per capita, more whites use illicit drugs than blacks, but fewer whites get arrested for using drugs and even fewer of them get sent to jail for using drugs than blacks.

Of all the modern countries in the world, the United States has more people in jail at any one time than any other country. According to U.S. Bureau of Statistics, there were 2. 3 million people in jail in the United States as of 2012.

The U.S. represents 5% of the world population and yet 25% of all people in jails around the world are found in the U.S. All together, there are 9 million people in the jail in the world and half of them are found in China, Russia and the U.S.

Though Blacks represent 13.6% of the United States population and Hispanics represent 16.3%, together thet represent 29.5%, of the U.S. population. In 2012, 43.91 per cent of those in jail were Blacks, 18.26 per cent of them were Hispanics, and 34.72 per cent were Whites. So, a total of 62.17 % of those in jail in the U.S. were a combination of Blacks and Hispanics, which is an outrageous number, although these two groups Blacks and Hispanics made up 29.5% of the total population of the U.S. of 312. 780, 968. 1 out 36 every Hispanics is in jail in the U.S. and 1 out of 15 Blacks is in jail in the US.

Overall 1 out every 100 people in the U.S. is in jail. In the year 2005, 7 per cent of those in jail in the U.S. were females. There were 107,518 Blacks in jail in the U.S. in 2005. A third of blacks who are in jail are there for drug-related offenses.

The overall rate of illicit drug use reported in United States black population, age 12 and older, was 11.9%. Relative to the total United States blacks population, Native Americans users of illicit drug are 19.8%, Puerto Ricans 13.3%, Mexican-Americans 12.7%, Asian Pacific Islanders 6.5%, Caribbean-Americans 7.6%, Central Americans 5.7% and Cuban-Americans 8.2%.

"The 2009 National Survey of Drug Use and Health reports that 39 percent whites used an illicit drug in the past year. For blacks, the rate was 34 percent."

According to the National Center on Addiction and Substance Abuse at Columbia University, 21.5 million blacks in the United States smoke, 4.5 million are alcoholics; 3.5 million blacks misuse prescription drugs and 3.1 million blacks use illicit drugs.

According to this important report, one out of every five pregnant woman smokes, drinks alcohol and abuses drugs, totaling more than 800,000 women.

The psychological and physical manifestations of drug addiction

The mindset that causes people the world over to abuse drugs is no doubt similar to the mindset of people all over the world. However, the circumstances of life that are associated with drug abuse are quite different in some measure different in minorities than they are in whites. Most whites who are drug addicts start out using marijuana recreationally.

They then gradually move on to harder drugs, such as amphetamines, LSD, other psychedelic drugs. As the addiction deepens, they move on to using cocaine, heroin and crack-cocaine. These people are financially able to support their addictions, because they have good jobs with good pay, which enables them to pay for these drugs. Some of these people are in the entertainment world (the sports world, the business world and the art world, a world that predisposes some of them to drug addiction). Minorities are in a different set of circumstances as whites, in that they do not have money to support their drug habits.

A significant percentage of people are addicted to prescription drugs and the most frequently abused prescription drugs are the followings:

1. Valium
2. Librium

3. Xanax
4. Ativan
5. Tranxene
6. Klonopin
7. Codeine
8. Vicodin
9. Demerol
10. Morphine
11. Hydrocodone
12. Ambien
13. Restoril
14. Methadone etc;

Some people become addicted to prescription drugs because of chronic pain associated with illness, such as cancer, arthritis, headaches, sickle cell disease, diabetic neuropathy and many other chronic diseases, which require chronic pain medications for relief.

Sometimes these individuals continue to get the prescription for these medications for a long time, but once they are no longer able to obtain these prescriptions, they resort to illicit drugs to ease their pain.

Some of these people become chronic drug addicts in this way. Drug addiction and all other addictions are psychological illnesses. The craving associated with drug addiction is controlled by neurotransmitters within the brain, in particular the dopamine center.

When the urge comes upon an addicted person to get a high, that person will do just about anything to get the money to buy the drug. Drug addiction is a mental illness and ought to be treated as such. Percentage-wise, IV drug addiction is more common among minorities, as compared to whites.

This is so, because this type of drug addiction is more closely associated with the inner cities where most poor people live around the world. Although it is a known fact, the incidence of IV drug use is on the rise in the middle class as well as in the upper class communities of the United States and the world. In other words, illicit drug use is also on Wall Street, Madison Avenue and most definitely in the suburbs and where rich people work and live all over the world.

The brain is affected by illicit drug use in many other ways. For example, heavy marijuana use is known to affect the brain in ways that lead to slow and slurred speech and memory loss. Both cocaine and heroin use are associated with seizures. When heroin and cocaine are used intravenously, sepsis and bacterial endocarditises can occur. Infected emboli can be thrown to the brain from the heart valve, resulting in brain abscesses. Most importantly, the brain is frequently affected by drug overdose causing coma and sometimes deaths.

Different illicit drugs affect the brain in different ways, examples include:
"Marijuana causes
Relaxation
Distorted sensory perception
Euphoria
Impaired coordination
Increased heart rate
Increased appetite
Impaired learning
Impaired memory
Anxiety
Panic attacks
Psychosis
Frequent respiratory infection
Addictioon
Possible brain damage"

Heroin affects the brain and the rest of the body in these ways:
Euphoria
Impaired coordination
Drowsiness
Dizziness
Confusion
Nausea
Vomiting
Sedation
Constipation
Respiratory failure
Hepatitis
Endocarditis
Addiction
Coma
Death"

Cocaine affects the brain and the rest of the body in these ways:
"Increase heart rate
Increase blood pressure
High tempature
Exhilaration
Mental alertness

Tremors
Poor appetite
Anxiety
Panic attacks
Paranoia
Violent behavior
Psychosis
Weight loss
Insomnia
Arrhythmias
Seizure
Stroke
Heart attacks
Addition
Coma
Death"

Other illicit drugs that frequently abused include:
Methamphetamine
Crystal
Sped
PCP
LSD
Dextromethorphan
Anabolic steroid
Nitrous oxide etc;

Source: National Institute on Drug Abuse (National Institutes of Health)

The lungs are affected by drug addiction in many ways as well. Addicts who use cocaine or heroin intravenously frequently develop symptoms of upper airway diseases such as coughing, wheezing, and bronchitis. Acute pulmonary edema (when the lungs become filled with fluid) can occur as an idiosyncratic reaction to heroin use. Another complication involving the lungs in heroin and cocaine use is pulmonary embolism (a clot to the lungs). This happens because the addicts use veins in their legs to infuse the drug and sometimes the vessels in the groin and legs get damaged and infected and become swollen.

These conditions can lead to stasis, which in turn can lead to clot formation, deep vein thrombophlebitis (DVT). The clots can then migrate through the blood vessels into the lung, causing acute pulmonary embolism. Infected emboli can also be thrown to the lungs from infected vegetation from the heart valves (a condition called bacterial endocarditis). Still another frequent pulmonary complication of the IV drug abuser is pneumonia, which occurs often in IV drug abusers because of their overall poor physical condition predisposing them to the development of different types of lung infection.

The incidence of AIDS is the highest among all minority groups in the U.S., and around the world. The incidence of the lung infection called pneumocystis carinii (PCP) is the highest among minority people with AIDS. PCP is a most serious lung infection and frequently is the cause of death of people with AIDS. The incidence of pulmonary tuberculosis has decreased in the general population over the last several years, but it has gone up in people with AIDS.

The effects of illicit drug use on the heart

The heart suffers immensely from illicit drug use, be it use of amphetamines, LSD, marijuana, prescription drugs, cocaine, crack-cocaine, heroin, etc. The heart is likely to become affected by any one of these drugs once in the bloodstream and is more so when used in excess. Once in the bloodstream, the drugs stimulate the heart, causing it to beat too fast and frequently, irregularly.

Cocaine use can cause sudden death due to acute myocardial infarction (heart attack). Other cocaine-associated complications of the heart include cardiac arrhythmias, which sometimes can be lethal, myocarditis (inflammation of the heart muscle), cardiomyopathy (enlargement of the heart), and coronary spasm (spasm of the vessel that carries blood around the heart). The heart can, at times, become very slow (bradycardia). The heart rate can also be slowed by cocaine.

At times, in the middle of acute cocaine intoxication, it has been reported that the heart can actually rupture abruptly, resulting in sudden death. It is believed that it is a metabolite (breakdown product) of cocaine that causes the toxicity to the heart.

Acute heroin intoxication can cause the heart to slow down (bradycardia) as well as suppression of the respiratory system, which can result in cardiopulmonary failure. Many things can happen to the heart of an intravenous drug abuser, but one of the most serious is a condition called bacterial endocarditis.

There are two forms of endocarditis: 1) acute bacterial endocarditis, 2) sub-acute bacterial endocarditis. Endocarditis occurs when bacterial organisms enter the bloodstream of the individuals, injecting drugs into their veins. Once in the bloodstream, the bacteria multiply, resulting in a condition called sepsis.

Bacteria then settle on the heart valve, damaging it, causing different types of cardiac decompositions. In drug addicts, the valve most frequently affected is the tricuspid valve (54% of the time), followed by the aortic valve (25%), then by the mitral valve (about 20%), and the rest (6%) can be mixed right-sided and left-sided endocarditis. The bacterial organism most frequently found in drug addicts is staphylococcus coagulase positive, followed by streptococci; fungi, such as candida and aspergillus, can also cause bacterial endocarditis.

Gram-negative organisms of different types can also settle on the heart valves, causing endocarditis. Staph coagulase negative can also settle on the heart valve, causing bacterial endocarditis in the drug addicts. In intravenous drug abusers, when the tricuspid valve is the affected valve, 80% of the time the Staph coagulase positive is the organism isolated.

They can also become infected with Methicillin-Resistant Staph Aureus.(MRSA). In acute bacterial endocarditis, the affected person becomes acutely ill with fever, chills, shortness of breath, chest pain, sometimes, cardiac arrhythmia and the development of an acute heart murmur, which was not there before with congestive heart failure.

Other physical findings may include distended neck veins, decreased blood pressure; fast pulse rate, increased respiratory rate, cardiac rub, and rales in the lungs can be heard. An enlarged and tender liver can occur and a large spleen can be palpated. Acute pain in the lower back is frequently present in an individual who is septic. Headache with nausea and vomiting can also occur.

Laboratory findings include a high white blood cell count, low red blood cell count, elevated erythrocyte sedimentation rate, low platelet count, positive ANA, and elevated liver function test.

A chest x-ray may show diffuse infiltrates in the lungs. EKG may show fast rate with regular rhythm or fast rate with irregular rhythm, a slow rate with decreased voltage indicating that the heart is being compromised with fluid around the sac, a condition called cardiac tamponade. Arterial blood gases may be grossly abnormal with low O2 SAT. An echocardiogram may show valvular abnormalities such as vegetation, and an enlarged heart may be seen.

A transesophageal echocardiogram may show the presence of vegetation on the heart valves if the regular echocardiogram does not show it. Sometimes, a transthoracic Echocardiogram can also be done if the technology is available in that particular institution. It is a much better test to detect heart valve vegetation than the regular echocardiogram.

The urine may show the presence of protein and red blood cells because of emboli to the kidneys. Septic emboli can also affect the skin, causing assorted skin lesions. Acute bacterial endocarditis is a severe medical emergency requiring the help of a cardiologist and cardiac surgeon to quickly take over the management of the patient, in order to try to replace the heart valve and save the individual's life. If any significant delay takes place, the chances of recovery may not be very good in acute bacterial endocarditis.

What happens is that the bacteria sit on the valve and literally eat it away and then blood flows back and forth, resulting in acute cardiac decomposition with impending deaths, because of the valve having been acutely destroyed. As for management, these individuals frequently have to be intubated if they are in acute congestive heart failure. They cannot breathe.

They need assistance to breathe and 100% oxygen has to be provided for them. Blood cultures ought to be taken and if they are positive, then clinical decisions must be made to provide appropriate antibiotic treatment for these patients. If staph is suspected, which it frequently is, Vancomycin IV is an excellent choice in antibiotic with coverage for gram-negative organisms. Vancomycin also covers MRSA.

Once the organism is identified, and then an appropriate antibiotic should be provided based on the sensitivity. In the case of enterococcus, Gentamicin, along with Ampicillin, will be the drug of choice; if pseudomonas, then Fortaz will be a very good medication and if it is staph and it is sensitive to pencillin, then Oxacillin IV will be switched, as the medication of choice and the Vancomycin will be stopped. If it is Methicillin-resistant staph, then the medication of choice clearly in this case is Vancomycin as stated above.

The other infection frequently involving the heart is sub-acute bacterial endocarditis. Sub-acute bacterial endocarditis can be more insidious and often is more insidious in its development, causing difficulty, at times, in arriving at a diagnosis. Sub-acute bacterial endocarditis manifests itself as a febrile illness with chills, general malaise, joint pain, low back pain, and headache.

At times, a person with sub-acute bacterial endocarditis might present with general weakness, pallor, intermittent low-grade fever, and a general feeling of unwellness.

In this instance, a high index of suspicion must be brought into play so as not to mistake the diagnosis for something else. The profile of the patient is of major importance, i.e., in an intravenous drug abuser who is prone to sub-acute bacterial endocarditis by virtue of her habit of using drugs and sharing dirty needles with other drug addicts, the index of suspicion is quite high. Sometimes, these individuals use water from the toilet bowl to prepare the drug, in this way injecting themselves with contaminated materials.

The liver is a frequently affected organ in drug addicts. For those who abuse prescription drugs, the liver may get sick from these drugs, in particular when alcohol is combined with these drugs, as is frequently the case. Intravenous drug abusers' livers get sick most frequently because of hepatitis B and hepatitis C. In rare circumstances, they can also be infected with hepatitis A and hepatitis D, but these types of viral hepatitis occur less frequently in intravenous drug users.

Hepatitis A, B and C can be sexually transmitted and many drug addicts, when they are high on drugs, have sexual intercourse with whomever, wherever and whenever. Some drug addicts prostitute themselves either for drugs or for money to buy drugs. These loose behaviors predispose the drug addicts to contracting sexually transmitted diseases, such as hepatitis A, B and C, syphilis, gonorrhea, chlamydia, genital herpes, human papilloma virus (HPV), HIV, etc.

Several of these sexually transmitted diseases, such as hepatitis A, B and C, syphilis, gonorrhea, and HIV can be spread to different parts of the body, resulting in all sorts of different symptoms and damage to the human body. In particular, hepatitis B and C can cause chronic liver disease such as chronic active hepatitis, chronic persistent hepatitis, and cirrhosis of the liver, with all its associated complications, including liver cancer and death.

Drug addicts can also get infected with hepatic a through needle sharing, Because of that, sub clinical, acute hepatitis A can develop as well as fulminant hepatitis resulting in acute liver failure. It is therefore a very good idea to do a complete hepatitis profile on drug addicts, to include hepatitis, A, B, and C including DNA-PCR for Delta hepatitis. Delta hepatitis virus needs the presence of hepatitis B to support its growth in the body.

An other very important to remember is that drug addicts must be vaccinated against the hepatitis viruses that they are not infected with, so as to prevent them from becoming infected with other hepatitis organisms on top of an already sick liver, which can have lethal clinical consequences.

The gastrointestinal tract is affected in drug addicts in several ways. One of the most common gastrointestinal symptoms that drug addicts suffer from is abdominal pain associated with craving for drugs.

Secondly, drug addicts suffer frequently from diarrhea. The diarrhea has two bases: 1) nervousness and anxiety associated with craving for drugs; 2) parasitic infestation, which they contract during anal intercourse, transmitting organisms such as amoebae and Giardia lamblia. Upper gastrointestinal bleeding can occur as well when these people become cirrhotic because of chronic hepatitis. The bleeding occurs because of esophageal varices.

The kidneys are affected by intravenous drug addiction in several ways. As part of the sepsis and septic shock, the kidneys frequently fail in drug addicts, who present to the hospital with bacterial sepsis. As part of sub-acute bacterial endocarditis, septic emboli because of septic vegetations being thrown from the heart valves to the kidneys can affect the kidneys. Nephrotic syndrome occurs in intravenous drug addicts. This is probably due to antigen-antibody complexes, which form and circulate in the bloodstream either because of low-grade chronic infection or as a result of the different materials that are used to cut and mix either cocaine or heroin that the addicts use.

These complexes settle in the tubules of the kidneys, causing nephrotic syndrome. Kidney abscesses can also occur in some IV drug addicts.

The female reproductive system is quite often affected by IV drug addiction. The most frequent problem that women drug addicts experience with their reproductive system is menstrual irregularity, which occurs because of drug addiction-related endocrine dysfunctions. Further, when the female's liver is sick with hepatitis, which has resulted from drug addiction, the sick liver is unable to properly break down estrogen, and the result is too much estrogen in the blood, which overstimulates the uterus, resulting in frequent breakthrough vaginal bleeding.

The men's genital organ is also affected by liver disease resulting in cirrhosis causing small and shiny testicles because of the inability of the liver to break down estrogen in cirrhotic men's liver, and ejectal dysfunction can also develop.

Intravenous drug addicts, because they having sexual intercourse with multiple sexual partners, have a high incidence of cervical cancer. Sexually transmitted disease is quite common in drug addicts. When these people are under the influence of drugs they have the propensity of engaging in risky sexual intercourse with multiple sexual partners without regard to barrier protection, exposing their genital organs to being infected with gonorrhea, chlamydia, herpes simplex virus, human papilloma virus, and HIV infection.

Pelvic inflammatory disease (PID) is extremely common in these women drug addicts, causing chronic lower abdominal pain and chronic vaginitis. HIV infection is the most serious and the most deadly infection that afflicts blacks drug addicts. The spread of the AIDS virus through the IV drug addicts is the main reason why there is such a high incidence of AIDS in drug addicts in the United States and all over the world. (see chapter on AIDS).

The blood is one of the most commonly abused systems by drug addicts. This is so because the blood is the entry point of most of the drugs that are used and abused by drug addicts. Once the drugs reach the bloodstream, it gets carried to all parts of the body.

Frequently, the blood of drug addicts gets infected with bacterial organisms such as staphylococcus aureus, staphylococcus epidermidis, streptococci pneumonia, pseudomonas, klebsiella pneumonia, E. coli, hemophilus influenza, and pneumococci. Other Methicillin-Resistant Staph Aureus (MRSA) and fungi such as candida, aspergillus, and viruses such as hepatitis A, B, C, D, E, and G can all enter the bloodstream through injection of drugs into the blood system.

As described earlier, all these different microorganisms have at one point or another caused infection in drug addicts. The blood cells of the body are all affected by drug addiction. Different drugs that are abused by addicts affect the bone marrow by suppressing it. The suppression of the bone marrow that these drugs can cause leads to anemia, leukopenia, or thrombocytopenia to occur acutely.

Leukocytosis can occur, reflecting the presence of the infection. Pancytopenia can also occur because of an acute infection such as sepsis, as well as hepatitis-induced cirrhosis of the liver, with secondary portal hypertension. When an IV drug abuser is infected with the AIDS virus, parvovirus #B-19 can enter the bloodstream, resulting in pure red cell aplasia. Hepatitis can at times cause aplastic anemia. Both hepatitis C and B have been described in aplastic anemia, and in some instances hepatitis A has been described in some part of the world as being responsible for aplastic anemia.

Bacteria also get into the blood through broken and rotten teeth. However, more often, the bacteria get into the blood through skin abscesses that drug addicts develop during skin-popping or infected veins or dirty needles that addicts use to inject drugs. Another disease that can occur in drug addicts in IVDA is bone infection (osteomyelitis), a condition that results when bacteria that are circulating in the bloodstream infect the bone.

Different bones can become infected in drug addicts, but the lumbar spine, the thoracic spine, the hip joints and the knees, etc. can frequently become infected. Often drug addicts present to the hospital with high fever, severe low back pain, or a swollen knee with effusion. When that happens, the back has to be evaluated with a CT scan and/or an MRI looking for the possibility of destruction of bones because of infection. Sometimes a bone scan might add some more information to the clinical presentation.

When the bone is discovered to be infected, an orthopedic surgeon must be brought into the picture to try to surgically remove the infected bone. In addition, the individual requires several weeks of IV antibiotics. That often is a problem because it is difficult to keep an IV drug abuser in the hospital for as long as six weeks; he or she oftentimes elopes so she or he can go back to continue his or her destructive habits of using drugs.

The skin is the most frequently abused organ by the intravenous drug addicts. The heroin or cocaine addicts who inject drugs have to go through the skin to get the veins or arteries to inject themselves. Frequently, the skin is dirty because of lack of proper cleansing. Some addicts, when they run out of veins to inject, inject drugs under their skin, a practice called skin-popping. Some addicts have multiple sores over their legs, abdomen, buttocks, neck, and arms with very little good skin left. These open sores represent a ready entry point for infection to enter into the bloodstream, resulting in blood infections of different types.

The blood is the main vehicle through which drugs are introduced into the bloodstream. Other routes through which illicit drugs are introduced into the body are smoking, snorting, and skin-popping. Once the drugs are in the bloodstream, and if the doses of the drugs are excessive, the result is frequently drug overdose, resulting in different degrees of mental aberration. Frequently, confusion, stupor, seizures and, oftentimes, coma can develop. Once coma develops, if immediate medical attention is not provided, death may result.

Treatment of drug addicts and drug addiction

Drug addiction is a serious mental illness that affects people in all segments of society. Some people are addicted to prescription drugs, some people are addicted to illicit drugs, and some people are addicted to a combination of illicit drugs and prescription drugs. Drug addiction treatment requires a multi-team effort. The mental aspect of drug addiction requires treatment from mental health professionals and drug counselors and these individuals ought to go to drug treatment clinics and hospitals, both on an outpatient basis and when necessary on an inpatient basis for long-term drug rehabilitation treatments.

The medical treatments of drug addicts must be both organs and systems directed. One of the key components of intravenous drug abuse treatment is Methadone treatment. Methadone is a synthetic drug that is used to relieve the drug craving of heroin addicts. There are roughly 3.8 million chronic and regular drug addicts in the United States. They represent about 20% of the total drug addicts in the United States, which means that there are about 19 million drug addicts in the United States. 25 million individuals are addicted to illicit drugs in the U.S in 2011 and worldwide 200 million people use illicit drugs.

Methadone use contributes greatly in reducing HIV infection in IV drug abusers.

It helps put people to work and to some degree; it helps to decrease the crime rate because these addicts do not have to commit crimes to find money to buy their drugs. According to published report, only 1.7 million drug addicts can get into a Methadone program in the United States. It is said that only 115,000 of the 800,000 chronic users of heroin are getting Methadone. In New York City, about 35,000 of the 200,000 hardcore drug users are able to get into a Methadone Program. Methadone according to some people is encouraging drug addiction.

This is untrue because Methadone is a form of medical treatment for heroin addiction. Drug addicts can abuse Methadone also. Some addicts take the Methadone from the clinic and sell on the street. Some people on purpose lie about the actual dose of Methadone and as a result too much Methadone is given to them and they can overdose on Methadone on that basis. Because of Methadone overdose, they can go into coma. Some addicts abuse the Methadone Program and stay on it permanently as a form of work disability.

These problems with the Methadone Program are not widespread, and overall the Methadone Program is useful and constructive. The hardcore drug users in the ghettos of the United States use a significant percentage of heroin, cocaine and crack-cocaine. However, according to recent reports, Whites and people in the middle class, upper middle class and celebrities in the sports and entertainment world use more cocaine, heroin and crack cocaine than people of color who live in the ghettos of the U.S.

Because Blacks, Hispanics and other minorities both in the U.S. and around the world are arrested, persecuted and put in jail more often than whites for drug offenses, there is a misconception that they use more of these drugs, than whites, that is, in fact, not the case.

As mentioned above, there are 2.2 million people in jail in the U.S. This is the highest rate of incarceration than any industrial country in the world. In 2009, 754 people per 10,000 were in jail in the U.S. One of 32 American adults is in jail, either on probation or on parole.

At anytime, there are 7 million people in the U.S. in jails, either on probation or on parol. "The U.S. has 5% of the world' population and 25% of the world's prison population" Sixty-five million people in the U.S. have a criminal record. Source: U.S Justice Department.

Many of the people in State prisons or Federal prisons are there for drug related offenses. "Currently, the United States houses over 500,000 prisoners for drug related offenses. The drug addiction subculture is associated with criminal behavior because it is illegal to distribute and to use illicit drugs; the trafficking of drugs is controlled by the criminal elements of society. Blacks and Hispanics are more frequently sentenced for drug related offenses. 23% of Blacks, 21% Hispanics, and 15% of whites are sentenced for drug related crimes. The trhee stikes, you are out send more blacks to jail than other racial groups.

"In 2007, 4,618 black males per 100,000, 1,747 Hispanics males per 100,000, and 773 white males per 100,000 were incarcerated in the U.S." As of April 2010, there were
211,455 people in Federal prisons in the U.S.

Poverty, racial discrimination, poor education, poor housing, lack of economic opportunities, and the chronic depressive state of mind associated with being in the underclass of society contribute to the factors that persist for the proliferation of drugs in the ghettos.

The dynamics for the penetration of drugs into the suburbs are altogether different from that which exists for the poor people's communities. Rich folks get into the drug use subculture for recreational purposes, or to be in with a particular crowd or to be "cool." Either way, drug addiction is drug addiction and a drug addict is a drug addict.

Providing treatment for drug addiction and addressing the multiple and different issues that make drug addiction what it is take a back seat to the building of jails, stiff sentences, and the "Three strikes, you are out" policies of the U.S. and different state governments. There are people in jail serving life sentences because they were arrested for possessing marijuana.

It is utterly absurd that an individual can be thrown in jail for life for using crack-cocaine and most frequently, these individuals happen to be people of color. Individuals in the upper echelon of the United States society can be arrested for using cocaine or heroin, and get away at times with just a slap on the back of the hand. It would seem clear that these laws are placed in the books specifically to punish people of color, simply to get them out of society and throw them in jail.

This seems to be grossly unfair, though no one should condone the use of drugs of any kind, because that is illegal. However, putting it in its proper context, clearly there is some inequity in the way the law is being used as it relates to blacks, versus blacks in the majority community. It is not hard to envision that these problems would be resolved rather promptly if the hardcore drug users in the United States were white middle class and the white community was being devastated by these drugs.

It is fair to say that a Marshall type of plan would have to be put into effect to deal with the drug problems, and as certain as the sun rises in the east and sets in the west, these problems would have been solved, if not completely, but certainly much better than they are being dealt with now. According to the International Centre for Prison Studies

At King's College in London England, "more people are behind bars in the United States than in any other country. China ranks second with 1.5 million prisoners, followed by Russia with 870,000."

The brain is frequently evaluated when drug addicts present with headaches, fever and seizures. Evaluation and treatment include brain CT, brain MRI, EEG, echocardiogram, CBC, SMA 18, PT, PTT, chest x-rays, urinalysis, blood cultures and lumbar punctures. Treatments directed towards possible acute brain disease in the IV drug abuser are based on any abnormal results the aforementioned tests may show. If all the tests are normal, or the results are pending, empirical treatments must be started promptly.

For the seizure, Valium IV followed by Dilantin IV or by mouth should be started. For the fever, broad-spectrum antibiotics are given IV. In this setting, Vancomycin IV is given to cover for gram-positive organisms, and Fortaz or other broad-spectrum gram-negative antibiotic is given to cover for gram-negative organisms. There are multitudes of other antibiotic combinations that can be used to cover both for gram-negative and gram-positive organisms in this setting.

Treatments of acute lung disease in IV drug abusers when they present with fever and shortness of breath are tailored to the findings on physical examination and/or chest x-ray. If the patient is afebrile but shows signs and symptoms of acute pulmonary disease, then arterial blood gas is done and oxygen is quickly started, and if the signs and symptoms are consistent with congestive heart failure, then treatment is given with IV Lasix right away.

If signs and symptoms are consistent with acute pulmonary embolism, then a lung scan must be ordered along with ultrasound of the lower extremities. If the suspicion is strong and these tests are not readily available, then the patient should be given IV Heparin, if there is no contraindication to anticoagulation. If all signs, symptoms and findings on chest x-ray and CBC are consistent with pneumonia, then broad-spectrum antibiotics with Vancomycin IV and with Fortaz ought to be started immediately. If the patient is able to cough up sputum, then the sputum ought to be sent to the laboratory for gram stain and culture prior to starting the antibiotics.

Infection of the heart is one of the most common infections seen in IV drug abusers. Anytime an IV drug addict presents to the hospital with fever, heart valve infection such, as acute bacterial endocarditis or sub-acute bacterial endocarditis must be suspected. Once the blood cultures have been obtained, broad-spectrum antibiotics with Vancomycin IV and Fortaz IV must be started to cover for the possibility of bacterial endocarditis.

In acute bacterial endocarditis, the patient's cardiopulmonary system can become decompensated quickly, resulting in acute shortness of breath and acute congestive heart failure (pulmonary edema) because of acute destruction of the heart valve. This happens because bacteria settle on the affected heart valve and destroy it.

As stated earlier, the most frequently affected valve in intravenous drug abuser is the tricuspid valve, followed by the aortic valve, followed by the mitral valves. This is an acute medical emergency necessitating evaluation by a heart surgeon for replacement of the affected valve surgically.

It is important when treating a patient for possible bacterial endocarditis to frequently listen to the patient's heart, looking for the development of a new heart murmur, which would be the first sign of possible cardiac decompensation. Sub-acute bacterial endocarditis can present with no definite cardiac symptoms.

Oftentimes, sub-acute bacterial endocarditis presents as part of sepsis with fever, chills, and low back pain. Sometimes infected vegetation can be seen on an echocardiogram.

Sometimes, sub-acute bacterial endocarditis presents and manifests itself with general malaise, weakness and intermittent low-grade fever and anemia. If serial blood cultures are drawn, a positive drug culture will eventually be found and the diagnosis of sub-acute bacterial endocarditis can be established.

The treatment of bacterial endocarditis is Vancomycin to cover for Staph coagulase, positive MRSA, ceftriaxone for other gram-positive cocci, and Fortaz to cover for organisms such as pseudomonas. There are other combinations of antibiotics, which can also be quite effective in treating this infection. The main reason to always give the patient Vancomycin at presentation is that there is significant percentage of Staphylococcus organisms that are resistant to penicillin-like medications, such as Nafcillin, Kefzol, MRSA, and Oxacillin.

Once the culture and sensitivity results are back from the lab, then Nafcillin can be switched for the Vancomycin, assuming that the patient is not allergic to penicillin and that the organism is shown to be sensitive to the Nafcillin. Vancomycin is much more expensive than Nafcillin. In addition to antibiotic treatment, proper fluid management, proper electrolyte management and antipyretic for fever and nasal oxygen must be included as part of the treatment.

Intravenous drug abusers must also be given medication such as methadone to forstall the development of drug withdrawal.

Many drug addicts use alcohol to supplement their drug addiction needs. These patients, when acutely ill, must be watched closely for seizures, which, if they develop, can complicate the patient's overall clinical picture.

Treatment of liver disease in drug addicts is dictated by the clinical condition of the individual patient. If the drug addict presents with acute hepatitis, fever, chills, nausea, vomiting, abdominal pain and elevated liver function tests, the patient ought to be placed in isolation with hepatitis precautions being adhered to. In this setting, the prothrombin time is most important.

This is so because the prothrombin time is a measure as to how well the liver is able to function. The sicker the liver, the higher the prothrombin time will be. If the prothrombin time is elevated, then 10 mg of Vitamin K SC ought to be given in the deltoid with applied pressure both as a test and as a treatment.

The prothrombin time should be repeated 6-12 hours later.

If the prothrombin time is corrected back to normal after the Vitamin K, it means that the patient still has good liver function left though the liver is tender and the liver tests are abnormal. Further, it also means that the patient though may have abnormal platelet count, and does not have DIC.

Treatments with IV fluids, anti-fever medications such as Tylenol, anti-itching medication, anti-vomiting medication ought to be provided to control these particular symptoms. If the patient is not vomiting, is able to eat, and the prothrombin time is normal, it is advisable to treat the patients who have hepatitis at home while monitoring his or her vital signs and liver function tests.

Chronic liver disease, such as chronic active hepatitis and chronic persistent hepatitis, are treated either aggressively or supportively in a conservative way. In the case of chronic active hepatitis, treatment will be provided after liver biopsy and based on the symptoms of the patient and the findings on the liver biopsy.

The most frequently used treatment for patients with chronic active hepatitis and symptoms of chronic active hepatitis with documented liver biopsy are alpha Interferon.

The degree of inflammation seen in the liver biopsy documents the severity of the liver disease. In chronic persistent hepatitis, there is minimal inflammation with no fibrosis in the liver and the liver tests are either slightly or moderately elevated chronically. In chronic lobular hepatitis there is mild to moderate inflammation and mild fibrosis. In chronic active hepatitis there is, as stated above, moderate severe inflammation and moderate to severe fibrosis of the liver.

Patients who abuse intravenous drugs can also develop acute hepatitis A because of intravenous drug use, though less so than hepatitis B and C, but it can occur. There are no chronic sequelae of hepatitis A. It is a good idea for patients who are chronic abusers of drugs to be vaccinated with the hepatitis virus A vaccine, which is available.

In addition, drug addiction is a major psychiatric disease that affects the mind in a very significant way. Once addicted to drugs, these individuals are mentally dependent and emotionally dependent on the drugs and become very preoccupied with when and where they are going to find money for their next fix and their entire preoccupation is related to their drug activities.

The behavior of individuals who are addicted to drugs is totally irrational, particularly when they are under the influence of drugs. They lose complete control of their humanity; they will do anything under the influence of these drugs. Under the influence of drugs, blacks and men are capable of engaging in a multitude of immoral and illegal activities that have negative impacts on them, their families, and society as a whole.

Individuals who are addicted to drugs are mentally dependent on these drugs. The addiction to drugs preoccupies them totally. Their humanities are no longer their own; their lives are controlled by the drugs that they are addicted to. They are constantly scheming, lying and committing crimes of different types to get money to buy the drugs that their brains crave. Getting the next fix to satisfy their craving is the most important thing in their lives because they have lost complete control of their beings. When under the influence of these drugs, they are capable of committing a multitude of illogical, irrational and illegal acts.

Drug addiction in blacks is a major problem in U.S. society, and it contributes to the destruction that occurs in the families of these blacks who fall victims to the awful power of drug addiction.

It is important for those in government to proactively undertake actions and create policies that are designed to get to the root causes of drug addiction problems in all their aspects. It is quite clear that present policies of building jails and throwing people in them and treating those people like animals are not working.

You cannot treat a psychological medical problem with jail or "three strikes, you are out" policies. Those policies are designed to get politicians, and district attorneys and judges elected at the expense of the people who are suffering from mental, medical, and physical problems. Those who commit crimes ought to be punished for the crimes they have committed. While in jail, they ought to be given treatments for their addiction and its associated problems.

They should be given a real chance of rehabilitating themselves and they ought to be taught trades of different types that would enable them to be wage earners once they have completed their sentence and back in society.

It is also important to realize that once a drug addict, always a drug addict and, that being the case, long-term psychological treatment ought to be made available to these individuals after they have left jail.

Treatments that are necessary are costly, but they are important, and drug prevention programs, educational programs dealing with the prevention of drugs are very important. Programs to prevent the dissemination of drugs within the communities where those blacks live are very important. The federal and state governments need to spend the billions of dollars that are necessary to fund those programs to help them to become successful.

It is important that drug addiction seminars begin at the earliest grades in schools across the country, so that children can become sensitized to the ravages that drug addiction can cause, as a way to let them know what the facts really are, so that when people approach them trying to get them involved in drugs, they will say "no".

As it is right now, the incidence of drug addiction in schools across the country is high and begins at the earliest age, in elementary school up through middle school and high school.

It is crucial that the educational system join forces with the government agencies to try to encourage drug prevention and drug education programs in elementary schools, middle schools, and high schools. In college, there is also a significant evidence of drug use going on, but these are young adults who choose to do these things to themselves. It is wrong, but they are at an age where they can make their own decisions.

They also should be encouraged to give up drug use or not to start at all, because once a person starts using drugs, it is very difficult to give it up because drug addiction is so overwhelming that these individuals are weakened by the force of the addiction. The colleges also ought to organize drug prevention seminars on their campuses for the benefit of students and faculty, and most definitely confidential drug treatment programs ought to be offered and must be made easily available for college students who are using illicit drugs, to help them give up their habits. It is hypocritical to sweep it under the carpet and pretend that it does not exist.

To help individuals who are addicted to drugs, it requires money, it requires better governmental involvement, and it requires better involvement of the educators, the clergy, and other members of society working as a team to attack a scourge that is destroying significant numbers of people in society.

Chapter 61
VIRAL HEPATITIS

There are five main types of viral hepatitis

Hepatitis A
Hepatitis B
Hepatitis C
Hepatitis D
Hepatieis E

HEPATITIS A

Hepatitis A is transmitted in stools to human when they eat contaminated foods with hepatitis A
Other Foods that are frequently contaminated with hepatitis A include
Raw shellfish
Fecal contaminated fruits
Fecal contaminated green vegetables
Fecal contaminated water etc;

Other ways to get infected with hepatitis A include:

Sexual contact
Blood transfusion (rarely)
Blood products (rarely)
Intravenous Drug addiction
Tatooing etc;

Worldwide 1.5 million people become infected with hepatitis A every year and 80,000 people become infected with hepatitis A every year in the U.S.

Once this virus enters into the body, the incubation period (the time it takes the virus to begin to cause symptoms) is 2-6 weeks.

Symptoms of hepatitis A include:
Weakness
Fatigue
Nausea

Vomiting
Diarrhea
Loss of appetite
General body aches
Fever
Chills
Right sided-abdominal pain
Evaluations of hepatitis A include:

History and Physical examination
Hepatitis A, B, C, D, E profile
CBC
Complete chemistry profile
GGTP
Urinalysis
PT/INR
PTT
Abdominal ultrasoundet c;

Signs of hepatitis A include:

Tenderness of the right of the upper abdomen
Enlarged liver
Enlarged spleen
Dark urine
Jellowness of the skin
Jellowness of the eyes
Abnormal liver function tests
Dark urine
Positive hepatitis blood test

Treatments for hepatitis A include:
Bed rest
Zofran or Kytril for nausea and vomiting
NSAID's for fever (if platelets count is normal)
Avoid Tylenol if the liver is failing
IV fluid with D5W1/2 (if the patient is too sick to eat he or she should admitted to the hospital)
If the PT/INR is elevated the patient must be admitted to the hospital because, the liver may be failling.

If the patient is able to eat and the PT/INR is positive, it is best to keep the patient at home to avoid spreading the virus to people in the hospital.

The patient's CBC, complete chemistry, and PT/INR should be monitored closely for several weeks.

Hepatitis A does not cause chronic liver disease.
Prevention of hepatitis A include (30million Americans travel every year to countries where hepatitis A is prevalent)
Proper hygiene
Avoid eating raw shell fish
Avoid drinking contaminated water
When traveling to developing countries get vaccinated against hepatitis A.

Vaiccines that are in use to prevent hepatitis A are:
Twinrix
Havrix
VAQTA.

Chapter 62
HEPATITIS B

Worldwide hepatitis B infectect two billion people and 1.5 million people die every year from hepatitis B. Source: WHO. Hepatitis B is the most common cause of liver disease in the world. In the U.S. 12 million people have hepatitis B and 1.2 million people have chronic hepatitis B and 5000 people die every year from hepatitis B. Hepatitis B is transmitted through infected blood, blood products, IVDA and other body fluids. There are 8 different genotypes of hepatitis B and different genotypes of hepatitis B are found in different parts of the world. All 8 getotypes of hepatitis B are common in the U.S.

Risk factors for hepatitis B include:

Blood and blood products transfusion
Intravenous drug abuse
Semen
Saliva
Unprotected sexual intercourse
Infants of mothers who are infected with hepatitis B (hepatitis B can be transmitted from infected mothers to infants during child birth)
Using tooth brush of people infected with hepatitis B
Babies born to mothers infected with hepatitis B

Once the hepatitis B virus enters into the bllod stream of the individual being infected, it takes 40-150 days or an average of 12 weeks for the first symptoms to appear. (Incubation period) Some people infected with hepatitis B never develop acute symptoms but may go on to be carrier of hepatitis B and some go on to develop chronic persistent hepatitis B.

Signs and symptoms of hepatitis B include:
Fatigue
Poor appetite
Nausea
Vomiting
Abdominal pain
Jaundice (Yellow color of the skin)
Itching
Fever

Chills

Headache

Dark urine

Abnormal CBC

Abnormal liver function tests (elevated SGPT, SGOT, Alkaline Phosphataste, PT, INR, PTT, and bilirubin)

Positive blood test for hepatitis B antibody

Evaluations of hepatitis B include:

History and physical examination

CBC

Complete chemistry profile

GGTP

PT/INR

PTT

Urinalysis

Blood test for hepatitis B antibody

PCR/RNA

Hepatitis B viral load

Abdominal ultrasound

Liver biopsy etc;

Treatments of hepatitis B include:

Zofran for nausea and vomiting

or

Kytril for nausea vomiting

or

Compazine for nausea and vomiting

Tylenol for fever (low dose only, and no Tylenol if the liver shows signs of failing)

NSAID's for fever (no NSAID's if the platelets count is low)

Benadryl for itching

IV fluid with D5W1/2 normal saline

or

IV with D5 normal saline

If the patient is not able to eat and vomiting, he or she should be admitted to the hospital

If the PT/INR and PTT are elevated, he or she should be admitted to the hospital because this is a sign of liver failure.

If the patient is able to eat, and the PT/INR is normal, the patient should be kept at home to avoid spreading the hepatitis to the hospital staff.

About 5-10% of individuals who develop acute hepatitis B goes on to develop chronic hepatitis B. Chronic hepatitis B causes cerrhosis of the liver and some people go on to have cancer of the liver.

Chronic persistent hepatitis is manifested mainly by persistent mild to moderate elevation of liver function tests, such as bilirubin, SGOT, SGPT, alkaline phosphatase and the GGTP (gamma glutamine transpeptidase) and no major physical findings nor symptoms. On the other hand, chronic active hepatitis is an active inflammatory liver disease with elevation of liver function tests, increased serum ferritin along with malaise, weakness, anemia, and sometimes-palpable liver with right-sided abdominal pain and at times persistent low-grade fever.

Sometimes chronic active hepatitis goes on to develop cirrhosis of the liver with portal hypertension, hypersplenism, pancytopenia, and esophageal varices. Once the esophageal varices develop, recurrent upper gastrointestinal bleeding can occur.

One of the many chronic complications of hepatitis B in these individuals who develop cirrhosis is hepatocellular carcinoma (cancer of the liver). This cancer in this setting occurs usually 10 to 30 years after the individual becomes sick with hepatitis B.

Fulminant hepatitis with acute liver failure can occur with hepatitis A, B, C, D, E or G. Acute management of hepatitis includes supportive care, careful IV fluid management, careful monitoring of liver function tests, including the prothrombin times, platelets, red blood cells and serum ammonia level.

Dietary management in acute hepatitis is very important, which includes a low-protein diet and low salt. Management of chronic liver disease also includes attention to diet with low protein, low salt, with close attention to liver function tests including the PT, platelet, red cell count and ammonia level. These individuals ought to be given anti-itching medications such as Benadryl, Periactin, etc.

The reason for the itching is because the liver is too sick to be able to properly get rid of bile salts, and these bile salts accumulate in the blood, causing severe itching. It is also important that individuals who have chronic liver disease stay away from antiplatelet medications such as aspirin, and NSAIDS.

It is also important not to give them too much Tylenol. Large doses of Tylenol have the propensity to make the liver disease worse. In patients who have cirrhosis of the liver, regardless of the cause of their cirrhosis. One has to be very careful to prevent bleeding from the gastrointestinal tract from occurring, because any amount of blood placed in the GI (blood contains protein) tract will be broken down into ammonia by actions of bacteria in the gut.

Because the ammonia cannot be picked up properly by the sick liver, the end result is elevated level of blood ammonia.

High elevated level of ammonia in the blood can cause the patient to become somnolent, confused at times, and if treated prmtely and properly can lead to the development of the comatose state.

High ammonia level is treated low protein diet and Lactulose to induce diarrhea and cleanse the bowel of the stools that contain too much ammonia and other toxic waste matters.

Neomycin 4-12 grams per day can be used to kill as many bacteria as possible to decrease the bacterial load in the gut thereby decreasing the production of ammonia to improve the state hepatic encephalopathy.

Medications in use to treat hepatitis B are

Alpha interferon-2a
PEGylated Interferon-2a (Pegasys)
Adefovir
Lamivudine
Enteccavir
Telbivudine
Tenofovir
Vaccines in use to prevent hepatitis B are
Recombivax B and Engerix-B

Chapter 63
HEPATITIS C

Worldwide 170 million people are chronically infected with hepatitis C and 350,000 peolple die every year from hepatitis C. About 3.2 million people in the U.S. are infected with hepatitis C and 15,000 people die every year in the U.S. from hepatitis C. 75% of adults American who are infected with hepatitis C are baby boomers born between 1945 and 1965.

There are 11 different geno types of hepatitis C, 1-6. Genotype is more common in the U.S. 70-90% of people infected with hepatitis C in the U.S. is infected with genotype 1a and 1b. People who are infected with genotype 1 of hepatitis C respond best to treatments and genotype 1b is highly associated with a high incidence of liver cancer.

Risks for hepatitis C include:

　　Contaminated blood
　　Contaminated blood products
　　Unprotected sexual intercourse with people infected with hepatitis C
　　Accidental needle sticks
　　Intravenous drug addiction
　　Sharing needles
　　Tattoos
　　Piercing
　　Acupuncture with contaminated instruments
　　Organ transplants
　　Long—term hemodialysis
　　HIV infection
　　Health care workers
　　Infants born to mothers infected with hepatitis C.

Once become infected, it takes 2 weeks up to 6 months before symptoms develop.

Signs and symptoms of hepatitis C include:

　　Fever
　　Chills
　　Fatigue

Decrease appetite
Nausea
Vomiting
Headache
Itching of the skin
Abdominal pain
Dark urine
Jaundice
Joints pain
Total body pain
Jellowness of the eyes
Jelloness of the skin

About 80% of individuals who become infected with hepatitis C have no symptoms.

About 75-85% of people who just become infected with hepatitis C go on to develop chronic hepatitis C and 70% of these people develop chronic liver disease; and 5-20% of them develop cirrhosis of the liver.

5% of people who develop cirrhosis of the liver because of hepatitis C die of cancer of the liver. Over all, hepatitis C is responsible for 25% of all people who die of cancer of the liver. Source: WHO

Evaluations of hepatitis C include:

History and physical examination
Blood test for hepatitis C antibody
Rapid diagnostic test (RDTs) this test is new
Point of-care tests (POCTs) this test is new
CBC
Complete chemistry profile
PT
INR
PTT
Urinalysis
Abdominal ultrasound
FibroScan
Hepatitis C RNA-PCR
Hepatitis C Viral load
Hepatitis genotype
Liver biopsy
HepaScore
HCV FibroScore

Treatments for hepatitis C include:

Bed rest

Kytril for nausea and vomiting
or
Zofran for nausea and vomiting

NSAID's for fever if platelets are normal
or
Tylenol for fever if PT/INR is normal

Benadryl for itching

If the PT/INR is normal and patient can eat, he or she should be treated at home

If he or she is vomiting and cannot eat, he or she should be hospitalized

If the PT/INR, PTT are elevated, this is an indication that the liver may be failing, he or she must be hospitalized

Once in the hospital the patient must be placed in isolation for the protection of other patients and the hospital staff.

At home the patient must used a personal bath room to avoid spreading the hepatitis to other people in the house or apartment.

Pegylated interferon
Ribavirin
Telaprevir
Boceprevir
Ritonavir 100mg with ABT-450 (experimental by Abbott's) Source: Wall Street Journal 10/16/12
Genotype 1 hepatitis C requires treatment for 1 year
Genotype 2 and 3 can be treated for 6 months.

Hepatitis D is contrated in the ways as do hepatitis B and C and causes the similar problems to the liver as do hepatitis B and C. However, hepatitis D requires the presence of of hepatitis B for its replication.

Hepatitis E is contracted in the same ways as do hepatitis A. There are 20 million people in the world who are infected with hepatitis E. Similar to hepatitis A, hepatitis E does not cause chronic liver diseases.

Other types of hepatitis include:

Alcoholic hepatitis
Drug induced hepatitis
Autoimmune hepatitis
Primary billiary cirrhosis
Primary sclorosing cholangitis
Primary hemochromatosis
Secondary hemochromatosis etc;

Chapter 64
CIRRHOSIS OF THE LIVER

Worldwide over 500 million people suffer from liver diseases and in the U.S. 5.5 million people have cirrhosis of the liver and every year 25,000 people in the U.S. die of cirrhosis of the liver.

Cirrhosis of the liver develops because different things happen to the liver that causes inflammation to develop. Once the inflammation becomes chronic, then scaring of liver tissues takes place resulting in the development of cirrhosis.

The different things that cause cirrhosis of the liver include:

Alchol abuse
Hepatitis B
Hepatitis C
Hepatitis D
Fatty liver disease
Primary biliary cirrhosis
Hemochromatosis
Primary sclerosing cholangitis
Biliary atresia
Cystic fibrosis
Wilson disease
Lupus erythematosus
Rheumatoid arthritis
Mixed connective tissue diseases
Glycogen storage disease
Parasitic infestation etc;

Signs and symptoms of cirrhosis of the liver include:

Fatigue
Poor appetite
Weight loss
Easy bleeding
Easy bruising
Nose bleed

Upper gastrointestinal bleeding (from esophageal varices)
Bleeding from the gums
Nausea
Abdominal pain
Jaundice
Jellowness of the eyes
Enlarged liver
Enlarged spleen
Itching
Spider angiomata
Redness in the palm of the hands
Break through vaginal bleeding
Enlarged breasts in men
Small and shiny testicles
Edema of lower legs
Fluid in the abdomen (ascites)
Anemia
Leukopenia (low white cells)
Thrombocytopenia (low platelets)
Low Folic acid level
Low B12 level
High reticulocytes count
Dark urine
Clay color stools
High aldosterone level in the blood
Erectal dysfunction etc;

Evaluations of cirrhosis of the liver include:

History
Physical examination
Vital signs
Body weight
CBC
Reticulocyte count
Complete chemistry profile
Hepatis B, C and D profile in the blood
Viral load for hepatitis B and C
PCR/RNA for hepatitis B and C
Genotype for Hepatitis C (there 11 known genotypes of hepatitis C)
Genotypes of hepatitis B (there 8 known genotypes of hepatitis B)
ANA
Rheumatoid factor

ESR
PT/INR
PTT
Urinalysis
GGTP
Serum folate level
Serum B12 level
Blood alcohol level
Serum Copper level
Stools for ova and parasites
HIV/AIDS 1 &2 blood tests
VDRL blood test for syphilis
Sweat test for cystic fibrosis
Genetic test for cystic fibrosis
Molucular genetic testing for collagen storage disease
Abdominal ultrasound
Abdominal CAT scan with contrast
Abdominal MRI with IV contrast
FibroScan
Liver biopsy
HepaScore
HCV FibroScore

Complications of cirrhosis of the liver include:

Portal hypertension
Hypersplenism
Esophageal variceal
Upper gastrointestinal bleeding
Anemia
Ascites
Swollen legs
Itching
Jaundice
Vaginal bleeding
Erectal dysfunction
Hepatic encephalopathy
High incidencer of infection
Cancer of the liver (cancer of the liver due the complications of hepatitis B kills up to 2 million people per year in the world and is the fourth leading cause of deaths in the world. In the U.S. 25,000 people die every from cirrhosis of the liver due complications of alcohol abuse and hepatitis B and C mainly.

Definitive treatment for cirrhosis of the liver is liver transplant.

Every year 6,000 liver transplants are done in the U.S. and 21,000 liver transplants are done worldwide annually.

Chapter 65

THE COMMON COLD

The common cold is the most common disease in the world.

Adults usally have two five colds per year and children have five to 10 colds per year. On an average Americans get 1 billion colds per year.

"In the U.S. colds results in about 100 doctor visits per year at a cost of $7.7 billion per year" "Americans spend $2.2 billion per year on over the counter drugs and $400 million on prescription medicines for symptomatic relief"

"An estimated 189 school days are missed annually and parents missed an estimated126 million work days to stay home to care for their children." In addition, "150 million work days are missed by employees suffering from colds." "The total economic impact of cold related work loss exceeds $20 billion per year" in the U.S.

In 2010, it was estimated that 230, 136, 966 people in the world had a cold every day or about 84 billion colds per year in the world. The worldwide economic of the common cold is known, but it is probably in the trillion of dollars.

The common is a viral infection and there more than 200 different viruses that can cause the common cold. The most viruses that cause colds are
Rhinovirus (80% of the time)
Coronovirus
Human parainfluenza virus
Human respiratory syncytial virus
Adeovirus
Enterovirus metapneumovirus

The viruses that cause colds are transmitted via airborne droplets or direct contact with objects infected with nasal sectretions. Hand shakes are frequent ways of tramsmitting colds from persons to persons. Coughing is also an easy of transmitting the cold virus from persons to persons.

Risk factors for getting include:
Cold temperature
Time of the (fall and winter)
Infants

Children
Exposure in schools
Exposure in day care centers
Immunosuppression
COPD
Asthma
Cystic fibrosis
Cold miners'lung
Smokers
HIV/AIDS etc;

Signs and symptoms of colds include:

Stuffy nose
Runny nose
Cough
Itchy throat
Sore throat
Body aches
Headache
Sneezing
Watery eyes
Fever
Chills
Fatigue
Sinus pain
Sinusitis
Redness in the eyes
Pain in the eyes
Ear ache
Hoarness
Enlarged lymph nodes
Stiff neck
Nausea
Vomiting
Ambominal pain
Shortness of breaths
Persistent crying in infants
Dehydration
Dizziness
Vertigo etc;

Complications of cold include:

Wheezing (specially in asthmatics and people with COPD/Emphysema)
Coughing greenish sputum
Coughing up yellowish sputum
Bronchitis
Ceoup in children
Pneumonia
Otitis media
Streptococcal pharyngitis

Evaluations people suffering with colds include:

History and physical examination
Throat culture for streptococcus when indicated
CBC
Mno spot when indicated
Complete chemistry profile when patients are dehydrated and not able to eat or dring well
Chest X-ray when indicated to rule out pneumonia

Treatments of the common cold include:

Symptomatic treatment is the preferred treatment for the common cold
Tylenol 650m four times per day for fever and body aches
Advil 2 tablets three times per day for fever and body aches
Motrin 400mg three times per day for fever and body aches
All NSAIDs work well to treat the symptoms of the common cold
Aspirin should be used in infants and young children
Aspirin 325mg 2 tablets three times per for fever and body aches in adults and adolescents
Claritin 10mg 1 tablet per day for nasal stuffiness
Zyrtec 10mg 1 tablet per day for nasal stuffiness
Allegra 180 mg 1 tablet per day for nasal stuffiness
Sudafed 120mg 1 tab twice per day for nasal stuffiness
There several other antidecongestant medications in use in the U.S. and around the world
Nasonex nasal spray 1 spray in each nasal passage twice per day for nasal congestion is quite effective
Cough syrups prescribed or over the counter are used to treat the cough seen in the common cold
Patients who are hypertensive should not take cough syrup over the counter without a physician advice, because most cough syrups contain ephedrine and ephedrine can cause the blood pressure to go up.

Other OTC cold medications in use include:
Clarinex
Claritin-D
Allegra-D
Actifed
Dimetapp
Chlor-Trimeton etc;

Frequently used cough syrups include:

Rubitussin CF
Rubitussin DM syrup
NyQuil
Phenegan Plain
Mucinex
Delsym suspension etc;
Coricidin HBP (good for people with hypertension)
Phenergan with codeine (needs a prescription from a physician)
Hycodan syrup (needs a prescription from a physician)
Tessalon perles is a very good cough suppressor medication and is most effective in diabetics, because it does not contain sugar.
There are several sugar free OTC sugar free cough syrups available.

In specific circumstances antibiotics can be used in the setting of a common cold infection and these are:

1. Asthmatics with a persistent common cold with yellowish/greenish sputum should be treated with an antibiotic to prevent triggering an acute an asthmatic attack.
2. COPD/Emphysema a persistent common cold with yellowish/greenish sputum should be treated with an antibiotic to prevent the decopemsation of the COPD/Emphysema.
3. People with any underline chronic lung disease should be treated with antibiotic in the setting of a common cold.
4. People with a common cold and a streptococcus throat infection should be treated with an antibiotic.
5. People with acute sinusitis in the setting of a common cold should be treated with an antibiotic.
6. People with otitis media in the setting of a common cold should be treated with an antibiotic.

7. People with painful conjunctivitis in the setting of a common cold should be treated with eye drop containing antibiotic and steroid.
8. People with bronchitis in the setting of a common cold should be treated with an antibiotic.
9. People with pneumonia in the setting of a common cold should be treated with an antibiotic in the office or inside the hospital.

People who have no chronic lung diseases and have a cold should not be treated with antibiotics, because cold is caused by viruses and viruses do not respond to antibiotics.

Frequently used antibiotics to treat upper air way infection include:

Amoxcillin
Zytrhomax
Cipro
Levaquin
Biaxin
Avelox
Erythromycin
Bactrim DS
Keflex etc;

Frequently used antibiotics to treat lung infection include:
All of the above plus
Ceftriaxone
Cetazadime
Cefuroxime
Cefoxitin
Vancomycin
Unasyn etc;

Over use of antibiotics to treat the common cold is ill advised and can lead to antibiotic resistance and should be avoided.

Chapter 66
ALLERGIC RHINITIS (HAY FEVER)

Allergic rhinitis or seasonal allergy occurs because IgE is attached to mast cells and basophils and when stimulated by allergens cause the release of histamine that causes inflammation in the nasal passages, sinuses, in the eyes and the throat resulting in mucus production.

About 50 million people in the U.S. suffer from hay fever/allergic rhinitis and worldwide 30% of the population suffers from hay fever/allergic rhinitis.

Risk factors for hay fever/allergic rhinitis include:

Grass pollen as seen in the spring and summer
Tree pollen as seen in the spring
Ragweed as seen in the fall
Spores from molds and fungi
Dust mites
Cockroaches
Dender from cats, dogs and birds
Asthma
Eczema
Flowers etc;

Signs and symptoms of hay frver/allergic rhinitis include:

Watery eyes
Itchy eyes
Swollen eyes
Conjunctivitis (redness of the eyes)
Sneezing
Itchy nose
Itchy throat
Hoarsness
Cough
Sinus pressure
Sinus pain
Dizziness
Vertigo

Labyrinthitis
Headache
Nausea
Vomiting etc;

Evaluations of hay fever/allergic rhinitis include:

History and physical examination
Patch test
Scratch test
Intradermal test
RAST blood test
IgE antibodies level
CBC with differential (looking for elevated eosinophil
CT of the sinuses when indicated
ENT consultation when indicted
Laryngospic examination when indicated etc;

Treatments of hay fever/allergic rhinitis include:

Flonase
Nasocort
Nasonex
Rhinocort
Benadryl
Claritin
Zyrtec
Allegra
Astelin
Afrin
Cromolyn
Singulair
Steroid by mouth or IV
Immunotherapy etc;

Complications of hay fever/allergic rhinitis include:

Poor quality of life
Imsonia
Tiredness
Coughing
Wheezing
Sinusitis
Otitis media
Acute asthmatic attacks etc;

Prevention of hay fever/allergic rhinitis includes:

Avoidance of allergen exposure
Take anti-histamine medications prior to being exposed to allergen etc;

Chapter 67
INFLUENZA (THE FLU)

The Flu is a very serious contagious respiratory disease that affects 20% of the U.S. population annually and worldwide about 5 million people are affected annually.

There are three different types of Influeanza A, B and C.
Types A and B are responsible for the seasonal annual flu epidemic all over the world.

Every year in the U.S. 200,000 people get hospitalized in the U.S. due to the flu and about 36,000-40,000 people die every year from the flu. Worldwide 500,000 people die from the flu every year.

The influenza viruses are transmited from persons to persons through sneezes mucus directly into the noses, eyes or mouths of the persons being infected, coughing, hand shakes and touching contaminated surcafes and kissing infected people etc;

Risks for getting the flu include:
Infancy
Young children
Age 65 and older
Immunossuppression (non-acquired)
Immunossuppression (acquired) HIV/AIDS
Cancer
Chemotherapy
Steroid treatment
Diabetes mellitus
Rheumatoid arthritis
Mixed connective tissue diseases
Lupus
Kidney failure
COPD
Emphysema
Asthma
Cystic fibrosis
Cirrhosis of the liver
Heart diseases
Pregnancy

Sickle cell disease
Beta-thalassemia
Alpha-thalassemia
Auto-immune hemolytic diseases
Hemochromatosis
Being a health care worker etc;
Signs and symptoms of the flu include:
Fever
Chills
Rapid pulse
Rapid respiration
Body aches
Sweating
Headache
Cough
Fatigue
Weakness
Nasal congestion

Complications of the flu include:
Bronchiitis
Pneumonia
Ear infection
Sinusitis
Deaths

Evaluations of the flu include:
History and physical examination
Nasal swab
Blood titers for influenza A, B and C
CBC
Complete chemistry profile
Blood culture
Urinalysis
Chest x-ray etc;

Treatments of the flu include:
Bed rest
Drink plenty of fluid
Tylenol, NSAIDs or aspirin for fever
Tamiflu or Relenza within the first 72 hours
Cough syrup for cough
Nasal decongestant etc;

Preventions include:
Influenza vaccine
Hand washings
Cover the mouth while coughing
Avoid being in a crowd
Avoid hand shakings
Wear mask
Wear gloves
Wear a gown etc;

Chapter 68
SINUSITIS

Sinustis occurs because of inflammation of the sinuses. Sinusitis can be caused by viruses, bacteria, fungus, allergy, or autoimmune diseases.

Thirty five million people in the U.S have chronic sinusitis yearly and I million people have acute sinusitis every year in the U.S. resulting in 16 million doctor office visits per year. Sinusitis that lasts more than 10-12 weeks is called chronic sinusitis.

Worldwide there are hundred of millions of people who suffer from both acute and chronic sinusitis.

The viruses that usally cause sinusitis include:
Rhinoviruses
Coronaviruses
Influenza viruses
Human parainfluenza viruses
Human respiratory syncycial virus
Adenoviruses
Metapneumovirus
Enteroviruses etc;

The bacteria that usally cause sinusitis include:
Streptococcus pneumoniae
Haemophilus influenza
Moraxella catarrhalis
Staphylococcus aureus etc;

Locations of sinusitis are:
Frontal sinus
Maxillary sinus
Ethmoid sinus
Sphenoid sinus

Risk factors for sinusitis include:
Hay fever/allergic rhinitis
Deviated nasal septum
Nasal polyps

Enlarged adenoids
Tooth infection
Cystic fibrosis
GERD
HIV/AIDS
Autoimmune diseases such as Wegerner granulomatosis, Sjogren's etc;

Signs and symptoms of acute sinusitis include:
Yellow discharge from the nose
Greenish discharge from the nose
Nasal congestion
Pain over the affected sinus
Tenderness over the affected sinus
Pressure around the eyes
Pain and pressure around the cheecks
Pain and pressure around the nose
Pain and pressure around the forehead
Aches and pain in the jaw
Aches and pain in ther teeth
Inability to smell well
Night time cough
Headache
Ear ache and pain
Sore throat
Fatigue
Fever
Bad breath
Double vision
Stiff neck
Shorness of breath
Comfusion etc;

Evaluation of sinusitis include:

ENT consultation
History and physical examination
Nasal endoscopy
CT of the sinuses
MRI of the sinuses etc;

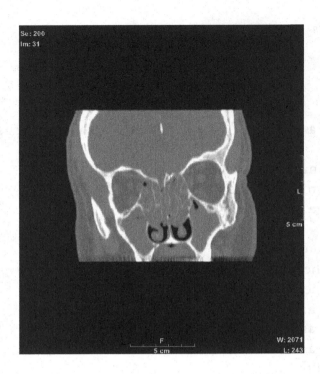

68:1 CT scan demonstrates severe maxillary and ethmoid sinusitis. There is nasal polyposis.

Treatments of sinusitis include:
Naasonex
Flonase
Rhinocort
Nasocort
Beconase AQ
Sudafed
Actifed
Afrin
Allegra
Xyrtec
Claritin
Claritin D
Allegra D
Amoxicillin
Zythromaxin
Bactrim
Cipreo
Levaquin
Ceftin
Avelox
Biaxin

Corticosteroid by mouth
Nasal saline wash
Antifungal medication if fungal sinusis is documented by culture
Immunotherapy when indicated.

Complications of sinusitis include:
Flare up of COPD/Emphysema
Flare up of asthma
Meningitis et;

Chapter 69
ASTHMA

One in 12 individuals in the U.S. has asthma. That represents 8% of the U.S population or 25 million Americans who suffer from asthma. Each day 11 people in the U.S. die of asthma and 4,000 individuals die annually of asthma.

Worldwide there are 300 million people with asthma and 250,000 people die every year from asthma.

Asthma is more common in Blacks Hispanics and other minorities than in whites and in 2011 there were 3000 blacks with asthma in the U.S. Ashma is more common in women than men and Black, Hispanic and other minorities women have the highest mortality rates from asthma than any other racial groups. The death rate is 2.5 times higher in Black, Hispanic and other minority women compared to white women.

Blacks, Hispanics and other minorities are hospitalized 3 times more often than whites are and blacks die of asthma three times more frequently than whites do. Each year 3 million people visit emergency room because of asthma, 500,000 get hospitalized because of asthma and 10 million out patient visits are made because of athma. Each year 14 million school days are missed because of asthma attacks in children.

About half of asthma cases develop before age 10 and about one-third of asthma cases develop before age 40. Most cases of allergic asthma begin in early childhood and frequently are associated with family history of asthma, rhinitis, eczema, hay fever, bronchitis, and emphysema.

Many cases of asthma are genetically transmitted. The other common form of asthma is called idiosyncratic asthma, meaning that the individuals who suffer with this type of asthma have no family history of asthma and no history of hay fever, negative skin types were tested, and there is normal IgE level in their blood.

There is still another group of blacks with a mixed form of asthma, with features of both allergic asthma and idiosyncratic asthma.

Risk factors for asthma in clude
Genetic
Children
Women

Men
Living in urban areas
Poor urban air quality
Poverty
Poor education
In door allergens
Out door allergens
Smoking
Dweling with roches, mice, rats, moles and old and pealing paints
Housedogs
House cats
House birds
High humidity in housing due lack fan and air condition during summer time
Dampness/cold in housing due to lack of heat during winter time
Stress
Obesity
Upper airway infection
Chronic sinusitis
Gastroesophageal reflux disease (GERD)
Racial discrimination
High unemployment
Inferior medical care etc;

Symptoms of asthma include:
Coughing
Wheezing
Shortness of breath
Thightness in the chest
Rapid heart rate
Sneezing
Stuffy nose
Runny nose
Sore throat
Head ache
Insomnia
Difficulty in speaking

What happens in asthma that causes the asthmatic patient to have trouble in breathing is that the bronchioles inside the lungs become obstructed to different degrees, because of being exposed to either one of several irritants. Bronchioles are tube-like structures that are located inside the lungs through which air is channeled in and out the lungs.

The irritants that affect the inside of the bronchioles cause swelling, inflammation and secretion of mucoid-like materials to develop. The result is that air gets trapped inside the bronchioles, resulting in shortness of breath, wheezing, marked difficulty in breathing and a feeling of an impending doom.

The wheezing sound that is heard when an asthmatic breathes is due to air fighting to get through the narrow passages that have been created by mucous plug, edema, and swelling inside the bronchioles. The inflammation that occurs at the cellular level is mediated by T lymphocytes that secrete type 2 T-helper cytokines like interleukins 4, 5, and 13. Interleukin 4 and 13 regulate the production of IgE. High-affinity IgE receptor on mast cells mediates the release of histamine, prostaglandins, leukotrienes and inflammatory cytokines, along with interleukins 5 mediation of eosinophils, result in an overall inflammatory process that starts off the asthmatic attack.

Many things can bring on acute asthma attacks; some are allergenic, environmental, infectious, occupational, and pharmacological and some are emotional.

The most frequent form of allergic asthma is seasonal and is associated with hay fever and pollens. Other allergens that can precipitate acute asthma attacks are such things as animal dander, feathers, dust, mites, molds, paints, roaches, mice, rats, and exposure to cats and dogs. Exercise and, in particular, breathing cold air can precipitate an acute asthmatic attack. It is believed that the high incidence of asthma seen in poor communities is the result of the poor living conditions associated with poverty.

Many of these individuals live in poorly ventilated, roach—and rat-infested apartments. The high level of crime seen in these communities' forces those who live there to stay behind closed doors to shield themselves from the daily problems associated with living in these communities and under these conditions.

Roaches carry over their body's irritants and materials that get carried by the air that, when breathed by the asthmatics, precipitate asthmatic attacks. Rats and mice that live in these apartments, no doubt, leave droppings that, when they get airborne, also can be inhaled and participate in bringing about most asthmatic attacks. All these outlined allergens, when inhaled, can precipitate asthmatic attacks.

Environmental factors associated with high incidence of asthma are seen in industrial areas where factories and industrial machines emit sulfur dioxide and nitrogen oxide combining with air, which, when breathed, causes pulmonary diseases of different types, including asthma. Upper airway infection is the most commonly associated precipitating factor triggering asthma attacks. The common infections that frequently precipitate asthmatic attacks are the common cold, which is brought on by rhinoviruses and parainfluenza viruses in adolescents, adults and in young children.

Other infections that can trigger acute asthmatic attacks are respiratory syncytial virus, bacterial infections, such as bacterial bronchitis, bacterial pneumonia, and bacterial sinusitis are all associated with the precipitation of asthmatic attacks. Different types of viral sinusitis, viral bronchitis, and viral pneumonias are also frequently associated with the precipitation of asthmatic attacks.

Occupational exposure plays a major role in both the causation and in the precipitation of asthma. The lists of precipitating materials that blacks can be exposed to that can cause asthmatic attacks are almost endless. Some of the known industrial materials that are associated with the causation and precipitation of asthma attacks are laundry detergents, different types of fumes, coffee beans, nickel, and platinum dust, etc.

A multitude of pharmacology product drugs, when used by asthmatics, can bring on an asthmatic attack. Some of the most common drugs that can set off an asthmatic attack are aspirin, beta-blockers, and some coloring medications, such as red dye number 3, and sulfur medications. There is a syndrome of asthma, nasal polyps, and aspirin allergy. Some of these people can also have a similar reaction when they ingest NSAIDs.

It is, therefore, always prudent to ask these folks the question, "Are you allergic to aspirin or NSAIDs or have ever taken those medications before with no problem?" before prescribing them for any person who suffers with asthma.

Another common precipitant of asthmatic attacks is exercise. Exercise-induced asthmatic attack seems to be associated with the coldness of the air being breathed in. It is, therefore, not a good idea for asthmatics to participate in sports such as skiing, ice-skating and ice hockey. Sports activity where the air is warm is fine. If an asthmatic person wishes to participate in these activities, he or she would be wise to get advice from his or her physician as to what to do to prepare himself or herself to partake in them.

Another frequent trigger of asthmatics is emotional stress. The mechanism for this form of asthmatic attack precipitant is not altogether clear, but the overall mental turmoil associated with stress is capable of triggering an asthma attack.

Before starting the evaluation, quickly listen to the lungs for air movement and the heart to check the rate and the rhythm of the heart, and give her nasal oxygen and an injection of epinephrine subcutaneously. Now proceed with the evaluation.

How to evaluate a person presenting with an asthma attack:

1. First the physician must take a history from the patient to find out several things.

2. It is important to watch how the patient is breathing.
3. Does he or she have labored breathing?
4. It is important to watch how the patient is speaking.
5. Can he or she hold a sentence and for how long?
6. How does he or she look?
7. Does he or she look tired?
8. Ask the question how many hours ago did the attack start?
9. What medication did he or she take before presenting?
10. Are the nasal passages stuffed up?
11. Is he or she coughing up sputum?
12. If yes, what color is the sputum whitish, yellowish, or greenish or bloody?
13. Does he or she have a fever, chills or body aches?
14. Ask whether he or she has just been exposed to any of the possible irritants outlined in the preceding paragraphs.
15. Is he or she wheezing
16. Does he or she has shorntness of breath
17. Is he or she gasping for air?
18. Does his or her lip looks bleu?
19. Do a peak flow test immediaitely
20. Do aterial blood gas (ABG)
21. Give him or her oxygen immediately
22. Give him or her dose of 0.5 cc of 1:1000 solution of epinephrine immediately SC
23. Begin nebulizer treatment immediately
24. Establish IV access immediately
25. Begin IV fluid

Then quickly do a peak flow, using the breathing meter. Try to ascertain the patient's previous known base peak flow. Do an arterial blood gas to determine whether she is retaining carbon dioxide or not. If so, quickly prepare for possible intubation of the patient to secure the airway, to prevent sudden respiratory arrest. Get a good IV line started to provide medications such as fluid and steroid.

Start Alupent nebulizer treatment immediately and continue these treatments every 4-6 hours until the patient is better. Steroid is the backbone and most effective treatment in asthma, but it takes about 6 hours before it starts to work. Get a chest x-ray; look for pneumonia, bronchitis, congestive heart failure, and pneumothorax, which, if present, will complicate the patient's management.

As part of the ER evaluation of the asthmatic patient, a CBC and SMA20 chemistry profile ought to be done. The decision as to whether to admit the patient who presents with an asthmatic attack depends on how the patient looks clinically, how good the peak flow is, and how improved is the examination of the lungs.

If after several hours in the ER with significant and appropriate treatments having been provided without significant improvement in the overall clinical state of the patient, then the patient ought to be admitted for more prolonged treatments. An improved peak flow is good objective evidence that the asthmatic patient has gotten better. One of the controversial issues of the treatment of acute asthma associated with upper airway infection is whether to add antibiotics, either by mouth or intravenously.

Some much respected experts in infectious diseases say, "Don't use antibiotics because the organisms responsible for the infection are viruses," yet there are some who say, "Yes, antibiotics ought to be used." The reason given is that the inflammation that the viral infection causes breaks down the protective membranes within the lining of the upper airway.

Once the protective membranes are broken down, local bacteria proliferate, resulting in a superimposed mixed bacterial-viral upper airway infection, precipitating and complicating the asthmatic attack. Even when the upper airway of the asthmatic is irritated with a noxious material, the resulting inflammation can cause the protective membranes to lose their integrity, allowing the bacteria that live in the upper airway to set up an acute asthmatic attack, requiring antibiotic treatment.

The way to diagnose asthma is by:

1. The history
2. Physical examination
3. The chest x-ray and
4. The FEV (forced expiratory volume in 1 second), after administration of 2 puffs of a beta-adrenergic medication and showing that the airway obstruction has been reversed by 15% or greater increase in the FEV. Examination of the chest of the asthmatic patient usually demonstrates different types of wheezes, both inspiratory and expiratory wheezes. Shortness of breath with a fast respiratory rate (normal respiratory 15-20 per minute), the heart rate/pulse rate is fast, 100 or greater per minute. Frequently, the patient uses her abdominal muscles to help to breathe.
5. The peak and ABG are crucial to show whether a person is retenting carbon dioxide or not. An asthmatic who is retaining carbon dioxide is n the process of dying and needs to be intubated immediately. Ordinarily, asthmatics have low carbon diaoxide because of rapid breating, so, when they are retainibng carbon dioxide, it means that either bronchospams and or mucus plugs are preventing exchange of oxygen causing carbon dioxide retention. This condition is called hypoxymia.

The chest x-ray shows hyperinflated lungs in asthmatic patients.

Treatments of asthma include

Some of the medications used to treat asthma:
Immediate response medications
1. Epinephrine 0.3-0.5 ml. of 1:1000 solution subcutaneously
2. Alupent inhaler
3. Proventil inhaler
4. Albuterol inhaler
5. Bronchodilators in aerosol solution 0.4%-0.6%
6. Xopenex inhaler
7. Maxair inhaler
8. Vantolent inhaler
9. Atrovent inhaler
10. Serevent
11. Prednisone
12. Theophylin
13. Theo-Dur
14. Medrol

Long acting asthma medications include:
1. Salmeterol inhaler
2. Beclovent
3. Vanceril
4. Azmacort
5. Flovent
7. Advair Diskus
8. Aerobid
9. Azmacort
10. Symbicort
11. Qvar
12. Flovant HFA

Leukotriene Modifiers is new family of medications being used to treat asthma. Among these medications are
Singulair
Zyflo
Zyflo CR
Zafirlukast

Asthma is a chronic inflammatory lung disease and, as such, requires different types of medications working via different mechanisms to treat it both acutely and chronically. One of the most common medications used to treat asthma are steroids.

Different types of steroid preparations are used to treat asthma intravenously, by mouth, or via inhalation technique. Steroid is indispensable in the treatment of asthma.

Frequently used intravenous steroids in the treatment of acute asthmatic attacks are
Solu-Medro
Decadron
Solu-Cortef
Prednisone by mouth and by inhalation is also frequently used in the treatment of asthma.
Different irritants, when inhaled, cause an acute inflammatory reaction to occur within the bronchioles (tubes that carry air through the lungs).

Steroid works to decrease that inflammatory reaction, thereby preventing the swelling, mucus production, and spasm within the bronchioles, tissues and other tubes inside the lungs. The spasm and the mucus plugs that occur within the bronchioles prevent air flow from getting in and getting out of the lungs.

The different medications used to treat asthma decrease the spasm, the inflammation and the production of mucus, allowing air to move easier within the lungs, relieving the acute symptoms will improve the overall incidence of asthma in blacks. The annual cost of asthma is 18 billion dollars in the U.S.

Chapter 70
EMPHYSEMA/COPD

Chronic Obstructive Pulmonary disease COPD/Emphysema is divided in 2 parts COPD and Emphysema. COPD occurs because of recurrent exposure of lung tissues and bronchioles to irritants from tobcco smoking such as cigarettes and cigars. In pure Emphysema, it is the alveolars that are damaged preventing air exchange to occur.

Every year tobacco smoking is responsible for 6 million deaths in the world.

Tere are 12 million people with COPD/Emphysema in the U.S. and probably an other 12 million people who have COPD/Emphysema do not yet diagnosed. Source: NHLBI March 31, 2011. Each year 120,000 people die of COPD/Emphysema in the U.S. and the yearly cost of COPD/Emphysema is 49.9 billion dollars Source: National Institute of Health.

Worldwide 600 million people have COPD/Emphysema and every year 2.74 million people die of COPD/Emphysema and COPD/Emphysema is the 5th leading cause of deaths in the world.

Risk factors for COPD/Emphysema are
Cigarette smoking
Cigar smoking
Air pollution
Industial exposure to pollution
Black lung/coal miners' lung
Gold mining
Alpha-1-antiprypsin deficiency (responsible for 2% of COPD)
Cystic fibrosis
Cotton textile workers
Exposure to cadmium
Exposure from welding fumes
Exposure to isocyanates
Exposure to silica dust
Exposure to asbestos
Sugar cane cutters
Sugar cane mills workers
Recurrent pneumonia etc;

In COPD, the inflammation that results due to the irriting effect of cigarette/ tobacco smoking or other pollutants from the air causes secretion of thick mucous that blocks the free flow of air in and out of the lungs, making very difficult for people with COPD to breath.

Emphysema and Chronic Obstructive Pulmonary Disease in Blacks in the US: Adult blacks in the U.S. who smoke by age and level of education are as follows:

Age 18 to 24 24.5 percent
25 to 44 25.6 percent
45 to 64 22.5 percent
65 and older 11.2 percent
Whites who smoke 23.6 percent
Blacks who smoke 21.6 percent
Hispanic blacks who smoke 13.3 percent
American Indian/Alaskan/Native blacks who smoke 38.1 percent
Asian/Pacific/Islander blacks who smoke 9.9 percent

10.7% of blacks with 8 years education or less smoke cigarettes.
34.3% of blacks with 9 to 11 years of education smoke cigarettes.
24.1% of blacks with 12 years of education smoke cigarettes.
22.8% of blacks with 13 to 15 years of education smoke cigarettes.
11.2% of blacks with 16 and more years of education smoke cigarettes.

Source: National Health Interview Survey, 1998, National Center for Chronic Disease Prevention and Health Promotion, Center for Disease Control Prevention.
Presently there are about 55 millions smokers in the U.S.

Tobacco smoking is a very dangerous habit. Cigarettes and other tobacco products contain chemical that cause diseases in people who use them and in those who are near them when they are smoking.
"Tobacco smoke contains over 4,000 different chemical, at least 50 are known to be carcinogens (cause cancer in humans), and many are poisonous." Source: Health Education Authority (UK) Life saver

The list of harmful chemicals found in cigarettes include
"Benzene
Formaldehyde
Ammonia
Acetone
Tar
Nicotine
Carbone Monoxide

Arsenic
Hydrogen Cyanide act;"
Source: Health Education Authority (UK) Lifesaver

Symptoms and complications of COPD/Emphysema include
Chronic cough
Sputum production (in chronic bronchitis)
Dyspnia
Wheezing
Tiredness
Weight gain in bleubloater
Weight loss in pinkpuffers
Pulmonary hypertension
Pulmonary embolism
Right heart failure-cor pulmonale

Left heat failure (when the right heart fails the left will eventually fail)
Cushing disease due to chronic steroid use
Osteoporosis due to chronic steroid use
Aseptic necrosis with arthritis due steroid use
Depression due in part due to steroid use
Psychosis due to steroid use
Elevated blood sugar due steroid use in pre-diabetics/diabetics
Peptic ulcer due to chronic steroid use
Acute exacerbation due to bacterial, and viral infections (usually 25% of the infections are bacterial, 25% are viral and 25% are a combination of bacterial and viral.

Cigarette smoking is the number-one cause of lung disease in blacks. There are two general forms of COPD/Emphysema: one form is the pink puffer and the other form is the blue bloater. The pink puffer type is the so-called dried emphysema. It is called dried emphysema because blacks with pink puffer cough a lot but no sputum comes up. These individuals are called pink puffers because they breathe with a pursed lip to force the air into their lungs and their lips look puffed.

In addition, they have barreled chests and they are usually thin in stature. Another distinct feature that differentiates pink puffers from blue bloaters is that pink puffers usually do not retain carbon dioxide because they are continuously puffing it out.

On the other hand, blue bloater COPD/Emphysema patients are usually obese; they cough up copious amount of sputum, their lips are blue and retain carbon dioxide. The toxic effects of the tobacco which the smokers inhale damage the substance of the lungs, resulting in a multitude of anatomical abnormalities causing trapping of air. It is the trapping of air and the stiffness of the lung that cause the patients with emphysema so much difficulty in breathing. Frequently, blacks with emphysema develop right-sided heart disease, complicating their overall cardiopulmonary state.

The incidence of tobacco use increased significantly in blacks in the last 40 years, and the result is that lung diseases of different types and severity have increased accordingly. Prominent among these lung diseases are chronic bronchitis, asthma, lung cancer and frequent pneumonia. Because the inner lining of the lungs are damaged by the effects of tobacco, bacterial growth is favored and frequent lung infections develop which can lead to different degrees of respiratory decompositions.

Very often, when people with COPD/Emphysema develop pneumonia, the respiratory system becomes decompensated, resulting in the need for the individuals to be placed on the respirator. The incidence of adult respiratory distress syndrome (ARDS) increases in blacks who smoke.

In the year 2011, 23,220 blacks will be diagnosed with lung cancer and 16,790 blacks will die of lung cancer in the U.S. Source: ACS facts & figures for African Americans 2011-2012. Ninety per cent of lung cancers are caused by tobacco smoking.

Lung diseases in people are associated with tobacco smoking, air pollution, exposure to industrial pollutants, exposure to asbestos and anti-trypsin deficiency etc.

Exposure to asbestos can lead to the development of a type of cancer called mesothelioma. Characteristic of asbestosis of the lungs is calcification of the lining of the lungs. Emphysema frequently results in end-stage lung disease. End-stage lung disease causes pulmonary hypertension, right ventricular heart failure, distended neck veins, swollen abdomen, swollen lower legs, large liver and cardiac arrhythmias of different types, which contributes, often times, to the death of affected people.

Exposure to several other noxious materials is also known to cause damage to the lungs that can lead to COPD/Emphysema in people. One well-known example is coal miner lung disease. Other examples include exposure to inhalation of cotton fibers by blacks who work in cotton mills; a similar lung disease can develop in people who work in sugar cane fields/factories as described above.

How to evaluate people with COPD/emphysema

The first thing to do is to take a good history from the person to ascertain his or her symptoms and what kind of noxious materials or environment she may have been exposed to. It is important to find if she smokes tobacco, if it is via cigarettes, cigars, or pipe. What type of work he or she does? If he or she does not smoke, it is important to find out whether his wife or her husband, boyfriend, girlfreind or significant other, with whom he or she is frequently in close contact, smokes tobacco.

It is also important to find out if he or she is exposed to tobacco smoke from his or her co-workers on the job.

The next thing to do is to carry out a complete physical examination, paying close attention to the following:

1. Is he or she very thin?
2. Is he or she fat?
3. Is he or she short of breath?
4. Is he or she constantly coughing?
5. Is the cough dry or productive of sputum?
6. Are his or her lips blue or pink?
7. Does he or she purses his or her lips when he or she breathes or not?
8. How hard is his or her breathing?
9. Can he or she carry a sentence through without stopping to catch his or her breath?
10. Is he or she using accessory abdominal muscles to help him or her to breathe?
11. Does he or she have clubbed fingers?
12. On listening to his or her lungs, how well is he or she moving air?
13. Are there rales or wheezes heard in his or her lungs?
14. On listening to the heart, are the heart sounds distant?
15. Are the heart sounds heard best below the breastbone?
16. Is the heart rhythm regular or irregular?

In people who have the dried type emphysema (pink puffer), the heart sounds are distant and very difficult to hear and the air movement is difficult to hear, as well.

The best way to hear the heart beats in these individuals is below the breastbone area. This is so because in this type of emphysema, the position of the heart is shifted to that area.

The heart frequently beats irregularly in emphysema patients because of an abnormal rhythm called atrial fibrillation. Other abnormal heart rhythms such as premature atrial and ventricular contractions are also quite common in patients with emphysema /COPD.

These cardiac abnormalities occur because of a combination of lung and heart malfunctions that emphysema causes. Rales are heard by listening to lungs because of heart failure, which causes fluid to accumulate within the lungs.

The most common chamber of the heart that fails in people who have emphysema/COPD is the right ventricle. When the right ventricle fails, the bulk of the work is left to the left ventricle, which ultimately fails as well, resulting in biventricular failure.

After the history and physical examinations are completed, several tests have to be done to document the fact the patient does have emphysema. The first tests to do are a chest x-ray, followed by spirometry, arterial blood gas, and pulmonary function test.

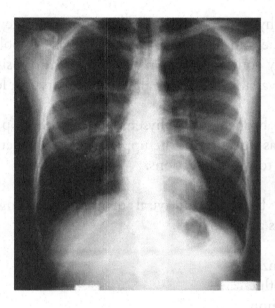

Figure 70:1—Normal chest X-ray in non-smoking female

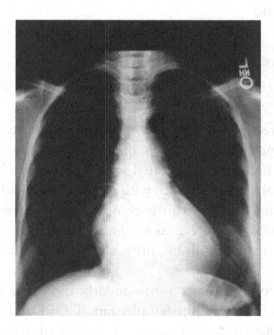

Figure 70:2—Abnormal chest X-ray in female smoker with emphysema

Chronic Obstructive Pulmonary Disease—COPD/Emphysema is the number forth cause of death in the U.S. There are 12 million individuals with COPD in the U.S. and there are about 12 million more individuals with COPD who are yet to be diagnosed.

Frequently both arterial blood gas and the pulmonary function tests are abnormal in COPD/Emphysema patients.

When COPD/Emphysema is discovered in a non-smoker with no exposure to secondary tobacco smoke and no exposure to industrial air pollution, etc., it is likely to be due to a hereditary condition known as alpha-1-antitrypsin deficiency. There is a commercial blood test available to test for alpha-1—antitrypsin level in the blood.

People with chronic bronchitis/emphysema/COPD develop infection in the lungs very frequently, as well as infection of the upper airway. The very nature of this disease predisposes these blacks to those infections.

The most frequent bacterial and viral organisms causing upper air way/lungs infections in these blacks are as follows:

Haemophilus influenzae
Haemophilus parainfluenzae
Streptococcus pneumonia
Moraxella catarrhalis
Klebsiella pneumoniae
Serratia marcescens and
Pseudomonas
Rhinoviruses
Corona virus
Influenza viruses

Frequently, these infections are mixed infections, associated with more than one bacterial organism causing the infection. Frequently, these upper airway infections start out with viral URI and become complicated with a secondary bacterial infection. Any infection affecting the airway of blacks with chronic bronchitis/emphysema/COPD usually causes their pulmonary status to become decompensated resulting in difficulty of breathing and anoxia. If the infection in the upper airway is not treated early and aggressively with antibiotic, the result oftentimes is the development of pneumonia.

Pneumonia and its complications are frequently the cause of death of individuals who suffer from chronic bronchitis/emphysema/COPD. The effects of tobacco smoking and other inhaled toxins damage the tissues of the lungs and the chronic nature of these diseases places these individuals in an immuno-suppressed state, which predisposes them to the development of pulmonary infections of different types and severity.

The micro-organisms that most frequently cause pneumonia in blacks with emphysema/COPD are the following:

Haemophilus influenzae
Haemophilus parainfluenzae
Streptococcus pneumonia
Moraxella catarrhalis
Klebsiella pneumoniae
Serratia marcescens
Pseudomonas
Staphylococcus aureus
Methecillin resistant staph aureus (MRSA)

Rhinovirusis and corona viruses are responsible for the majority of upper airway infections. Influenza viruses also cause a significant percentage of URI. URI causes exacerbation of COPD/Emphysoma. All these microorganisms can cause pneumonia further worsening the clinical status of COPD/Emphysema.

How to evaluate a patient with emphysema for pneumonia

The first thing to do is to take a good history from the patient. Ask him or her, are you coughing and for how many days? Is the cough productive? What is the color of the sputum? Is the sputum yellow, green, dark green, bloody, or whitish? Do you have a fever? Are you having chills? Does your chest hurt when you cough? Are you having headaches? Is your nose stuffed? Do you have a runny nose? Do you have generalized body aches and pain? Who else is sick in your household? Do you have birds in the house? Have you traveled recently out of the country or to other states in the USA? Do you have night sweats? Have you lost weight? Do you have poor appetite? The next thing to do is a physical examination.

When a physician suspects pneumonia in a patient, the most important parts of the physical examination are as follows:

1. The respiratory rate: Is it greater than 20?
2. The pulse rate: Is it 100 or greater?
3. Is the blood pressure normal or is it abnormally low?
4. Is the patient using abdominal muscle to help in breathing?
5. Does the patient look pale? Is the skin warm and moist?
6. How sick does the patient look?
7. Is the temperature below 98.6°F or 100 .4°F or greater?

8. How fast is the heart rate?
9. How do the lungs sound?
10. Is the patient moving air well?
11. Are there pneumonia sounds (rales) in the lungs? If so, where are they located in the lungs?
12. Is the patient wheezing?

Once the physical examination is completed, the next step is look at the chest x-ray. Are there infiltrates in the lung fields? What do those infiltrates look like? What does the arterial blood gas look like? Is the patient hypoxic (low oxygen)? In the case of the patient with emphysema, is he or she retaining carbon dioxide? If so, how much? Is the patient producing sputum? What is the color of the sputum? Is it yellow? Is it green? Is it bloody? Alternatively, is it whitish? On the other hand, is it a mixture of all these colors?

Once the physical examination has been completed, the next thing to do is to order some tests.

The most appropriate tests to order are the following:

1. Chest x-ray
2. ABG
3. Spirometry
4. EKG
5. CBC
6. Chemistry profile (SMA 20)
7. 2 sets of blood cultures
8. Sputum gram stain
9. Sputum culture and sensitivity

Once these tests have been ordered, treatment for pneumonia/COPD can be started.

1. The type of IVand amount of fluid that is given to these patients depends on the level of dehydration that the patient presents with. Usually Dextrose with normal saline or half normal saline, either alone or with dextrose at a reasonable rate of 125 cc per hour can be started. If the patient is a diabetic, half normal saline or normal saline can be given at the same rate.
2. Oxygen can be given via nasal canals of 2-3 liters per minute in patients who have pneumonia and no emphysema. If the patient has emphysema/COPD and pneumonia, it is best to give oxygen via venti-mask, to prevent too much oxygen from being administered, since, in a patient who is suffering from emphysema, such as a blue bloater who retains carbon dioxide, too much oxygen can cause

more carbon dioxide to be retained. The higher the level of carbon dioxide in the body, the sicker he or she will become.

If this high concentration of carbon dioxide is allowed to persist, several major complications, including inability of the heart and brain to function properly, can develop. Frequently, patients with emphysema who have pneumonia develop respiratory failure, necessitating placement on the respirator for breathing assistance.

The next step is to administrate antibiotics intravenously. If the patient comes from home, then a protocol that provides antibiotic coverage for community-acquired pneumonia is put into place. Examples of the intravenous antibiotics that can be used are the following:

a. Ceftriaxone, 1 or 2 grams every 24 hours, or
b. Levaquin, 500 mg. IV every 24 hours, or
c. Penicillin G, 10 to 20 million units daily in divided doses of IV, or
d. Ampicillin, 2-4 grams every 6 hours IV or,
e. In penicillin-allergic patients, Cipro, 400 mgs. IV daily, or
f. Erythromycin, 500 mg. IV every 6 hours or
g. Tequin, 400 mg IV daily for 7-10days
h. Ceftazadine 1 gram IV q8h plus
I. Vancomycin 1 gram IV q12h plus
J. Zosyn 3.375 grams IV q6h
k. Doribax 500mg IV q8h
l. Cefepime 2 grams IV daily
m. Zyvox 600mg IV q12h (MRSA)
n. Bactrim IV in Pneumocystis carinii 15-20 mg/kg/day q6-8h for 14 days
p. Zythromax 500 mg per day has recently been found to be very effective in COPD patients to prevent pulmonary decompasation

Even though the patient is coming from the community, the health profile of the patient determines whether the patient gets started on one or more antibiotics. The types of work the patient does for a living, as well, where the patient may have been prior to getting sick, also determines whether she gets started on one or more antibiotics and what type of antibiotics are used to start treatment.

Erythromycin is an excellent antibiotic to use, especially in the setting where atypical pneumonia and organisms such as legionella is suspected. Once the result of sputum gram stain/culture is back, antibiotic treatment is adjusted according to the results of these two tests.

People who are coming from a nursing home or who are in the hospital, and who develop pneumonia, are treated with different antibiotics, because bacterial organisms such as pseudomonas and staphylococcus for which specific antibiotics are required for treatment, frequently colonize these blacks.

The best antibiotic to use to treat pseudomonas is Ceftazidime and the best antibiotic to use to treat staphylococcus/methicillin resistant staphylococcus-MRSA is Vancomycin. Examples of IV antibiotics that can be used to treat hospitalized patients with pneumonia and their usual doses are as follows:

1. Ceftriaxone, 1-2 grams IV every 12 to 24 hours
2. Cefotaxime, 1-2 grams IV every 8-12 hours
3. Cefuroxime, 750 mg IV every 8 hours
4. Cipro, 400 mg IV every 24 hours
5. Erythromycin, 500 mg IV or by mouth every 6 hours
6. Imipenem, 500 ml IV every 6 hours
7. Nafcillin, 2 grams IV every 4-6 hours
8. Penicillin G, 2 million units every 6 hours IV
9. Vancomycin, 1 gram IV every 12 hours
10. Flagyl, 500 ml IV every 6 hours
11. Clindamycin, 600 ml IV every 8 hours
12. Levaquin, 500 ml IV once per day
13. Ceftazidime, 1gram IV every 8 hours
14. Tequin, 400mg IV every 24 hours
15. Bactrim DS, one tablet 2 times per day or IV Bactrim when the situation calls for it.
16. Doribax 500mg IV q8h
17. Cefepime 2 grams IV daily

In the office setting, Levaquin, Tequin, Zithromax, Cipro, Avelox, Biaxin, and Bactrim DS can be used as a single antibiotic, to treat appropriate individuals for pulmonary infection.

Other medications that are used to treat patients with pneumonia and emphysema include: steroid IV or by mouth; Ventolin inhaler; Albuterol inhaler Alupent treatment; Maxair inhaler; Serevent; Flovent; and Singulair by mouth, etc. together with oxygen, IV fluid, cough syrup and pulmonary toilet.

Viral pneumonia is treated with IV steroid, Alupent treatment, IV fluid, oxygen; cough syrup, and pulmonary toilet. In patients with chronic lung disease and viral pneumonia, broad-spectrum antibiotics must be added to their treatments to cover for the possibility of secondary bacterial infection which inevitably always becomes part of the pulmonary infection. If it is determined that the clinical picture is that of pure viral pneumonia, then the antibiotics can be stopped.

This determination can sometime be made through viral titers.

As for fungal infection of the lung, this diagnosis is more appropriately established with specimen taken during bronchoscopic examination with biopsy/brushing, then treatment can be started with Amphotericin B or Fluconazole.

Pneumocystis carinii pneumonia (PCP) is more commonly seen in patients with AIDS. The diagnosis is usually made by the history, the clinical picture with breathing difficulty, hypoxemia, fever, chills, night sweat, weight loss, the chest x-ray characteristics, the propensity for oxygen desaturation on exercising, O2 concentration under 70, alveolar-arterial oxygen gradient over 35, elevated LDL and the recovering of the PCP organism on pulmonary washing or on lung biopsy.

Acute PCP is treated with IV Bactrim and IV steroid or steroid by mouth for 21 days. Pentamidine IV can also be used in patients who are allergic to Bactrim. Pentamidine has serious cardiac, kidney, and pancreatic complications, including severe hypoglycemia (low blood sugar).

Chapter 71
PNEUMONIA

Pneumonia is an infection of the lung that can be caused by bacteria, virus, fungus, protozoa and sometime by aspiration of chemichal materials.

The most common bacterium that causes pneumonia is Streptococcus pneumoniae.
Streptococci include
Alpha hemolytic streptoccus
Beta hemolytic streptococcus
Pneumococcus

These organisms come from people's throats where they live or people get pneumonia
When people cough near them and they inhale the organism causing the pneumonia into they lungs.

Staphylococcus is another bacterium that frequently causes pneumonia.
Staphylococcus include
Staphylococcus Aureus
Staphylococcus epidermidis
Methicillin-resistant staphylococcus Aureus (MRSA)
Vancomycin Resistant Staphylococcus aureus (VRA)
MRSA is resistant penicillin and penicillin like antibiotics
VRA is resistant to Vancomycin
Both Streptococcus and Staphylococcus are gram negative organisms.

Other bacteria that frequently cause pneumonia are gram negative bacteria.
These Gram negative organisms that frequently cause pneumonia include
Haemophilus influenza
Pseudomonas aeruginosa
Klebsiella pneumoniae
Escherichia coli
Moraxella catarrhalis
Serratia
Legionella etc;

Atypical bacteria that can cause pneumonia include:
Chlamydophilia pneumoniae

Coxiella burnetii mycoplasma pneumoniae

Once the bacteria enter into the lung tissues through inhalation, they mulityply causing an acute inflammatory reaction inside the lungs. The inflammation inside the lungs interferes with the exchange of oxygen, resulting in a state of hypoxemia.

The elderly, infants, and people with diseases such as cancer, diabetes COPD, Asthma, cystic fibrocysis and AIDS or otherwise immunosuppressed are prone to getting pneumonia. In addition people who are in the hospitals or live in nursing homes are at high risk of getting pneumonia.

Signs and symptoms of pneumonia include
Cough (productive of greenish or yellowish sputum)
Fever
Chills
Headache
Chest pain
Rapid breathing
Rapid heart rate
Sweating
Weakness

Evaluations of pneumonia include:

History and physical examination (rales/pneunmonic sounds are heard in the lung affected by pneumonia during examination of the lung with the stethoscope)
Chest Xray
CBC
Sputum Gram stain
Sputum culture
Blood culture
Nasal swab for MRSA
Complete chemistry profile
ABG
EKG
Chest Xray of a patient with bacterial pneumonia

Treatments of bacterial pneumonia include:

Nasal Oxygen
Intravanous fluid with DW5/normal saline or DW5 with ½ normal saline, or normal saline or ½ normal saline

Antibiotics treatments are dictated by the underline medical condition or conditions of the patient, or whether the patient is coming from the community, nursing home, in the hospital, the age of the patient or whether the patient is immunosuppressed or not.

In clinical practice, when a patient presents with pneumonia broad spectrum antibiotics are given empirically until result of the sputum culture is back from the bacteriology laboratory. Result of the sputum Gram stain gives important information by letting the physician know whether the bacterium causing the infection is Gram negative or Gram positive but, this information is not enough to be used to make a definitive antibiotics treatment.

The best antibiotics to treat these patients are:

Cetazidime 1 gram IV qh 8 hours and Vancomycin 1 gram IV Q12 hour
Or
Ceftriaxone 1 gram IV q12 hour and Vancomycin 1 gram IV q 12 hour
Or
Levaquin 500mg IV q 24 hours and Vacomycin 1 gram IV q 12 hour
Or
Cipro 400mg IV q 12 hour and Vancomycin 1 gram IV q 12 hour
Or
Zoszyn 3.375 grams IV q 6 hour and Vancomycin 1 gram IV q 12 hour
Or
Nafcillin 1 gram IV q 6 hour and Vancomycin 1 gram IV q 12 hour
Or
Penicillin G 600,000 to 1 million units per day and Gentamin 1.5 mg/kg q 12 hour

Other antibiotics that available to treat pneumonia in combination or singly include
Cubicin
Erythormycin (very good to treat Ligionair pneumonia)
Pipercillin
Zithromax
Biaxin
Avelox
Keflex
Ceftin
Imipenem
Meropenem
Primaxin
Augmentin
Ampicillin
Amoxicillin

Bactrim DS (good to treat MRSA as well)
Clindamycin
Flagyl
Doxycycline etc;
Zyvox for VRA or MRSA (this medication is very expensive and Vacomycin is used more frequently for MRSA).

Patients in the hospital who develop pneumonia must be treated for Pseudomonas till proven otherwise. The same is true for patients residing in nursing home and other health care facilities. Nursing home patients must also be treated for MRSA till proven otherwise. Nasal swab can easily rules out MRSA.

People living at home who present to emergency rooms with pneumonia must also get tested for MRSA with nasal swab because there have been several cases of MRSA pneumonia reported in the medical literature.

In addition, patients being treated for pneumonia should have blood test to rule out TB in particular, if these patients come from areas where TB is prevalent or if they are immunosuppressed.

All patients with HIV/AIDS, who have pneumonia, should be evaluated for Pneumocystis caranii pneumonia (PCP).

Viral pneumonia is a very common type of pneumonia in all age groups.
The viruses that can cause pneumonia include
Influenza A
Influenza B
Parainfluenza virus
H1N1 virus
Respiratory syncitial virus RSV
Herpes simplex virus
Varicella-zoster virus
Adovirus
Measles virus
Rubella virus
Cytomegalovirus (CMV)
Corinavirus (Severe acute respiratory syndrome virus (SARS)

Signs and symptoms of viral pneumonia include
Cough
Fever
Chills

Body aches
Chest pain
Weakness
Shortness of breath
Flu like symptoms
Headache
Rapid heart rate
Rapid respiratory rate (breathing fast)
Runny nose
Sore throat
Poor appetite
General malaise
Rales/Pneumonic sounds on examination of the lungs (may or may not present)
Inflitrate seen on chest Xray

Evaluation of viral pneumonia include
History and physical examination
Chest Xray
CBC (the white cells count may be slightly high, normal, or low and the number of lyphocytes and monocytes may be high, and atypical lymphocytes may be present)
Nasal swab for influenza A or B
Viral titers in the blood for influenza A, B, herpes, Adeno virus, Varicella virus and for H1N1 virus depending on the clinical setting
Complete chemistry profile
ABG
EKG

Treatments of viral pneumonia include
IV fluid with D5W/normal saline or D5W1/2 normal saline or plain normal saline
Nasal Oxygen
Tylenol for fever
Non-steroidal anti inflammatory drugs (NSAID's) don't give Aspirin to children with pneumonia
Cough syrup
Amentadine
Tamiflu
Rimantadine
Ribavirin
Acyclovir (for herpes simplex virus)
Gancyclovir (CMV)

The best way to prevent Viral pneumonia is to be vaccinated against adenovirus, herpes simplex, herpes zoster, measles, adeovirus, rubella, influenza A an B, SARS, H1N1, and the flu virus.

People who are sixty or older, young children and those who are immunosuppressed should get the flu shot every year.

Chapter 72
SARCOIDOSIS

Other chronic common lung diseases that afflict people include:

1. Sarcoidosis
2. Pulmonary hypertension
3. Pulmonary embolism
4. Hypersensitivity pneumonitis
5. Eosinophilic pneumonitis
6. Cystic fibrosis
7. Interstitial lung diseases
8. Asbestosis etc.,

Sarcoidosis is a very common disease of unknown etiology that frequently affects the lungs of blacks. The lungs are the most frequently affected organs with sarcoidosis and most definitely the most important organ to be affected by this disease. Sarcoidosis is much more common in blacks and other minorities than whites are.

The most frequent symptoms of pulmonary sarcoidosis are the following:

1. Shortness of breath
2. Coughing
3. Wheezing
4. Fever
5. Night sweats
6. Weight loss

Infiltrates and nodules of different sizes can be seen on chest x-ray. The pulmonary function test is abnormal in pulmonary sarcoidosis. In time, there will be the development of pulmonary fibrosis.

The diagnosis of sarcoidosis is usually established by taking a biopsy of a pulmonary nodule during a bronchoscopic examination or by biopsying a palpable lymph node. The characteristic histopathological finding on tissues taken from a person with sarcoidosis is non-caseating granuloma. The angiotensin-1-converting enzyme blood test is usually elevated in blacks suffering from sarcoidosis. Sarcoidosis is a multi-system disease that affects many organs in the human body

Clinical manifestations of sarcoidosis

Sarcoidosis has the potential to affect all organs in the body and its manifestations may be felt throughout the body.

The organs most frequently affected are the following:

1. The lungs
2. The lymph nodes
3. The eyes
4. The skin
5. The upper respiratory tract
6. The liver
7. The spleen
8. The bone marrow
9. The kidney
10. The heart
11. The nervous system
12. The endocrine system
13. The gastrointestinal tract
14. The exocrine glands and
15. The musculoskeletal system; etc

The most frequent symptoms of sarcoidosis include:

1. Shortness of breath and wheezing
2. Cough
3. Fever
4. Night sweats
5. Weight loss
6. General weakness
7. Difficulty seeing
8. Kidney stones
9. Swollen joints
10. Hoarseness
11. Irregular pulse
12. Palpitations
13. Facial paralysis
14. Seizures
15. Excessive urination

About 90% of people with sarcoidosis have their lungs involved with the disease process. Approximately, 50% of these individuals develop permanent lung abnormalities and about 15% develop pulmonary fibrosis, and a significant percentage of these people go on to die of respiratory failure.

Fever of unknown origin is frequently due to sarcoidosis. Weight loss, night sweats, general weakness, and poor appetite can be seen in sarcoidosis.

Blurry vision and bleeding into the eyes can also occur in sarcoidosis 25% of the time.

The usual types of the eye problems that are frequently seen in sarcoidosis are uveitis, detached retina, etc. When the eyes are affected, sore eyes and dryness of the eye can develop and if left untreated, blindness is the usual result.

Kidney stones with acute back pain and kidney stones in the urine can occur in sarcoidosis because of high serum calcium. Sarcoidosis is frequently associated with hypercalcemia (high serum calcium), and when the calcium is high in the blood, it can precipitate in the kidneys, resulting in calcium kidney stones.

Multiple and different joints and muscles can get involved in sarcoidosis, resulting in severe pain, arthralgias, arthritis, and different bone abnormalities. Carpal tunnel syndrome can also be seen in sarcoidosis. Muscle weakness, such as polymyositis, has also been described in sarcoidosis.

Sarcoidosis can involve the heart 5% of the time. The parts of the heart most frequently affected by sarcoidosis are the left ventricle, the conductive system causing complete heart block, etc. Both congestive heart failure and different types of cardiac arrhythmias can also occur in sarcoidosis.

The neurological system is commonly affected by sarcoidosis and in about 5% of the time a neurological finding is documented. Damage to the nerve resulting in Bell's palsy (paralysis of one side of the face) can be seen in sarcoidosis. Damage to the liver and spleen can also occur in sarcoidosis resulting in enlargement of both the liver and spleen, causing significant abnormalities in liver functions and white blood cells, red blood cells, as well as platelets.

The bone marrow is involved in about 40% of cases of sarcoidosis.

The manifestation of the bone marrow involvement with sarcoidosis is reflected by anemia, leukopenia, and thrombocytopenia.

The skin is commonly involved in sarcoidosis in up to 20%-25% of the cases.

Among the most commonly seen skin lesions in cases of sarcoidosis are erythema nodosum and alopecia. Enlargement of the lymph nodes is quite frequently seen in sarcoidosis. Mediastinal nodes are enlarged in about 90% of patients with sarcoidosis. Other nodes that are frequently enlarged in sarcoidosis are axillary notes, cervical nodes, inguinal nodes, etc.

Several laboratory tests can be abnormal in sarcoidosis; examples are low white blood cells, low red blood cells, low platelets, high serum calcium, and high sedimentation rate. Steroid is the treatment of choice for all forms of sarcoidosis. Cytoxan can also be used in cases where the side effects of steroid are too bothersome.

Pulmonary failure leading to death can be the result of pulmonary sarcoidosis in many people who suffer from sarcoidosis.

Chapter 73
THROMBOPHILIA

Thrombophilia is a condition that when it exists in a person blood causing the blood to become thick. The tickness of the blood (hypercoagulable state) can result from many conditions.

The conditions that can cause hypercoagulable state include:

Cancer (Trousseau's sign/Trousseau's syndrome)
Elevated homocysteine level
Anti-thrombin III deficiency
Protein C deficiency
Protein S deficiency
Elevated lipoprotein-a
Prothrombin mutation G 20210A screen
Factor V Leiden mutation screen
Lupus anticoagulant
Anti-cardiolipin antibody
Elevated Fibrinogen
Elevated Factor VIII
PA1-1 mutation
Taking birth control pills
Taking estrogen as treatment for post monopaul symptoms
Taking estrogen to treat prostate cancer

Other conditions that predispose people to the development of DVT are:

Travelling long distances by planes or by cars
Lying in bed in the hospital after surgery

Anyone of the things listed above when abnormal can cause the affected person to have a thrombophilia and thus becomes hypercoagulable. Thrombophilia predisposes a person to the development of DVT and pulmonary embolism.

All types cancers can cause Trousseau's disease (clot formation) but the most cancers that more frequently associated with the development of DVT/Pulmonary embolism are:

Cancer of the pancreas
Cancer of the stomach
Cancer of the colon
Cancer of the prostate
All hematological malignancies etc;

The way cancer causes DVT/Pulmonary embolism is that the cancer cells secrete a series of procoagulant proteins, and once these procoagulant proteins enter into the blood stream, they create a state of hypercoagubilty resulting in the formation of clots.

Sometimes the first presentation of cancer is DVT/Pulmonary embolism. So, if a person presents with DVT/Pulmonary embolism and no obvious cause or causes can be found, then an evaluation ought to be carried out looking for the presence of cancer in the body.

Chapter 74
DEEP VEIN THROMBOPHLEBITIS

Every year 600,000 individuals in the U.S. develop pulmonary embolism, resulting in 300,000 deaths. About 60,000 individuals die yearly in the U.S. because of undiagnosed pulmonary embolism whose diagnosis are determined at autopsy.

Most of the time pulmonary embolism occurs because a person develops deep vein thrombophlebitis (DVT) in an extremity or extremities and a piece of the clot brakes off and migrates to the lung causing pulmonary embolism to occur.
Every year in the US 2.5 millions individuals develop DVT.

DVT occurs because of a thrombus (clot) that develops in the venous system (low flow system). The thrombus that develops in the venous system is a red thrombus (red clot). This red thrombus is composed of red blood cells and debris.

Thrombi that develop in the high flow system (arterial system) are white thrombi. White thrombi are composed of white blood cells and platelets.

How to evaluate a person for DVT

History
Physical examination
Ultrasound of the affected area
D-dimer
CBC
Complete metabolic profile
PT, INR
PTT
Chest Xray
EKG

Treatments of DVT

The mechanism that causes clot formation leading to DVT and pulmonary embolism and other clotting problems are:
Clots form in both the arterial system (high flow system)

692

venous system (low flow system)

The clots that form in the arterial system are called white clots because they are composed of white cells and platelets mainly. The clots that form in the venous system are called red clots because they are composed of red cells debris mainly.

Knowing that they are red clots and white clots and what they compositions are and where they develop in the body is of utmost importance because these different clots are treated with different medications.

Clots that are composed mainly of white cells and platelets in the arterial system are treated with Aspirin, heparin, and coumadin mainly. Clots that are composed mainly of red cells and debris are treated with heparin, Lovenox, and coumadin.

Aspirin and Plavix are not very effective in preventing clots in the venous system (low flow system) because these types of clots are deficient in platelets. Aspirin and Plaavix prevent clot formation by preventing the aggregration of platelets.

Other medications in use to treat and to prevent clots include:

Xarelto
Pradaxa
Apixaban
Argatroban
Fondaparinux
Idraparinux etc;

These medications are good to prevent clot formation in the arterial and venous systems. Inferior venacava filter is used to prevent pulmonary embolism in certain clinical settings.

Once it is established by ultrasound that the person has DVT, then anti-coagulation must be started first with heparin IV. The reason why it is preferable to begin anti-coagulation with heparin is because heparin has anti inflammatory property that helps to decrease the inflammation that DVT causes.

While on heparin, it is important to monitor daily PTT and CBC and stool hemoccult. The reasons for daily PTT and CBC are to monitor the the levels of red blood cells and platelets. If the red blood cells dropped from baseline, it means that the person is bleeding from the heparin. If the PTT is elevated near 70 second, 80, or 90 second, it does not matter much. Because, once the PTT is elevated at the level 45-50, it means that all the factors in the intrinsic pathway are already affected maximally.

What is most important is when the PPT remains in the normal range eventhough the patient is on full dose of. In case case, this case it means that the person so actively that he or she is secreting massive amount of platelet factor IV. Platelets factor IV is anti-heparin. In this case, the dose of heparin needs to be increased.

If the platelets dropped by 50% from baseline, it means that the person has developed Heparin induced thrombocytopenia and the heparin must be stopped immediately.

In this case, the person must be started on Argatrobin as per protocol and at the appropriate time, the person can be started on Coumadin to complete the course of treatment.

Individuals who developed heparin induced thrombocytopenia must never again be treated with heparin and Lovenox.

DVT is treated for a total 12 weeks. However, if it is determined that a person develops DVT because of a Thrombophilia, then that person must remain on prophylaxis anticoagulation for life.

When DVT or Pulmonary embolism develops in the setting of Trousseau's sign/ syndrome, namely because the person is suffering from cancer, Coumadin should never be given to treat the DVT/Pulmonary embolism because it will not work.

Coumadin does not work in Trousseau's syndrome because the cancer cells overwhelm the blood system by damping massive amount of procoagulant proteins into the blood that are constantly causing clotting to occur.

The way to treat DVT/Pulmonary embolism in the setting of Trousseau's syndrome is to use heparin or lovenox as anticoagulant.

Better still, is to treat the cancer. Once the cancer is treated, the hypercoagulable state /Trousseau's syndrome should resolve. It is important to keep in mind that DVT/ Pulmonary embolism may be the presenting sign of cancer.

Therefore, when cause cannot be found to explain why someone has DVT/ Pulmonary embolism, a full and complete work up ought to be carried out looking for cancer in that person.

Chapter 75
PULMONARY EMBOLISM

Every year 600,000 individuals in the U.S. develop pulmonary embolism, resulting in 300,000 deaths, and many of these individuals are blacks. About 60,000 individuals die yearly in the U.S. because of undiagnosed pulmonary embolism whose diagnosis are determined at autopsy.

Most of the time pulmonary embolism occurs because a person develops deep vein thrombophlebitis (DVT) in an extremity or extremities and a piece of the clot brakes off and migrates to the lung causing pulmonary embolism to occur.

Every year in the US 2.5 millions individuals develop DVT.

Conditions that predispose people to DVT or pulmonary embolism include:

1. Obesity
2. Birth control
3. Hormone replacement therapy
4. Post-surgery immobilization
5. Multiple trauma
6. Immobilization after a stroke
7. Hypercoagulable state due to cancer of different types
8. Deep vein thrombophlebitis (DVT)
9. Polycythemia vera
10. Post-partum state
11. Elevated homocysteine level
12. Anti-thrombin III deficiency
13. Protein C deficiency
14. Protein S deficiency
15. Elevated lipoprotein-a, etc.

The most frequent symptoms of pulmonary embolism consist of:

1. Shortness of breath
2. Tachycardia (rapid pulse rate)
3. Pleuritic chest pain
4. Sweating
5. Paleness
6. Restlessness

7. Coughing
8. Coughing up blood
9. Pain in calf muscle
10. Syncopal episode
11. In massive pulmonary embolism, sudden death can occur

Following the history and physical examination, the most important tests to do to confirm the presence of pulmonary embolism consist of:

1. Arterial blood gas (ABG)
2. d-Dimer
3. Chest x-ray
4. Ultrasound of the lower extremities
5. Lung scan

The most definitive test to do to establish the diagnosis of pulmonary embolism is the pulmonary angiogram, but this test is hardly ever necessary nowadays because d-Dimer; ultrasound of the lower extremities and the high probability lung scan are sufficient to arrive at the diagnosis of pulmonary embolism. The d-Dimer blood test is extremely important because when pulmonary embolism is present, this test is positive.

Whenever a clot is formed anywhere in the body, the clots release plasmin in the blood stream which in turn causes d—Dimer to become elevated. D-Dimer is not specific for DVT or pulmonary embolism because, it is also elevated in pregnancy, sepsis, and DIC.
However, if the lung scan is read as high probability for pulmonary embolism, the d-Dimer is elevated, and if the ultrasound of the extremity shows a DVT, the possibility that the patient has pulmonary embolism is greater than 90%.
Computed Tomographic Pulmonary Angiography is also a very good test that can show the presence of pulmonary embolism.

Treatment for pulmonary embolism:

The treatment choice for pulmonary embolism is intravenous heparin. However, before starting heparin, several blood tests must be done:

1. Prothrombin time (PT)
2. Partial thromboplastin time (PTT)
3. Hematocrit
4. Platelet count
5. Stool for hemoccult

The importance of the PT and PTT is to ensure that the patient's coagulation system is working normally, so as not to precipitate bleeding. The importance of the platelet count is 1) to make sure the platelet count is not too low prior to starting heparin; 2) to have a baseline normal platelet count. The rationale for establishing that the baseline platelet count is normal is that in the event that if the platelet count drops to 50% of the baseline platelet count that means that the patient is developing platelet-induced thrombocytopenia.

Therefore, the heparin administration must be stopped immediately.

Lovenox and other high molecular weight heparin can also cause heparin induced thrombocytopenia sometimes therefore, are not good alternative to regular heparin.

Heparin induced thrombocytopenia occurs because an antigen/antibody reaction.

The best way to evaluate HIT is to test for anti-platelets antibodies. However this test takes several days to come from the lab and is not always positive eventough HIT exists. Drop in the platelets count by 50% from base is much more important in making the diagnosis of HIT because daily platelets count can be done.

HIT can cause thrombosis to occur in about 2-5% of people causing stroke or acute myocardial infartction (heart attack).

Once HIT is suspected, heparin must be stopped immediately. The anticoagulant Argatrobin must started IV to anticoagulate the person.

In the setting of HIT, Coumadin must never be used. Doing so can lead to major clinical catastrophy such as acute cold limb syndrome and possibly death. The reason this happens is because the HIT causes an acute hypercoalugable state and giving Coumadin to patient makes the hypercoagulable worse resulting in diffuse clotting.

Everyone who gets Coumadin becomes hypercoagulable immediately because the ½ life of factor VII is 4-6. Factor X ½ life is 48 hours, and Factor II ½ life is 72 hours. These factors are vitamin K dependent factors, Coumadin decreases them sequentially, and while this process is going on, the person on Coumadin remains hypercoagulable until all of these factors are depleted. Once all of them are depleted coagulation occurs.

That is why adding Coumadin to acute HIT is contraindicated.

The only medication approved in the U.S. to treat HIT is Argatroban.

This medication is given IV. Once the platelets count becomes normal, then and only then can coumadin be given to complete the course of anticoagulation treatment.

The reason why it is necessary to check the hematocrit every day in a patient receiving heparin is that the heparin can cause bleeding to occur and a drop in hematocrit would document that.

697

Checking the stool for blood every day is important, because if the stool is positive for blood, it means that the patient is bleeding and the heparin must be stopped.

Once these tests are done, then heparin can be infused as a 5000 units bolus IV, followed by 1000 units per hour intravenously. While on heparin, the patient must be monitored with daily PTT and CBC.

It is a good idea to keep the patient with pulmonary embolism on heparin for 7 to 10 days. If a woman is not pregnant, then Coumadin ought to be started while the patient is still on heparin. After 5 days of the Coumadin by mouth, the heparin can be stopped if the prothrombin time and the INR (international normalized ratio) are therapeutic. This protocol of treating with heparin for 7-10 days and begin Coumadin as just described applies to male patients as well.

The Coumadin is continued for 6 months to 1 year. Anticoagulation may need to be continued for life, if the pulmonary embolism is associated with a hereditary hypercoagulable state (thrombophilia).

Heparin can be used during pregnancy, but Coumadin cannot be used during pregnancy because of its negative effects on the fetus (Coumadin causes fetal malformation).

Prevention of DVT/Pulmonary embolism:

It is very important that people make sure they are screened for the presence of thrombophilia as part of their routine medical evaluation. Knowing whether or not an individual has does not a thrombophilia dictate what medication he or she can or cannot take? As mentioned before, there are several common medications such as birth control pills and other estrogenic medications that anyone with any type of thrombophilia should avoid, because these medications can precipitate clots formation ina thrombophilic person.

In addition, if a thrombophilic person must travel long distances either by air plane or by car, he or she should be anticoagulated daily with Lovenox while traveling to prevent DVT/Pulmonary embolism.

One of the most frequent complications of anticoagulation treatments is bleeding.
To avoid bleeding people should be tested before any aniticoagulation treatment is started with.
PT/INR
PTT

Platelet count

Once bleeding is detected, the anticoagulation medications or antiplatelets medications must be stopped immediately. And if necessary, Fresh frozen plasma (FFP) should be given if heparin/lovenox is responsible for the bleeding. Vitamin K IV should be given if
Coumadin is responsible for the bleeding. In certain cases where the bleeding is profuse and excessive, FFP should be given.
FFP works in 2-3 hours to stop bleeding, while vitamin K takes 12-24 hours to stop bleeding.

If Aspirin/Plasvix or NSAIDs is responsible for the bleeding, Desmopressin (DDAVP) should be given to stop the bleeding. DDAVP 20mcg in 50cc of normal saline over ½ hour stops the bleeding in 1 ½ hour. DDAVP works to stop the bleeding by increasing the factor VIII Von Willebrand by 15-20% and this enough to transiently correct the qualitative platelet abnormality caused by the antiplatelets medication.

The effects of Aspirin/Plavix on the platelets last 7-10 days in the body, the effects of NSAIDs on the platelets last only 6 hours in the body.

Chapter 76
PULMONARY HYPERTENSION

Another lung disease that can afflict people is primary pulmonary hypertension. The root cause of primary pulmonary hypertension is due to an increase blood pressure in the pulmonary artery, pulmonary vain or pulmonary capillaries in lungs.

According to the WHO, there are five different groups of pulmonary hypertension.

Group 1: Idiopatic, familial, which can be associated with scleroderma, congenital shunts between the systemic and pulmonary circulation, HIV infection, portal hypertension due to cirrhosis of the liver, drugs such as cocaine, methamphetamine, alcohol or chronic hepatitis C or B causing cirrhosis of the liver resulting in portal hypertension etc;

Group II Pulmonary hypertension due to left heart disease, such as Ventricular or atrial disease, valvular heart disease such as mitral stenosis etc;

Group III Pulmonary hypertension due to lung diseases such as hypoxemia, COPD, interstitial lung disease, sleep apnea, chronic exposure to high altitude, developmental lung abnormalities etc;

Group IV Pulmonary hypertension due to chronic emboli to the lungs
Other causes of pulmonary hypertension are Sickle cell disease, Sarcoidosis, parasites invasion of the pulmonary arteries, cancer invasion of the pulmonary arteries, HIV infection, black lung disease etc;

The most common symptoms of primary pulmonary hypertension are
Shortness of breath on exertion
Fatigue
Weakness
Chest pain
Syncope
Physical findings include
Distended jugular veins
Rales in the lungs
Different abnormal heart sounds such as loud S2

Stenal heave
Pedal edema
Clubbing
Ascites
Hepatojugular reflux etc;

Swelling of lower leg and ankles may represent evidence of right heart failure, causing right lung symptoms. Pulmonary hypertension can also cause pulmonary embolism.

Evaluations of pulmonary hypertension include
History and physical examination
ABG
CBC
Complete chemistry profile
Hemoglobin electrophoresis
HIV test
Angiotensin-1-convertenting enzyme
D-dimer
PT, INR, PTT
BNP
Stool for ova and parasite
Chest xray
EKG
Echocardiogram
Chest CT
Lung scan
Lung biopsy (if sarcoidosis or interstitial lung disease is suspected)
Abdominal sonogram/Abdominal CT.

Treatments of pulmonary hypertension include:
Nasal Oxygen
Lasix IV/by mouth
Bumex IV
Digitalis IV/by mouth
Anticoagulation by mouth with either Coumadin, or Pradaxa
Heparin IV
Lovenox SC
Phosphodiesterase type 5 inhibitors (Viagra, Levetra, or Cialis) to relax the smooth muscle inside blood vessels in the lungs
Surgical repair of valvular heart diseases

The most preventable lung diseases that people suffer from are COPD/emphysema and lung cancers; both of them are, in most part, due to tobacco smoking. About 55 million individuals in the U.S. smoke tobacco. Smoking tobacco is a deadly habit, which accounts for roughly 430,000 deaths per year in the United States; all these deaths are preventable if people would stop smoking.

Chapter 77
TUBERCULOSIS

Tuberculosis is one of the world's most common infections that affect the lungs.

"In 2010, a total of 11,181 tuberculosis (TB) cases were reported in the United States." MMWR 2010 More than two billion people, equal to one third of the world's population, are infected with TB bacilli. "Each year, over nine million people around the world get infected with TB and almost two million TB related deaths are recorded worldwide. TB is a leading killer among people living with HIV." Source: WHO
Source: WHO

Blacks and other minorities are 8 times more frequently affected with tuberculosis than whites are. "In 2007, TB was reported in 4,470 blacks in the U.S." the World Health Organization reported that 9 million cases of tuberculosis occurred worldwide each year and that 1.6 million people died in the world from tuberculosis during that same period.

A significant percentage of the people who died of TB were also infected with HIV/AIDS. About 98% of these cases of tuberculosis occurred in the developing countries of the world.

About 10% of new tuberculosis cases that occur in the U.S. occur in individuals who were skin-test positive for TB, (latent TB) therefore this group of individuals serves as a reservoir for new TB cases.

The organism that causes tuberculosis is mycobacterium tuberculosis. Infected individuals can transmit the TB organism to uninfected people through droplets that come from the lungs when they cough.

Once the TB organism enters into the lungs of the person being infected, it locates itself in the upper/posterior part of the lung, where the oxygenation of that area of the lung favors its growth.
Symptoms of pulmonary tuberculosis include:

1. Fever
2. Chills
3. Weight loss
4. Loss of appetite
5. Night sweats

6. Cough
7. Hemoptysis (coughing blood)
8. Shortness of breath

Findings on physical examinations may be positive for enlarged lymph nodes, large spleen, large liver, fever, and evidence of weight loss.

Evidence of fluid in the lungs may show evidence of fluid around the heart (cardiac tamponade pericardial effusion). X-ray findings frequently seen in tuberculosis include:

1. Infiltrate seen on chest x-ray
2. Cavity seen on chest x-ray

Non-specific laboratory tests that may be abnormal in pulmonary tuberculosis:

1. Low white blood cells
2. High white blood cells
3. Low red blood cells (anemia)
4. Low platelet count
5. High platelet count
6. High serum calcium
7. High alkaline phosphatase
8. High serum protein
9. Low serum albumin
10. High LDH (lactic dehydrogenase)
11. Low serum sodium due syndrome of inappropriate antidiuretic hormone (SIADH)

Specific laboratory tests that are positive in pulmonary tuberculosis are as follows:

1. Acid fast bacteria (AFB) seen on stain of sputum coughed up by the patient.
2. Acid fast bacteria (AFB) seen on stain of washing/tissues taken during bronchial examination of the lungs/pleural biopsy of pleural fluid.
3. M. tuberculosis organism grown on AFB culture six weeks after it is plated on appropriate culture medium.
4. AFB organism seen on lymph node biopsy from patients suspected of suffering with tuberculosis
5. AFB DNA probe (PCR) This test can confirm M Tuberculosis quickly.

The pathological finding seen on tissue specimens taken from an individual suspected of suffering from tuberculosis is caseating granuloma.

Positive sputum for AFB does not necessarily mean that the person has M. tuberculosis because mycobacterium avium intracellulare (MAI) also stains positive for

AFB. However, using DNA probe test, MAI can be differentiated from M. tuberculosis quickly.

How to test the skin for TB

When an individual has been exposed to a person infected with tuberculosis, the first thing to do is to plant a PPD 5TU on the person's arm. If the PPD is positive and the person being tested has not been vaccinated with BCG this then raises the possibility that the individual may in fact have been exposed to TB. This finding has an even stronger meaning if the person being tested is known to have had a negative PPD in the past.

The PPD test must be read within 48 hours to 72 hours from the time it was planted.

The Interferon-Y release Assays (IGRA), T-SPOT.TB and QuantiFEROn-TB Gold are new quicker and more accurate tests to diagnose diagone TB that are clinically available.

The FDA has approved a new test for TB called Xpert MTB/RIF. This test is an assay and is able to identify M tuberculosis with 98.1% accuracy and is simultaneously able to diagnose Revamping resistant TB 97.6% of the time. In addition, this test provides results in 2 hours, while the old Tb test takes up 3 months to give a result. Source: FDA, 7/26/2013

Four percent or 360,000 of the 9 million new cases of TB around the world are resistant Rifampin. Source: WHO

When any of these tests are positive, the next thing to do is a chest x-ray. If the chest is positive for TB, then the person is treated for TB. If on the other hand, the chest x-ray is negative, the person then is to be given prophylaxis with Isoniazid (INH) 300mg daily for 6 months together with Vitamin B6 one tablet per day, or Rifampin 300mg twice perday for 4 months.

TB can affect all organs in the human body and Symptoms can mimick many diseases. Therefore, it is always prudent for physicians to include TB in their differential diagnoses when evaluating individuals with complicated symptoms.

Treatment for tuberculosis

The medications that are used to treat M. tuberculosis are Rifampin, Isoniazid, Pyrazinamide, Ethambutol, and Streptomycin. The usual period of time that individuals are treated for TB is 9-12 months. The usual adult doses of these medications are: 1) Isoniazid 150 mg by mouth twice a day; 2) Rifampin 300 mg by mouth twice per day; and 3) Pyrazinamide 2 grams per day by mouth and Ethambutol 15 mg/kg body weight per day by mouth and Streptomycin 10-15 mg/kg body weight per day. Usually after the first month of treatment the sputum becomes negative for AFB.

During treatment for TB, complete blood count and liver function tests must be done every 6-8 weeks to monitor for possible low platelets, low white blood cells, low red cells count, and medication-induced hepatitis with elevated liver function tests.

Chapter 78
MALARIA

It is estimated that 300-500 million people worldwide become infected with malaria each year and 1 million people in the world die of malaria of malaria yearly: Source CDC

Malaria is a parasite that is carried by mosquitos and humans get infected with malaria when they are bitten by mosquitos carrying the malarial parisites. Malaria can also be transmitted by blood transfusion in rare occasions.

Malaria is develops mainly in tropical and subtropical countries.
The countries where malaria is often found are
Africa
Asia
The Americas
South East Asia

Malaria is common in these countries because these countries have high humidity and rain, conditions which are perfect for malaria to grow.

Malarial disease is highly associated with poverty.
The people who are mastly affected by malaria live in poor conditions that predispose them to being infected by malaria.

Most of them live in poorly constructed houses that offer no protection from malaria.
To be protected from malaria requires living inside nets that shield them from being bitten by malaria. In addition, certain repellents that can kill malaria are needed to be used to spray areas that harbor malaria. In addition, using nets to shield people from being bitten from malaria is necessary. Tavelers to malaria infested countries are at high risk of becoming infecected with malaria.

The five commonly known malarial organisms are
Plasmodium falciparum
Plasmodium vivax
Plasmodium ovale
Plasmodium malariae
Plasmodium knowlesi (more prevalent in South East Asia)

P. falciparum is the most virulent malarial parasite and the severe form of malarial disease.

Once a person becomes infected the malarial parasites/sporozoites,
the sporozoites travel from the through the blood to the liver. In the liver the
sporozoites mature into mezoites. From the liver the parasites re-enter the blood stream and infect red blood cells. They remain inside the red blood cells for 48-72 hours.

After 72 hours, the red blood cells birst open (hemolyze) releasing more infecting more
red blood cells with malarial parasites. This process goes on and on for as long as the infected person remains infected with malaria.

After infecrion symptoms of malaria infection ussuasly develops within 10 days to 4 weeks. However, symptoms can develop up to 1 year after infection. Symptoms occur in a cycle of 48 to 72 hours.

Symptoms of malaria include:
Fever
Chills
Sweating
Headacche
Nausea
Vomiting
Muscle cramps/pain
Anemia
Bloody stools
Jaundice
Seizure
Coma etc;

Evaluations of malaria include:
History
Physical examination
CBC with differential count
Malarial blood smear
Complete chemistry profile
Reticulocytes count
Serum LDH
PT/INR, PTT
Urinalysis
Chest x-ray

EKG

Abdominal ultrasound (to look at the liver and spleen)

Treatments of malarial infection depends of the type of malarial parasites responsible for the infection and the severity of the infection.

Acute P. faciparum infection is a medical emergency and needs hospitalization for treatments to be given.

Treatments for acute malaria infection include:

Bed rest

Vital signs

Nasal Oxygen

IV fluid with D5 Normal saline at 150cc per hour

Blood transfusion if necessary

IV Quinidine or Quinine plus IV Doxycycline or Doxycycline by mouth

or

Clindamycin IV

Monitor Fibrinogen, PTT to rule out DIC

Monitor renal profile

Monitor peripheral blood smears to look schistocytes

Prevention of malaria is extremely important.

Many people who live in countries and areas of the world where malaria is common have antibodies to malaria, but travelers to these countries and areas do not have antibodies to malaria. Therefore, people who are going these countries and areas where malaria is endemic, need to take anti-malaria medications 1-2 weeks before traveling and 4 weeks upon returning.

Different anti-malaria medications are used for different countries.

People traveling to Africa, South America, Latin America, Central America, the Caribbean, Asia, Indian sub-continent, and the South Pacific should take either Mefloquine, Chloroquine, Doxycycline, Malarone, or Hydroxychloroquine.

Anti-malaria prophylaxis medications should be taken 1-2 weeks before traveling and Once per week while in that country and for once per week for 4 weeks upon returning.

Before taking anti-malaria medications, people should be tested for G6-PD deficiency and women of child bearing age should have either blood or urine pregnancy test done.

Chapter 79
DENGUE FEVER

According to WHO, Dengue is responsible about 100 million infections and 500,000 hospitalizations and 25,000 deaths worldwide annually. According to the WHO, as many as 390 million people are infected with dengue fever annually and roughly two-third of people who are infected with dengue fever has only mild symptoms.

The number of people who live in the subtropical and tropical countries of the world where Dengue fever is prevalent is in the range of 2.5 billion.

Dengue fever occurs when a person is bitten by mousquitoes Aedes. These mousquitoes bite during daytime. Dengue is virus and it belongs to the family of flaviviruses. There are 4 types of Dengue viruses DENV-1, DENV-2, DENV3, and DNV-4.

Dengue fever is found in Africa, South America, Central America, Mexico, the Caribbean, the US Virgin Island, and Puerto Rico, American Samoa and in some parts of Asia.

In most cases Dengue fever is asymptomatic but in about 20% of cases people
can develop fever, abdominal pain, nausea, vomiting, fluid in the lungs and bleeding from the gums and nose, rash, joints pain, melena, hematemesis, hematuria, vaginal bleeding etc;

In some cases one can see sore throat, enlarged lymph nodes, and headache, back and groin pain can occur. Some people can go into shock with acute Dengue fever.

Evaluation of Dengue fever includes:

History and physical examination
CBC
Complete metabolic chemistry profile
Chest Xray
EKG
Serum antibody for Dengue fever DENV-1, DENV,-2 DENV-3, and DENV-4
DENV-1-4 real Time PCR Assay (This is a new test created to diagnose Dengue fever within the first 7 days after infection, before antibody is formed). Source CDC
Blood culture

Urine Culture
Stool culture
Stool for Ova and parasite
Malarial smear

Treatments for Dengue fever include IV fluid
Electrolytes replacement
Anti-emetic
Tylenol by mouth or by suppository to control fever
Do not use Aspirin or NSAID's because thsese medications can make the bleeding worst.

If possible avoid traveling from Dengue fever infested areas of the world and for people who reside in these places and for those who must travel to these places, appropriate precautions must be taken to avoid being infected by the mosquitos that carry the Dengue viruses.

Chapter 80

PARASITIC INFESTATION

Parasitic infestation is the 6ᵗʰ most common disease in the world and parasitic diseases outrank cancer as the number one killer in the world. Source: WHO

About ½ to 1/3 of the world 7 billion people are infested with one type of parasites or an other.

Some of the most common parasites that infest humans are:

Toxoplasma Gondii 3-3/12 billion people in the world are infested
Ascaris 807 million people
Hook worm 740 million people in the world are infested
Round worm (Trichuris trichiuria) 1 billion
Tape worm 50 million
Pin worm 200 million
Whip worm 1.5 billion
Schistosomiasis 230 million people are treated yearly for this worm Source: WHO
Entamoeba histolytica 500 million people in the world
Giardia lamblia 200 million
Cryptosporidium causes about 748,000 infections yearly and worldwide is one of the common diarrheal diseases in the world. This infection is most common in people with AIDS worldwide.
Other intestinal infections seen in AIDS causing diarrhea include
Cytomegalovirus, Ttospora Belli
Other enteric parasitic infections include Cyclospora, Microsporidia, and Toxoplasma etc.

Intestinal parasitism is quite common in people who originate or travel to the tropics or who live in the rural parts of the southern United States. Intestinal parasitism is also commonly seen in people who migrated to the United States from Southeast Asia and other third world countries where poor sanitation and poverty are prevalent.

Parts of the world where parasitic infestation is include

Africa
Southeast Asia
North Africa
India

China
Indonesia
The Americas
The Middle East etc;

It is estimated that hookworms infest about 740 million in the world and the daily blood loss is estimated at 7 million liters. Two million people in the United States are infected with hookworm. Ascaris infestation is a very common parasitic infestation.

The Signs andsymptoms of intestinal parasitic infection are many and can manifest as

Nausea
Vomiting,
Constipation
Diarrhea
Weakness
Dizziness
Headache
Chronic
Cough,
Skin rash
Generalized itchiness
Bloody stools
Iron deficiency anemia
Bloating
Hematemesis (Chinese Flukes)
Flu like symptoms
Fever
Cramping and Gas
Weight loss
Itching around the anus (mostly at night)
Foul smelling stools
Passing worms in the stools
Irritable bowel syndrome
Joints pain
Musdcles aches
Elevated IGg
Eosinophelia on peripheral blood smear
Allergy dermatitis
Nervousness
Anxiety
Insomnia

Headaches

Seizures (due to Cysticercosis of the brain dueTaenia Solium-Pork Tape worm)

Transverse Myelitis of the spinal cord (due Schistosomiasis mansoni's eggs in the spinal cord)

B12 deficiency

Depression

Poor memory (due to B12 deficiency)

Dementia (due to B12 defiency)

Intestinal obstruction (due large worms)

In recent years, there has been a greater increase in intestinal parasitism brought about by the AIDS epidemic. People who are immunosuppressed are more prone to be infested by parasites of all types including Giardia lamblia, amoeba, etc.

Strongyloides stercoralis a round worm whose larvae can get into the venous system of the blood stream and migrate to the lungs. They recycle in lungs and can spread to multiple organs including the brain, the heart etc causing fever, chills, abdominal pain and shock and often time death. People infected with strongyloides when placed on steroid for one reason or another, can develop acute systemic strongyloides. Therefore, before placing a person at high risk for strongyloides on steroid, stools for ova and parasites or serum antibody for strongyloidis should be done.

Evaluations of intestinal parasitic infestation include:

Physical examination

CBC

Complete chemistry profile

Stools for ova and parasite

Toxoplasma titer

Strongyloides titer

HIV test

Urinalysis

Serum B12

Chest xray

Brain CT

Brain MRI

EEG

EKG etc;

Medications available to treat intestinal parasitic infestation include:

Mebendazole

Albendazole

Diethylcarbamazine
Ivermectin
Praziquantel
Pyrantel pamoate
Piperazine citrate
Flagyl
Levamisole
Metrifonate
Oxamniquine

These different medications are recommended by the WHO to use to treat different individual intestinal parasites.

It is up to the treating physicians to choose which medications to use to treat which worm.

Some of these people, due to poverty, walk barefooted, exposing their feet to fecal materials, permitting parasites to enter into their bloodstream and, with no water available to wash hands after bowel movements, hands soiled with parasite-contaminated stool that provides an entry point for intestinal parasitism and all its serious medical complications.

Proper hygene with hand washing with water and soap and walking with shoes or sandals

and eating properly coked foods will help to decrease the incidence of intestina parasitism.

However since there is so much poverty in the world forcing people to live

in deprorable conditions, it is doubdtful that intestinal parasitic infestation will ever be eliminated.

Another common parasitic infestation that causes a lot of people to suffer throughout the world is tape worm (Taenia solium) disease of the brain known as neurocysticercosis. According to the WHO, there are about 2 million people in the world who are suffering from this condition. The countries where neurocysticercosis is prevalent include Africa, Asia, Latin America and other developing countries. The people who have neurocysticercosis (Tape worm brain disease) have recurrent seizures. The available medications to treat Tape worm of brain disease include Albendazole to kill the worms and Dexamethasone to reduce the inflammation and anti seizure medications. Source: JAMA, May 15, 2013—Vol 309, No 19.

Chapter 81
TICK BORNE DISEASES

The most common thick born diseases in U.S. are

Lyme disease
Babesiosis
Ehrlichiosis
Rocky Mountain spotted fever
Anaplasmosis
Rickettsia parkeri rickttsiosis
Southern tick-associated rash illness (STARI)
Tickborne relapsing fever (TBRF)
Tularemia
364D rickettsiosis Source: CDC

Tickborne diseases abroad
Crimean-congo hemorrhagic fever
Imported tickborne spotted fevers
Tickborne encephalitis (TBE) Source: CDC

The different ticks that cause tickborne diseases are
Rocky Mountain spotted fever (American dog tick, Rocky Mountain Wood tick, Lone star tick, Brown dog tick
Brown dog tick (Rickettsia parkkeri rickettsiosis)
Blacklegged tick (Ixodes scapularis) deer tick (anaplasmosis, babesiosis, and Lyme disease)
The lone star tick (ehrlichiosis, tularemia)

Signs and symptoms of tickborne diseases include:

Skin rash (macular, popular, erythema migrans, Bull's eye rash, (Lyme disease)
Muscle aches
Headache
Fatigue
Fever
Chills
Fatigue
Joints pain

Heart block (Lyme disease)
Pericarditis
Myocarditis
Meningitis (Lyme disease)
Hepatitis
Anemia
Seizure
Arthritis
Bell's palsy (Lyme disease)
Memory loss (Lyme disease)
Paralysis (Lyme disease)
Chronic fatigue (Lyme disease)
Depression (Lyme disease)
Insomnia (Lyme disease) etc;

Evaluations for tickborne diseases include
History and physical examination
CBC
Complete chemistry profile
Blood titers/ Western blot for the suspected tickborne disease
Blood culture
Malarial smear
Blood tiers for babesiosis
VDRL
Urinalysis
ESR
Chest Xray
Brain CT
EKG
24 Hour Holter monitor
EEG
Dermatology consultation etc;

Antibiotics in use to treat tickborne disease include
Doxycycline
Mepron
Amoxicillin
Erythromycin
Tetracycline
Azythromycin
Ceftriaxone IV
Cefuroxime IV

Other treatments are provided for individual complications.

Prevention of tickborne diseases include
Dress with light color cloths so that the tick can be seen
Wear socks up to knees
Wear high booths
Remove shoes and socks before entering the house
Make dogs and cats do not bring ticks in the house
Use repellents with DEET to kill ticks
Individuals with fair skin must examine their skins looking for tick when they come from
Tick infested areas. In particular, look for the baby tick called Nymph (it is white and as such can be missed easily). It is very infectious.

If a tick is found on the skin, use a tweezer to remove it without breaking it.
You should check with your physician immediately to seek treatment, and anyone who thinks he or she has tickborne disease should seek medical treatment for his or her physician immediately.

Chapter 82
HEADACHE AND MIGRAINE

Head ache is one of the most common maladies that has affected mankind since the beginning of time. Head ache is much more common in blacks and other minorities than whites. In the U.S. 28 million individuals suffer from head ache.

World wide there several hundred millions people who suffer from head ache. Nine out of 10 people in the world suffer from head ache sometime in their lives.

Some of the most common head aches are:

1. Tension
2. Migraine head ache
3. Cluster head ache
4. Sinus head ache
5. Cervical spine arthritic disease headache

Some of the medical conditions that can cause head ache are:

1. High blood pressure
2. Brain aneurism
3. Severe anemia
4. Polycythemia
5. Lyme disease
6. Lupus (SLE)
7. Rheumatoid arthritis
8. Mixed collagen vascular disease
9. Viral meningitis
10. Fungal meningitis
11. Neuro syphilis
12. Sepsis
13. Temporal arteritis
14. Cryptococcal infection of the brain
15. Toxoplasma infection of the brain
16. Histoplasma infection of the brain
17. Herpes simplex infection of the brain

18. Cytomegalovirus infection of the brain
19. Parasitic infection of the brain
20. Malarial infection of the brain
21. Encephalitis
22. Brain abscess
23. Vasculitis of the brain
24. Stroke
25. Cancer of the brain
26. AIDS brain disease
27. Osler, Weber, Rendu disease of the brain (AVM) causing bleeding
28. Sub-dural hematoma
29. Multiple Sclerosis
30. Viral syndrome; etc

Tension headache is the most common form of headache.

Tension headache is more common in blacks and other minorities than whites. It affects 90 percent of blacks and other minorities and 70 percent of whites. It affects people between the ages of 20-50.

Symptoms of tension head ache are:

Tension headache can cause a dull pain around the forehead and some time the pain can radiate to the back of the neck and shoulder.

1. **The evaluation of patients with tension head ache includes:**
2. A complete history and physical examination
3. CBC
4. Erythrocyte sedimentation rate (ESR)
5. SMA 20 chemistry profile
6. Urinalysis
7. ANA
8. VDRL blood test for syphilis
9. HIV/AIDS blood test
10. Lyme disease blood test
11. Chest X-ray
12. CT scan of the brain with or without IV contrast
13. MRI of the brain with or without contrast
14. MRI of the cervical spine

The most common medications used to treat tension headache are:

Aspirin Non-steroidal anti-inflammatory drugs NSAID (such as ibuprofen, Naproxen, Advil etc.)

Some patients respond to muscle relaxant or tricyclic antidepressant.

The next most common head ache is Migraine head ache.

Risks of migraine headache include:

Female sex Genetic transference, if both parents suffer from migraine, there is a 75 percent chance that an offspring will also suffer from migraine. If one parent suffers from migraine, there is a 50 percent chance an offspring will also suffer from migraine.

Migraine usually begins in childhood, adolescent and in early adulthood.

It is believe that migraine is caused by a combination of vascular dilatation and constriction of blood vessels in the brain.

Some of the things that known to be able to bring on symptoms of migraine are:

1. Fatigue
2. Hunger
3. Changes in the whether
4. Menstruation
5. Emotional stress
6. Foods such as
7. Nuts
8. Cheese
9. Chocolate
10. Birth control pills
11. Avocados
12. Alcohol consumption; etc

Symptoms of migraine include:

1. Throbbing pain in the head
2. Nausea
3. Vomiting
4. Sensitivity to light
5. Numbness in the face
6. Tingling of the face and lip

7. Weakness of arm or leg; etc
8. An attack of migraine headache can last for several hours and up to several days.
9. Close to 60% of people who suffer with migraine can have one or more attacks per month, 28 million individuals suffer from migraine in the U.S.
10. 11 million of them are made disabled by the severity of these migraine attacks.
11. Roughly, 175 million work days are lost yearly as a result migraine attacks in the U.S. impacting the economy greatly.

The evaluation for migraine headache includes:

1. A history and physical examination
2. CBC
3. Erythrocyte sedimentation rate (ESR)
4. SMA-20 chemistry profile
5. Urinalysis
6. VDRL for syphilis
7. HIV/AIDS blood test
8. Lyme disease blood test
9. Chest X-ray
10. CT scan of the brain with or without IV contrast
11. MRI of the brain with or without IV contrast

Medications in use to treat migraine headache include:

1. Aspirin
2. NSAID
3. Cafergot
4. Midrin
5. Imitirx
6. Replax
7. Zomig
8. Beta Blocker such as Inderal
9. Calcium channel blocker such as Procardia
10. Compozine or Zofran for nausea and vomiting

Another form of headache is cluster headache.

The pain associated with cluster headache usually comes on suddenly and frequently subsides just as quickly.

The evaluation for cluster headache includes:

A complete history and physical examination
1. CBC
2. ESR
3. SMA-20 chemistry profile
4. Urinalysis
5. ANA
6. VDRL blood test for syphilis
7. HIV/AIDS blood test
8. Lyme disease blood test
9. Chest x-ray
10. CT scan of the brain with or without IV contrast
11. MRI of the brain with or without IV contrast

Medications in use to treat cluster headache include:

1. IM Imitrex
2. Zomig
3. Dihydroergotamine either IM, IV or intranasal

Some people respond to surgery to cut the trigeminal nerve to relieve symptoms of chronic cluster headache

Cervical spine arthritic headache results from severe arthritis of the cervical spine or, herniated cervical disc.

Evaluation of cervical arthritis headache includes:

1. History and physical examination
2. CBC
3. SMA-20 chemistry profile
4. ESR
5. ANA
6. Serum uric acid level
7. MRI of the cervical spine
8. Referral to a neurologist/neurosurgeon/orthopedist

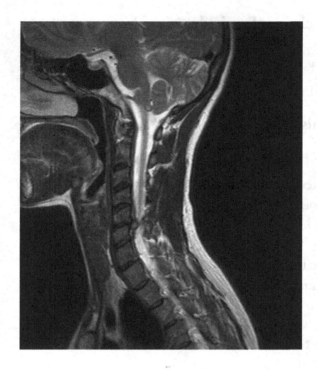

82:1 MRI *of cervical spine demonstrating an extruded disc herniation at C5-C6 (see arrow):*

Treatments of cervical arthritis headache include:

1. NSAID
2. Heat pad
3. Neck collar
4. Analgesia as necessary to control pain

How to detect, evaluate, and treat the medical conditions that can cause headache

To detect hypertension as a cause headache:
1. Take the person's blood pressure using the blood pressure cuff.
2. Do a CBC, SMA20, Urinalysis, Chest X-ray, and EKG

To treat the hypertension associate headache:

1. Use a thiazide diuretic if the person's kidney function is normal.
2. Add either an ARB such as Cozaar or a calcium channel blocker such Cardizem if the diuretic is not sufficient to control the blood pressure.
3. Decrease salt intake to a between 3-4 grams sodium per day.

4. Exercise and weight management is important in controlling blood pressure.

How to detect brain aneurism associated headache:

To detect brain aneurism associated headache:

Take a complete history from the patient.

Do a complete physical examination

Do Brain MRI with IV contrast

If an aneurism is detected, the patient must be referred to a neurosurgeon for surgical

intervention to treat the brain aneurism and relieve the headache.

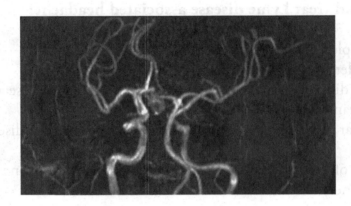

84:2 MR *Angiogram demonstrating an aneurysm of the anterior communicating artery (See arrow):*

How to detect anemia associated headache:

1. Take care a history from the patient
2. Do a complete physical examination
3. Do CBC

(see chapters on anemia for evaluation and treatments of different anemias)

If severe anemia is found, such as a hematocrit of between 15-20 per cent, the patient, cannot deliver oxygen properly to the brain which, can cause headache to occur.

How to detect Polycythemia associated headache:

1. Take a history from the patient.
2. Do a complete physical examination
3. Do a CBC

4. Do a SMA20 chemistry profile
5. If the hematocrit is found to be 60% or above, the polycythemia evaluation ought to be carried out to determine whether the polycythemia is primary or secondary.
6. Polycythemia causes the red blood cells level to be too viscous preventing blood
7. and oxygen from moving with ease through blood vessels to deliver oxygen to the brain and other organs in the human body.
8. The viscosity of the can cause both headache and stroke to occur.
9. Treatments of polycythemia are complex and is determined based on the type of polycythemia and the cause.

How to detect and treat Lyme disease associated headache:

1. Take a complete history from the patient
2. Do a complete physical examination
3. Do a Lyme disease Elisa and Western blot blood test and these are positive
4. Do a CT scan of the brain
5. Do a lumbar puncture and send the spinal fluid for Lyme disease antibody test and culture
6. Treatments of Lyme disease meningitis include IV Ceftriaxone and Doxycycline by mouth and pain medication.

How to detect and treat Lupus (SLE) associated headache:

1. Take a complete history from the patient
2. Do a complete physical examination
3. Do a CBC
4. Do an SMA20 chemistry profile
5. Do a ESR
6. Do an ANA
7. Do a double stranded DNA
8. Do a brain CT scan
9. Do a lumbar puncture
10. Send the spinal fluid to the lab for ANA, double stranded DNA, glucose. Protein and
11. Cell count, Gram stain, and culture.
12. Treatments for lupus associated head (meningitis) include usual medications used to
13. Treat lupus plus steroid and pain medication.

How to detect and treat Rheumatoid arthritis associated headache:

1. Take a complete history from the patient
2. Do a complete physical examination
3. Do CBC
4. Do SMA20 chemistry profile
5. Do a ESR
6. Do an ANA
7. Do a Rheumatoid factor
8. Do double stranded DNA
9. Do MRI of the cervical spine
10. Do CT scan of the brain
11. Do a lumbar puncture

Send the spinal fluid for ANA, Rhuematoid factor, glucose, protein, cell counts, Gram stain and culture.

Treatments of Rheumatoid arthritis associated headache include the usual medications used to treat RA (see chapter 13) plus steroid.

If the headache is due to herniated cervical spine, then, the patient needs to be evaluated by a neurosurgeon. In addition, the patient needs treatment with NSAID plus pain medication.

How to evaluate and treat Mixed Conective Tissue Diseases associated headache:

1. Take a complete history from the patient.
2. Do a complete physical examination
3. Do a CBC
4. Do SMA20 chemistry profile
5. Do ERS
6. Do ANA
7. Do ENA
8. Do RNP
9. Do rheumatoid factor
10. Do double stranded DNA
11. Do CT scan of the brain
12. Do MRI of the cervical spine
13. Do lumbar puncture
14. Send spinal fluid for ANA, rheumatoid factor, double stranded DNA, glucose, protein, cell counts, Gram stain and culture.

How to evaluate and treat temporal arteritis associated headache:

1. Take a complete history
2. Do a complete physical examination
3. Get the Eye doctor to do complete eye examination
4. Do an ESR
5. Start patient on Steroid immediately to prevent blindness.
6. Doing surgery to section the temporal artery to diagnose temporal arteritis is very inaccurate.

How to evaluate and treat viral meningitis associated headache:

1. Take a complete history
2. Do a complete physical examination
3. Do CBC
4. Do an SMA20 chemistry profile
5. Do an ESR
6. Do blood tests for viral profile
7. Do HIV1/HIV2 blood tests
8. Do Blood culture
9. Do Chest X-ray
10. Do brain CT
11. Do a lumbar puncture
12. Send spinal fluid for cell counts, Gram Stain, both bacteria, viral and fungal cultures,
13. Glucose and protein
14. Start treating patient with Ceftriaxone IV and Vacomycin IV if he or she is not allergic to penicillin.
15. If the patient is allergic to penicillin, Levaquin IV can be added to IV Vancomycin till the results of microbiological tests are back from the laboratory.

How to evaluate and treat bacterial meningitis associated headache:

1. Take a complete physical examination
2. Do a complete physical examination
3. Do CBC
4. Do an SMA20 chemistry profile
5. Do Urinalysis
6. Do an ESR
7. Do Blood culture
8. Do Urine culture

9. Do HIV1/HIV blood tests
10. Do chest x-ray
11. Do EKG
12. Do brain CT
13. Do a lumbar puncture
14. Send spinal fluid for cell counts, Gram stain, bacterial culture, viral culture, fungal culture, TB culture, AFB stain, glucose, and protein.
15. Start treatment with Ceftriaxone IV and Vacomycin or Penicillin G IV, Fortaz and Vacomycin. Rifampin plus Ampicillin IV can also be used depending on the patient's profile and age till the results of the microbiological laboratory are back.

How to evaluate and treat fungal meningitis associated headache:

1. Take a complete history
2. Do a complete physical examination
3. Do a CBC
4. Do an SMA20 chemistry profile
5. Do urinalysis
6. Do ESR
7. Do blood culture
8. Do urine culture
9. Do HIV1/IHV2 blood tests
10. Do VDRL
11. Do blood test for CMV
12. Do blood tests for herpes simplex type 1 and type 2
13. Do blood test and blood smear for malaria
14. Do PPD skin test for TB
15. Do chest x-ray
16. Do EKG
17. Do brain CT
18. Do MRI with IV contrast
19. Do a lumbar puncture
20. Send spinal fluid to the lab for cell counts, Gram stain, fungal culture, bacterial culture,
21. viral culture, TB culture, AFB stain, HIV1/HIV2 tests, Cryptococcal antibody, Toxoplasma antibody, Histoplasma antibody, Candida, Aspergillus, India ink test, do tests for protozoa, Herpes simplex, Cytomegalovirus and VDRL. parasitic organisms, glucose and protein.
22. Start treatment with IV Amphotericin B or Fluconazole and provide treatments based on the results of laboratory and x-ray results.

These types of infections are most frequently seen in individuals who are inmmunosuprssed, such as people who have AIDS or people who have been treated with chemotherapy.

How to evaluate and treat brain cancer associated headache:

Take a complete history
Do a complete physical examination
Do MRI of the brain with IV contrast

The different brain tumors that can be found include:

1. Glioma
2. Astrocytoma
3. Meningioma
4. Acoustic neuroma
5. Oligodendroglioma
6. Glioblastoma multiforme
7. Medulloblastoma etc
8. Metastatic cancer frequently occurs in the brain as well.

Some of the most common cancers that can metastasis to brain include:

1. Lung cancer
2. Breast cancer
3. Colon cancer
4. Prostate cancer
5. Melanoma
6. Lymphomas
7. Leukemias etc.

If a tumor is found in the brain, the patient needs to be referred to a neurosurgeon for a brain biopsy.

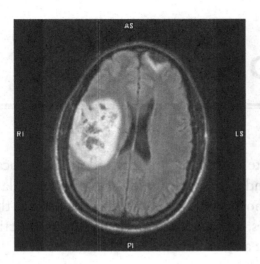

8:3 Axial MRI image demonstrates a glioblastoma multiforme of the right cerebral hemisphere. There is also evidence of old traumatic injury at the left frontal pole:

At times it may be necessary to obtain a consult from a neurologist to examine the patient and do a lumbar puncture, using a thin needle to avoid herniation of the brain.

The spinal fluid obtained from the patient must be sent to the laboratory for
1. Cytology
2. Glucose
3. Protein
4. LDH
5. Cell counts
6. Gram stain and culture.

Treatments of brain cancer associated headache include:

1. Surgical resection
2. Radiation therapy
3. Chemotherapy
4. Steroid IV or by mouth
5. Pain medication etc.

Chapter 83
THYROID DISEASES

Thyroid diseases are quite common. The thyroid gland is located in the neck and its normal functions are under the control of the pituitary gland which produces the thyroid-stimulating hormone, which is located at the base of the brain. The hormones, which the thyroid secretes, are necessary for proper body functions. The most common diseases of the thyroid are as follows:

1. Thyroid goiter
2. Hypothyroidism
3. Hyperthyroidism
4. Grave's disease
5. Acute thyroiditis
6. Chronic thyroiditis
7. Hashimoto's thyroiditis
8. Thyroid nodules
9. Thyroid cancer

There are three different types of goiters: simple goiter, nontoxic goiter and, toxic goiter. Simple goiter is quite common and is due to lack of iodine in the water and diet of those who are affected. Simple goiter causes enlargement of the thyroid gland. Toxic goiter occurs when the thyroid gland is enlarged because of either an acute inflammation of the thyroid gland or thyroid cancer.

Hypothyroidism occurs because of failure of the thyroid gland to produce enough thyroid hormone. The most frequent causes of hypothyroidism consist of:

1. Surgical removal of the thyroid gland, due to disease
2. Destruction of the thyroid gland with radioactive iodine as treatment for hyperthyroidism
3. Hashimoto's thyroiditis with resulting hypothyroidism.

Hyperthyroidism is sometimes seen in association with lupus, vitiligo, rheumatoid arthritis and pernicious anemia. Sometimes the neck becomes painful and a person may think he or she has an ordinary sore throat, and sometimes it occurs with no symptoms at all. Both acute and sub-acute thyroiditis can lead to either transient or permanent hypothyroidism.

Hyperthyroidism is divided in two major parts:

1. Hyperthyroidism due to excessive production of thyroid hormones, resulting in the clinical hyperthyroid state
2. Grave's disease with its three parts:

   a. A large goiter
   b. Large protruding eyes (exophthalmus)
   c. Skin abnormalities (dermatopathy)

Cancer of the thyroid

Most thyroid nodules are not malignant.

There are two types of thyroid nodules, hot nodule and cold nodule. Hot nodules are usually benign and are not cancerous. Cold nodules are not always associated with cancer, but when local thyroid cancers develop, frequently, they arise from a cold nodule.

Because the thyroid gland is extremely vascular, a lot of blood passes through it, and consequently metastatic cancer of the thyroid from lung, breast, melanoma, and esophagus occur frequently. Lymphoma of the thyroid also occurs and represents about 5% of all thyroid cancers.

The most common form of thyroid cancer is papillary carcinoma, which is 70% of thyroid cancers. Follicular carcinoma represents 15% of thyroid cancer, and anaplastic cancer of the thyroid occurs 5% of the time. The most malignant and aggressive type of thyroid cancer is the follicular type.

Among the risks for the development of thyroid cancer are being female and exposure to radiation. People who have had radiation treatment to their tonsils as a child have high incidence of thyroid cancer when they become adults.

To diagnose thyroid cancer, the first thing to do is to:

1. Take history from the patient.
2. Palpate the thyroid gland, looking for a nodule.
3. Examine carefully the anterior and posterior cervical areas of the neck, looking for enlargement of nodes.
4. Do a thyroid scan.
5. Do a thyroid ultrasound.
6. Do thyroid function tests (T4 and TSH).

7. Do a fine-needle aspiration biopsy of the thyroid nodule (this is done usually by an endocrinologist) or by a surgeon.

Once biopsy documents that thyroid cancer is present, surgical removal of the thyroid gland must be carried out. The extent of the surgical incision depends on the cell type of the cancer.

Following resection of the thyroid cancer, radioactive iodine must be administered to destroy all remaining thyroid tissues.

The other necessary treatment is Synthroid by mouth, both for suppression and treatment for life. There is no effective chemotherapy available for thyroid cancer except for VP16 which has shown some response. Blacks with thyroid cancer must remain under the care of an endocrinologist for many years.

Symptoms, physical findings, evaluation, and treatment of thyroid goiter

The first sign of goiter is a swelling in the neck, either on both sides or on one side. On palpitation of the neck, the goiter can be felt.

On auscultation with a stethoscope, a bruit sometimes can be heard. Sometimes the goiter may be located under the collarbone and is seen only during x-ray test of the upper chest. Sometimes the first indication that a person has goiter is difficulty swallowing or breathing, due to pressure on the trachea and upper esophagus, and at times hoarseness can occur due to pressure on the vocal cords.

To evaluate a thyroid goiter, the tests that are done are ultrasound of the neck along with a thyroid scan. Treatment of thyroid goiter consists of surgical removal or suppressive treatment with Synthroid to try to shrink the size of the gland.

Symptoms, evaluations, and treatment by hyperthyroidism

The symptoms of hyperthyroidism (overactive thyroid gland) are as follows:

Weight loss
Diarrhea
Agitation
Insomnia
Palpitations
Cardiac arrhythmia
Chest pain
Shortness of breath
Poor appetite
Weakness

Depression
Nervousness
Sweatiness
Warm feeling
Psychosis
Mental confusion
Poor memory
Dementia
Thyroid storm etc;

The usual findings on physical examination of people who are suffering from hyperthyroidism/Graves' disease includes:

1. Large thyroid gland, tender or non-tender
2. Protruding eyes
3. Fine, smooth skin
4. Sweaty palms
5. Fast pulse rate
6. Irregular heartbeat
7. Fluid in the lungs
8. Heart murmur.

Laboratory evaluations in hyperthyroidism consist of:

1. Serum T4, TSH, free T4 and T3
2. ANA, serum B12
3. CBC
4. Reticulocytes count
5. Liver Function Tests
6. Anti-thyroid antibody and anti-microsomal antibodies
7. Thyroid scan
8. Thyroid ultrasound

In hyperthyroidism, serum T4, T3 and free T4 are high and serum TSH (thyroid-stimulating hormone is low).

There is a subgroup of hyperthyroidism called apathetic hyperthyroidism (or T3 thyrotoxicosis) with high serum T3 and low serum TSH, seen often in elderly people.

These people usually become bed-bound and show no obvious signs of overactive thyroid, except for a fast heart rate, weakness, poor appetite, and poor memory. The fast heart rate and the apathetic look in the patient's face are the red flags that overactive thyroid is responsible for the patient's total body weakness which, if left untreated, can lead to the death of the affected person.

Graves' disease is a form of hyperthyroidism (overactive thyroid) state, during which the thyroid gland is enlarged and tender. The eyes are markedly enlarged (exophthalmus), the skin areas that are affected are thickened and edematous. The swelling around the eyes is due to infiltration by lymphocytes and mononuclear cells. Graves' disease occurs commonly. Graves' disease may be an autoimmune disease.

There exists a link between Graves' disease, Hashimoto's disease, hypothyroidism, pernicious anemia and vitiligo, etc.

The evaluations of Graves' disease (hyperthyroidism) are as described earlier. The treatments of Graves' disease are the same as that of other forms hyperthyroidism.
The different types of treatments used to treat hyperthyroidism are as follows: high

1. Surgical removal of part of the thyroid
2. Medication to suppress the thyroid glands' ability to produce thyroid hormone
3. Steroid IV or PO
4. Radioactive iodine to destroy the thyroid glands

Treatments that are preferable to treat hyperthyroidism in women who are pregnant are surgical removal of the thyroid gland or administering Propylthiouracil by mouth. In women who are not in childbearing age or who are elderly, radioactive iodine is preferable.

For people who present with hyperthyroidism and a fast heart rate, Inderal by mouth is given to slow the rate of the heart down to prevent cardiac decompensation and possible cardiac arrhythmia that can develop if the heart rate is allowed to remain fast.

Whether or not the treatment is given inside the hospital or in the office setup depends on the judgment of the treating physician and or how sick the patient looks.

The next thing to do is to give medication to shut down the production of thyroid hormones. The most frequently used anti-thyroid medications are Propylthiouracil and Tapazole. The usual dose of Propylthiouracil is 100 to 150 mg every 6 or 8 hours, by mouth. Propylthiouracil works to decrease the symptoms of hyperthyroidism by preventing the conversion of T4 to T3 in the bloodstream. Tapazole works to decrease the symptoms of hyperthyroidism by inhibiting the production of thyroid hormone by the thyroid gland. The usual dose of Tapazole is 30-40mg in divided doses 2-3 times per day by mouth.

In the acute hyperthyroidism state to prevent the so-called thyroid storm, large doses of Dexamethasone 2 grams every 6 hours can be given in addition, to reduce the level of T4 in the body, thereby improving the overall condition of the affected person. Either Propylthiouracil or Tapazole can be used for up to 2 years, while a decision is being made regarding a long-term modality of treatment. During the administration of these medications, a complete blood count must be done every month or so, because leukopenia and low platelet count can develop.

When it is decided based on clinical facts and the appropriate patients that radioactive iodine is the treatment modality, an endocrinologist will administer the proper dose of radioactive iodine to the patient to destroy the thyroid gland.

Following the administration of the radioactive iodine, the patient will be monitored for many years, waiting for the development of the hypothyroidism state, which is guaranteed to develop in time. When the T4 and TSH evaluation indicates that the patient has developed hypothyroidism, then Synthroid by mouth for life will be given to her.

Hypothyroidism is much more common in women than in men. Some of the conditions that can cause hypothyroidism include:

1. Surgical removal of the thyroid gland
2. Treatment with radioactive iodine to treat overactive-state thyroid gland
3. Hashimoto's thyroiditis

Hashimoto's thyroiditis is a chronic inflammatory/autoimmune disease that, when present, causes the thyroid gland to hypo-function, resulting in the state of hypothyroidism. Hashimoto's thyroiditis is frequently seen associated with pernicious anemia, rheumatoid arthritis, systemic lupus erythematosus, diabetes mellitus, and adrenal defficiency.

Sometime Hashimoto's thyroiditis can present with a goiter, but frequently there are no obvious physical findings in the thyroid gland.
Symptoms of Hypothyroidism:

1. Weight gain
2. Tiredness
3. Sleepiness
4. Hair loss
5. Depression
6. Slow heart rate
7. Anemia
8. Dry skin

9. Swollen legs
10. Irregular menstrual periods
11. Bleeding between menstrual periods
12. Loss of eyebrows, etc.

The diagnosis is usually made when a patient presents to the doctor with complaints of not feeling well, feeling tired, and other vague complaints, and an evaluation is carried out which includes T4 and TSH blood tests. If the T4 is low and the TSH is high, that establishes a diagnosis of hypothyroidism. If the T4 is normal and the TSH is high that also establishes the diagnosis of normal T4 hypothyroidism.

This is called normal T4 hypothyroidism.

Other tests to order are anti-thyroid antibody and anti microsomal antibody, ANA, B12, rheumatoid factor, ESR, and fasting blood sugar. If the anti-thyroid is positive, the diagnosis of Hashimoto's thyroiditis is established.

The next thing to do is a thyroid scan, to look at the anatomy of the thyroid gland. Once these tests have been done, then treatment with Synthroid can be started.

Hashimoto's thyroiditis may be responsible for 90% of the cases of hypothyroidism.

It does not matter what causes the state of hypothyroidism; once it occurs, the treatment choice is thyroid hormone replacement, and most of the time for life.

The dose of Synthroid that is used to treat hypothyroidism in mcg must be individualized from patients to patients, while monitoring the serum T4 and TSH to adjust the dose.

Chapter 84
HYPERPARATHYROID DISAESES

There are 4 parathyroid glands in the human body and they are located in the neck.

The role of the of the parathyroid glands are to secrete parathyroid hormone (PTH) to keep a proper level of calcium and phosphorus in the body.

Parathyroid hormone (PTH) plays a key role in both Vitamin D and magnesium levels in the human body.

When one or more of these glands developd an adenoma (a bening) tumor, or when hyperplasia develops in these glands, the serum calcium becomes elevated. On rare occasions, cancer can develop in the parathyroid gland causing elevated serum calcium as well.

"Primary hyperparathyroidism is caused by a solitary adenoma in 80% to 85% of cases and genetic endocrine disorder in 10 % to 15% of cases, less than 1% of primary hyperparathyroidism is due to parathyroid cancer." Source: American Journal of Medicine October 2011, volume 124 Number 10

Primary hyperparathyroidism develops in 1 in 1000 people in the U.S. secondary Hyperparathyroidism develops when the level of vitamin D is low in the body.

Risks for primary hyperparathyroidism in clude:

Menopause
Multiple endocrine neoplasia type 1
Treatment with lithium
Radiation treatment to the neck etc;

Many patients with primary hyperparathyroidism are asymptomatic. Those with symptoms usually have serum calcium in the range of 12 mg/dL or 14 mg/dL. Serum calcium higher than 15 mg/dL can cause serious symptoms.

Symptoms of primary hyperparathyroidism in clude:

Fatigue
Weakness
Seizure

Cardiac arrhythmias
Osteoporosis
Abdominal pain
Frequent urination
Kidney stones
Bone and joint pain
Depression
Loss of appetite
Nausea
Vomiting
Muscle soreness
Constipation
Dementia
Increase thirst
Dyspepsia
Peptic ulcer
Anemia
Osteitis fibrosa cystica

Parathyroid hormone increases serum calcium by the actions it has on bone, gut, and kidneys. In addition, there is increased calcium absorption from the diet, as well as increased kidney reapportion of calcium caused by a high level of 1,25-hydroxy vitamin D.

The evaluation of a person suspected of having hyperparathyroidism include:

History and physical examination
CBC
Complete metabolic (chemistry) profile including serum calcium
Urinalysis
24 hour urine calcium
Serum IGG, IGM, IGA, IGD
Serum immuno electrophoresis
Urine immuno electrophoresis
Serum PTH
Serum Phosphorus level
Serum magnesium level
EKG
Chest Xray
Chest CT
Ultrasound of the neck
Sestamibi Scan
Endoscopic examination of the stomach

Surgical Consult

If the parathyroid hormone is elevated or nomal, and serum calcium is high along with low serum phosphorus, the diagnosis of primary hyperparathyroidism is confirmed. The next most important non-surgical test to do to fully establish the diagnosis is to show parathyroid adenoma on the Sestamibi nuclear test.

Once these things are done, the next step is surgical intervention to remove the adenoma from the parathyroid gland or glands.

If the parathyroid glands are found to have hyperplastic tissues in them, the surgeon will remove some of glands as a treatment. Surgeons always leave on parathyroid gland so that the patient can have parathyroid endocrine function. If the patient refuses surgery and is not able to have surgery, Sensipar (cinacalcet) can be used to treat patients with high calcium due to primary hyperparathyroidism. The usual dose of Sensipar is 30 mcg per day by mouth.

People with primary hyperparathyroidism seem to suffer more serious complications because there are always delays in making their diagnoses due to lateness in presentation for medical evaluations and treatment.

Secondary hyperparathoidism is more common in blacks and other minorities than in their white counterparts because blacks and other minorities suffer more from hypertension and diabetes mellitus than do whites.

Hypertension and diabetes frequently cause chronic kidney failure, and kidney failure causes secondary hyperparathyroidism.

Secondary hyperparathyroidism is due to low serum calcium in the body.
Conditions that cause low calcium and secondary hyperparathyroidism include:

Kidney failure
Diatery calcium deficiency
Vitamin D deficiency
Malabsorption
Lactose intolerance (75% of blacks have lactose intolerance. People with lactose intolerance are able to tolerate dairy products in their diets. Dairy products contain vitamin D and calcium.
Dark skin (vitamin D is made in the body under the skin by the action of the rays of the sun and the darker the skin the more difficult it is for the rays of the sun to penetrate the skin to stimulate the production of vitamin D). 90% of blacks have low vitamin D.

Parathyroid hormone (PTH) is needed for calcium metabolism and the concentration of calcium in the blood stream controls the secretion of parathyroid hormone. When the circulating calcium is low and the level of phosphate is high the parathyroid is left unchecked and over secretes parathyroid hormone.

The over secretion of PTH leads to removal of calcium from bones causing osteomalacia, low phosphorus, low magnesium. This complex of abnormalities can cause renal tubular acidosis (kidney disease) because of excretion of excess magnesium and phosphorus in the urine.

Magnesium is needed in normal amount in the blood stream in order for the parathyroid gland to function normally. Low serum magnesium, low phosphorus, low calcium and low vitamin D cause over activation of the Parathyroid glands leading to secondary hyperparathyroidism, osteomalacia and if severe Rickets.

Rickets/Osteomalacia is treated with vitamin D, magnesium, and neutrophos by mouth.

The treatments of secondary hyperparathyroidism include:

Calcimimetic is approved by the FDA to treat hypercalcemia due to cancer of the parathyroid gland and secondary hyperparathyroidism.

Sensipar 60mcg per day is used to treat people with primary and secondary hyperparathyroidism and kidney failure.

Chapter 85
MULTIPLE SCLEROSIS

Multiple sclerosis affects 2.5 million people in the world and 400,000 Americans Multiple Sclerosis is an imlammatory condition that affects the myelin sheats that cover the axons in the brain and in the spinal cord causing damage and scarring of the myelin sheats. The damage that occurs in the myelin sheats covering the nerves causes interference in the communication systems of the nerves between the brain, the spinal cord and other parts of the body.

These abnormalities can lead to severe disabilities in individuals who are afflicted with MS. MS occurs two times more often in women than men. However, MS is much severe in men than in women. MS occurs in all age groups but, it occurs more often in the age groups 20-40. MS affects people in all racial groups but, people of Norhtern European descent such as New Zealand, southeastern Austrealia, Canada and northern U.S. are affected more often. People from Africa, Asia and Native Americans are affected much less by MS. MS can runs in famililies.

The cause of MS is not known but there appears to be an association with Epstein-Bar viruses herpes 6 and 8 and MS.

Signs and symptoms of MS include:

Tingling and pain in different parts of the body
Double vision
Blurry vision
Tremor
Unsteady gait
Electrical sshock sensations
Slurred speech
Dizziness
Fatigue
Headache etc;

Evaluations of MS include:

History
Physical examination
Blood pressure

Pulse
Respiratory rate
Temperature
Weight

Laboratory evaluations include:

CBC
Complete chemistry profile
Urinalysis
VDRL
Lyme disease Western Blot blood test
ANA
RF
ESR
T4
TSH
Vitamin B12 level
Serum IGG, IGA, IGM, IGD
Serum Immuno electrophoresis
HIV 1 and HIV II blood tests
Blood to screen for Herpes #6 & #8
Radiological evaluations include:

Chest X-ray
MRI of the brain with IV contrast
MRI of the spinal cord with IV contrast
Lumbar puncture
Evaluation of CSF for oligoclonal bands (OCBs)
Evaluation of CFS for WBC, bacteria with gram stain, AFB stain and fungal stain
Bacterial culture
TB culture
Fungal culture
CSF for protein
CSF for sugar
CSF for LDH
CFS for Lyme disease
CSF for HIV 1 and II
CSF for Syphillis
PPD TB skin test
EEG
Electroencephalographic examination
Visual evoked potentials (VEPs)

Somatosensory evoked potentials (SSEPs)
Brainstem auditory evoked potentials (BAEPs)
EKG
Echocardiogram
Neuological consultation

Medications in use to treat MS include:

Corticosteroid
Azathioprine
Methotrexate
Cytoxan
Mitoxantrone
Ampyra
Inteferon beta-1a
Interferon beta-1b
Tysabri
CopaxoneTecfidera
Gilenya
Aubagio
Symmetrel
Dantrium
Baclofen

There are many complications associated with MS and among them are:

Abnormal urinary bladder function
Abnormal bowel function
Abnormal sexual function
Muscle spasms
Muscle stiffness
Paralysis of the legs
Poor memory
Difficulty concentrating
Depression
Seizure etc;

Physical therapy treatment as well as psychiatric treatment plays a major in the management of individuals with MS.

Chapter 86
PSORIASIS

Psoriasis is very common skin condition. Worldwide 125 million people have psoriasis. In the U.S. 7.5 million people have psoriasis.

Psoriasis is the most common autoimmune disease in the U.S., about 10-30% of people with psoriasis develops psoriatic arthritis. Psoriasis is prevalent in 1.3% African Americans and 2.5% in whites.

Risk factors for psoriasis include:
Bacerial infection
Viral infection
Insect bites
Cuts on the skin
Skin burn
Medications
Too much unlight
Not enough sun light
Stress
HIV/AIDS
Non HIV auto immune disease
Chemotherapy

Symptoms of psoriasis include
Dry skin
Flaky skin
Pink/red color skin
Thick and raised skinLesions in the male genital area of men
Scaly/redish lesions over elbows
Scaly/redish lesions over knees
Scaly/redish lesions over abdomen and chest wall
Severe dandruff on the scalp
Thick plaques and red patches over multiple parts of the body
Joints pain

Evaluation of psoriasis in clude
History and physical examination
CBC

ESR
ANA
HIV 1 and 2 bloods test
Complete chemistry profile
VDRL test for syphilis
Rheumatoid factor
Lactic dehydrogenase (LDH)
Skin biopsy
Chest xray
Abdominal CT
Chest CT etc;

Treatments of psoriasis include

Streroid ointments
Steroid Creams
Steroid lotions
Ointments that have Vitamin D and vitamin A
Shampoos
Enbrel
Humira
Amevive
Remicade
Phototherapy etc;

ABOUT THE AUTHOR

Valiere Alcena M.D., M.A.C.P. is a practicing physician, medical scholar, medical educator, and author.

He is a Clinical Professor of Medicine at the Albert Einstein College of Medicine, Bronx NY and Adjunct Professor of Medicine, New York Medical College, Valhalla N.Y.

He is an attending physician at Montefiore Hospital Center in the Bronx, NY.

He is also an attending physician at White Plains Hospital Center in White Plains, NY.

On May 15, 2008, Dr. Alcena was inducted into the American College of Physicians as MASTER-MACP in a ceremony held in Washington, D.C. (Mastership in Medicine is the highest level in the profession of Medicine that any physician in the world can achieve).

On October 19, 2010, Dr. Alcena was elected Fellow of the Royal Society of Medicine in London, England (Royal Society of Medicine was founded in 1773).

Dr. Alcena is a TV Producer and TV Journalist. He is the producer and host of the award winning weekly TV program Discussing Problems and Issues of Health with Dr. Alcena (The longest running TV health show in the New Tri-State region—on the air since 1994)

He is also the producer and host of the weekly TV program: White Plains Community Health Fair Speaks.

Dr. Alcena is the Chairman Emeritus of the White Plains Cable Access Commission.

Dr. Alcena founded the Minority medical Students Affair Committee (MAC) at Albert Einstein College of Medicine in 1969 and is still the Chairman of that Committee.

This was the first such committee of his kind in the U.S.

Dr. Alcena created the first Community Health Fairs in the State of New York and in the U.S.

He has published numerous articles in the scientific literature.

Dr Alcena published the article that first recommended the creation of community health centers in the U.S.

Dr. Alcena is credited as the physician who originated the idea that male circumcision would decrease the incidence of HIV/AIDS. Dr. Alcena wrote the article about AIDS and circumcision in August of 1986 in the NY State Journal of Medicine. This idea has prevented several million people from becoming infected with HIV/AIDS (6.3 million" between" 2006-2007). Close to 1 million deaths have also been prevented during that time because of male circumcision. Time Magazine named the idea of "Male circumcision #1 among the Top 10 medical breakthroughs for the years 2007".

In 2007, Dr. Alcena was named ICM teacher of the year at Albert Einstein College of Medicine. In 2000, Dr. Alcena received "The Community-Based Excellence in Teaching Award" by the American College of Physicians.

In 1996 he was the winner of the "Ten Year Community-Based Outstanding Teacher Award" from the American College of Physicians.

Dr. Alcena first published the idea of the need for the creation of community health centers in the United States to serve the Ghetto Poor while a medical student at Albert Einstein College of Medicine in the Bronx N.Y.

Dr. Alcena has made many major discoveries, come up with, and published many other ideas and concepts that have made major contributions to the field of Medicine in the 20th and 21st centuries and have saved countless lives throughout the world.

Dr. Alcena is recognized as the pioneer who first exposed the health care disparity that existed and still exists in minorities in the United State of America. He wrote about it in 1994 in his first book. Dr. Alcena is the recipient of the PIONEER HEATH CARE DISPARITY AWARD—THE VOICE FOR THE ELIMINATION OF HEALTH CARE DISPARITY PRESENTED BY WESTCHESTER, PUBLIC, PRIVATE PARTNERSHIP FOR AGING SERVICES at a ceremony held at Pace University Law School in White Plains, NY on June 11, 2005.

In addition, Dr. Alcena has received several dozen other awards over the years from many academic, governmental and, community organizations. Dr. Alcena has his medical office in White Plains, New York where he practices General Internal Medicine, Hematology, and Medical Oncology.

The followings are the many Books that Dr. Alcena has written

1. The Status of Health of Blacks in the States of America—A Prescription for Improvement (1994)
2. The Third World Tropical Diet, Health Maintenance, and Medical Management Program (1994)
3. African American Health Book (1994)
4. AIDS the Expending Epidemic, What the Public Needs to know: A Multi Cultural Overview (1994)
5. African American Women's Health Book (2001)
6. Women's Health and Wellness for the Millennium (2002)
7. Men's Health and Wellness for the New Millennium (2007)
8. The Best of Women's Health (2008)
9. Health Care Disparity in the United States: An Urgent Call for Universal Health Insurance & A Public Health Insurance Plan (2009)
10. Triumph and Tragedies of Haiti and Its People (2010)
11. Health Care Disparity in the United States of America. (2011)
12. THIRD WORLD HEALTH CARE IN A FIRST WORLD COUNTRY (2011)